Intracranial Pressure IX

Edited by
H. Nagai, K. Kamiya, and S. Ishii

With 371 Figures and 116 Tables

Springer-Verlag
Tokyo Berlin Heidelberg New York London
Paris Hong Kong Barcelona Budapest

Hajime Nagai, m.d.
Emeritus Professor, Department of Neurosurgery,
Nagoya City University Medical School,
1 Kawasumi, Mizuho-cho, Mizuho-ku, Nagoya, Aichi, 467 Japan

Ken Kamiya, m.d.
Department of Neurosurgery, Nagoya City University Medical School,
1 Kawasumi, Mizuho-cho, Mizuho-ku, Nagoya, Aichi, 467 Japan

Shozo Ishii, m.d.
President, Juntendo University,
2-1-1 Hongo, Bunkyo-ku, Tokyo, 113 Japan

ISBN 4-431-70146-X Springer-Verlag Tokyo Berlin Heidelberg New York
ISBN 3-540-70146-X Springer-Verlag Berlin Heidelberg New York Tokyo
ISBN 0-387-70146-X Springer-Verlag New York Berlin Heidelberg Tokyo

Printing and binding: Kobunsha, Tokyo

Proceedings of the Ninth International Symposium on Intracranial Pressure
Held in Nagoya, Japan, May 16–19, 1994

Contributors

Preface

This book is a compilation of the papers submitted and presented at the Ninth International Symposium on Intracranial Pressure (ICP IX) held from 16 to 19 May, 1994, in Nagoya, Japan.

This symposium was subtitled "ICP & its related problems," which we believe proves that the triennial ICP symposia have focused increasingly on research in broader clinical fields. As a matter of fact, the 111 oral presentations and 134 poster presentations given during the scientific sessions at ICP IX covered a wide range of aspects pertinent to ICP matters including microdialysis and imaging.

This symposium consisted of 20 oral sessions and 12 poster sessions, during which topics were heatedly discussed and expertise was exchanged. It played the role of formally introducing advanced medical research and technologies as well as of providing an occasion to make new acquaintances and renew old friendships.

The ICP IX meeting was of great significance to scientists and researchers in Asia not only because of its scientific fruits and the opportunity for all participants to benefit from each other's progress but also because it was the second conference in Asia (subsequent to the ICP V held in Tokyo in 1982, which was presided by Prof. Shozo Ishii, Juntendo University) to have the honor of hosting an ICP meeting.

Since the very start of these symposia in Hanover in 1972, through the other eight ICP meetings in Lund (1974), Groningen (1976), Williamsburg (1979), Tokyo (1982), Glasgow (1985), Ann Arbor (1988), Rotterdam (1991), and Nagoya, we have ascertained more and more that the advances in understanding gained from these conferences have been providing important contributions to our daily medical practices and clinical applications and we believe that the proceedings of this most recent symposium will be of great value as well.

The organizers of ICP IX would like to take this opportunity to thank all the members of the Honorary Board, the Advisory Board, the Organizing Committee, and the Local Arrangement Committee. Their efforts and advice provided helpful guidance and encouragement to all participants. The outstanding contributions made by all the Chairmen of the sessions were also an inspiration and were heartily appreciated by the organizers.

The Tenth Symposium on Intracranial Pressure will be held in Virginia, U.S.A. in 1997.

Nagoya, Japan
May 1994

The Editors

Preface

This book is a compilation of the papers submitted and presented at the Ninth International Symposium on Intracranial Pressure (ICP IX) held from 16 to 19 May, 1994 in Nagoya, Japan.

[illegible]

Contents

Session IV: Causes of Increased or Decreased ICP (1)
Chairmen: J.T. Hoff and M. Furuse

Session V: Causes of Increased or Decreased ICP (2)
Chairmen: J. Ekstedt and S. Matsumoto

Session VI: Causes of Increased or Decreased ICP (3)
Chairmen: D.A. Hovda and T. Ohta

Session VII: Effects of Increased ICP (1)
Chairmen: A. Marmarou and T. Ohmoto

Session VIII: Effects of Increased ICP (2)
Chairmen: R.M. BULLOCK and H. KANAYA

Session IX: Biophysics (1)
Chairmen: A. MARMAROU and S. ISHII

Session X: Biophysics (2)
Chairmen: A. Unterberg and H. Nagai

Session XI: Treatment for Abnormal ICP (1)
Chairmen: A. Baethmann and N. Kodama

Session XVII: Effects of Increased ICP (3)
Chairmen: P. Reilly and H. Yamada

Session XVIII: Effects of Increased ICP (4)
Chairmen: M.J. Rosner and K. Hashi

Session XIX: Drugs and Anesthetic Agents (1)
Chairmen: M. Brock and T. Sakabe

Session XX: Drugs and Anesthetic Agents (2)
Chairmen: G. Teasdale and S. Nagao

Poster I: Methodology
Chairman: M. MAEDA

Poster II: Monitoring
Chairman: J. GOFFIN

Poster IX: Edema and Others
Chairman: M. Brock

Poster X: Effects of Increased ICP
Chairman: J.T. Hoff

Poster XI: Imaging and Others
Chairman: K. UEMURA

Session I: Methodology

Chairmen: C.J.J. Avezaat and T. Tsubokawa

Evaluation of a Microsensor Intracranial Pressure Transducer

SHANKAR P. GOPINATH, CLAUDIA S. ROBERTSON, RAJ K. NARAYAN, and ROBERT G. GROSSMAN

Department of Neurosurgery, Baylor College of Medicine, One Baylor Plaza, Houston, TX 77030, USA

INTRODUCTION

Elevated intracranial pressure (ICP) is a common complication of severe head injury, intracranial hemorrhage, and neoplasms. Following the pioneering work of Lundberg,[1] interest in ICP monitoring has grown steadily. ICP monitoring is being increasingly utilized in many neurosurgical units since aggressive management of the elevated ICP has been shown to significantly decrease mortality.[2] Improvement in the technology and the ease of handling of the ICP monitors has significantly contributed to the overall increase in utilization.

A recent laboratory evaluation of a new microsensor transducer (MicroSensor™,Codman and Shurtleff, Inc., Randolph, Mass., USA) has shown accurate ICP readings compared to a fluid coupled catheter over a wide range of pressures, and excellent *in vitro* stability that exceeds that of previously available transducers.[3] The purpose of the present study was to compare ICP measured in the intensive care unit with an intraventricular microsensor transducer and with an intraventricular catheter fluid-coupled to an external transducer.

MATERIALS AND METHODS

Patients Characteristics

Twenty-five patients (19 males, 6 females; average age 42 ± 19 years) with a clinical indication for intracranial pressure monitoring were studied after obtaining an informed consent from a relative. The etiology of the neurological injury requiring intracranial pressure monitoring included closed head injury (n=13), gunshot wound (n=5), subarachnoid hemorrhage (n=6), and hydrocephalus (n=1). The average Glasgow Coma Score on admission to the hospital was 7.8±3.0 (range 3-14).

Measurement of ICP

The microsensor ICP monitoring system consists of two parts: a disposable microsensor transducer and a monitor interface that can be connected to any commercially available monitor (Fig. 1 and 2). The microsensor transducer has a microchip pressure sensor at the tip of a 0.7 mm diameter flexible nylon cable. The cable connecting the transducer to the monitor interface is 100 cm in length and can be bent or kinked without disturbing the function of the transducer. The natural frequency response of the microsensor pressure transducer is greater than 10 kHz. The version used in this study was enclosed in a silastic ventriculostomy catheter. The ventriculostomy catheter can be connected to an external transducer or to a drainage bag.

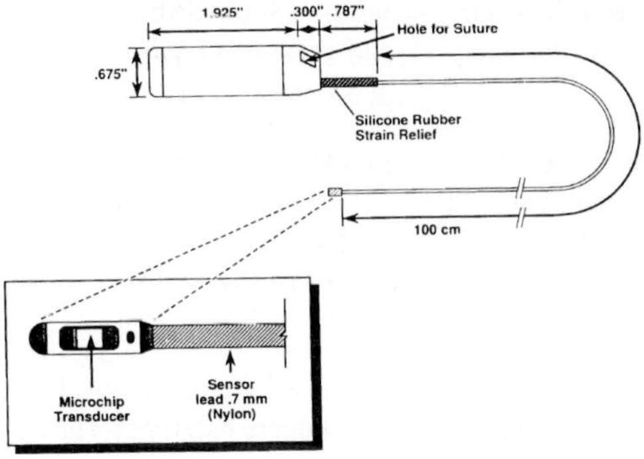

Fig. 1. Diagram of the microsensor transducer (from Gopinath et al., J Neurosci Meth 49:12,1993).

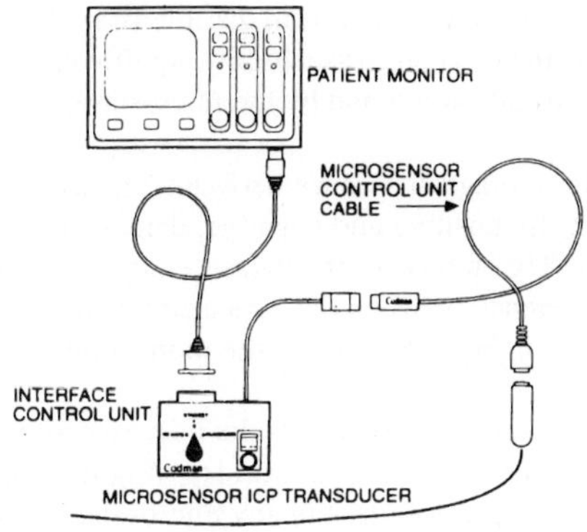

Fig. 2. Diagram of the interface control unit attaching the microsensor transducer to the patient monitor.

Prior to inserting the ventriculostomy catheter, the microsensor transducer was positioned approximately one centimeter from the end of the catheter to prevent injury to the transducer during insertion. The tip of the catheter was moistened with saline and the microsensor transducer was zeroed at ambient pressure. Then the ventriculostomy catheter was inserted using standard procedures. After proper insertion in the lateral ventricle, the ventriculostomy catheter was fluid-coupled to an external transducer, which was connected to a Hewlett-Packard monitor and zeroed at the level of the foramen of Monro. Subsequently, the ventriculostomy was rezeroed every 8 hour or whenever there was more than 3 mm Hg difference from the microsensor transducer value.

For the time that ICP monitoring was required for clinical purposes, ICP was observed continuously by both the ventriculostomy catheter and by the microsensor transducer, and simultaneous values were recorded every hour by the bedside nurse. At the end of monitoring, the value of the microsensor transducer at ambient pressure was recorded after removing the catheter.

Statistical Analysis

Summary data are expressed as the mean $\pm$ the standard deviation. Simultaneous values of ICP measured by the ventriculostomy and by the microsensor transducer was compared by linear regression analysis.

RESULTS

Thirty microsensor transducers were evaluated in 25 patients (1-3 catheters/patient). No problems occurred during insertion of the ICP monitor, and the only complication associated with the ICP monitor was one case of ventriculitis (incidence of 3%). The patients were monitored for up to seven days, the average duration being 3.8 $\pm$ 1.6 days.

A total of 2218 simultaneous measurements of ICP were obtained. The average ICP by the ventriculostomy catheter was 15.4 ± 10.1 mm Hg (range = -9 to 104) and the average ICP by the microsensor transducer was 15.9 ± 10.0 mm Hg (range = -3 to 104). The size and the shape of the ICP waveform recorded from the microsensor transducer and the ventriculostomy was observed to be identical. There was a highly significant correlation over the wide range of pressures measured by the ventriculostomy and by the microsensor transducer ($n = 2218$, $r = 0.97$, $p < 0.001$).

The average difference between 2 measurements of ICP was -0.5 ± 2.6 mm Hg. The differences were equally positive and negative, demonstrating no consistent bias. The 2 values for ICP were within 2 mm Hg on 63% of the measurements, and within 4 mm Hg on 89% of the measurements. The average difference between the 2 measurements of ICP did not consistently change over time, and was -1.0 ± 2.6 mm Hg at the end of the monitoring period.

The average zero drift of the microsensor transducer, measured at ambient pressure after removal of the catheter, was 0.2 ± 0.5 mm Hg. Eighty-one percent of the microsensor transducers had 0 mm Hg drift, and the greatest drift in any microsensor transducer was 2 mm Hg.

DISCUSSION

The intraventricular catheter, fluid-coupled to an external transducer is the most reliable method for measuring ICP, against which newer systems have been compared [4]. The ventriculostomy catheter has the advantage of providing a method for calibration *in vivo*, and the ability to drain ventricular CSF for reduction of elevated ICP. It has the disadvantage of penetrating the meninges and brain, with the possibility of transmission of bacteria through the system. In addition, placement of ventriculostomy catheter can be difficult in presence of compression and shift of the ventricles.

Compared to the gold standard ventriculostomy, the microsensor transducer reliably measured ICP, and had remarkably little drift during the average monitoring time of 4 days. The microsensor may be a useful alternative to the ventriculostomy.

ACKNOWLEDGMENTS

This work was supported by a grant from Codman and Shurtleff, Inc., and by NIH grant #PO1-NS27616.

REFERENCES

1. Lundberg N (1960) Continuous recording and control of ventricular fluid pressure in neurosurgical practice. Acta Psychiatr Neurol Scand 36(Suppl 149):1-193
2. Marshall LF, Smith RW, Shapiro HM (1979) The outcome with aggressive treatment in severe head injuries. 1. The significance of ICP monitoring. J Neurosurg 50:20-29
3. Gopinath SP, Cherian L, Robertson CS, Narayan RK, Grossman G (1993) Evaluation of a microsensor intracranial pressure transducer. J Neurosci Meth 49:11-15
4. Allen R (1976) Intracranial pressure: a review of clinical problems, measurement techniques, and monitoring methods. J Med Eng Technol 10:299-320

Comparison Between Indirect and Direct Measurements of the Intrasinus Pressure in Humans

A.Y. Razumovsky[1], S.S. Gasparian[2], E.F. Nekipelov[2], and A.R. Shakhnovich[2]

[1] Department of Neurology, Johns Hopkins Medical Institutions, Meyer 8-141, 600 N. Wolfe Street, Baltimore, MD 21287, USA
[2] N.N. Burdenko Neurosurgical Institute, 5 Fadeev Street, 125047 Moscow, Russia

An accurate clinical method for determining the intrasinus pressure (P_{is}) without catheterization of the cerebral sinuses is desirable, but still not realized. Direct method of the cerebrospinal fluid (CSF) formation rate measurement based on the CSF drainage, when further reduction of the cerebrospinal fluid pressure (P_{csf}) fails to reduce the outflow rate is well known [1]. Our indirect method for P_{is} measurement is based on the assumption that during direct measurement of CSF formation rate, the CSF absorption arrests due to the lack of the gradient between P_{csf} and P_{is}. At this level of the CSF drainage the P_{csf} becomes equal to P_{is} and, hence, it is possible indirectly to measure P_{is} during P_{csf} drainage (Fig. 1). To prove the adequacy of this assumption we compared the results of the indirect method with the results of direct P_{is} measurements during catheterization of the cerebral venous system.

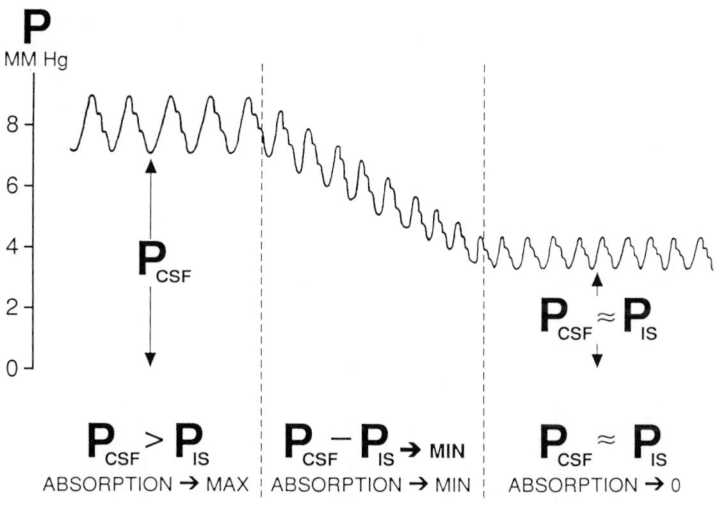

Fig. 1 Theoretical scheme of the P_{csf} and P_{is} changes during CSF drainage

CLINICAL MATERIAL AND METHODS

Seven patients (4 male, 3 female) with meningiomas were studied at the N.N.Burdenko Neurosurgical Institute, Moscow, Russia. Sinusography with catheterization of transverse or sigmoid sinuses via jugular vein was performed for diagnostic purposes. None of the patients had occlusion of the sagittal sinus. At the same time a lumbar puncture at the level L4-5 was performed and about 10 ml of the CSF was drained. Lumbar catheter for P_{csf} and sagittal sinus catheter for P_{is} measurements were connected to a single pressure transducer. Alternating P_{csf} and P_{is} measurements were performed to minimize error of the measurements. During CSF drainage a point is reached when further reduction P_{csf} fails to reduce the CSF outflow rate. According to Portnoy et al. when P_{csf} is slightly below then desired steady state pressure level it is possible to obtain only 1-2 drops of CSF per minute. After that the number of drops increases until a constant CSF flow is attained. At this point the CSF outflow rate is equal to the CSF production rate [1] and this P_{csf} will be equal to P_{is}. All results were analyzed with a 2-tailed paired t-test with significance level set at $p \leq 0.05$. Results are shown as mean $\pm$ 1 standard deviation.

RESULTS

At rest before CSF withdrawal the mean P_{csf} was 13.9 $\pm$ 6.4 mm Hg and mean P_{is} was 5.3 $\pm$ 2.1 mm Hg. There was statistically significant difference ($p \leq 0.01$) and no correlation ($r=0.239$) between mean P_{csf} and mean P_{is} at rest. At the end of CSF drainage the mean P_{csf} (i.e. indirect P_{is}) was equal 5.3 $\pm$ 1.4 mm Hg and mean direct P_{is} was equal 4.4 $\pm$ 1.8 mm Hg. The results shows coincidence of the P_{is} values obtained by direct and indirect methods (table 1). At the CSF drainage equilibrium point coefficient of correlation between absolute values of the P_{csf} and P_{is} was 0.867 and there was a statistically significant difference between the P_{csf} and P_{is}.

Table 1 Values for P_{is} (mm Hg) measured by direct and "indirect" methods

Patient	Indirect Method	Direct Method
1	6.2	6.5
2	5.9	3.4
3	5.7	4.4
4	2.6	1.5
5	4.2	3.6
6	6.7	6.7
7	5.5	4.6
Mean $\pm$ S.D.	5.3 $\pm$ 1.4	4.4 $\pm$ 1.8

DISCUSSION

The results demonstrate that indirect P_{is} measurement coincide with direct P_{is} measurements. although the direct P_{is} was nearly always less than the indirect P_{is}. The 1 mm Hg difference between the two methods is not physiologically significant despite the statistical difference between the means. Direct P_{is} method assess pressure in the posterior region of the sagittal sinus. On the other hand, indirect P_{is} method determine a pressure that integrates the pressure characteristics of all cerebral venous sinuses. Despite these methodologic differences, we conclude that indirect P_{is} measurement is accurate, less invasive than direct method, and therefore may be safer for patients. A limitations of the indirect method is that P_{is} cannot be measured indirectly in the presence of the block between cranial and spinal compartments of the brain. The data concerning the relationship between CSF pressure fluctuations, ventricular changes, and cerebral venous pressure may be useful in clarifying the complex interaction of these parameters and their significance in the development of the intracranial hypertension and hydrocephalus.

REFERENCES

1. Portnoy HD, Croissant PD. (1976) A Practical Method for Measuring Hydrodynamics of Cerebrospinal Fluid. Surg Neurol 5:273-277

ACKNOWLEDGMENTS

The author (A.Y.Razumovsky) very grateful to Drs. Daniel F. Hanley, M.D. and Michael A. Williams, M.D. for helpful comments and editorial review of this manuscript. The authors gratefully acknowledge the excellent secretarial assistance of Ms. Yarvis Simmons in the preparation of this manuscript.

An Intracranial Pressure Arithmetic System Using Ultrasound and Results in Healthy Adults

H. Kuchiwaki[1], S. Inao[1], K. Yoshida[1], M. Yamamoto[1], K. Sugita[1], N. Ishii[2], and Y. Ogura[3]

[1] Department of Neurosurgery, Nagoya University School of Medicine, Japan
[2] Department of Electronic and Computer Engineering, Nagoya Institute of Technology, Japan
[3] FA Division, Hitachi Construction and Machinery Co. Ltd., Japan

SUMMARY

Our noninvasive method of intracranial pressure (ICP) measurement was earlier reported in animal models. In the present study, we introduced data on the changes in dural thickness using our revised algorithm of Fast Fourier Transform-cepstrum for human study. Changes in dural thickness were evaluated in the supine position, sitting position, and Valsalva's maneuver in seven volunteers. By the Valsalva method the thickness of the dura mater decreased significantly compared to the other positions ($p<0.05$). Our results show that our novel method of ICP measurement is useful in human study.

INTRODUCTION

Measurements of intracranial pressure (ICP) are much time-consuming because of the aseptic condition and invasive surgical techniques involved. Numerous noninvasive methods have been proposed for the measurement of ICP. Measurement of ICP using ultrasound method has been presented with different ideas to obtain the relations between intensities or waveforms of ultrasound echoes and levels of ICP [1,2,3].

Jeppson's method of ICP measurements has attracted many researchers' interest [1]. However, the data obtained by his method are available in far higher ranges than useful for clinical use. ICP levels have not yet been determined by an ultrasound method of tissue characterization in different pathologies in the cranium [3]. We earlier reported our novel method of ICP measurement using ultrasound [4-9]. This method is based on signal processing of interference echo from a thin layer, an approach frequently used in measuring thin layer as a nondestructive method in a non biological system [10]. The relation between ICP and the dural thickness has also been presented elsewhere in our animal studies [4,5,9]. In applying our method to human study, the difficult problem has been obtaining reproducibility and reliability. In the present study, we obtained data from healthy volunteers by means of our revised algorithm for the detection of a relation between ICP and the dural thickness on the scalp, and then evaluated its clinical usefulness.

SUBJECTS AND METHODS

The present investigation was performed in seven male volunteers (22 to 51 y.o.) after a complete explanation of our aims and ultrasound method, and obtaining their informed consent. A circular flat probe (5 MHz) with a 25 mm diameter was brought in contact with an acrylate plate with a known thickness, and the reflected waves were inputted into a computer. Then a base echo was inputted to the computer before attachment to anything for normalization of ultrasound echoes. Next, the probe was placed on the scalp of the temporal region of the subject using ultrasound paste and a hair band, and the reflected waves obtained were inputted into the computer. The R wave from the electrocardiogram of the volunteer was then used as a trigger to start the system. The trigger time was 200 msec after the R wave. The reflected waves between delay time 0 and 20 μsec were sampled in each volunteer. Each volunteer assumed the supine positioned on a bed. The ICP was varied with the supine position (n=10), Valsalva's method (n=4), and the sitting position (n=4). An algorithm that cuts the reflected waves on the scalp was produced, and the delay time of the peak of the reflected wave was made clear on the quefrency axis by the fast Fourier Transform (FFT)-cepstrum analysis with maximum entropy method (MEM) [11,12]. The thickness of the dura (μm) was calculated from the time difference between the peak of the reflected wave from the incidence plane of the dura and that from its back side (nsec) x 1,600 m /sec (sound speed of the dura mater) X 1/2. Results were analyzed by Wilcoxon signed rank test at a significance level <0.05. Reproducibility was estimated using Kolmogorov-Smirnov test.

RESULTS AND DISCUSSION

The thickness of the dura in the healthy adults was 880 ± 130.5 μm in the supine position, 894 ± 40.3 μm in the sitting position, and 640 ± 46.7 μm by Valsalva's method. The thickness significantly decreased by Valsalva's method ($p<0.05$). Reproducibility was good in each subject. Findings were quite similar to those reported for the canine experiments [4,5,8,9]. The human study indicates a decrease in thickness with increasing ICP by Valsalva's method.

Our previous animal experiments showed a negative linear correlation between the thickness of the dura and ICP levels [4,5,9]. The present results from human study are similar, although we could not measure the levels of ICP. Our previous study indicated that our transcranial method is possible where the thickness of the skull is less than 5 mm [6,7]. In that study we could present continuos measuring method that is another ultrasound method of our ICP measurement in the human study.

In application of the method to human study, there are multiple echoes after FFT-cepstrum with MEM. An initiation of Most of them originate from the scalp. In this study, we set two time gates to eliminates the echoes from the scalp in the revised algorithm. We could define echo time by inserting an echo from an acrylate plate with a known thickness in echoes on time series from the probe on the scalp. Each power spectrum after FFT-cepstrum was normalized by the base echo obtained before attachment of the probe to the scalp. By processing we could clearly determine three echo peaks that indicate the surface of the skull, complex echoes from the back of the skull and the surface of the dura mater, and the back of the dura mater. These three echo peaks appeared on the quefrency axis according to the delay time.

In conclusion, present results shows our ultrasound method to be applicable and useful in human study.

REFERENCES

1. Jeppson S (1964) Echoencephalography V: A method for recording the intracranial pressure with the aid of the echoencephalographic technique. Acta Chir Scand 128:218-224
2. Richardson A, Eversden ID, Sterngergh Jr WCA (1972) Detecting intracranial pressure waves with ultrasound. Lancet 1:355-357.
3. Pranevicius O, Bertasius K, Pranevicius M, Jarzemskas E (1992) Noninvasive dynamic assessment of the elasticity of intracranial structures. Acta neurol Scand 86:512-516
4. Kuchiwaki H, Itoh J, Ishiguri H, Andoh K, Ogura Y, Sakuma N, Takishita T (1989) An approach to non invasive analysis of intracranial pressure (ICP) using an ultrasound probe. In: Hoff JT, Betz AL (eds), Intracranial Pressure VIII, Springer-Verlag, Berlin, Heidelberg, pp 22-26
5. Itoh J, Kuchiwaki H, Inao S, Kageyama N, Sakuma N, Takishita T, Ogura Y (1991) A study of signal processing in changes of intracranial pressure (ICP) using an ultrasound probe. Theoretical and experimental aspects. Artères et Veines 10:42-45.
6. Kuchiwaki H, Andoh K, Itoh J, Inao S, Sugita K, Sakuma N, Takishita T, Ogura Y (1991) An approach to a signal processing of intracranial pressure using ultrasonic probe. A preliminary report of continuous recording in a clinical use. Artères et Veines 10:48-51
7. Kuchiwaki H, Inao S, Andoh K, Itoh J, Sakuma N, Takishita T, Ogura Y (1992) Continuous recording of changes in intracranial pressure using interference echoes of ultrasonic wave: A preliminary report of practicality and clinical evaluation. J Clin Ultrasound 20:447-455.
8. Kuchiwaki H, Inao S, Andoh K, Sugita K, Sakuma N, Takishita T, Ogura Y (1992) Intracranial pressure measurements using ultrasound. Part 1. Results from continuous recordings of interference echoes. In: Oka M, von Reutern G -M, Furuhata M, Kodaira K (eds), Resent Advances in Neurosonology, Excerpta Medica, Amsterdam, London, pp 239-243
9. Kuchiwaki H, Inao S, Kanaiwa K, Sugita K, Zhu H, Ishii N, Sakuma N, Takishita T, Ogura Y (1992) Intracranial pressure measurement using ultrasound. Part 2: Experimental results from signal processing for determining pressure levels. In Oka M, von Reutern G -M, Furuhata M, Kodaira K (eds), Recent Advances in Neurosonology, Excerpta Medica, Amsterdam, London, pp 245-249

10. Sakuma N, Ogura Y,Takishita T (1989) Application of MEM-Cepstrum analysis to nondestructive measurements of thin layer thickness using ultrasonics. In: Boogaard J, van Dijk GM (eds), Non-Destructive Testing (Proc. of the 12th World Conf.), Elsevier Science Publisher BV, Amsterdam, pp1590-1592
11. Akaike H, (1974) A new look at the statistical model identification. IEEE Transaction on Automatic Control AC19:716-723
12. Kamerait RC, Childers DG (1972) Signal detection and extraction by cepstrum technique. IEEE Transaction on Information Theory 17-1:745-759.

Non-Invasive Pressure Measurement and Flow Regulation Device in Shunt System

TAKUO HASHIMOTO[1], SATOSHI IKEUCHI[1], TSUTOMU KOYAMA[1], TOSHIAKI ABE[2], HIDEAKI SHIMAZU[3], TOSHIAKI TAMAI[4], and MASAKATSU GONDOH[4]

[1] Department of Neurosurgery, Jikei University School of Medicine, Kashiwa Hospital, Chiba, Japan
[2] Department of Neurosurgery, Jikei University School of Medicine, Tokyo, Japan
[3] Department of Physiology, Kyorin University School of Medicine, Tokyo, Japan
[4] MDM Co. Ltd., Tokyo, Japan

INTRODUCTION

The ideal shunt system would release excessive CSF only and prevent shunt complications completely. Recently, pressure or flow controlled shunt systems have been used. However, as various types of hydrocephalic patients exist, shunt revision may be required due to malfunction of the shunt such as the obstruction of a shunt tube, hypofunction or hyperfunction. Since such malfunction can be detected by the periodic monitoring of the intracranial pressure(ICP), a new shunt system to allow the non-invasive measurement of ICP and the regulation of CSF flow has been developed in our department. In this paper, we report the principle of pressure measurement, flow regulation and its usage in a shunt system.

PRINCIPLE AND METHODS

We have developed a multipurpose shunt system to allow non-invasive measurement of ICP and regulation of CSF flow(5).The device for pressure measurement,which is implanted subcutaneously, is a dome shaped silicone reservoir with a diameter of 17mm, height 6mm and thickness 0.4mm. This reservoir is connected between the ventricular port and the flow regulatory device. The principle of pressure measurement is the collapse method which is similar to the coplanar theory. The pressure measurement system consists of a pressure transducer and a pusher dome. The surface of the reservoir collapses when the external pressure exceeds the internal pressure as the pusher dome percutaneously presses on the reservoir via the skin. Surface restoration occurs during the reverse process. The point of restoration or of collapse reflects the ICP, thus providing an indirect measurement of ICP(Fig. 1). The error can be set to be constant and they are adjusted automatically in the system. To calculate the ICP, the system takes the point of restoration.

The flow rate changeable device contains two slit valves and two titanium balls. One of the slit valves is with high resistance and the other is with low resistance. The flow rate is different between two valves. The flow rate is regulated through two slit valves by the location of two titanium balls. The flow rate can be set at four stages of off, low, medium and high flow.

RESULTS

A pressure devices was implanted on the thoracic wall in anesthetized dogs. Pressure within the reservoir was created artificially using a water tank, and was measured percutaneously. The pressure by changing the height of the water tank to change in pressure inside the reservoir. The difference between the actual pressure and the measured pressure by a sensor percutaneously was examined. The point of restoration was taken as the measuring point and the error adjusted. The pressure was measured once every two weeks for 6 months. A good correlation was obtained within the range of 0−40 cmH_2O. A total of 214 observations was collected. The relationship between the actual and measured pressures showed a linear regression; $Y=0.993X+0.557$, correlation $r=0.98$. The error of $+0.6$ cmH_2O caused by the characteristics of the silicone dome must be compensated for. The measurement of pressure by collapsing technique was reproducible and reliable in experimental studies(Fig.2). To evaluate the pressure measurement device clinically, we used it in conjunction with the Sophy programmable pressure valve in 20 patients with hydrocephalus. Measurement can be performed any time after the shunt operation. The device must be positioned at the level of the external auditory meatus. The pressure readings obtained were as anticipated. Five out of 20 cases required an adjustment of the pressure setting. These patients showed improvement. However, the ICP measurements were considered to be lower than expected. The patient's clinical condition, the measurement of ICP and the pressure setting of the Sophy shunt system did not always correlate. Obstruction of the shunt tube, hyperfunction and hypofunction may be evident by the ICP obtained percutaneously. The flow control device which we developed can have the flow rate set off, low, medium and high flow. The pressure-flow characteristics indicated that this flow control system can be applied to different pressure which occur in hydrocephalus. The multipurpose shunt system were used in 21 patients with hydrocephalus. Flow change was required in a few cases by moving the titanium balls percutaneously,when hyperfunction or hypofunction occurred after shunt operation. The authors have not experienced any major complications using a multipurpose shunt system(Table 1).

DISCUSSION

Infection and obstruction of the shunt tube are the main problems requiring shunt revision, while complications such as hypofunction and hyperfunction are also common. Conditions such as slit ventricle, craniostenosis and subdural hematoma caused by dysfunction require shunt revision (1,2,3,4,6,8). A shunt revision is sometimes required due to under or over drainage using the conventional shunt systems. Recently, pressure or flow controlled devices such as the Sophy programmable pressure valve, the Orbis Sigma shunt system or the multipurpose shunt system (MDM. Japan) are clinically used to prevent these complications (5,9). We can manage hyper- or hypofunction by changing the pressure control setting of the programmable pressure valve percutaneously. However, the patients may not show symptoms of either hyperfunction or hypofunction. We also observed that no symptom was seen in some patients even though a slit ventricle was apparent on their CT scan. Whether the shunt system is functioning properly or not can be obtained from the patient's clinical condition or by compression of the flushing device. Pumping of flushing device is not as reliable as we had previously thought. Imaging of the ventricle may be used even though the injection of isotope, contrast medium etc. into flushing device to check the flow may sometimes be required (10). Other methods such as Doppler technique and thermography can be used but they are not non-invasive. A sensor can be implanted for non-invasive measuremen (7). In practical, because the method is not easy, it is not often used clinically. The principle of pressure measurement we have applied here is called the collapse technique, a modification of coplanar theory. The core of the system is dome shaped pressure device made of silicone. A pressure sensor was used externally to obtain ICP measurements, and proved to be simple and provide reproducible data. Thickness of the skin did not influence the results. The error, which needed to be adjusted, was within $+0.6$ cmH_20. It was possible to evaluate the intracranial pressure in a shunt system within range of ± 3.0 cmH_2O. In a clinical study, our pressure device with Sophy programmable pressure valve has been used. We have experienced some cases with hyperfunction or hypofunction in these cases. It is also possible to use this pressure device with other conventional shunt system. The multipurpose shunt system were used in 21 cases with hydrocephalus. When the change of flow is required in a situation of hyperfunction or hypofunction, reasonable flow rate can be adjusted in the shunt system by moving the two titanium balls can non-invasively. The ICP could be obtained from the pressure device immediately following shunt operation, and the values were reproducible. Although data is preliminary, it appears that suitable ICP involves evaluation of the individual patient. Obstruction of the shunt tube, or its hypofunction and hyperfunction can be detected by periodically monitoring the ICP using this pressure device. We have not experienced major complications using multipurpose shunt system. These studies indicated that non-invasive monitoring of ICP was useful to prevent complications after shunt operation. It was possible to regulate CSF flow and evaluate ICP non-invasively in the multipurpose shunt system.

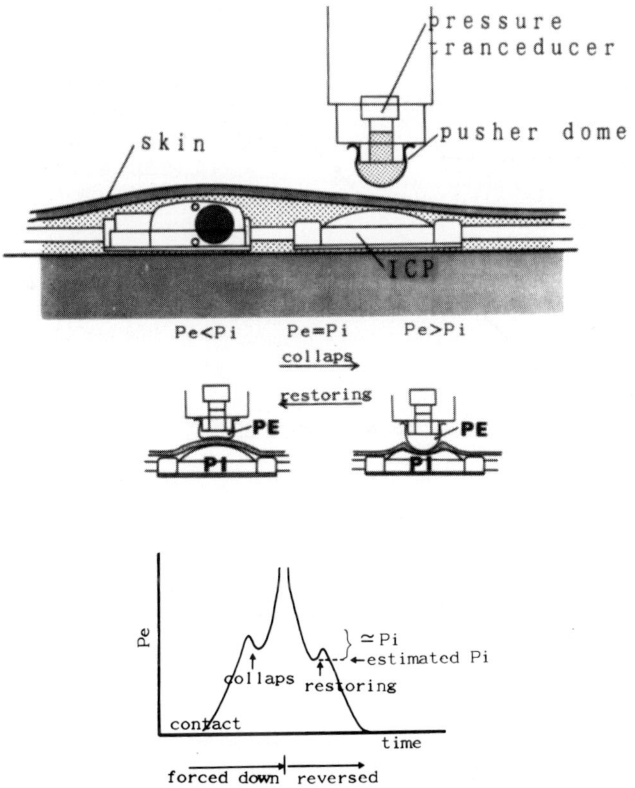

Fig. 1; Collapse and restoration of reservoir dome in response to the pressure difference between the internal and external domes. Elucidation of recognition of the collapse and restoration of the domes.

Multipurpose shunt system (MDM, Japan)

Case	Age	Sex	Cause of Hydrocephalus	MDM Flow	Pressure Meas. (cmH_2O)	Complication
1	51	F	SAH	Low flow	14.8	None
2	77	F	SAH	Low flow	12.3	None
3	62	F	SAH	Low flow	9.6	None
4	75	M	SAH	High – Medium	8.5	Effusion - None
5	55	M	SAH	High flow		None
6	19	M	Tumor	Low flow	11.2	None
7	65	M	Tumor	Medium flow	3.4	None
8	60	F	SAH	High flow	10.8	None
9	61	M	ASDH	Low flow		Infection
10	6	F	Congenital	Medium flow	15.3	None
11	7	M	Tumor	High flow	9.5	None
12	52	F	Obstructive	Low flow	8.6	None
13	40	M	Tumor	Low flow	10.3	Effusion - None
14	18	M	Tumor	Low flow	16.8	None
15	50	M	Tumor	Medium - Low	7.8 - 13.6	CSDH - None
16	76	F	SAH	Medium flow	8.9	None
17	50	F	SAH	Medium flow		None
18	44	F	SAH	Medium flow	10.2	None
19	67	F	SAH	Medium flow	9.4	None
20	58	F	Trauma	Medium flow	8.7	None
21	36	M	Tumor	Low flow	11.5	None

SAH;Subarachnoid hemorrhage,ASDH;Acute Subdural Hematoma
CSDH:Chronic Subdural hematoma

Table 1;Multipurpose shunt system was used in 21 patients with hydrocephalus

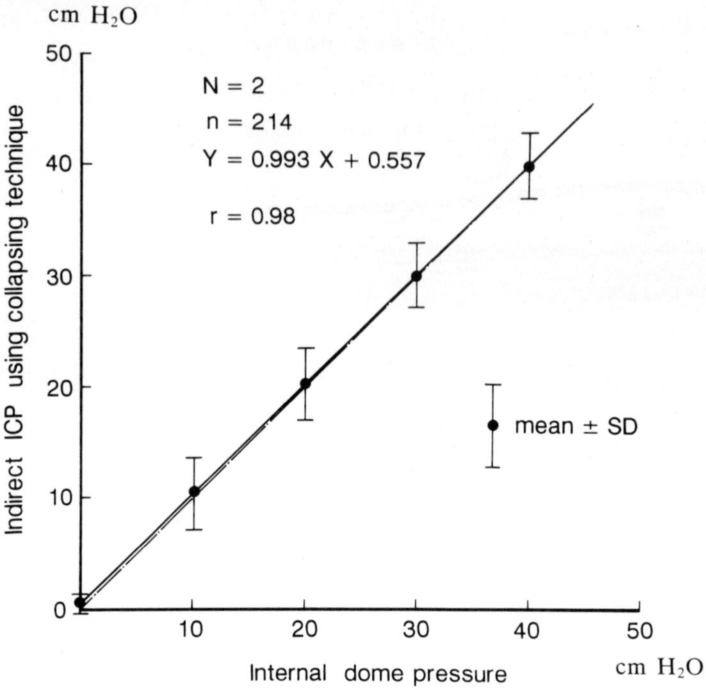

Fig.2; Correlation of the intracranial pressure estimated indirectly by the dome collapse technique and direct pressure of the internal dome implanted subcutaneously in a dog.

REFERENCES

1. Carteri A, Longatti PL, Gerosa M, Mazza C, Pasqualin;Complications due to incongruous drainage of shunt operations. Adv. Neurosurgery 8; 199-203, 1980
2. Engel M, Carmel PW, Chutorian AM; Increased intraventricular pressure without ventriculomegaly in children with shunt; "Normal volume" hydrocephalus. Neurosurgery 5; 549-552, 1979
3. Epstein F, Lapras C, Wisoff JH; Slit ventricle syndrome etiology and treatment. Pediatr Neurosci 14; 5-10, 1988
4. Faulhauer K, Schmitz P; Overdrainage phenomena in shunt treated hydrocephalus. Acta Neurochir (Wien) 45; 89-101, 1978
5. Hashimoto T, Nakamura N, Kanki T, Shimazu T, Yamakoshi K, Gondoh K, Tamai T; A new shunt systemm with non-invasive flow regulation and pressure measurement. in Matsumoto S, Tamaki N (Eds.); Hydrocephalus -Pathogenesis and treatment- Springer-Verlag 1991 pp422-431
6. Kiekens R, Mortier W, Pothmann R et al; The slit ventricle syndrome after shunting in hydrocephalic children. Neuropediatrics 13; 190- 194, 1982
7. Numoto M, Hara M, Sakai T et al;A non-invasive CSF flow meter. J. Med Eng Technol 5; 218-220, 1984
8. Samuelson S, Long DM, Chou SN; Subdural hematoma as a complication of shunting procedures for normal pressure hydrocephalus. J Neurosurg 37; 548-551, 1972
9. Sante-Rose C, Hooven MD, Hirsch JF; A new approach in the treatment of hydrocephalus. J Neurosurg 66;213 - 226, 1987
10. Sato O, Ohya M, Tsugane R et al;Quantitative measurement of cerebrospinal fluid shunt flow. Monogr Neural Sci 8;34-38, 1982

Experimental Evaluation of a New Solid State ICP Monitor

ANTHONY MARMAROU, OSAMU TSUJI, and JANA G. DUNBAR

Division of Neurosurgery, Medical College of Virginia, Richmond, VA, USA

INTRODUCTION

At present, the most utilized method for ICP measurement in our setting is the conventional ventricular catheter as originally described by Lundberg. [1] Clearly, this technique has limitation in those circumstances where brain swelling has occurred and there is difficulty in ventricular cannulation. Currently, there is no solid state device that is used uniformly as an alternate method as performance of these new products vary among investigators. The objective of this study was to evaluate the accuracy , drift, and dynamical response of a new solid state ICP sensor by Codman and compare the performance of this device with conventional measurement techniques.

MATERIALS AND METHODS

Protocol description

To accomplish these objectives four protocols were designed to evaluate the new Microsensor. The first protocol was restricted to bench testing and evaluated drift characteristics in a controlled fluid environment. (Protocol 1) In the second protocol, the output of the Microsensor placed in brain tissue of anesthetized adult cats was compared with ventricular fluid measurement of ICP. In the third and fourth protocols, similar comparisons were made with placement of Microsensors in the subdural and ventricular fluid and Microsensor pressure (MP) at these sites compared to conventional ventricular fluid pressure.(VFP)

Drift Testing Methods

Microsensors (n=4) were submersed in water baths (20 x 20 x 10 in.) filled with deionized water and maintained at 37 degrees Centigrade. The depth of immersion equaled 2 cm. As it was expected that pressure readings would vary with depth of immersion, water baths were covered by aluminum wrapping to minimize evaporation.

One Microsensor output was connected to the Codman ICP module which provided a direct reading of ICP. The remaining three Microsensors were connected to Hewlett Packard Pressure monitors (Model 78205D) which were known to have minimal electronic drift. This allowed us to evaluate the drift of the Microsensor and Codman Electronic Module independently.

Microsensor outputs at controlled temperature were monitored continuously by computer and manual readings were obtained from the digital monitors at 2 hour intervals. After obtaining the 2 hour reading, the Microsensor was immersed to a depth of 20 cm in order to test the sensitivity at the same temperature and returned to the 2 cm position.

To measure Codman electronic module drift independently, the zero calibration position on the Codman interface was activated at 0 and 100 mmHg every 12 hours and the readings were followed by computer.

Animal preparation

All animal protocols were approved by our internal review board and procedures in compliance with NIH guidelines. Adult cats (n=6) weighing 2.5 to 5.8 Kg were initially anesthetized with pentobarbital (30 mg/kg) and maintained with a mixture of Halothane (1-2%), nitrous oxide (60 %) and oxygen (38-40 %) . Animals were positioned on a stereotaxic apparatus and femoral vein cannulated for administration of fluids and femoral artery for measurement of blood pressure. A 25 gauge needle was placed in the ventricle stereotaxically and connected to a conventional fluid catheter and strain gauge for measurement of VFP.

Similarly, cisterna magna fluid pressure was also measured utilizing conventional strain gauge devices. Microsensor output for each type of placement was connected to the Codman Pressure Module.

When all pressure devices were in place and zeroed, computer monitoring was initiated and after 1 hour of baseline measure, the ICP was elevated by fluid infusion into the cisterna magna up pressures of 60 mmHg. Pressure was maintained at this level for approximately 5 minutes and pumps were turned off allowing pressure to recover.

RESULTS

Drift tests indicated that the MS devices were quite stable and had a small negative drift coefficient which was monotonic and averaged -0.00523 mmHg /hr or -0.125 mmHg per day (S.D.= 0.0875) at the 2 cm depth. At the 20 cm depth, the drift was less and equal to 0.110 mmHg/day (S.D. =0.0541). The drift characteristics over a period of 144 hours are shown in Figures 1a and 1b for the 2 cm and 20 cm depth of immersion respectively.

Fig. 1a

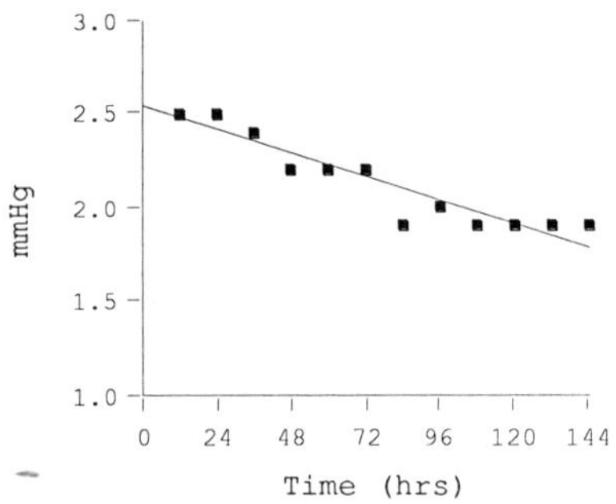

Fig. 1b

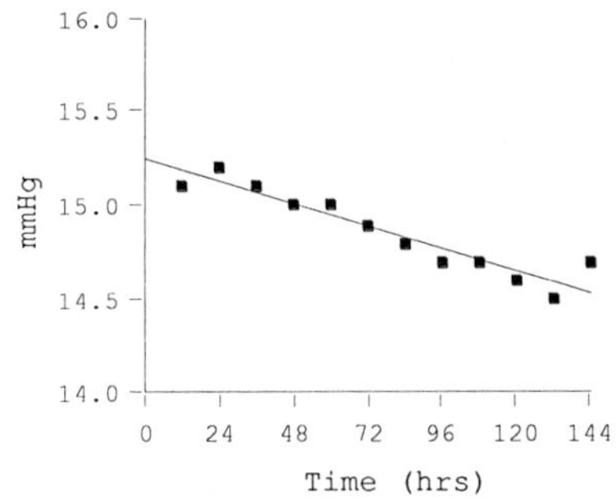

Fig.1 : Drift Characteristics of the Codman Microsensors at 2cm depth (a) and 20cm depth (b). Average Drift was always negative and equaled 0.005 mmHg/hr or -0.110 mmHg/day.

Comparison of Microsensor and VFP

The pulsatile characteristics of the Microsensors placed in brain tissue were of high fidelity and of greater magnitude than the corresponding ventricular fluid pressure pulse indicating a wide dynamic range. (Fig 2a) The same fidelity was experienced in all placements. The similarity between VFP and MP pressures during a typical pressure cycle is shown in Fig 2b. Note the increased pulsatile component of the MP device.

Fig. 2a

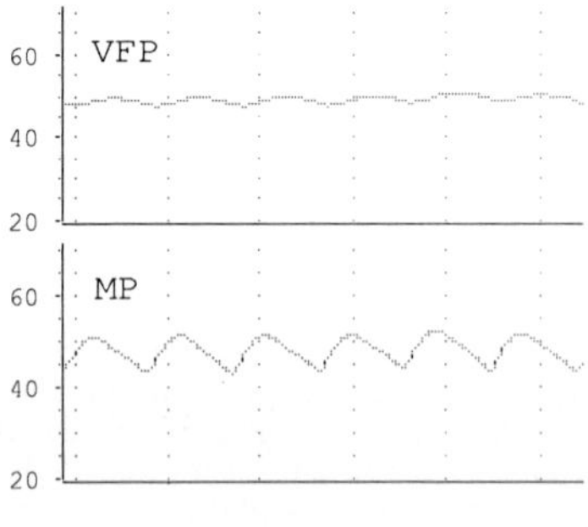

Fig. 2b

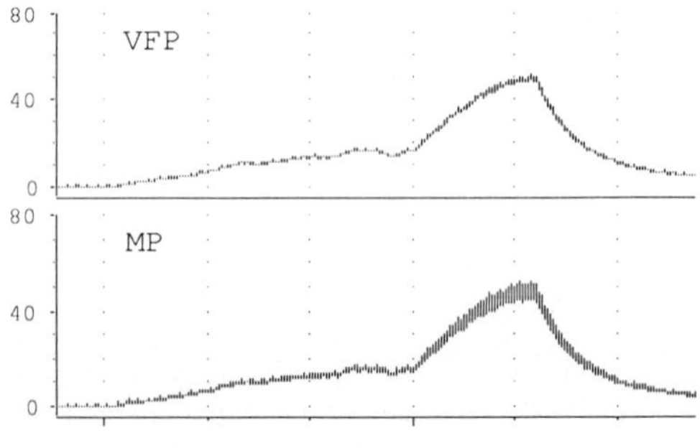

The comparison of data points for all pressure cycles are shown in figures 3. Figure 3a compares the tissue placement of the MP with VFP, figure 3b shows the comparison of the subdural site with VFP and figure 3c compares MP positioned in the ventricle compared to VFP. With subdural placement, it is necessary to insure that the sensor is placed facing the brain tissue. These comparisons indicate a good correlation between fluid and sensor pressures. Linear regression of the MP in parenchyma resulted in the equation ; MP = 0.98 * VFP - 0.69, r^2 = 0.994 (n = 5). Similarly, a close correlation of MP measure in the subdural space (sensor facing brain tissue) resulted in the equation ; MP = 0.93 * VFP + 0.96, r^2 = 0.993. Finally, the correlation of MP placed in the ventricle with fluid measured VFP was also very good and equaled MP = 1.04 * VFP - 0.046, r^2 = 1.000.

Fig. 3a Fig. 3b Fig. 3c

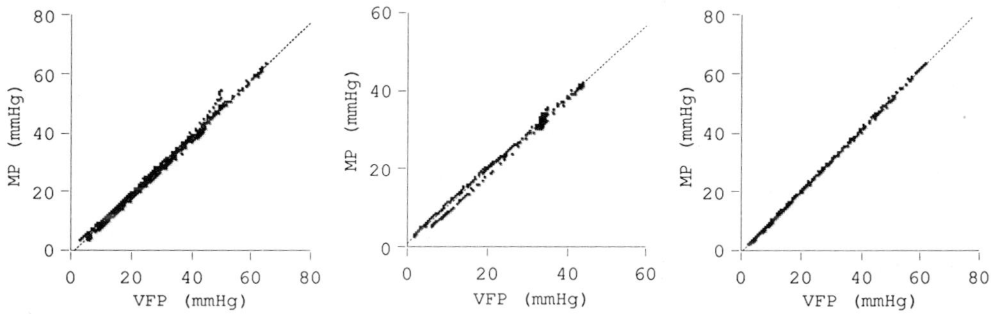

Figure 3 : Comparison of Microsensor pressure placed in the parenchyma (a), subdural space (b) and ventricle (c) compared to ventricular fluid pressure.

DISCUSSION

These studies show that this new device provides a reliable measure of pressure in parenchyma or the subdural space when compared to ventricular fluid pressure. Moreover, the drift studies show that the device is very stable over long periods of time with a relatively small temperature coefficient and is consistent with findings by other investigators using this device.[2] In general, although our experience has been limited to the experimental setting, we found the device and instrumentation to be easily used with little training required. Following our drift tests, our focus was to compare the performance of this unit placed in the parenchyma with fluid pressure measured by conventional disposable strain gauge. In this regard, it was our experience that the pulsatile levels measured by the Microsensor were always greater than the fluid pressure pulses which attests to the sensitivity and fidelity of the transduction by this new unit. To our surprise, this high level of performance was reproducible with subdural placement. In this regard, for greater accuracy, it is necessary to insure that the device is positioned so that the active surface is facing brain. This only applies to subdural placement as the device is not position sensitive when implanted in tissue. In summary, in our hands, the Microsensor is a reliable, drift free device which provides an accurate measure of ICP with high pulsatile fidelity.

REFERENCES

1. Lundberg N (1960) Continuous recording and control of ventricular fluid pressure in neurosurgical practice. Acta Psychiatr Scand [Suppl 149] 36:1-193

2. Gopinath SP, Cherian L, Robertson CS, Narayan RK, Grossman RG (1993) Evaluation of a microsensor intracranial pressure transducer. J Neurosci Methods 49:11-15

Multicenter Clinical Evaluation of a New ICP Device

ANTHONY MARMAROU[1], OSAMU TSUJI[1], JOHN MYSEROS[1], TIMOTHY HARRINGTON[2], LAWRENCE PITTS[3], and DUNCAN MCBRIDE[4]

[1] Department of Neurosurgery, MCV, Richmond, VA, USA
[2] Barrows Institute, Phoenix, AZ, USA
[3] UCSF, San Francisco, CA, USA
[4] UCLA, Los Angeles, CA, USA

INTRODUCTION

The recent advent of fibre-optic devices (FOD) has resulted in the development of transducers capable of sensing pressure in either brain parenchyma or fluid. The use of FOD's in contrast to the conventional fluid pressure strain gauge for measurement of ICP offers distinct advantages to the clinician in terms of ease of insertion and continuous wave form availability. The disadvantage of these devices are that they cannot be calibrated in-vivo and as a result the drift characteristics are of great importance. In a previous report, the laboratory experience in the evaluation of a new FOD by Innerspace Company indicated that the sensitivity, bandwidth and drift characteristics were suitable for potential use in the clinical setting.[1] This report describes the clinical evaluation of the new fibre optic catheter (OPX) in four head injury centers where efforts were made to test the performance in brain parenchyma, subdural and ventricular spaces.

METHODS

The patient population consisted of 50 brain injured patients undergoing ICP monitoring in the intensive care unit. OPX catheters with an outer diameter of 1.3 mm were positioned in parenchyma (n=12), subdural (n=14) or ventricle (n=22) (3.0 mm i.d. with drainage port) space after having been zeroed to atmosphere. OPX catheters placed in these sites were compared to ventricular fluid pressure (VFP) measured by conventional strain gauge systems. OPX catheters placed in the subdural space were compared to fluid pressures measured via the drainage port. Using procedures developed by the traumatic coma data bank, end hour ICP measurements from the FOD and the fluid device were recorded on forms and transferred to Medical College of Virginia for analysis.

RESULTS

There were no complications during the insertion of the OPX devices and the temporal pressure course derived from the OPX devices compared favorably with the ICP measures from conventional fluid pressure. A histogram analysis was utilized to provide a measure of the deviation of the OPX device from fluid pressures over a wide range of pressure for the respective sites. (Fig. 1a, 1b, 1c)

Fig. 1a : Ventric

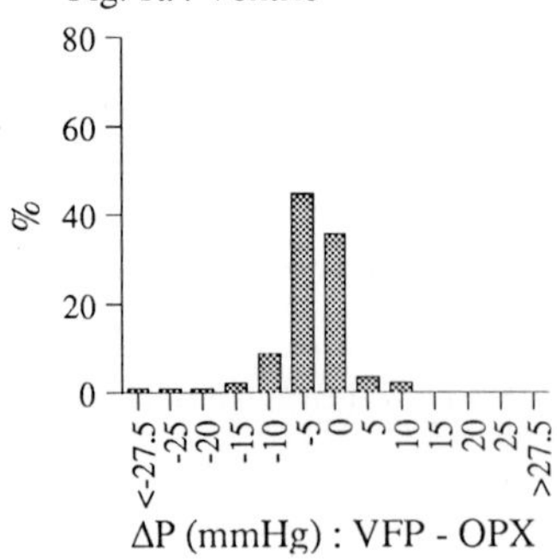

Fig. 1b : Parenchymal

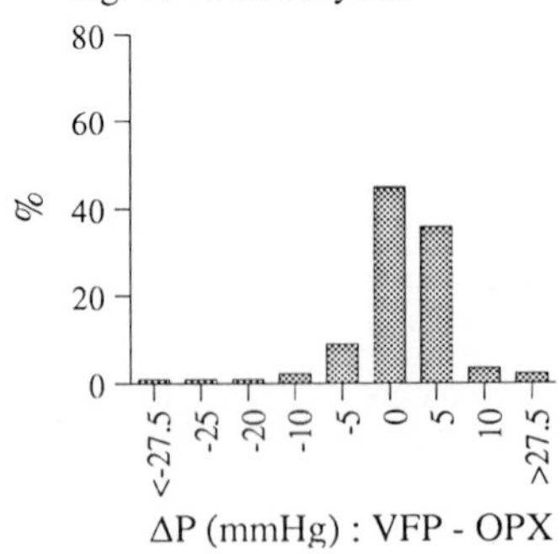

Fig. 1c : Subdural

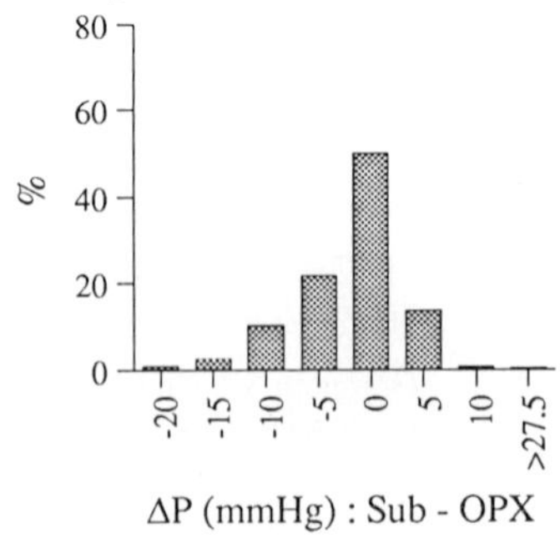

The percentage of OPX readings within a mean of +/- 5 mmHg of the respective fluid pressure standard are summarized in Table 1.

Table 1. Percentage of OPX readings within +/- 5.0 mmHg of fluid pressure

Site	ICP < 15	ICP > 15	Overall
OPX VFP vs VFP	85.7 %	92.8 %	87.7 %
OPX Sub vs FSub	90.9 %	87.3 %	89.6 %
OPX Parenchyma vs VFP	81.0 %	95.1 %	85.3 %

DISCUSSION

ICP measured by the new OPX device in 3808 hours of testing compares favorably with respective fluid pressures. The comparison of differences at high and low pressures (Table 1.0) shows that the correspondence seems greater at high pressures when positioned in the ventricle and parenchyma while the differences between OPX positioned subdurally with the fluid subdural pressure is equally distributed above and below 15 mmHg. With regard to parenchymal placement, manipulation of ventricular fluid pressure by occasional drainage precludes a direct comparison of parenchymal placed catheters. However, we would conclude that transient pressure gradients in parenchymal placed catheters occur similar to those observed by other FOD devices. The ICP measured by the OPX catheter in the ventricle and subdural sites correlates closely with the respective fluid pressures as was observed in previous laboratory studies. The flexibility, small size, ease of insertion and non-directional sensitivity is of clinical advantage.

REFERENCES

1. Yoshihara M., Marmarou A., Dunbar, J. et al.; A fibreoptic device suitable for subdural pressure measurement.: In Intracranial Pressure VIII, C.J.J. Avezaat, J.H.M. van Eijndhoven, A.I.R,Maas and J.T.J. Tans (eds); (1991) Intracranial Pressure VIII Springer Verlag Berlin, Heidelberg, pp 20-24

Session II: Monitoring (1)

Chairmen: L. Symon and S. Nakazawa

Cerebral Autoregulatory Threshold Assessed Using Transcranial and Laser Doppler Flowmetry in Anesthetized Rabbits

H.K. Richards, M. Czosnyka, P.J. Kirkpatrick, and J.D. Pickard

MRC Cambridge Centre for Brain Repair & Academic Neurosurgical Unit, University of Cambridge, UK

INTRODUCTION

Transcranial Doppler (TCD) recording of blood flow velocity in the basal cerebral arteries is widely used clinically for monitoring the cerebral blood supply. There are suggestions derived from both clinical and experimental observations that the pulsatile component may be used as an index of cerebral autoregulatory reserve.

In 70 head injured patients, the Pulsatility Index (PI, defined as the amplitude divided by flow velocity time average) increases as cerebral perfusion pressure (CPP) decreases below 70 mmHg. [1] This occurrs in parallel with a progressive increase in arterio-venous oxygen difference indicating the global decrease in cerebral blood flow (CBF). In experimental investigations in anaesthetized rabbits, Nelson et al. [2] showed that the amplitude of the flow velocity pulse wave started to increase before CPP reached the lower limit of autoregulation as defined by intermittent measurement of local CBF by hydrogen clearance technique. We have decided to investigate this phenomenon by comparing changes in the pulsatile component of flow velocity in the basilar artery of the anaesthetized rabbit with continuous monitoring of cortical perfusion using laser Doppler flowmetry. Continuous assessent of these CBF parameters should lead to a better understanding of the mechanisms responsible.

MATERIAL AND METHODS

Twelve New Zealand rabbits of both sexes (weight from 2.8 to 4.3 kg) were studied under the UK Animals Act (Scientific Procedures), 1986. Anaesthesia was induced using intravenous alphaxalone/alphadalone (Saffan, 3mg/kg) and maintained using 1-3% halothane in 3:1 nitrous oxide/oxygen. Body temperature was maintained using a warming blanket. The animals were subsequently paralysed (pavulon, 0.5 mg/kg/hr) and ventilated to maintain PaCO2 at 30-38mmHg. Blood pressure was recorded from the common carotid artery and a cannula placed in the left femoral artery to control arterial blood pressure by haemorrhage. The animals were then supported in a Sphinx position using a head frame with three-point skull fixation.

Ultrasound Doppler spectra were obtained from the basilar artery using an 8Mz pulsed Doppler probe positioned over the dura exposed by a posterior frontal burr hole. Another burr-hole was made to insert the Laser Doppler probe intraparenchymally (in 6 cases) or on the surface of dura (in 6 cases). Adjustment of the laser probe was performed to ensure that a parallel decrease in blood flow velocity and flux occurred during a brief Valsalva manoeuvre (of 3-5 seconds) at the end of preparatory period.

Waveforms from arterial blood pressure monitor, Doppler ultrasound blood flow velocity and flux from laser Doppler flowmeter (Flux) were fed to an analog-to-digital converter fitted into an IBM compatible personal computer, sampled with a frequency of 150 Hz and saved digitally on hard disk using a program designed by W.Zabolotny, Warsaw University of Technology. Digital signals were then analyzed using our own software for clinical data processing (ICMR, M.Czosnyka, University of Cambridge). All parameters were saved as time trends for individual processing or statistical analysis.

Laser Doppler flux was corrected by subtracting biological zero level measured post mortem. Changes in FV and Flux were normalised relative to their baseline values - average FV and Flux over 2-5 minute period before induced hypotension. All data was imported to a PC statistical package and relationships between the recorded variables and mean ABP have been evaluated using analysis of variance.

Baseline values of signals were assessed within 2-5 minute periods and then arterial blood pressure was gradually reduced by controlled haemorrhage over an average time of 9 min (ranging from 7 to 17 minute).

RESULTS

Basilar artery blood flow velocity was well correlated with Laser Doppler flux. The correlation coefficient between flux and time average flow velocity was R= 0.748; $p<10^{-6}$, between flux and systolic FV was R=0.805; $p<10^{-6}$ from data samples taken from all animals (Fig. 1)

The averaged amplitude of the flow velocity waveform was calculated and plotted on the same graph as mean FV systolic and diastolic (Fig. 2). The amplitude is increasing significantly ($p<0.05$) when ABP decreases below 70 mmHg, as a consequence of gradual divergence between FV diastolic and systolic. This results in a progressive increase in Pulsatility Index (PI) and Standardized Pulsatility Index (SPI) with ABP decreasing until 30 mmHg- (Fig 3).

DISCUSSION

A close relationship between Laser Doppler Flux and Transcranial Doppler Flow Velocity during deep hypotension shows that in healthy rabbits TCD can be used to estimate dynamic changes in cerebral

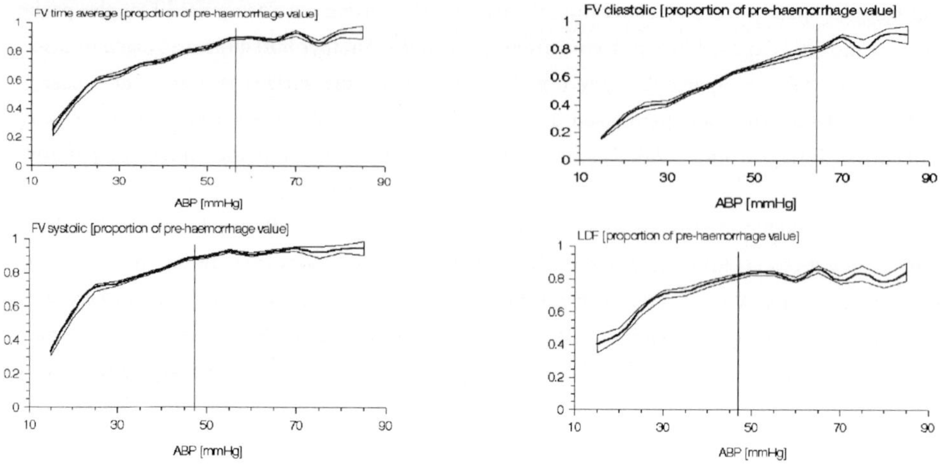

Fig. 1 The relationships between Flux, FV, FVs, FVd normalised by baseline values and mean arterial blood pressure during hypotension. The graphs show the mean with 95% confidence interval. Vertical lines show the limits below which the dependent variable starts to decrease significantly ($p<0.05$) with ABP falling in steps of 5 mmHg.

blood flow. These results confirm other reports where CBF and FV were measured simultaneously [3,2].

Our objective was to interpret the changes in flow velocity pulsatility when arterial blood pressure was decreasing below the limit of autoregulation. The mean lower limit of autoregulation, as assessed using analysis of variance for Flux versus mean ABP, did not differ significantly from the limit below which FV systolic started to decrease (45 mmHg - see Fig 1). However, flow velocity diastolic started to decrease when ABP fell below 65 mmHg - significantly higher ($p<0.0001$) than thresholds for FV systolic and Flux. FV time average had an autoregulatory threshold at approximately 60 mmHg. This discrepancy between the behaviour of systolic and diastolic flow velocities constitutes the key to understanding the increase in amplitude of TCD flow velocity with hypotension. When the systolic value is stable and FV diastolic is decreasing, amplitude increases, therefore, the pulsatility index, being the ratio of amplitude to time average FV, increases.

The gradual divergence between FV systolic and diastolic can be seen from the very beginning of hypotension, below ABP of about 70 mmHg. This phenomenon confirms the clinical observations of Chan et al. [2], who reported an increase in PI in head injured patients for cerebral perfusion pressure below 70 mmHg. In a previous experimental study the hydrogen clearance technique was used to measure CBF. These measurements required a period of steady state in cerebral perfusion pressure, which was technically difficult to achieve at low cortical flow. That study suggested that FV amplitude increase prior to any significant fall in CBF with falling CPP. Our present work based on laser Doppler which has better temporal resolution also demonstrates that the amplitudes of flow velocity and flux

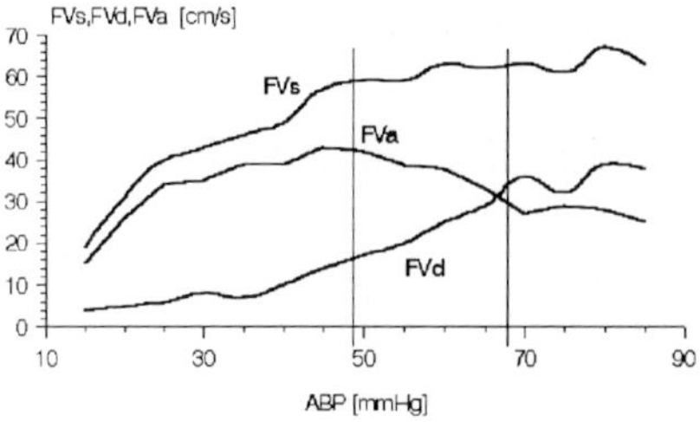

Fig.2 Averaged amplitude of the flow velocity waveform, FVa, flow velocity systolic, FVs and flow velocity diastolic, FVd

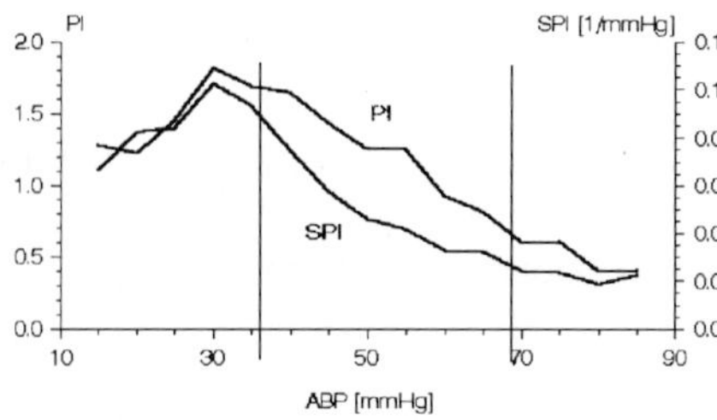

Fig.3 Flow velocity Pulsatility Indices demonstrates the relationship between amplitude of arterial blood pressure waveform (ABPa) and mean ABP.

increased before there was any fall in mean flux.

We have observed, that when FV diastolic falls, the pulsatile component of cerebral blood supply increases. Previously we have demonstrated experimentally [4] that the resistance to the continuous component of cerebral blood supply is higher than the resistance to pulsatile inflow (approximately three times in rabbits). Perhaps by increasing the pulsatile component of blood inflow, the pulsatile component of microflow may be augmented.

The increase in pulsatility of the cerebral circulation precedes the lower limit of autoregulation as ABP falls. Further studies are needed to elucidate the role of augmented flow pulsatility as a factor responsible for maintaining brain perfusion when the autoregulatory reserve is nearly exhausted.

REFERENCES

1. Chan KH, Miller DJ, Dearden M, Andrews PJD, Midgley S: The effect of changes in cerebral perfusion pressure upon middle cerebral artery blood flow velocity and jugular bulb venous oxygen saturation after severe brain trauma. J. Neurosurg 77:55-61, 1992

2. Nelson RJ, Czosnyka M, Pickard JD, Maksymowicz W, Perry S, Martin JL, Lovick AHJ: Experimental aspects of cerebrospinal haemodynamics : the relationship between blood flow velocity waveform and cerebral autoregulation. Neurosurgery 31:705-710, 1992

3. Barzo P, Doczi T, Csete K , Buza Z, Bodosi M : Measurements of Regional Cerebral Blood Flow and Blood Flow velocity in Experimental Intracranial Hypertension: Infusion via Cisterna Magna in Rabbits, Neurosurgery 28: 821-25, 1991

4. Czosnyka M, Richards H, Pickard JD, Harris N, Iyer V : Does the resonance of cerebral blood flow exist? Experimental study in anaesthetized rabbits. Ultrasound in Medicine and Biology (in press, 1994)

Laser Doppler Flowmetry in Head Injured Patients

P.J. Kirkpatrick, M. Czosnyka, P. Smielewski, S. Piechnik, and J.D. Pickard

University Department of Neurosurgery, Addenbrooke's Hospital, Cambridge CB2 2QQ, UK

Introduction

In conditions of low cerebral perfusion pressure (CPP), varying degrees of impaired cerebrovascular autoregulation occur which alters oxygen and substrate delivery to the brain parenchyma. Such events are believed to be important in the generation of ischaemic lesions seen after severe head injury [1]. The recognition of a changing state of CPP in head injured patients has required the continuous monitoring, recording, and computer processing of data derived from reliable intracranial and arterial pressure measuring devices [2].

Laser Doppler flowmetry (LDF) is a technique which provides a continuous measure of relative microcirculatory flow [3]. Using a rigid LDF probe, we have developed a relatively simple and safe procedure for monitoring cortical flux in the neurointensive care unit. The data derived from long-term monitoring in 22 severely head injured patients is presented, and the potential sources of artefact identified. The LDF signal changes occurring during changes in CPP, pCO2, mannitol infusion, and spontaneous hypoxic events are demonstrated.

Methods

Patients: Over a nine month period, 22 patients (aged 19 - 69yr) with a moderate to severe head injury (GCS 3 - 12) were entered into the study. All patients were sedated with midazolam (2-10mg/Hr infusion) and fentanyl (0.1 - 0.5mg/Hr), paralysed with atracurium (0.3 - 1.2mg/Kg/Hr infusion), and ventilated to a pCO2 of 3.5 - 4.0kPa.

Monitoring: Invasive and continuous monitoring of arterial blood pressure and ICP (Camino) were undertaken in all patients. At the time of insertion of the ICP device, a second bolt (Camino) was sited approximately 3cm further lateral to the ICP bolt to support a pre-calibrated rigid LDF probe (Moor's Instruments MBF3D, P3 probe) passed through the dural and positioned 2-3mm above the cortical surface. In 10 patients, long-term monitoring of middle cerebral artery flow velocities (MCA FV) was also undertaken using transcranial Doppler (Scimed), and in 6 of these recordings from jugular venous oximetry (Oxymetrix 3, Abbot) and cerebral oximetry (Hamamatsu 1000) were simultaneously carried out.

Signal analysis: Signals of CPP (mmHg), FV (cm/sec) and LDF (AU) were sampled at a frequency of 40Hz, and digitised using an 12 bit analog-to-digital converta. Signals were processed using specific software (ICM; M Czosnyka, University of Cambridge) and averaged over consecutive 3 second periods. The relationships between LDF signal and mean CPP were evaluated using analysis of variance (ANOVA) within a CPP range of 30 - 80mmHg. Breakpoints for decreases in the LDF signals were defined at CPP levels below which the LDF signals started to fall significantly ($p < 0.05$).

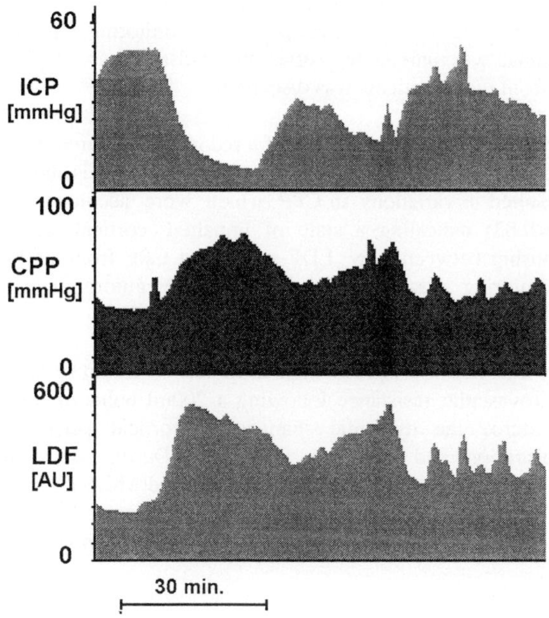

Fig.1
Continuous recordings of ICP, CPP and LDF signals during waves of raised ICP in a patient with a diffuse head injury. Variations in cortical perfusion measured with LDF were closely coupled to changes in CPP.

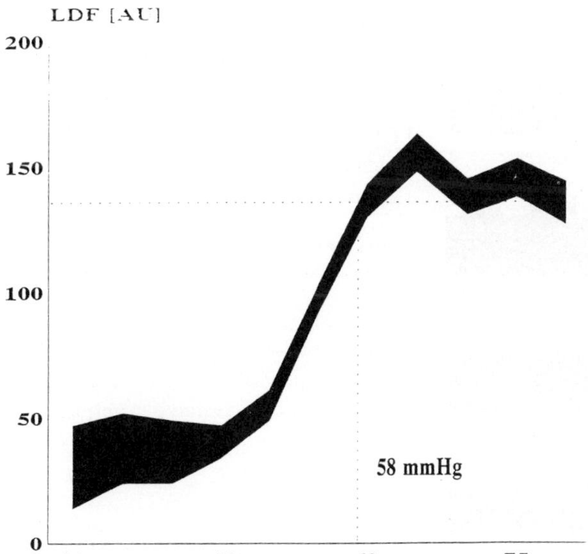

Fig. 2
Graph showing the upper and lower limits of standard deviation for the mean LDF signal versus CPP derived from analysis of raw data from long term recordings in 16 patients. The mean LDF signal demonstrates a breakpoint at a CPP of 58mmHg below which cortical perfusion falls significantly ($p<0.05$).

Results

No complications resulted from either ICP or LDF probe insertion . In 16 patients, a continuous pulsatile LDF signal was obtained throughout the period of monitoring. In the remaining 6 patients the LDF signal was unreliable, often non-pulsatile, and highly dependant on probe position. Data from these patients was discarded.

Relationship between cortical flux and CPP: An example of a recording captured from one patient with a severe diffuse head injury during spontaneous changes in CPP is shown in Figure 1. Fluctuations in ICP resulted in variations in CPP which were accompanied by changes in the LDF signal (r=0.83) indicating a state of impaired cortical auto-regulation. Analysis of the relationship between raw LDF signal and CPP from all 16 patients in whom long term monitoring was achieved indicated an autoregulatory breakpoint at a CPP of 58mmHg (Figure 2) below which cortical perfusion fell.

Relationship between cortical flux and MCA FV: The high temporal resolution of LDF helped characterise the fall in cerebrovascular resistance following a 200ml bolus of 20% mannitol (5%, $p<0.04$), and registered the dymamic changes of cortical perfusion associated with dopamine administration and changing pCO_2. During transient spontaneous episodes of decreased CPP, a close coupling between LDF and MCA FV was usually (Figure 3) but not always apparent (Figure 4). Spontaneous episodes of hypoxia were also invariable associated with a fall in CPP, MCA FV and cortical perfusion (Figure 4).

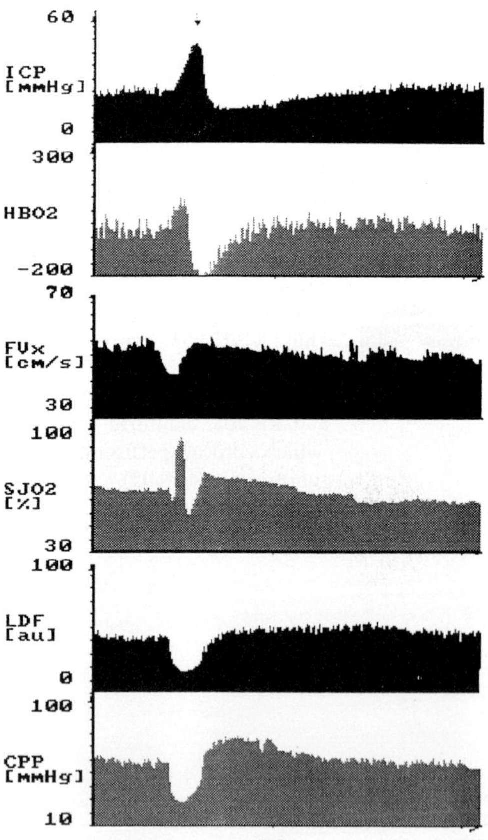

Fig. 3
Simultaneous recordings of middle cerebral artery flow velocity (Fvx), oxygenated haemoglobin (Hb02), jugular venous saturation (SJ02) and LDF during a transient increase in ICP which compromised CPP.

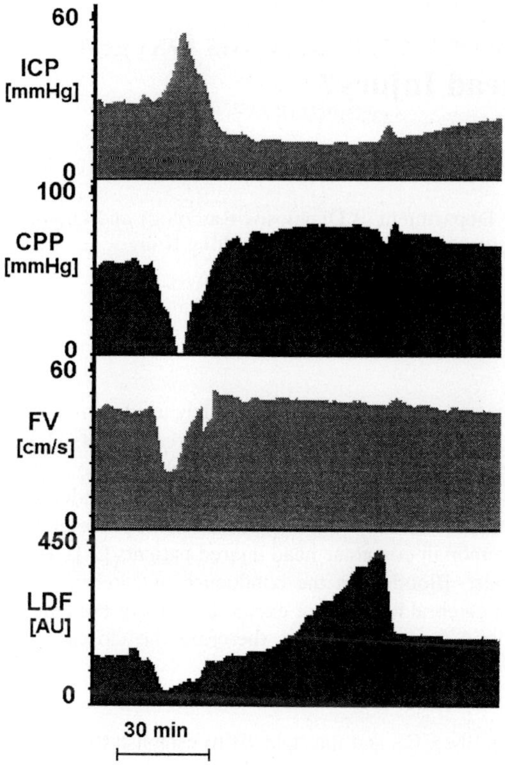

Fig. 4
Middle cerebral artery flow velocity (FV) and LDF signal changes during fall in CPP induced by an attempted withdrawal of dopamine support. A dramatic increase in ICP caused a fall in both FV and microcirculatory flux. After restarting dopamine, a transient hyperaemia was recorded by LDF only.

Conclusions

The advantage of LDF over other methods adopted for measurement of blood flow is the high temporal resolution provided LDF registers rapid changes in cortical perfusion in response to a falling CPP and hypoxia, and provides an additional method for monitoring the cerebrovascular response to therapeutic manipulation. Although cortical perfusion was usually closely correlated with MCA FV, uncoupling between the two variables did occur. The method of adopting a rigid LDF probe provided long-term pulsatile signals in a large proportion of patients. By comparing variations in CPP with the flux signal, a real time assessment of the autoregulatory state of the cortical microcirculation is possible. Further, such recordings may prove of value when considering general therapeutic manoeuvres to improve cortical flow. Alterations in probe design and the methods of placement may help to improve signal reliability further.

References

1. Bouma GJ, Muizelaar PJ, Stringer WA et al. Ultra-early evaluation of regional cerebral blood flow in severely head injured patients using xenon-enhanced computerised tomography. J Neurosurg (1992) 77:360-368.

2. Chan KH, Miller JD, Dearden NM, et al: The effect of changes in cerebral perfusion pressure upon middle cerebral artery blood flow velocity and jugular bulb venous oxygen saturation after severe brain injury. J Neurosurg (1992) 77:55-61.

3. Stern MD, Lappe LD, Bowen PD: Continuous Measurement of tissue blood flow by laser-Doppler spectroscopy. Am J Physiol (1977) 232: H441-H448.

Does Jugular Bulb Venous Oxygen Saturation Accurately Reflect Confluence of Cerebral Sinus Oxygen Saturation in Patients with Head Injury?

JOSEPH M.K. LAM[1], MICHAEL S.Y. CHAN[2], and WAI S. POON[1]

[1] Neurosurgical Unit, Department of Surgery, [2] Department of Diagnostic Radiology and Organ Imaging, Prince of Wales Hospital, The Chinese University of Hong Kong, Shatin, Hong Kong

INTRODUCTION

Continuous monitoring of the jugular venous oxygen saturation ($S_{JB}O_2$) is widely used in monitoring for adequacy of cerebral perfusion and cerebral oxygen metabolism in head injured patients [1][2]. Jugular bulb (JB) venous oxygen is considered representative of mixed cerebral venous blood (MCVB). Anatomically, however, there is no single venous outflow from the brain. In addition to anastomosis of the intracerebral and extracerebral venous system, significant hemisphere and / or regional cerebral blood flow differences are common in comatose head injured patients [3]. Hence, true mixed cerebral venous blood does not exist. Blood from the confluence of cerebral sinuses (CCS) is a mixture of venous drainage from the cerebral hemisphere except for part of the temporal lobes, the brainstem and the cerebellum. Blood from the CCS is therefore the closest to the theoretical MCVB.

We compared venous blood oxygen saturation in the CCS and the right JB to establish the accuracy of $S_{JB}O_2$ to reflect that of "MCVB".

CLINICAL MATERIALS AND METHODS

The blood oxygen saturation at the confluence of the cerebral sinuses ($S_{CCS}O_2$) was compared with that at the jugular bulb ($S_{JB}O_2$) in ten head injured patients. All these patients were managed in the intensive care unit (ICU), fully sedated and ventilated, with continuous arterial blood pressure and intracranial pressure (ICP) monitoring. The arterial oxygen saturation was monitored by pulse oximetry and intermittent arterial blood tests. The right JB was cannulated 1 cm lateral to the carotid pulse at the level of the cricoid cartilage. A 6F angiographic sheath was introduced retrograde into the right internal jugular vein using the Seldinger technique. The tip of the sheath was positioned at the JB as confirmed on angiography. A 4F angiographic catheter was introduced through the sheath. The tip of the catheter was then navigated into the CCS under angiography guidance. The catheter and the sheath were kept patent by heparinised saline infusion at a rate of 4 ml per hour.

Intermittent blood samples were taken simultaneously from the JB and CCS for oxygen saturation measurement using a cooximeter (Instrumentation Laboratories 482 Cooximeter, Instrumentation Lax., Lexington, MA). The tests were repeated at intervals of 15 minutes to 2 hours, depending on the clinical condition of the patients.

RESULTS

In a one year period between February 1992 and January 1993, 10 head injured patients had dual CCS and JB monitoring, with a mean monitoring duration of 58 hours (range from 10 to 122 hours). One hundred and fifty pairs of blood samples were collected. The range of $S_{JB}O_2$ was 19.0% to 91.2%. All except one case (Case 10) had good corresponding rates between $S_{JB}O_2$ and $S_{CCS}O_2$. For the nine cases that had good corresponding rate, the corresponding rate within 5% O2 saturation was 97.6% (123/125): $[S_{JB}O_2]=0.98[S_{CCS}O_2]+1.8$ where the correlation coefficient (r) was 0.97 and $p < 0.001$ (Fig. 1). In one patient (Case 10), $S_{CCS}O_2$ was persistently lower than $S_{JB}O_2$ (Fig. 2). This patient developed brain death due to intractable intracranial hypertension as a result of right hemisphere injury, despite a generous decompressive craniectomy. The CCS was 2.5 cm on the right side of the midline with a dominant right JB. The AVDO at CCS was consistently higher than that at the JB.

Only one patient had left JB dominance where no significant difference in $S_{JB}O_2$ (at the right JB) and $S_{CCS}O_2$ could be demonstrated (fig. 3).

Accidental puncture of the carotid artery occurred in one case and was treated with temporary compression. There was no clinical evidence of serious complications such as line sepsis or thrombosis of the sinuses.

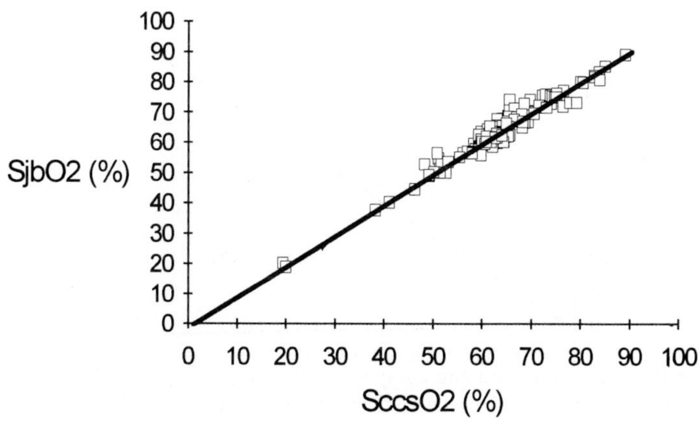

Fig. 1: $S_{JB}O_2$ versus $S_{CCS}O_2$ in 9 cases (all cases except Case 10)

$[S_{JB}O_2]=0.98[S_{CCS}O_2]+1.5$

$r=0.97$; $p<0.005$

Corresponding rate within 5% oxygen saturation = 97.6% (123/125)

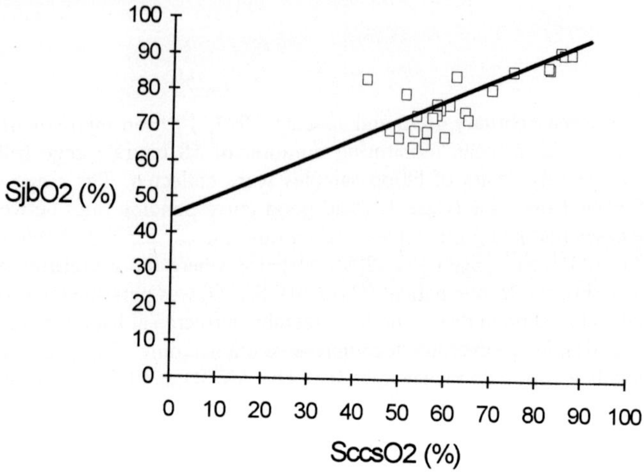

Fig. 2: $S_{JB}O_2$ versus $S_{CCS}O_2$ (Case 10)
$[S_{JB}O_2]=0.51[S_{CCS}O_2]+45.4$
$r=0.78$; $p<0.005$
Corresponding rate within 5% oxygen saturation = 8.0% (2/25)

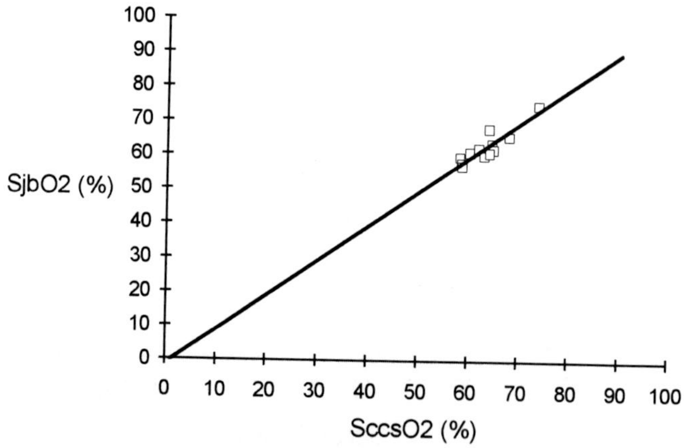

Fig. 3: $S_{JB}O_2$ versus $S_{CCS}O_2$ in the case with left JB dominance
$[S_{JB}O_2]=0.98[S_{CCS}O_2]+0.6$
$r=0.89$; $p<0.005$
Corresponding rate within 5% oxygen saturation = 100% (12/12)

DISCUSSION

Good correlation between $S_{JB}O_2$ and $S_{CCS}O_2$ was demonstrated in 9 of the 10 cases we studied. In case 10, there was a consistent difference between $S_{JB}O_2$ and $S_{CCS}O_2$. The reason for the discrepancy is not clear: it may be due to anatomical variation of the venous drainage of brain, or the pathological changes on the injured brain. The discrepancy is unlikely to be artefactual because when cerebral perfusion pressure fell, AVDO increased until the patient developed brain death. The severity of ischaemia of the cerebral cortex would have been underestimated if cerebral venous oxygen saturation monitoring was based on JB and not CCS in this particular case.

Simultaneous blood sampling of both right and left JB in normal individuals shows that oxygen saturation at the internal jugular vein ($S_{JV}O_2$) is equal on both sides.[4] More recently, however, significant side-to-side difference in $S_{JB}O_2$ was demonstrated [5]. From our study, eight of the nine cases with right-sided dominance of jugular vein and nine of the ten cases with cannulation of the right jugular veins had good correlation between $S_{JB}O_2$ and $S_{CCS}O_2$. Hence, monitoring $S_{JB}O_2$ at the dominant jugular vein or the right side is a reasonable empirical choice. The key question of how one could identify cases with discrepancy between $S_{JB}O_2$ and $S_{CCS}O_2$ remains unresolved and requires more work. Cannulation of CCS should not replace continuous $S_{JB}O_2$ monitoring because our data suggested that $S_{JB}O_2$ and $S_{CCS}O_2$ corresponded in the majority of cases. Dual CCS and JB cannulation may be helpful in cases where $S_{JB}O_2$ is normal or high, whereas other parameters such as cerebral perfusion pressure and cerebral blood flow are suggestive of an ischaemic state.

CONCLUSION

Cannulation of the confluence of cerebral sinuses in 10 head injured patients was shown to be a safe procedure for mixed cerebral venous oxygen monitoring. $S_{JB}O_2$ correlated well with $S_{CCS}O_2$ in 9 of the 10 cases we studied, suggesting that $S_{JB}O_2$ monitoring reflected reliably "MCVB" oxygen saturation in the majority of cases.

REFERENCES.

1 Chan KH, Dearden NM, Miller JD, Andrews PJD, Midgley S (1993) Multimodality Monitoring as a guide to treatment of Intracranial Hypertension after Severe Brain Injury. Neurosurgery, 32 (4):547-552.

2 Sheinberg M, Kanter MJ, Robertson CS, Contant CF, Narayan RK, Grossman RG (1992) Continuous monitoring of jugular venous oxygen saturation in head-injured patients. J Neurosurgery 76:212-217.

3 Obrist WD, Langfitt TW, Jaggi JL, Cruz J, Gennarelli TA (1984) Cerebral blood flow and metabolism in comatose patients with acute head injury. J Neurosurg 61:241-253.

4 Gibbs EL, Lennox WG, Gibbs FA (1945) Bilateral internal jugular blood. Comparison of A-V differences, oxygen-dextrose ratios and respiratory quotients. Am J Psychiatry 102:184-190.

5 Stocchetti N, Paparella A, Bridelli F, Bacchi M, Piazza P, Zuccoli P (1994) Cerebral venous oxygen studied with bilateral samples in the internal jugular veins. Neurosurgery 34:38-43.

Monitoring of Cerebral Oxygenation by Near Infrared Spectroscopy (NIRS) Versus Jugular Venous Oxygen Saturation (SJVO2) in Comatose Patients

A. ROSENTHAL, G.H. SCHNEIDER, A. UNTERBERG, and W.R. LANKSCH

Department of Neurosurgery, Rudolf Virchow Medical Center, Free University of Berlin, 13353 Berlin, Germany

SUMMARY

Monitoring of cerebral oxygenation is an important guide to therapy of comatose patients. While jugular venous oximetry (SJVO2) invasively measures oxygen saturation in the jugular bulb, near infrared spectroscopy (NIRS) can be used to monitor oxygenation of brain tissue non-invasively. Little is known about the significance of this new technology in comatose patients, e.g. following severe head injury. Thus, cerebral oxygenation was monitored in comatose patients by NIRS and SJVO2 simultaneously. In addition, intracranial pressure (ICP), blood pressure, cerebral perfusion pressure, arterial oxygenation and endtidal CO2 were recorded.

When SJVO2 was within normal limits (60-80%), regional tissue oxygenation as measured by NIRS ran parallel to jugular bulb oxygen saturation. There was a trend towards higher tissue oxygenation values compared to SJVO2 of about 5-10%. When SJVO2 fell below 55% - mostly associated with periods of intracranial hypertension - however, NIRS did not reflect the desaturation. Moreover, a significant number of technical disturbances rendered NIRS-measurements more difficult. Thus, further technological refinements and validation studies are needed before NIRS may become clinical routine in monitoring cerebral oxygenation.

INTRODUCTION

During the last years, monitoring of cerebral oxygenation has become widely accepted to guide the therapy of comatose patients, in particular following severe head injury (7). At the moment, monitoring of jugular venous oxygen saturation (SJVO2) represents the technique mostly used (7). While this is an invasive technique, near infrared spectroscopy (NIRS) has been proposed to monitor brain tissue oxygenation non-invasively (1 - 6). This new technology has been validated experimentally and under special clinical conditions, like in new-born infants, healthy humans and intraoperatively (1, 2, 4, 5, 6). So far, little is known, however, about its use and significance in intensive care, especially in severely head injured patients. Also, there are no reports on comparing SJVO2 and NIRS monitored cerebral oxygenation under these conditions.

MATERIALS AND METHODS

Cerebral oxygenation was monitored in 15 comatose patients, mostly due to severe head injury with a Glasgow Coma Score of 7 or less, by NIRS and SJVO2 simultaneously. Regional frontal tissue oxygenation was monitored by the INVOS 3100 cerebral oximeter (Somanetics); SJVO2 by the Oximetrix 3 system (Abbott). Simultaneously, intracranial pressure, mean arterial blood pressure, cerebral perfusion pressure, endtidal CO2 and the arterial oxygen saturation were monitored.

Two generations of NIRS-probes were used in the study. The main difference of these probes is the geometry of the optodes which was changed in order to reduce the influence of extracerebral blood of scalp and scull. The probes were always placed above the right frontal region as proposed by the manufacturer.

RESULTS AND DISCUSSION

Technical Considerations of NIRS-Measurements:

Following positioning of the NIRS probes above the right frontal region, tissue oxygenation ranged between 60 and 80%. In many cases, the monitoring-system had breakdowns and stopped to yield values of oxygen saturation soon afterwards. In some cases these errors could be solved by restarting the system, or replacements of the sensor. The duration of measurements of 10 consecutive patients is given in figure 1. The graph depicts the time periods where the monitor reportet tissue oxygen saturation values regardless whether these values were reliable or not. In all 10 cases the measurements were stopped because of a dysfunction of the system. In only 3 patients monitoring was possible for more than 48 hours. Monitoring with the second generation of probes was even more prone to disturbances than the first generation.

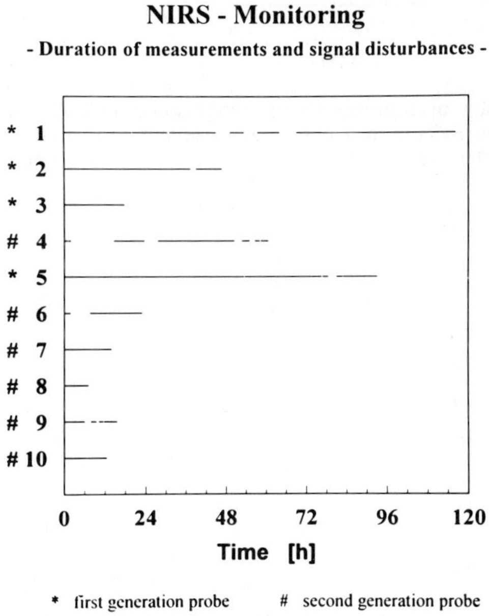

Figure 1: Duration of NIRS-measurements and periods of signal disturbances (blanc spots) of 10 consecutive patients

Comparison of NIRS versus SJVO2:

Figure 2 represents an original tracing comparing oxygen saturation as measured by NIRS, or in the jugular bulb together with ICP-monitoring. In this case as in most other cases, tissue oxygenation saturation was approximately 5% higher than jugular bulb oxygen saturation. If the SJVO2 was between 60 and 80%, NIRS-RSO2 was running more or less parallel.

In most cases, increases of jugular bulb oxygen saturation were sufficiently reflected by NIRS while decreases were insufficiently or not at all reflected by NIRS (Figure 2 and 3). The sensitivity of the near infrared measurements to reflect marked decreases of SJVO2 is summarized in Figure 3. Of 30 episodes of marked SJVO2 decreases (more than 10% of its actual value) only 6 episodes (20%) of NIRS data reflected a decrease, though these events were mostly due to an increased intracranial pressure and a consecutive decrease in cerebral perfusion pressure.

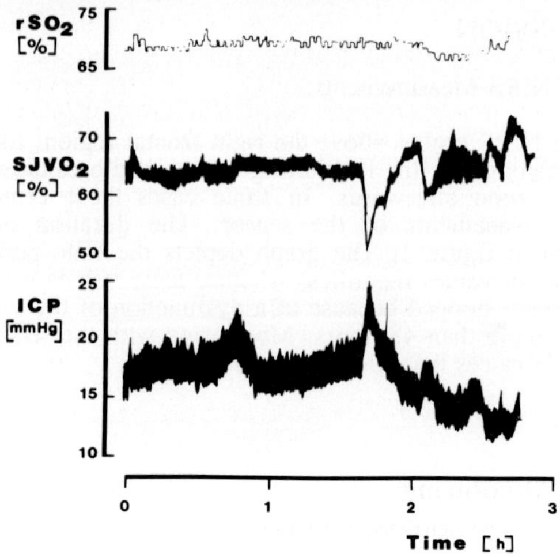

Figure 2: Original tracings of monitoring of regional tissue oxygenation (RSO2) by NIRS and global cerebral oxygenation by SJVO2 in a patient with severe head injury. Intracranial pressure is moderately elevated. While ICP sharply increases and SJVO2 decreases, RSO2 does not change.

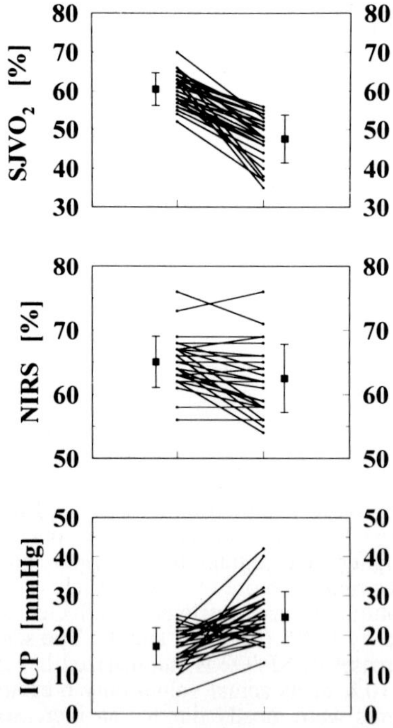

Figure 3: Synopsis of episodes in which SJVO2 markedly decreased due to an increase of intracranial pressure.

Taken together, the limited experience with near infrared spectroscopically monitored regional tissue oxygen saturation is ambiguous. Though a general correspondence of cerebral oxygenation monitored by NIRS and SJVO2 in the range of 60 to 80% was observed, marked decreases of jugular bulb oxygen saturation below 55% were insufficiently reflected by NIRS. Moreover, periods of signal disturbances and system breakdowns limited the use of the NIRS monitor.
Thus it is mandatory to introduce technological refinements and to perform additional validation studies, before this new technology becomes clinical routine for monitoring of cerebral oxygenation.

REFERENCES

1. Ausman JI, McCormick PW, Stewart M, Lewis G, Dujovny M, Balakrishnan G, Malik GM, Ghaly RF (1993)
   Cerebral oxygen metabolism during hypothermic circulatory arrest in humans.
   J Neurosurg 79: 810-815

2. Brazy JE, Lewis DV, Mitnick MH, Jöbsis FF (1985):
   Noninvasive monitoring of cerebral oxygenation in preterm infants: preliminary observations.
   Pediatrics 75: 217-225

3. Jöbsis FF (1977):
   Noninvasive, infrared monitoring of cerebral and myocardial oxygen sufficiency and circulatory parameters.
   Science 198: 1264-1267

4. McCormick PW, Stewart M, Goetting MG, Dujovny M (1991):
   Noninvasive cerebral optical spectroscopy for monitoring cerebral oxygen delivery and hemodynamics.
   Crit Care Med 19: 89-97

5. McCormick PW, Stewart M, Goetting MG, Dujovny M (1991):
   Regional cerebrovascular oxygen saturation measured by optical spectroscopy in humans.
   Stroke 22: 596-602

6. Smith DS, Levy W, Maris M, et al. (1990):
   Reperfusion hyperoxia in brain after circulatory arrest in humans.
   Anesthesiology 73: 12-19

7. Unterberg AW, Schneider GH, Lanksch WR (eds) (1993):
   Monitoring of Cerebral Blood Flow and Metabolism in Intensive Care.
   Acta Neurochirurgica Suppl. 59, Springer, Wien, New York

ACKNOWLEDGEMENT

The technical and secretarial assistance of Ms. R. Duisberg, C. Dürre and A. Riede is highly appreciated.

Clinical Utility of Jugular Bulb Oximetry in Severe Head Injury

S.B. Lewis[1], J.A. Myburgh[2], and P.L. Reilly[1]

[1] Department of Neurosurgery, Royal Adelaide Hospital, North Terrace, Adelaide, South Australia 5000, Australia
[2] Department of Intensive Care, Royal Adelaide Hospital, North Terrace, Adelaide, South Australia 5000, Australia

INTRODUCTION

The concept of primary and secondary injury has proved useful in understanding the pathological changes associated with brain trauma. The ability to influence primary injury processes thereby improving outcome is limited, however recent studies analysing the influence of neuroprotective agents in modifying the actions of neurotoxic substances are encouraging [1]. Secondary brain injury comprises a spectrum of hypoxic and ischaemic insults that occur subsequent to the initial trauma. These range from mass lesions (e.g. extradural haematoma) and raised intracranial pressure to subtle hypoxic / ischaemic insults resulting from suboptimal cerebral oxygen delivery. Following neurotrauma, autoregulatory mechanisms for maintaining cerebral perfusion may be embarrassed, thus rendering cerebral tissue particularly vulnerable to secondary insults. Accurate and continuous monitoring of cerebral oxygen utilisation may aid in the detection and prevention of these insults during this period of vulnerability.

Cerebral monitoring after head injury usually includes measurement of intracranial and arterial pressure. Cerebral perfusion pressure, while clearly important, does not give any indication of the capacity of cerebral perfusion to meet metabolic demand. Importantly, there is no continuous clinical measurement of cerebral blood flow or cerebral metabolic rate. The recent development of continuous jugular bulb oximetry may offer an opportunity to identify episodes of compromised cerebral blood flow and thus help to identify and prevent secondary injury [2, 3, 4].

The aim of this prospective observational study was to evaluate the clinical utility of jugular bulb oximetry in detecting secondary insults in patients with severe head injury as determined by jugular bulb oxygen desaturation and relating these episodes to other continuously monitored variables.

MATERIALS AND METHODS

Patients admitted to the Royal Adelaide Hospital Intensive Care Unit with a closed head injury and a Glasgow Coma Score < 9 following resuscitation were studied. All patients were mechanically ventilated to achieve moderate hypocapnia (35 - 40 mmHg) and to maintain arterial oxygen tension (PaO2) greater than 100 mmHg. Patients were sedated with combined narcotic and benzodiazepine infusion and nursed at 30 degrees head elevation.

Monitoring

Routine haemodynamic monitoring included systemic arterial pressure via radial artery cannulation (Arrow Radial Artery Catheter Set 20G, Arrow International Inc, Reading, PA, USA), central venous pressure and continuous heart rate via electrocardiography. Respiratory monitoring included continuous pulse oximetry (Criticare Systems Inc, 504 Pulse Oximeter), end - tidal capnography (Datex Normocap, Instrumentation Corp, Helsinki, Finland), minute ventilation and lung compliance (Servo 900C, Siemens Systems, Helsinki, Finland). Intracranial pressure (ICP) was monitored by a frontal intraparenchymal fibreoptic pressure tip transducer (Model 110-4B Camino Laboratories San Diego, California, USA).

Jugular Bulb Oximetry

Jugular bulb oxygen saturation was monitored by a 4-French fibreoptic oxygen saturation catheter (40cm Shaw Opticath. Abbott Laboratories, North Chicago, Illinois USA). The catheter was inserted in the dominant internal jugular vein as determined by alternate jugular compression. If the intracranial pressure rise was equal, then the side of greater trauma as determined by CT was chosen. If the CT indicated a diffuse injury then the right side was chosen. Following insertion the catheter tip was verified radiologically to be above the lower border of C1. Calibration against a laboratory oximeter (IL - 482, Instrumentation Laboratories, North Chicago, Illinois, USA) was performed eight hourly. If the catheter or laboratory oximeter values differed by more than 3%, the catheter was recalibrated in accordance with the laboratory oximeter saturation. Jugular bulb oxygen desaturation was defined as an oxygen saturation less than 55% lasting more than ten minutes under conditions of normal catheter light intensity. The following physiological parameters were recorded during an episode of desaturation: end-tidal carbon dioxide (ETCO2), cerebral perfusion pressure (CPP), ICP and pulse oximetry (SpO2). Abnormal variation of these measures were defined as follows: (1) hypocapnia (ETCO2 < 30 mmHg); (2) cerebral hypoperfusion due to arterial hypotension in the absence of raised intracranial pressure where CPP is less than 60 mmHg; (3) intracranial hypertension (ICP > 20 mmHg); (4) hypoxia (SpO2 < 90%). Continuation of these pertubations for ten or more minutes during an episode of desaturation was considered an association.

RESULTS

Sixteen patients (11 male, 5 female) with a mean age of 28 years (14 to 64) were studied. The mean delay from the time of head injury to arrival at hospital was 7 hours while the mean delay from arrival at hospital to jugular bulb oximetry was 8 hours. There were 36 episodes of jugular bulb oxygen desaturation in 16 patients, from 10 minutes to 9 hours with a mean of 89 minutes. 78% of these desaturations, occurred within 48 hours of the head injury (fig. 1).

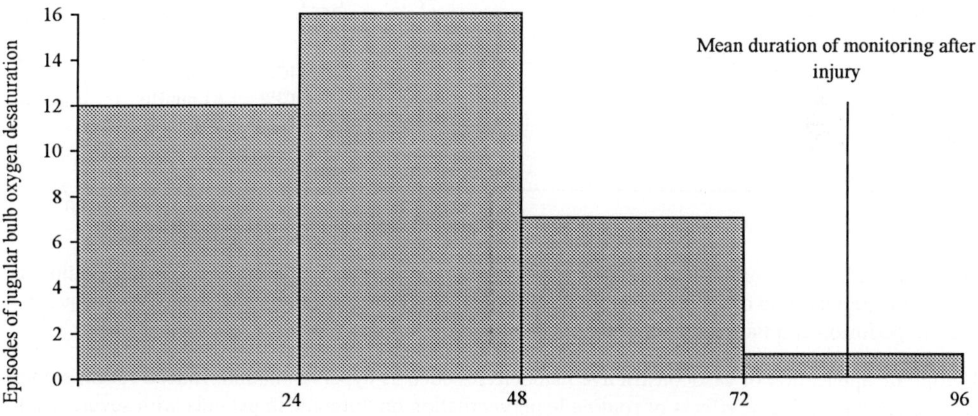

Fig. 1 Distribution of episodes of jugular bulb oxygen desaturation in relation to time elapsed since injury.

Jugular bulb oxygen desaturation was most frequently associated with hypocapnia which occurred as the only association in 47% (17/36) of episodes. Hyperventilation during periods of raised intracranial pressure was associated with reversible jugular bulb oxygen desaturation in two patients. Cerebral hypoperfusion due to arterial hypotension in the absence of intracranial hypertension was the only association in 17% (6/36). Intracranial hypertension was the only association in only 11% (4/36). Combinations of the above insults were present in 24% (9/36) of episodes (fig. 2). 22% (2/9) of these combinations were due to raised ICP associated with cerebral hypoperfusion.

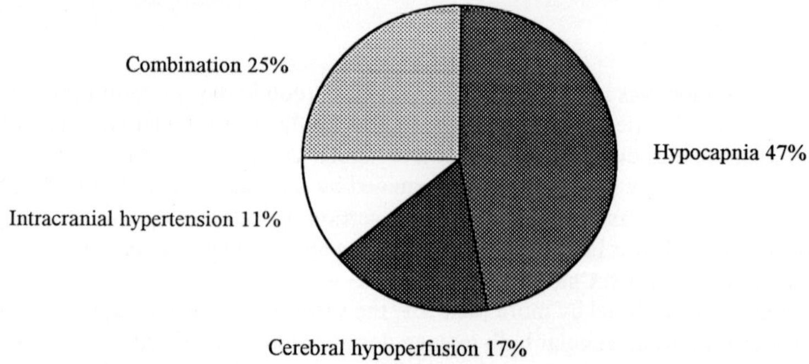

Fig. 2 Frequency of jugular bulb oxygen desaturation occuring in association with hypocapnia, cerebral hypoperfusion, intracranial hypertension and a combination of these.

DISCUSSION

Neuromonitoring of severe head injury should be able to detect potentially harmful secondary ischaemic / hypoxic insults early. This study highlights, as have others [3], the frequency of episodes of cerebral circulatory compromise which would not be detected without jugular bulb oximetry.
The commonest cause of jugular bulb oxygen desaturation was hypocapnic vasoconstriction due to hyperventilation used as standard therapy for acute head injury. The cerebral vasoconstrictive effects of hypocapnia are illustrated in fig. 3. These episodes of cerebral oligaemia would not have been detected by monitoring intracranial pressure or cerebral perfusion pressure alone. This may allow more selective and

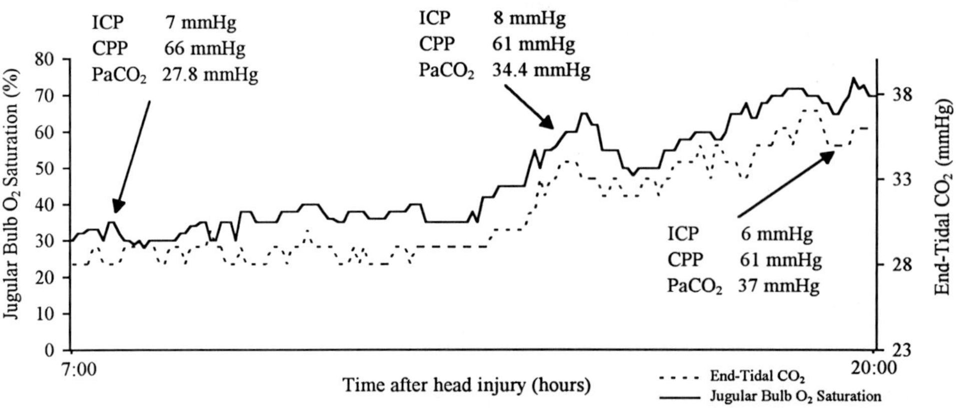

Fig. 3 Jugular bulb desaturation associated with hypocapnia. As $PaCO_2$ increased following ventilator adjustment, jugular bulb oxygen saturation rose in parallel reaching a value consistent with adequate cerebral perfusion at a $PaCO_2$ of 37 mmHg.

appropriate application of vasoconstrictive manoeuvres such as hyperventilation. Indeed recent studies have reported the adverse effects of routine hyperventilation on outcome in patients with severe head injury [5].

ICP monitoring alone does not reflect cerebral oxygen utilisation. Changes in ICP occured late or not at all in the presence of jugular bulb oxygen desaturation associated with cerebral hypoperfusion (fig. 4).

The delay in transfer from trauma site to hospital is readily explained by the large geographical area (4000 sq. kilometers) served. Of concern was a mean 8 hour delay from time of hospital admission to intensive care monitoring. The primary reason for this delay was the treatment of patients with multiple injuries prior to reaching the intensive care unit. The longest delays occured in patients who underwent fixation

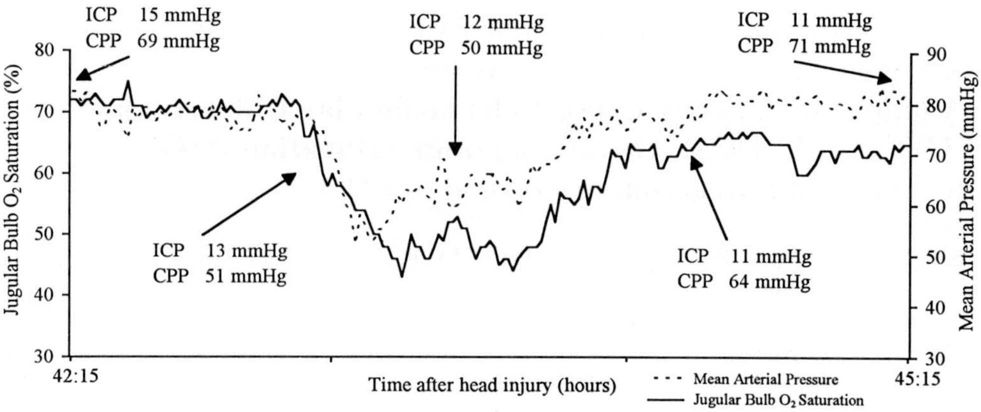

Fig. 4 Cerebral hypoperfusion due to arterial hypotension associated with a decrease in jugular bulb oxygen saturation to a critical level. No change in ICP was noted.

of long bone fractures. This is of particular importance as the majority of jugular bulb oxygen desaturations occurred within the first 48 hours following head trauma and recent work suggests that the frequency of episodes of jugular bulb oxygen desaturation is closely correlated with poor outcome [6]. These observations emphasise the need to institute appropriate intracranial monitoring as soon as possible once resuscitation is completed and the treatment of non - life threatening conditions must be carefully judged in the light of the patients intracranial injury.

In conclusion, jugular bulb oximetry provides information regarding the complex relationship between cerebral metabolic rate and cerebral blood flow hitherto undetected by conventional ICP and CPP monitoring [3, 7]. It identifies preventible secondary insults which occur frequently even in the presence of advanced neuro-intensive care. As our understanding and physiological monitoring capabilities improve then not only will intracranial pressure monitoring alone be insufficient to adequately monitor the traumatised brain but many of the standard therapies employed today may be found to do more harm than good under certain circumstances.

REFERENCES

1. Bullock R, Fujisawa H (1992) The role of glutamate antagonists for the treatment of CNS injury. J Neurotrauma; 9:S443-S462.
2. Andrews PJD, Dearden NM, Miller JD (1991) Jugular bulb cannulation: Description of a cannulation technique and validation of a new continuous monitor. Br J Anaesthesia 67:553-558.
3. Sheinberg M, Kanter MJ, Robertson CS, Contant CF, Narayan RK, Grossman RG (1992) Continuous monitoring of jugular venous oxygen saturation in head-injured patients. J Neurosurgery 76:212-217.
4. Cruz J, Miner ME, Allen SJ, Alves WM, Gennarelli TA (1990) Continuous monitoring of cerebral oxygenation in acute brain injury: injection of mannitol during hyperventilation. J Neurosurgery 73:725-730.
5. Muizelaar JP, Marmarou A, Ward JD, Kontos HA, Choi SC, Becker DP, Gruemer H, Young HF (1991) Adverse effects of prolonged hyperventilation in patients with severe head injury: a randomised clinical trial. J Neurosurgery 75:731-739.
6. Roberston CS (1993) Biochemical and metabolic monitoring of the head injured patient. Presented at the 2nd International Neurotrauma Symposium, Glasgow, Scotland.
7. Cruz J, Raps EC, Hoffstad OJ, Jaggi JL, Gennarelli TA (1993) Cerebral oxygenation monitoring.Critical Care Medicine 21:1242-1246.

Is There Agreement Between the Different Methods We Use in Monitoring Brain Ischemia? A Comparative Study Using Arterio-Jugular Differences of Oxygen ($AVDO_2$), Oxyhemoglobin Saturation (SjO_2) and Cerebral Extraction of Oxygen (CEO_2)

J. Sahuquillo[1], M.A. Poca[1], A. Garnacho[2], M. Baguena[2], L. Campos[2], M.D. Pellegri[3], and E. Rubio[1]

[1] Neurosurgical Department, [2] Neurotraumatology Intensive Care Unit, [3] Biochemistry Department, Vall d'Hebron University Hospital, 08035 Barcelona, Spain

Measurements of oxyhemoglobin saturation and/or derived parameters sampled through a catheter introduced into the jugular bulb has become a widely used method to monitor the adequacy of the brain supply/demand ratio of oxygen. Some authors have also suggested that in the absence of increased anaerobic metabolism, estimations of cerebral blood flow (CBF) are feasible using $AVDO_2$ [1]. Although there are still some controversies about the optimal methodology, this approach seems to be quite reliable in patients without mass lesions. However, various authors have suggested the use of different jugular blood-derived parameters to detect and monitor ischemia. Continuous or intermittent jugular venous saturation of the oxyhemoglobin (SjO_2), cerebral extraction of oxygen (CEO_2) (SaO_2 - SjO_2) and intermittent calculated $AVDO_2$ with or without simultaneous measurements of arterio-jugular differences of lactates (AVDL) have been alternatively used in clinical practice and research. Our objective in this study is to analyze agreement between these different methods of monitoring ischemia.

PATIENTS AND METHODS

This study was undertaken in a consecutive series of 60 severe head injury patients (post resuscitation GCS $\leq$ 8) and a diffuse brain injury in the admission CT scan (no deviations of the midline above 3 mm and no focal lesions above 25 ml). Immediately after admission to the ICU a 14 G catheter was inserted percutaneously in the internal jugular bulb. The catheter was placed in the right side in all but 8 cases. X-ray verification of the catheter position was obtained in each patient before obtaining jugular blood samples. A total of 328 technically satisfactory samples were obtained in these 60 patients. Arterio-jugular differences of oxygen ($AVDO_2$) were calculated by the following equation: $AVDO_2 = 1.34 \times Hb [SaO_2 - SjO_2]$. $AVDO_2$ were expressed in μmol/milliliter uncorrected for pCO2. Cerebral oxygen extraction (CEO_2) was calculated as the arterio-jugular difference in oxyhemoglobin saturation (SaO_2 - SjO_2) [2]. In a separate analysis of 52 cases and 108 samples of the same study group, patients were classified according to the categories proposed by Robertson et al. using LOI and $AVDO_2$ [1]. The ranges of normality for SjO_2, CEO_2 and $AVDO_2$ were obtained from the raw data of Gibbs' et al. study [3]. For SjO_2, values below 55 % were considered as ischemic and values above 70 were suggestive of hyperemia. The normal range for CEO_2 was considered to be 24 - 40 % [3]. According to the $AVDO_2$ patients were classified as hyperemic when $AVDO_2$ were below 2.2 μmol/ml and as ischemic when $AVDO_2$ values were above 3.7 μmol/ml. To calculate

[1] **Supported by Grants 93/1257 and 94/0688 from the Fondo de Investigaciones Sanitarias de la Seguridad Social (FISS).**

agreement, each measuring process (SjO_2, CEO_2 and $AVDO_2$) was viewed as an 'independent observer'. According to the above reported cut-off levels, patients were classified by each method as ischemic, hyperemic or with a CBF adequate for brain metabolism. Interobserver agreement beyond chance was calculated for the three methods using the unweighted overall Kappa statistic (True Epistat Software v 3.0, Epistat Services, Richardson, Texas). After overall agreement was obtained, agreement in hemodynamic diagnosis among the three possible different pairs of measurements was calculated.

RESULTS

The mean age of our series was 25.7 ± 15.8 years (mean ± SD). Of the 60 patients, 53 (88 %) were injured in a road traffic accident. Of the 328 samples, normal supply/demand between $CMRO_2$ and CBF was detected in 148 cases according to the SjO_2 method (45 %), in 164 cases with the CEO_2 method (50 %) and in 138 (42 %) with the $AVDO_2$ method **(Fig.1)**. The method that gave a higher number of hyperemic episodes was the $AVDO_2$ (57.3 %) while the lowest rate of hyperemia was detected by the CEO_2 (34.8 %). Overall agreement for the three methods and the three diagnostic categories was quantified by a Kappa value of 0.44. The agreement varied among the three diagnostic categories from a Kappa of 0.13 for ischemia to a Kappa of 0.59 for hyperemia **(TABLE 1)**. Unweighted overall Kappa calculated between pairs of methods, gave the highest agreement for $SjO_2/AVDO_2$ and the lowest for $CEO_2/AVDO_2$. In each pair of methods, the best agreement was in diagnosing hyperemia while the worst agreement was observed in the diagnosis of ischemia. Agreement between $SjO_2/AVDO_2$ and $CEO_2/AVDO_2$ when diagnosing ischemia was extremely poor, and no better than chance. Of the 108 sample set in which analysis of AVDO2/AVDL was performed, in 47 instances a LOI above or equal to 0.08 was detected (43.5 %) and therefore and ischemia/infarction pattern according to Robertson's classification. In 61 samples LOI was below 0.08 and considered as non-ischemic. In the analysis of ischemia/infarction group, mean $AVDO_2$ was 1.8 ± 0.97. Forty cases would have been considered as normal or hyperemic if AVDL and LOI had not been known **(Fig.2)**.

TABLE 1

Overall agreement between the three methods of hemodynamic monitoring

	Kappa	SjO_2/CEO_2	$SjO_2/AVDO_2$	$CEO_2/AVDO_2$
Normal CBF	0.37	0.37	0.52	0.23
Ischemia	0.13	0.35	- 0.01	-0.01
Hyperemia	0.59	0.60	0.61	0.57
Overall Kappa	0.44	0.46	0.54	0.35

$AVDO_2$: Arterio-jugular differences of oxygen, **SjO_2**: Oxyhemoglobin saturation, **CEO_2**: Cerebral extraction of oxygen

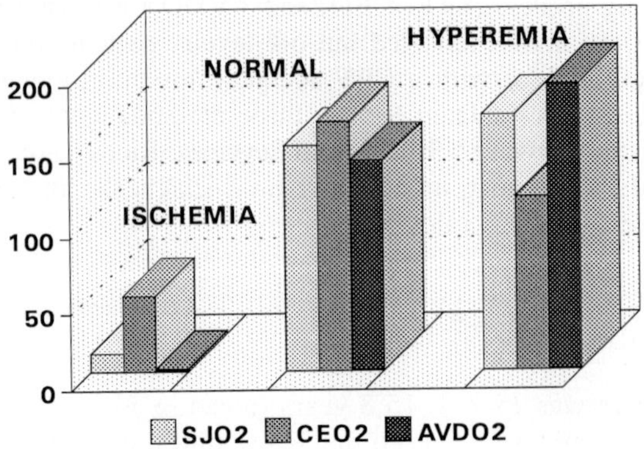

FIG.1: Bar chart showing the number of samples (vertical axis) with the diagnosis of normal CBF, hyperemia or ischemia according to the three different methods of estimating metabolism/cerebral blood flow coupling.

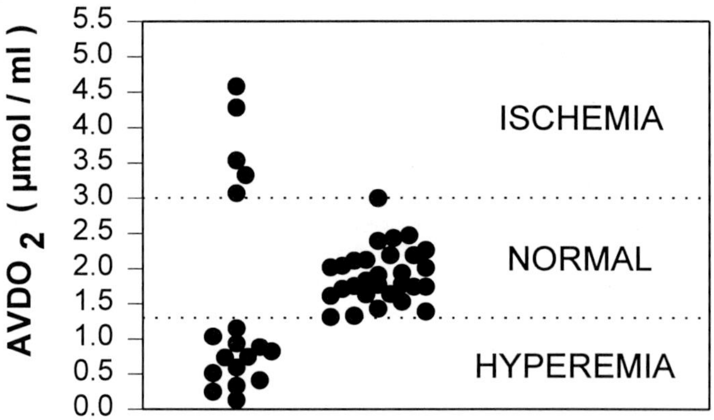

Fig.2: AVDO2 of the 47 patients with a LOI ≥ 0.08 (ischemia/infarction pattern). In this group three cerebral hemodynamic patterns were considered according to the estimated CBF: **1) Normal cerebral blood flow**, in those patients with $AVDO_2$ ranging from 1.3 to 3 μmol/ml, **2) Hyperemia**, in patients with $AVDO_2$ below 1.3 μmol/ml and **3) Compensated hypoperfusion**, in those cases with $AVDO_2$ above 3.0 μmol/ml [1].

DISCUSSION

Agreement in the diagnosis of ischemia, the target in head injury management, was very poor. Overall Kappa in the entire group was 0.39 for all diagnostic categories. Although a Kappa between 0.21-0.40 is considered representative of fair agreement, values below 0.61 are not acceptable in monitoring head injured patients. Agreement between the three methods was variable but generally poor. The lowest agreement was for ischemia diagnosis. Intermethod (interobserver) agreement was not better than chance for SjO_2/AVDO2 and CEO2/AVDO2 and less than acceptable for SjO_2/CEO2. $AVDO_2$ showed a very low prevalence of ischemia (0.6%), in contradiction to a prevalence of 3.7 % with the SjO_2 and of 15.2 % with the CEO2 method. This is surprising if we considered the elevated prevalence of increased anaerobic metabolism in the 108 samples analyzed in this study (43.5 %). Recently published results from our center using Robertson's method demonstrate a similar 46 % ischemia/infarction pattern within the first 24 hours of the accident [5].

CONCLUSIONS AND SUGGESTIONS FOR IMPROVEMENT

- Remarkable disagreement exists among different methods used at the bedside for monitoring adequacy of brain metabolism to cerebral blood flow, especially between those that use hemoglobin (AVDO2) and those that do not (SjO_2 an CEO2). The worst concordance between methods was found in the 'ischemia' category, where agreement was no better than chance.

- For continuous monitoring of $CMRO_2$/CBF coupling in the ICU setting, cerebral extraction of oxygen is perhaps the 'best' method although SjO_2 is a good alternative. Both CEO2/SjO_2 seem more reliable than the confounding AVDO2, especially in the presence of anemia. Furthermore, continuous monitoring of SjO_2 and SaO2 through jugular and arterial oximeters integrated in more complex computerized neuromonitoring systems can continuously assess CEO2. Periodic evaluation of AVDL and/or LOI could be helpful in this context to detect situations of infarction where CEO2 or SjO_2 could be misleading in estimating CBF.

- To be clinically useful, sensitivity, specificity and predictive value of AVDO2, AVDL and LOI should be analyzed before using this method for the diagnosis of ischemia/infarction patterns in the acute phase of head injury.

- A consensus should be attained for normal reference values and cut-off levels in identifying ischemia and hyperemia from hemometabolic variables. New studies with a higher number of normal volunteers, wider age ranges and reliable methods (Co-oximeter) are probably necessary before consensus can be reached. In the case of AVDO2, some methodological problems such as the 'best' oxyhemoglobin constant to use (1.31, 1.34 or 1.39) and the inclusion or not of the dissolved O2 in the equation should be addressed. Having standardized all of these points, we can look forward to obtaining a more comprehensive and reliable method of monitorization.

REFERENCES

1. Robertson, C.S., Narayan, R.K., Gokaslan, Z.L., Pahwa, R., Grossman, R.G., Caram, P., Allen, E. (1989): Cerebral arteriovenous oxygen difference as an estimate of cerebral blood flow in comatose patiens. J.Neurosurg. 70:222-230.

2. Cruz, J., Jaggi, J.L., Hoffstad, O.J. (1993): Cerebral blood flow and oxygen consumption in acute brain injury with acute anemia: An alternative for the cerebral metabolic rate of oxygen consumption. Crit.Care Med. 21:1218-1224.

3. Gibbs, E.L., Lennox, W.G., Nims, L.F., Gibbs, F.A. (1942): Arterial and cerebral venous blood. Arterial-venous differences in man. J.Biol.Chem. 144:325-332.

4. Cruz, J., Jaggi, J.L., Hoffstad, O.J. (1993): Cerebral blood flow and oxygen consumption in acute brain injury with acute anemia: An alternative for the cerebral metabolic rate of oxygen consumption. Crit.Care Med. 21:1218-1224.

5. Sahuquillo, J., Poca, M.A., Garnacho, A., Robles, A., Coello, F., Godet, C., Triginer, C., Rubio, E. (1993): Early ischaemia after severe head injury. Preliminary results in patients with diffuse brain injuries. Acta Neurochir.(Wien) 122:204-214.

Session III:
Monitoring (2)

Chairmen: G. Teasdale and T. Asakura

Interhemispheric Supratentorial ICP Gradients in Head Injury Patients: Are They Clinically Important?

J. Sahuquillo[1], M.A. Poca[1], L. Monforte[2], L.L. Sanchez-Massa[2], L. Campos[2], E. Rubio[1], and P. Zapater[2]

[1] Department of Neurosurgery, [2] Neurotraumatology Intensive Care Unit, Vall d'Hebron University Hospital, Paseo del Vall d'Hebron s/n, 08035 Barcelona, Spain

The classical concept about intracranial pressure (ICP) monitoring is that the intracranial space behaves as a unicameral compartment with pressure uniformly distributed. Experimental models have demonstrated that cranio-spinal and supra-infratentorial gradients exist, especially when subarachnoid spaces are partially or completely obliterated. However, the existence of interhemispheric gradients in the presence of space-occupying lesions is still controversial. In head injuries, Weaver et al. using subarachnoid catheters observed unilateral ICP gradients in patients with space-occupying lesions [1], while Yano et al. concluded that in patients with head injuries and mass lesions intracranial pressure is identical throughout the supratentorial intracranial space [2]. The purpose of our study is to reexamine the issue of interhemispheric supratentorial ICP gradients in head injured patients and their clinical relevance in the clinical management of these patients.

CLINICAL MATERIAL AND METHODS

Forty-seven patients with a Glasgow coma scale score below or equal to 12 were studied after admission or post-operative CT scan. In each case a concurrent bilateral frontal intraparenchymatous Camino transducer (Camino Laboratories, San Diego, CA, USA) was implanted within 6 hours of the CT scan. Both transducers were inserted 12 cm from the nasion and 3 cm to each side of the midline. Insertion depth was 2 cm. The analog output of both monitors was connected to a strip chart recorder. To avoid contamination of the results by the appearance of new lesions and to elude methodological problems with the zero drift, only the first 24 hours of monitoring were included in the analysis. Because at the end of the study only one intraparenchymatous device was removed, mean ICP was not corrected for the zero drift detected after monitoring.

CT scan classification

Every focal lesion was measured in the CT scan and the results summed up for each hemisphere. Each patient was included in one of the following groups: 1) **Diffuse lesions**, when hemispheric volumes above 25 cc were not present and the midline shift was below or equal to 3 mm, 2) **Focal F1**: When added hemispheric volumes of one hemisphere were above

---

[3] **Supported by Grant 94/0688 from the Fondo de Investigaciones Sanitarias de la Seguridad Social (FISS).**

25 cc and midline shift was less or equal to 3 mm and 3) **Focal F2**, when patients had a midline shift above 3 mm independently of the total measured volume for each hemisphere. Mean ICP was calculated in both hemispheres in 15 minutes periods using the method suggested by Price et al. [3]. The bilateral recording was visually examined to look for transitory ICP gradients that could have been overlooked when comparing only ICP means. The duration of each transitory episode was measured, the time of each one summed up and their whole duration expressed as a percentage of the total recording time. Differences between means in both hemispheres were analyzed using the paired t-test. Differences were considered statistically significant if $P < 0.05$. Every pair of measurements in each case were also evaluated using a simple linear regression model. In diffuse lesions, the independent variable was arbitrarily considered as the left hemisphere. In focal lesions the hemisphere with the highest estimated volume was considered as the independent variable. ICP gradients between hemispheres below or equal to 3 mm Hg were considered as clinically non-significant in spite of their actual statistical significance.

RESULTS

The mean age of our series was 34 ± 14.4 years. The type of lesion according to the above-mentioned criteria is summarized in Table 1. In the diffuse group, 3 patients had a bilateral swelling with compressed or absent basal cisterns. The analysis of the results allowed us to classify ICP findings in four different patterns: **Pattern I**: The intracranial compartment behaved as a true unicameral space with similar mean ICP in both hemispheres. To include a patient in this group, mean difference between hemispheres should be ≤ 3 mm and differences in global ICP amplitude should be ≤ 2 mm Hg. Spontaneous or therapeutically induced ICP increases and decreases were perfectly congruent in this group **(Fig.1A)**, **Pattern II**: Different mean ICP (> 3 mm Hg) and/or global amplitude (> 2 mm Hg) was observed, although in each case, ICP increases and spontaneously or therapeutically induced decreases were highly congruent **(Fig.1B).** In this pattern, the ICP profile of the intracranial compartment behaved as if both hemispheres had 'different compliance', **Pattern III** (true bicameral pattern): We included those patients with different mean ICP > 3 mm Hg and/or different ICP amplitude (> 2 mm Hg) and no congruent ICP increases or decreases. Those patients with transitory gradients in more than 25 % of the recording time were also included in this group, **Transient gradients**: Each patient with transitory gradients (congruent or not) in less than 25 % of the total recording time was considered separately. In each case the duration of the transitory differences in ICP were recorded.

A summary of the ICP pattern and the type of lesion is shown in **Table 1**. Mean correlation coefficient for pattern I was 0.95 ± 0.04 while mean difference between hemispheres was 1.8 ± 1.1 mm Hg (95 % CI 1.3 to 2.2) **(Fig.2)**. The mean correlation coefficient in ICP pattern II ranged from 0.49 - 0.99 and the mean ICP gradient between hemispheres was 7.5 ± 6.4 (95 % CI 4.2 to 10.8). Only one case in the entire group presented a type III ICP pattern. In 8 cases transient gradients (14 episodes) were found. These gradients ranged from 15 minutes to 3 hours in duration. The repeated CT scan showed, in 7 of these cases, a variable increase in the volume of the focal lesion, while in three no significant differences were observed.

Table 1. **Type of lesion and ICP pattern**

	I	II	III	T
Diffuse	14	0	0	0
Focal F1	4	5	0	0
Focal F2	13	10	1	8

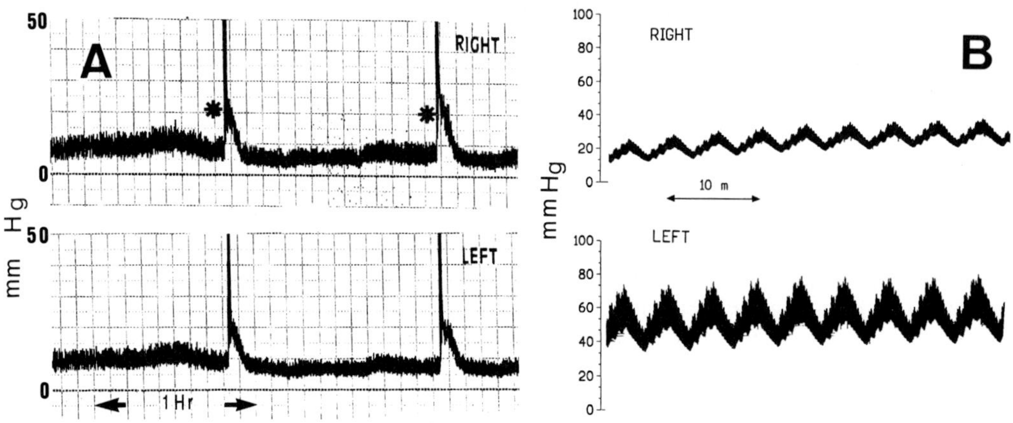

Fig.1: A) ICP pattern I. 44-year-old male in whom the CT scan showed small bilateral frontal contusion with an estimated volume of 15 ml and no midline shift. Mean ICP gradient was 0.5 mm Hg. Asterisks indicate endotracheal aspirations. **B)**: ICP pattern II. 27-year-old male injured in a motor vehicle related accident. The CT scan showed a small non-evacuated subdural hematoma with a severe associated unilateral hemispheric swelling and a midline shift of 13 mm. Mean ICP gradient was 27 mm Hg in spite of perfect congruent ICP changes in both hemispheres.

DISCUSSION

In our study, no patient with a diffuse brain lesion presented a clinically significant supratentorial ICP gradient. Small statistically significant interhemispheric gradients may exist, but they probably reflect methodological differences rather than true gradients. In about half the patients with a focal lesion, interhemispheric ICP gradients were detected. In almost fifty percent of these patients, those differences were clinically significant because they would have changed the therapeutic management based on ICP monitoring. A true bicameral pattern was exceptionally observed in one case with a severe midline shift. In this case, the incongruent bilateral recording could be generated by the complete block of the subarachnoid spaces and/or by important differences in the perfusion pressure of the brain tissue. Our findings agree with Gambardella's study in that transient gradients can exist in focal lesions that tend to dissipate with time [5]. In these cases, a transitory bicameral model of intracranial compartment is observed. Our findings suggest that to optimize ICP monitoring in patients with a mass lesion above 25 ml, the sensor should be implanted preferably in the brain parenchyma and in the side of the mass. In patients with a diffuse lesion we can assume that intracranial space behaves as a unicameral compartment and therefore, ICP is equal in both hemispheres. Bilateral cerebral tissue pressure monitoring could probably be justified in a highly selected group of patients with focal lesions and midline shift. In this group, brain tissue monitoring could detect the increase of volume of a mass lesion or the development of a new lesion and therefore help to anticipate neurological deterioration.

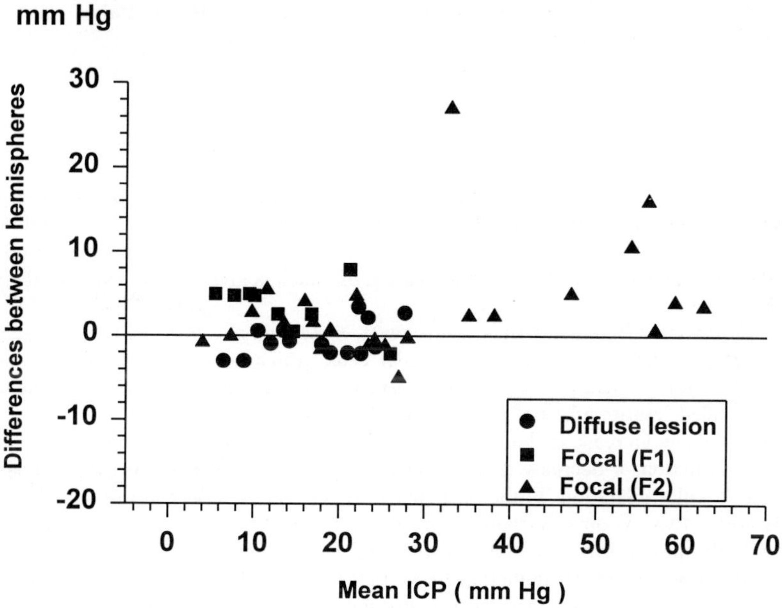

Fig.2: Agreement between ICP measurements in both hemispheres according to the method suggested by Altman [4]. ICP gradient between both hemispheres is plotted against mean ICP (right hemisphere ICP + left hemisphere ICP/2).

REFERENCES

1. Weaver, D.D., Winn, H.R., Jane, J.J. (1982): Differential intracranial pressure in patients with unilateral mass lesions. J.Neurosurg. 56:660-665.

2. Yano, M., Ikeda, Y., Kobayashi, S., Otsuka, T. (1990): Intracranial pressure in head-injured patients with various intracranial lesions is identical throughout supratentorial intracranial compartment. Neurosurgery 21:688-692.

3. Price, D., Driscoll, P. (1986): The problems of averaging ICP records by eye. In: *Intracranial Pressure VI*, edited by J.D. Miller, et al, pp. 705-712. Springer-Verlag, Berlin, Heidelberg, New York, Tokyo.

4. Altman, D.G., Bland, J.M. (1983): Measurements in medicine: The analysis of method comparison studies. Statistician 32:307-317.

5. Gambardella, G., D'Avella, D., Staropoli, C., Toscano, S., Tomasello, F. (1993): Bilateral intraparenchymal pressure in patients with unilateral supratentorial mass lesions. In: *Intracranial Pressure VIII*, edited by C.J.J. Avezaat, et al, pp. 82-84. Springer-Verlag, Berlin, Heidelberg.

Cerebral Perfusion Pressure Indirect Estimation. An Experimental Study

C. Anile[1], A. Mangiola[1], R. Gaspari[2], F. Della Corte[2], D. Catapano[1], F.F. Angileri[1], P. Santini[1], and G. Maira[3]

Institutes of [1] Neurosurgery and [2] Anesthesiology, Catholic University, Rome, Italy
[3] University of Perugia, Italy

INTRODUCTION

Since the pioneristic works of Ingvar and Larsell, it is a well known fact that the cerebral blood flow (CBF) remains relatively constant within a large range of variation in the so-called "cerebral perfusion pressure" (CPP), that is the difference between the distrectual carotid blood pressure (BP) and the distal cerebral venous pressure, the best approximation of which is given by the value of the intracranial pressure (ICP).

To explain this property different theories, neurogenic, metabolic and miogenic, have been advanced. Among these, the capability of the smooth muscular cells, which constitute the arterial and arteriolar walls, of adapting "automatically" the vascular diameter in relation to variations in the trans-mural pressure (the so-called "autoregulation"), has acquired a greater importance [1].

In other words, while an increase in the trans-mural pressure stimulates the vascular muscular cells and produces vasoconstriction, a decrease in the transmural pressure induces a muscular relaxation and, consequently, a vascular dilatation. In the intracranial system the trans-mural pressure is equivalent to the CPP; this means that, as already reported in literaturc [2], we may expect to observe an arterial vasodilatation both during systemic hypotension and/or intracranial hypertension when the CPP decreases because of a carotid BP reduction or an ICP increase. This vasodilatation, by reducing the cerebrovascular resistances, which are mainly located at the arterial and arteriolar level, should compensate the CPP decrease, thus maintaining a constant CBF, at least until this vasodilatatory action remains active. In this way an indirect ICP evaluation could be provided by analysing CBF velocity in the major cerebral vessels, as already proposed by Aaslid et al. [3]. Recently, however, some criticism to this theory has been advanced by these same authors [4] based on the observation that the lag between CPP variations produced by abrupt systemic BP decrease and CBF restoration is too short to be compatible with the time of response to the stimulus by the smooth muscle vascular cell, as demonstrated in "in vitro" preparation as well as in "in vivo" experimental condition, and consistent, on the contrary, with that expected if the cerebral autoregulation was mediated by a metabolic mechanism.

Whichever the CBF autoregulatory mechanism is, however, miogenic, metabolic or purely hydraulic, the vascular response is always associated to changes in the trans-mural pressure. This study was planned in order to investigate the possibility of obtaining a reliable ICP evaluation by non-invasive methods employing ultrasonic applications.

MATERIALS AND METHODS

Following our previous studies, an experimental reversible condition of intracranial hypertension was produced by infusing saline into a lateral ventricle until ICP approached arterial BP. In this new experimental series eight domestic pigs (all female) weighing between 20 and 25 kg were used. The animals were tranquilized with 5 mg/kg ketamine, paralyzed with 0.4 mg/kg/hr pancuronium bromide and mechanically ventilated with a gas mixture of 0.5 - 1% halothane, 50% N_2O, the rest oxygen. The respiration of the animals was adjusted to yield a $PaCO_2$ of about 35 mmHg and a PaO_2 of more than 100 mmHg.

ICP was measured through the same 18G epidural needle utilized for the infusion; arterial BP through a

16G catheter inserted into the right common carotid artery in the neck. CBF variations were analyzed by evaluating CBF velocities measured by utilizing two ultrasound 8 and 4 MHz continuous wave probes located intracranially at the sagittal sinus and at the left internal carotid artery level through two adequately tailored skull windows positioned respectively in the posterior part of the middle vertex and in the left temporal bone. The anatomy of the intracranial cerebral arterial and venous system in pig is quite similar to that found in man; the sagittal sinus, in particular, is devoted to drain exclusively from cortical and bridging veins to systemic circulation. Furthermore, the characteristic feature of this structure, delimited by rigid walls, permits us to regard the measurement of the blood flow velocity variations, recorded by doppler technique at this site, as a reliable evaluation of the global CBF variations. On the contrary, diameter variations of the internal carotid aretry at intracranial level associated with CPP changes could hinder the acquisition of reliable information on CBF. Both these methods, however, if considered together, should be very useful in evaluating the cerebral vascular reactivity.

Four different methods have been utilized for an indirect estimation of CPP: two based on the correlation between arterial BP and CBF velocity as suggested by Aaslid et al. in 1986 [3] and recently at the Fifth Meeting of the Neurosonology Research Group on the basis of the application of the concept of the critical closure pressure (CCP) as already described by Dewey et al. in 1974 [5]; the other two calculating the resistance index (RI = systolic - diastolic / systolic velocity) and the pulsatility index (PI = systolic - diastolic / mean velocity) of the intracranial carotid blood flow velocity in an attempt to explore the reliability of an indirect measurement of the CPP obtained exclusively by means of intracranial arterial blood flow velocity evaluation.

The integrity of the skull was reconstitued with dental acrylic cement.

Electrocortical activity was recorded by 4 screw electrodes located on the skull in symmetrical bilateral fronto-parietal position at distance of about 4 cm; electrocardiac activity by spindle electrodes at the extremities.

All signals were continuously recorded both on chart and on magnetic tape for delayed automatical data processing and storage utilizing self-developed software based on the Fourier frequency analysis.

Saline was infused at a progressively increasing rate, starting from 12 ml/hr, until a condition of brain tamponade was reached as documen - ted by the observation of a reverberating blood flow velocity wave pattern both at internal carotid artery and sinus level with a mean value of zero. This condition was maintained for 15' in 4 animals, 30' in 3 and 60' in the last one. At the end of the infusion the experimental observation was prolonged until an electrocortical activity was again clearly evident.

Statistical analysis was carried out by utilizing linear and non-linear correlation methods.

RESULTS

In our model in basal condition the CBF mean velocities at sagittal sinus and, respectively, at intracranial carotid artery level ranges from 8 to 12 and from 18 to 22 cm/sec. The CBF velocity, both at sagittal sinus and at intracranial carotid level, showed a typical pulsatile pattern synchronous with arterial and intracranial pulsation.

During the infusion the progressive reduction in CPP, still above the so-called "autoregolatory" limit (about 40 mmHg), was immediately associated with a typical modification of the pulsatile pattern in the carotid CBF velocity which showed a decrease both in diastolic and systolic values with a slight increase in the amplitude of the pulsation. No significant variation in the sagittal sinus CBF velocity was observed in this range of CPP reduction.

As soon as the CPP dropped below 40 mmHg, at carotid level the systolic CBF velocity remained relatively stable and the diastolic value became negative, while at sinus level both the diastolic and systolic blood flow velocity reduced until reverberating waves were observed simultaneously at arterial and venous level when CPP ranged between 0 and 25 mmHg, 0 value being observed only in two animals.

At the end of the intraventricular infusion the ICP immediately decreased and the brain became reperfused as demonstrated by the contemporary increase in the CBF velocity both at sagittal sinus and carotid artery level. In all the animals this increase reproduced in an almost specular fashion the

decrease observed during the infusional phase; no difference between the animals was noticed with regard to the duration of the brain tamponade condition (15', 30' or 60').
A statistically significant CPP estimation was found in 7 animals utilizing both the two methods proposed by Aaslid et al. and the RI. For the former ones the correlation was linear (Figs. 1 and 2), for the latter one of mixed exponential type (Fig. 3).

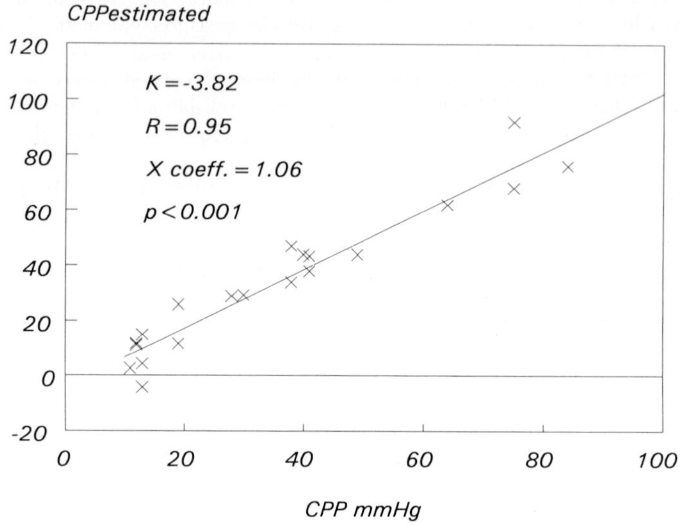

Fig. 1: An example of linear correlation between CPP and CPPestimated utilizing the formula proposed by Aaslid et al. in an experimental condition of intracranial hypertension.

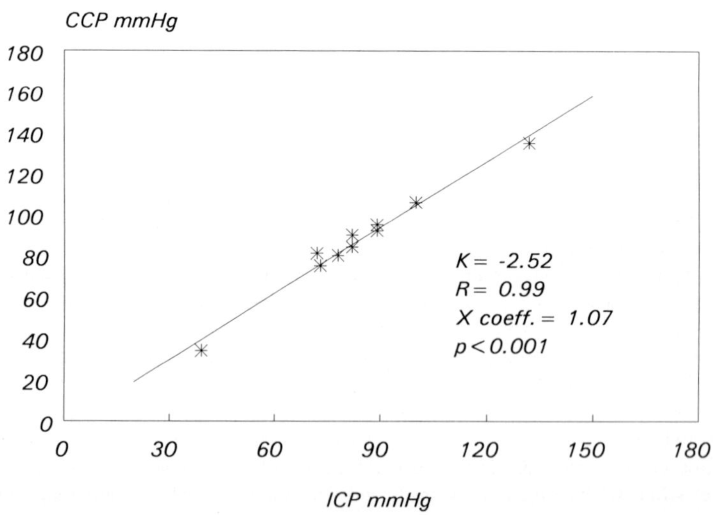

Fig.2: An example of linear correlation between intracranial presssure and critical closing pressure in an experimental condition of intracranial hypertension.

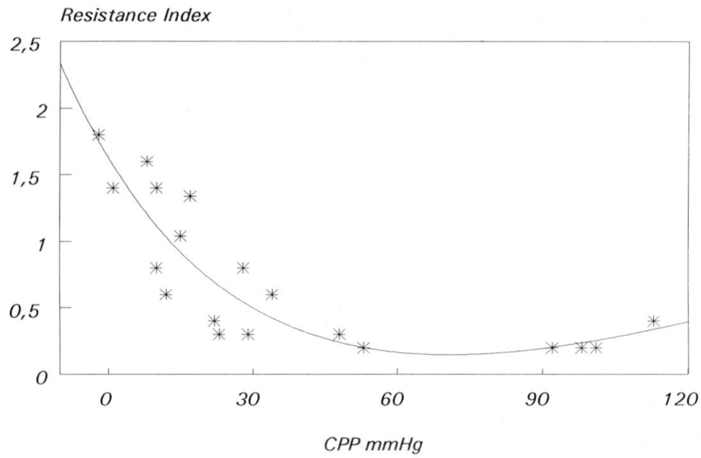

Fig. 3: An example of mixed exponential correlation between CPP and resistance index in an experimental condition of intracranial hypertension.

The PI calculation provided a good correlation in 2 animals only. Concerning the three first methods, the best fitting was observed for ICP values > 60 mmHg; in particular, above/below this limit an ICP over/underestimation, respectively, resulted from the CCP evaluation. Furthermore, for the first three methods a statistically significant correlation was also found considering all the data collected in all the experimental trials with a shape similar to that observed for each individual series.

DISCUSSION

Among the different methods investigated, the RI and the CCP evaluation seem to be the most promising for clinical application. However caution is still necessary: RI needs to be mathematically transformed for easier utilization and the CCP calculation requires a simultaneous invasive carotid blood pressure recording, as in our experimental model, which may be ethically unacceptable, at least for routine practice.

REFERENCES

1. Portnoy HD, Chopp M, Branch C, Shannon M (1982) Cerebrospinal fluid pulse waveform as an indicator of cerebral autoregolation. J Neurosurg 56:666-678.
2. Auer LM and Ishiyama N (1986). Cerebrovascular response to elevated intracranial pressure. In: Miller JD, Teasdale GM, Rowan JO, Galbraith SL, and Mendelow AD (eds) Intracranial Pressure VI. Springer-Verlag, Berlin Heidelberg, pp 399-403.
3. Aaslid R, Lundar T, Lindegaard K-F, and Nornes H (1986) Estimation of cerebral perfusion pressure from arterial blood pressure and transcranial doppler recordings. In: Miller JD, Teasdale GM, Rowan JO, Galbraith SL, and Mendelow AD (eds) Intracranial Pressure VI. Springer-Verlag, Berlin Heidelberg, pp 226-229.
4. Aaslid R, Newell DW, Stooss R, Sorteberg W, Lindegaard K-F (1991) Assessment of cerebral autoregulation dynamics from simultaneous arterial and venous transcranial doppler recordings in humans. Stroke 22:1148-1154.
5. Dewey RC, Pieper HP, Hunt WE (1974) Experimental cerebral hemodynamics. Vasomotor tone, critical closing pressure, and vascular bed resistance. J Neurosurg 41:597-606.

Plateau Waves in Acute Hydrocephalic Cats

Katsuji Shima and Hiroo Chigasaki

Department of Neurosurgery, National Defense Medical College, Tokorozawa, Saitama, 359 Japan

SUMMARY

We have previously reported that plateau waves were successfully produced in hydrocephalic cats and monkeys during calcium-induced sleep [1-3]. In the present study, plateau waves were spontaneously observed in a cat with kaolin-induced hydrocephalus. The plateau waves developed during the waking state under spontaneous respiration. These plateau waves did not disappear by artificial respiration and immobilization. The results suggest that plateau waves may be caused by cerebral vasoparalysis elicited from some neuronal dysfunction.

INTRODUCTION

There have been many experimental and clinical reports on the development of plateau waves associated with intracranial hypertension. However, this mechanism is not fully understood, because typical plateau waves are difficult to reproduce experimentally in animals. We have previously reported a reliable experimental model of plateau waves initiated by a sleep-like state induced within the hypothalamus in hydrocephalic cats and monkeys [1-3]. In clinical observations, plateau waves are observed most frequent during REM sleep, but also occur during the waking state in patients with intracranial hypertension. The present study was designed to produce typical plateau waves without any chemical [1-3] and electrical [4-6] induction of brain stem and to investigate the accompanying changes in systemic blood pressure (BP), respiration, EEG and cerebral blood flow (CBF).

METHODS

Seventeen adult cats, weighing 2-4 kg, were anesthetized with intravenous ketamine hydrochloride (20 mg/kg). Hydrocephalus was induced by injection of sterile kaolin suspension into the cisterna magna. At the acute stage of hydrocephalus between 5 and 8 days after kaolin injection, the animals were anesthetized, tracheostomized and placed on a stereotaxic frame. Intracranial pressure (ICP) was recorded using a 22-gauge needle inserted stereotaxically into the lateral ventricle through a burr hole and connected to a strain gauge transducer. BP was monitored from the femoral artery using a catheter connnected to a transducer. EEG was recorded from a cortical electrode on the frontal region, and the recordings were analysed by a frequency analyzer (MAF-5, Nihon Kohden). Horizontal components of ocular movements (OMG) and EMG of the nuchal muscle were recorded. Respiratory rate was measured using a thermister in the tracheal tube. Cerebral blood flow (CBF) in the frontal cortex was measured by means of the cross thermocouple technique. Continuoue monitoring of the ICP, BP, EEG, OMG, EMG, respiration and CBF were carried out under sontaneous breathing.

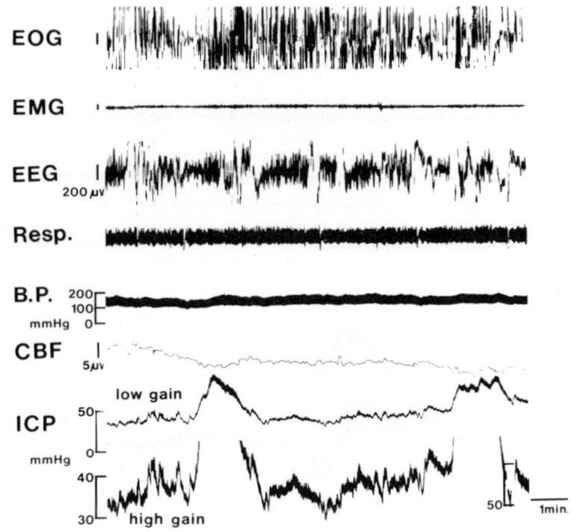

Fig. 1 Polygraphic recording of OMG, EMG, EEG, respiration, systemic BP, CBF and ICP at low and figh gains. Note the plateau waves during the waking state.

Fig. 2 A Recording under artificial respiration at 40 min after record shown in Fig.1. Horizontal bars (a-c) correspond to EEG tracings at faster paper speed. B The EEG records were taken (a) at the rapid rise phase of plateau wave, (b) during the plateau phase and (c) at the rapid fall phase.

A

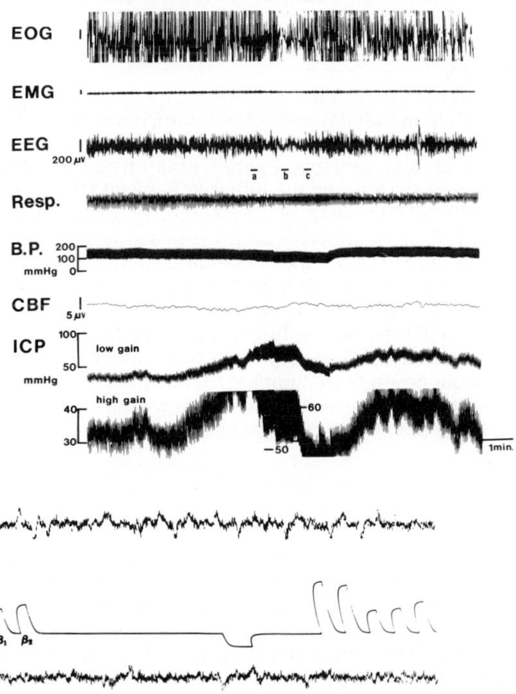

B

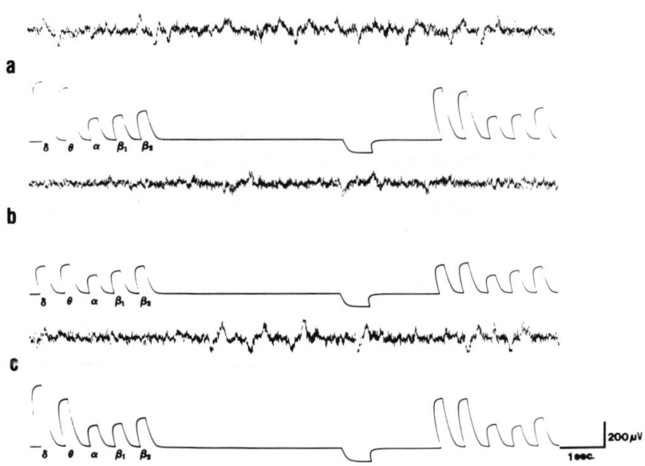

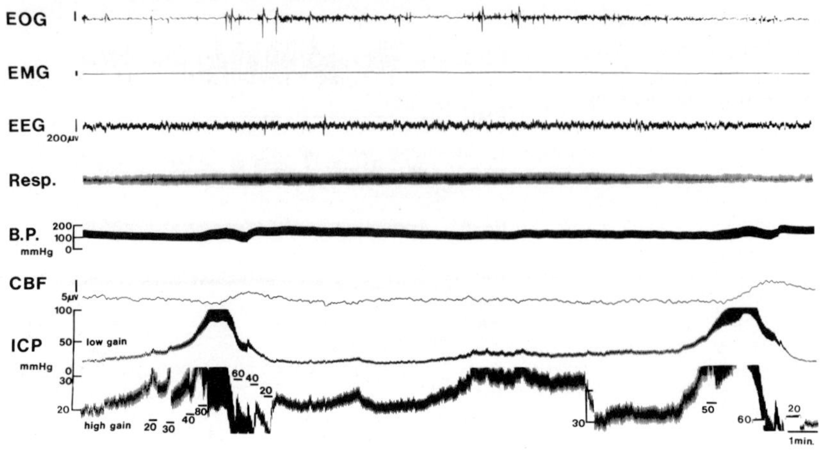

Fig. 3 Recording of plateau waves after immobilization under artificial respiration.

RESULTS

On the fifth to eighth days after kaolin injection, the initial ICP was increased to 13.4 ± 9.3 mmHg, and 10 (60%) of 17 animals had moderately dilated ventricles. Typical plateau waves occured in only one animal which had developed papilledma on the sixth day after the injection. On the eighth day, the recording was started, and the initial ICP, mean BP and cerebral perfusion pressure (CPP) were 30 to 40 mmHg, 130 to 140 mmHg, 90 to 100 mmHg, respectively. During the plateau waves, ICP suddenly rose to levels of 80 to 90 mmHg within 1 min and lasted from 2 to 3 min (Fig. 1). The CPP dropped to levels of 30 to 45 mmHg. After the cessation of the second plateu wave, the animal was ventilated with room air. After an interval of 40 min, plateau wave with a height of 70 mmHg and a duration of 4 min was recorded under artificial respiration (Fig. 2A). There were a decrease in CPP up to 30 mmHg and an increase in CBF corresponding with the plateau wave. The EEG during the plateau phase showed a dominant activity of low-amplitude fast wave component. Then, the animal was received intravenous panchronium bromide (0.2 mg/kg). Three plateau waves were recorded during which the ICP increased to 92.3 ± 12.8 mmHg and the CPP decreased to 20.1 ± 1.1 mmHg (Fig.3). There was no significant change in the blood gases during the plateau waves and their intervals.

DISCUSSION

Previous studies have shown that plateau waves are caused by the change of hypothalamic function closely related to sleep in animals with ICP higher than 15 mmHg and above [1-3]. The plateau waves were accompanied by a decrease in high-amplitude slow activity of EEG, the appearance of rapid eye movements and irregular breathing pattern, which were similar to those observed during REM sleep in patients with intracranial hypertension [3,7]. In the present study, we recorded the same changes in physiological variables except ocular movements during the waking state. This observation suggests that actual sleep per se is not necessarily essential for the occurrence of plateau waves. We have also observed that there is no causal relationship between the occurrence of plateau waves and changes in blood gases and respiration. Changes in BP and CBF associated with plateau waves may account for cerebral vasodilatation regardless of respiratory patterns. Previous studies in our laboratory have shown an increase in the metabolic rate for glucose in the hypothalamus and certain nuclei of brain stem during the induced sleep in hydrocephalic monkeys [2]. The findings in this study confirm that the plateau waves are correlated with some intrinsic neuronal mechanism in the brain stem during increased ICP [4-6].

REFERENCES

1. Shima K, Akiyama I, Ueno H, Ishii S (1980) Intracranial pressure changes during experimental sleep in cats and primates. Neurol Med Chir (Tokyo) 20:1215-1222

2. Ishii S (1983) Oscillation of intracranial pressure and local cerebral metabolism. In: Ishii S, Nagai H, Brook M (eds) Intracranial Pressure V. Springer, Berlin Heidelberg New York Tokyo, pp893-900

3. Shima K, Ueno H, Chigasaki H, Ishii S (1989) Comparative study with experimental and clinical plateau waves relating to sleep. In: Hoff J, Betz AL (eds) Intracranial VII. Springer, Berlin Heidelberg New York London Paris Tokyo Hong Kong, pp.241-244

4. Katayama Y, Nakamura T, Becker DP, Hayes RL (1984) Intracranial pressure variations associated with activation of the cholinoceptive pontine inhibitory area in the unanesthetized drug-free cat. J Neurosurg 61:713-724

5. Hayashi M, Ishii H, Handa Y, Kobayashi H, Kawano H, Kabuto M (1987) Role of the medulla oblongata in plateau-wave development in dogs. J Neurosurg 67:97-101

6. Maeda M, Takahashi K, Miyazaki M, Ishii S (1986) The role of the central monoamine system and the cholinoceptive pontine area on the oscillation of ICP "Pressure Waves". In: Miller JD, Teasdale GM, Rowan JO, Galbraith SL, Mendelow AD (eds) Intracranial Pressure VI. Springer, Berlin Heidelberg New York Tokyo, pp.151-155

7. Cooper R, Hulme A (1966) Intracranial pressure and related phenomena during sleep. J Neurol Neurosurg Psychiat 29:564-570

Correlation of Continuous Measures of Autoregulation and Compensatory Reserve with Cerebral Perfusion Pressure and ICP

D.J. PRICE[1], M. CZOSNYKA[2], Z. CZOSNYKA[2], and J.R. PRICE[1]

[1] Neurosurgical Department, Pinderfields Hospital, Wakefield, UK
[2] MRC Cambridge Centre for Brain Repair and Academic Neurosurgical Unit, Addenbrooke's Hospital, Cambridge, UK

INTRODUCTION

Continuous waveform analysis of the intracranial pressure (ICP) signal has been used to augment the monitoring of patients who have sustained severe head injury in the neurosurgical intensive care unit at Wakefield since 1977.
In a continuing search for an on-line method of estimating a patient's current position on the flat part of the pressure-volume curve, we have used software developed in Poland which displays changes in the regression coefficient of the amplitude/mean relationship every 14 seconds (RAP) [1]. A rise in this coefficient proved to be a more reliable warning of a rise in ICP than the amplitude/mean gradient [2].
In a recently reported preliminary study of the combined ICP data of 80 head injured patients [3] there was a significant decrease in the RAP when the ICP rose from 45 to 70mmHg. This correlated well with a break point in the ICP/AMP relationship with a rapid increase in amplitude when the ICP rose to 65mmHg with a sharp decrease above that level.
The purpose of this study is to ascertain as to whether the breakpoint which may well represent a breakdown of autoregulation occurs at a lower threshold ICP in those whose outcome is poor as compared with those who survive with minimal disabilities.

METHODS

139 patients admitted to the neurosurgical intensive care unit at Pinderfields Hospital Wakefield between March 1990 and December 1993 were studied. They had all sustained severe blunt head injury and were in coma prior to intubation, ventilation and transfer to the neurosurgical unit. Coma was defined as no obedience to commands, no understandable verbal response and no eye opening even to pain. ICP monitoring was initiated after evacuation of any intracranial haematoma. The ICP monitoring was used primarily to alert us to the development or re-expansion of haematomas or contusions. We attempted to ensure that the cerebral perfusion pressure (CPP) was above 70mmHg by the use of Mannitol, Propofol, vasopressor agents and very adequate fluid load to maintain vascular expansion and a normal osmolality. At times, this proved very difficult in practice. On many occasions, ICP instability with pressure waves was eliminated as soon as the CPP was artificially increased to above 80mmHg confirming Rosner and Becker's observations of 10 years ago [4].
Both the ICP and arterial pressure wave forms were continuously analysed. The amplitude of the fundamental harmonic components of ICP (the cardiac pulse wave - AMP) was calculated every 8 seconds using a 128 Fast Fourier Transform sampled at a frequency of 18 Hz. The mean ICP, AMP and arterial pressure from each 8 second transform were stored in a circular buffer to allow the generation of one minute averages for the last 7 samples. Every 2 minutes, 15 sample pairs of ICP and AMP were used for a linear regression and the correlation coefficient (RAP) was sampled and displayed along with the cerebral perfusion pressure, ICP, AMP and heart beat as trend graphs.

RESULTS

Of the 139 patients who had been followed up for a minimum of 6 months, 73 (52%) made a reasonably good recovery with at the worst moderate disability but allowing them to live independently (GOS 1 and 2). 22 (16%) were severely disabled and dependent on their family for them to be cared for at home (GOS 3). Four (3%) remained in a persistent vegetative state for several months (GOS 4) and 3 of these eventually died and the remaining 40 (29%) died within a week or so of the injury (GOS 5).
During a total artefact free recording time of 275 days (6,600 hours) the ICP was less than 50mmHg for 98.7% of the time, less than 40mmHg for 94.8% of the time, less than 30mmHg for 87.3% of the time and less than 20mmHg for 62.4% of the time. Unfortunately, for 10.8% of the time, the CPP was less than 40mmHg but some recordings had continued after we had abandoned our attempts to maintain it. The CPP was more than 50mmHg for 81.1% of the time, more than 60mmHg for 64.2% of the time and more than 70mmHg for 41.5% of the time and more than 80mmHg for 21.2% of the time.
In the preliminary series of the first 80 patients, we found that as the CPP decreased from 45mmHg to 30mmHg, there was a rapid rise in amplitude until a break point was reached (5). In this larger series of 139 patients, they were divided into three outcome categories GOS 1 and 2 (73/139), GOS 3 (22/139) and GOS 4 and 5 (44/139). For those with the best and worst outcomes, the CPP breakpoint was 35mmHg and the relationship between CPP and amplitude for those who were severely disabled was quite different with a more gradual increase in amplitude as the CPP fell until a modest breakpoint was reached at 45mmHg (Fig.1). These graphs are generated as empiric regressions. The conditional averages of the dependent variable (i.e. AMP or RAP) are plotted against the independent variable (i.e. ICP or CPP) in data bins 5mmHg wide. 95% confidence limits (+ or - 2 standard errors) are shown in either thinner lines or vertical bars.

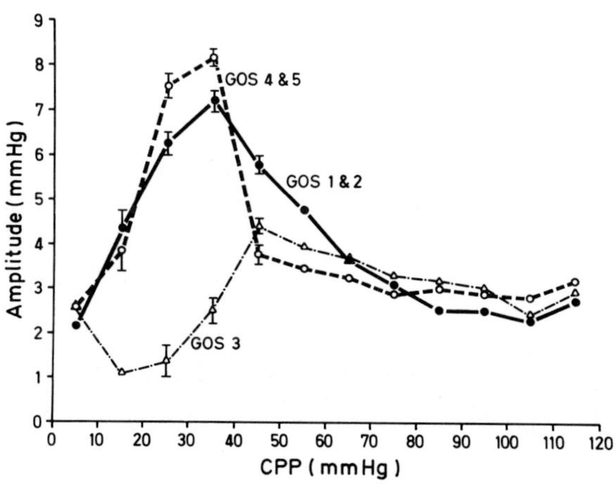

Fig.1 The relationship between CPP and Amplitude for 3 outcome groups

When the data was used to compare those who made a reasonably good recovery with those who died (Fig.2), the rise and fall in RAP with increasing ICP is quite dramatic with overall higher RAP in those who recover. The differences in the outcome groups becomes more obvious when the amplitude versus ICP empiric regression curve is seen (Fig.3). This demonstrates that those who die have a break point of 35-45mmHg suggesting a loss of autoregulation at relatively low pressure. Those who survive with a severe disability have a break point between 45 and 50mmHg and those who recovery sufficiently to be dependent do not lose autoregulation until 60mmHg is reached.

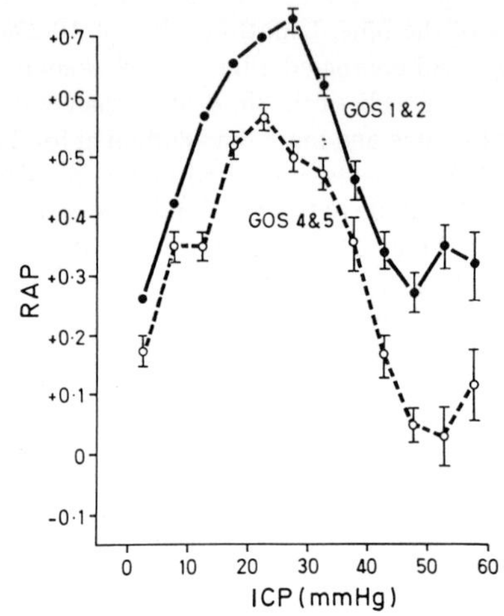

Fig. 2 Regression curves of the rise and fall of RAP with increasing ICP for 2 outcome groups

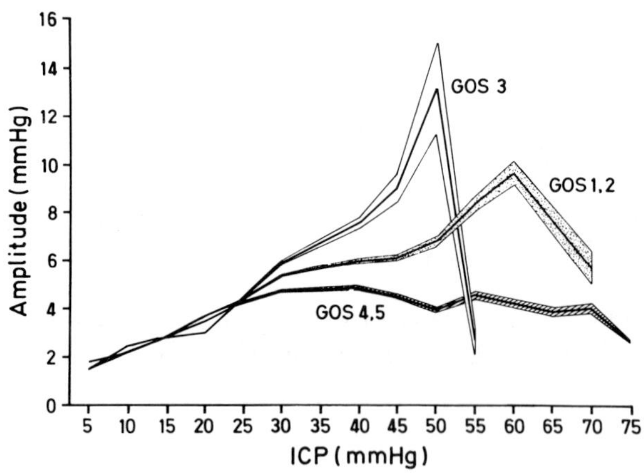

Fig. 3 Regression curves of Amplitude versus ICP for 3 outcome groups

DISCUSSION

The gradual increase in amplitude with increasing ICP up to 45mmHg (Fig.3) or with CPP steadily decreasing from 100 to 55mmHg (Fig.1) is often interpreted as due to the exponential cerebrospinal pressure-volume relationship [5]. Cardiac-related pulsatile changes in cerebral blood volume may produce higher pressure responses with increasing gradients on the pressure-volume curve with increasing ICP. Piper and his colleagues have suggested that the compliance of the cerebral arterial bed increases with the reduction of CPP. As a result, there may then be an increase in the transmission of arterial pressure wave to the CSF compartment [6]. If the CPP falls below 40mmHg suggesting a loss of autoregulatory control, some survive and some die (Fig.1). Further research is needed to ascertain as to why some tolerate this insult and others do not. The peak of the RAP intracranial pressures of between 20 and 30mmHg suggests that compensatory reserve does gradually become compromised at pressures as low as 20mmHg in both those who do well and those who die (Fig.2). There is surprisingly more relationship with outcome on the association of amplitude and ICP than with the association with amplitude and CPP (Figs. 1 and 3). Those who may be predetermined to die lose autoregulation at lower ICPs than those who will make a good survival.
The autoregulatory threshold in each individual may well merely reflect the severity of injury to the brain and its vasculature.

REFERENCES

1. Czosnyka M, Laniewski P, Batorski L, Zaworski W (1988) A system for ICP processing and interpretation in intensive care. In: Advances in Biomedical Measurement. Plenum Publ.Corp. pp 101-109

2. Williamson M, Price DJ, Czosnyka M (1993) Further attempts to anticipate post-traumatic intracranial hypertension by on-line analysis. In: Avezaat CJJ, vvan Eindhoven JHM, Maas AIR, Tans JThJ (eds). Intracranial pressure VIII. Springer-Verlag, Berlin, Heidelberg, New York pp 67-70.

3. Czosnyka M, Price DJ, Williamson M (1994) Monitoring of cerebrospinal dynamics using continuous analysis of intracranial pressure and cerebral perfusion pressure in head injury. Acta Neurochir (Wien) 126:113-119

4. Rosner MJ Becker DP (1984) The origin and evaluation of plateau waves: experimental observations and a theoretical model. J. Neurosurg 60:312-324

5. Marmarou A, Shulman K, Rosende R (1978) A non linear analysis of the cerebrospinal fluid system and intracranial pressure dynamics. J Neurosurg 48:332-344

6. Piper I, Miller JD, Dearden M (1990) System analysis of cerebrovascular pressure transmission: an observational study in head injured patients. J Neurosurg 73:871-880

Receiver Operator Characteristic (ROC) Curve Analysis Applied to CPP, ICP and Outcome in Severely Head Injured Patients

I.R. CHAMBERS[1] and A.D. MENDELOW[2]

[1] Regional Medical Physics Department, Newcastle General Hospital, England, UK
[2] Department of Surgery (Neurosurgery), University of Newcastle upon Tyne, England, UK

INTRODUCTION

It is well known that intracranial pressure (ICP) and cerebral perfusion pressure (CPP) correlate with outcome in patients with severe head injury although the optimal levels are still a matter of debate [1-4]. We have applied Receiver Operator Characteristic analysis to a series of patients to evaluate the predictive levels of CPP and ICP in relation to outcome.

METHODS

One hundred and eighty patients admitted to the Regional Neurosciences Centre, Newcastle General Hospital with severe head injury (GCS $\leq$ 8) who required ICP monitoring as part of their management were studied. ICP and CPP were continuously monitored and recorded [5]. For each patient minimum CPP and maximum ICP values for any two minute period and any 60 minute period of recording were calculated. Outcome was determined at six months and was divided into "Independent" (Good or moderate disability) and "Poor" (severely disabled, vegetative or dead).
If it is postulated that a CPP below a certain value is associated with a poor outcome then a two-by-two table for evaluating the validity of the test can be created.

Table 1: Derivation of Sensitivity and Specificity

	Outcome		
	Poor	Independent	
CPP $\leq$ x	a	b	a + b
CPP > x	c	d	c + d
	a + c	b + d	N

a, true positives (TP)
b, false positives (FP)
c, false negatives (FN)
d, true negatives (TN)

Sensitivity is defined as the proportion of poor outcomes who have a CPP less than or equal to the test value and specificity as the proportion of independent outcomes who have a CPP higher than the test value.

Thus:

$$Sensitivity = \frac{TP}{TP + TN} = \frac{a}{a + c} \quad and \quad Specificity = \frac{TN}{TN + FP} = \frac{d}{d + b}$$

For values of CPP from 30 to 130mmHg and for values of ICP from 0-100mmHg the sensitivity and specificity of incremental values as a predictor of outcome were calculated (ie the likelihood of producing an independent outcome) and by plotting the sensitivity on the y-axis against 1-specificity on the x-axis a Receiver Operating Characteristic (ROC) curve is produced [6].

RESULTS

Of the 180 patients 49 made a good recovery, 50 had a moderate disability, 29 a severe disability, 4 remained in the persistent vegetative state and 48 died. Because of the very small number of Vegetative outcomes we have grouped them together with those that died. The average age of the "Goods, moderates and severes" were very similar and the Vegetative + Dead group had a higher mean age (Table 2).

Table 2

Outcome	Number	Average Age (years)	Recording length (hours)
All	180	29.4	55.2
Good recovery	49	25.0	52.5
Moderate disability	50	28.8	56.5
Severe disability	29	26.8	74.2
Vegetative + Dead	52	35.3	46.6

The recording intervals were similar other than in the severe disability group where there was a considerably longer monitoring period.
The ROC curves (Fig 1) for CPP and ICP show that for example, at a CPP of 50mmHg the specificity is 0.8 but the sensitivity only 0.37. For CPP values below 40mmHg and ICP values above 68mmHg the specificity is unity; ie there are no independent outcomes. Likewise the sensitivity only approaches 1 at levels of 85mmHg for CPP and 4mmHg for ICP.

The curves for mortality (i.e. comparing death with all other outcomes, Fig2) are shifted upwards and to the left and ICP would appear to be a slightly better indicator of mortality than CPP. The specificity of CPP is 1 at 40mmHg. The specificity of ICP is 1 at 55mmHg.

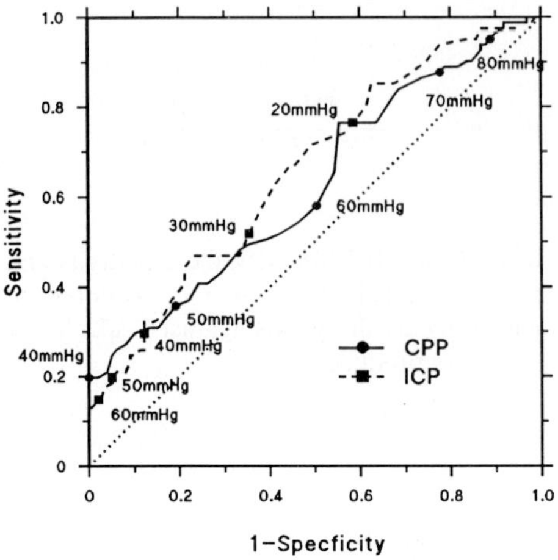

Fig 1 CPP, ICP and Independent/Poor outcomes

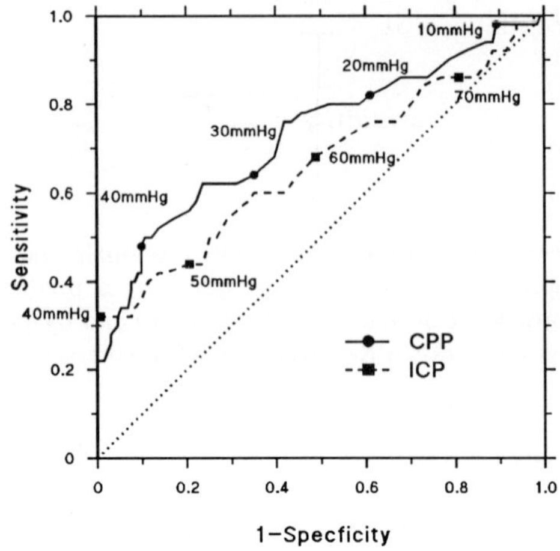

Fig 2 ICP and CPP and mortality

A previous study of head injury admissions in Newcastle had already determined that the age of forty was one of several important indicators associated with outcome [7]. If this is then added into the criterion and the ROC curves recalculated, there is a striking change in their appearance. For those patients in the over 40 age group, there would appear to be no association between CPP or ICP and mortality. By contrast in the under 40 age group both CPP and ICP are much more accurate at predicting outcome (Figs 3,4).

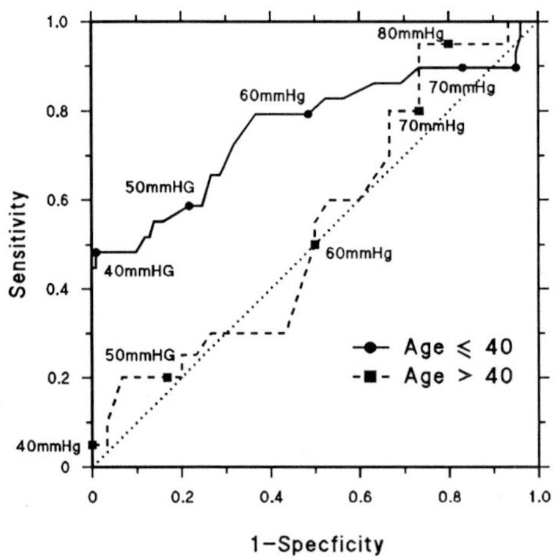

Fig 3 CPP, mortality and age

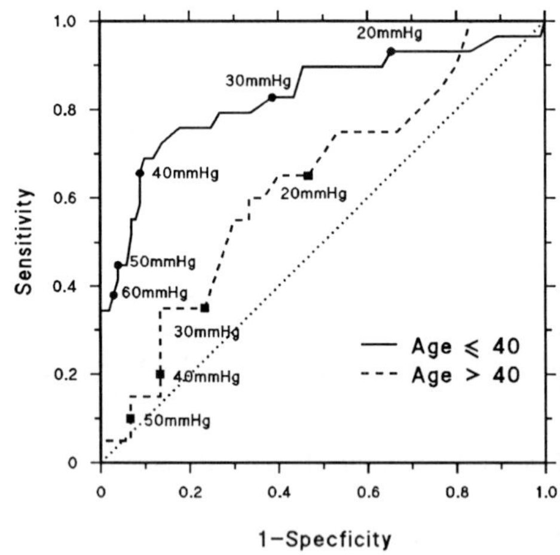

Fig 4 ICP, mortality and age

There is a minimum number of "wrong" readings (false negatives + false positives) for CPP at 54mmHg and for ICP and 36mmHg.

CONCLUSION

ROC curves are an interesting new way of looking at ICP and CPP data. They utilise the raw data and can demonstrate the validilty of tests without the need to resort to complex statistics. In conjunction with age a CPP of below 54mmHg and an ICP of above 36mmHg are strong predictors of mortality in head injured patients.

REFERENCES

1 Contant CF, Robertson CS, Gopinath SG, Narayan RK, Grossman RG (1993) Determination of clinically important thresholds in continuously monitored patients with head injury. J. Neurotrauma 10, Suppl 1, S57
2 Rosner MJ and Rosner SD (1993) Cerebral perfusion pressure management of head injured patients. In: Avezaat CJJ, van Eijndhoven JHM, Maas AIR and Tans JTJ (eds) Intracranial Pressure VIII. Springer Verlag, Berlin, pp540-543
3 Jones PA,Andrews PJD, Midgley S, Anderson SI, Piper IR, Tocher J, Houseley A, Corrie J, Slattery J, Dearden M, Miller JD (1993) Assessing the burden of secondary insults in head injured patients during intensive care. J. Neurol. Neurosurg. Psychiatry 56: 571-572
4 McGraw P. (1989) A cerebral perfusion pressure greater than 80mmHg is more beneficial. In: Hoff JT and Betz AL (eds) Intracranial Pressure VII. Springer Verlag, Berlin, pp 839-841
5 Chambers IR, Clark A, Kane PJ, Allcutt DA, Mendelow AD (1993) Continuous monitoring and recording of cerebral perfusion pressure. In: Avezaat CJJ, van Eijndhoven JHM, Maas AIR and Tans JTJ (eds) Intracranial Pressure VIII. Springer Verlag, Berlin, pp57-60.
6 Kramer MS (1988) Clinical Epidemiology and Biostatistics. Springer Verlag Berlin, Heidelberg New York, pp204-208
7 Treadwell L, Mendelow AD and the Head Injury Audit Team (1994) Audit of head injury in the Northern Region. Br.J.Nursing 3: 136-140

Session IV: Causes of Increased or Decreased ICP (1)

Chairmen: J.T. Hoff and M. Furuse

A Thrombin Antagonist, Hirudin, Inhibits Brain Edema Formation in a Model of Intracerebral Hemorrhage

KEVIN R. LEE, RICHARD F. KEEP, A. LORRIS BETZ, and JULIAN T. HOFF

Section of Neurosurgery, University of Michigan, Ann Arbor, MI, USA

INTRODUCTION

In the United States, 15% of deaths due to cerebrovascular disease (20,000 cases) are due to spontaneous intracerebral hemorrhages[1]. In addition, intracerebral hemorrhage is commonly associated with head trauma. The pathophysiology of brain edema formation with intracerebral hemorrhage remains unclear. The hematoma and secondary brain edema frequently combine to cause intracranial hypertension. The mass effect produces destructive brain shifts and causes compression of the vasculature leading to ischemia. The total mass effect is determined by the sum of the clot volume and the reactive edema. Many patients with intracerebral hemorrhages deteriorate further following the hemorrhage because of the progressive accumulation of edema fluid. This secondary decline in brain function due to edema is potentially preventable. Toxic mediators from the blood are hypothesized to be involved in secondary brain injury and edema formation.

Thrombin is a component of the blood present only in the setting of injury which may be toxic to the brain. Under normal conditions the inactive precursor, prothrombin, circulates in the blood in significant quantities. With hemorrhage into the brain prothrombin is converted rapidly to thrombin which interacts with the brain in ways that are unique to the central nervous system. Studies have shown that exogenous thrombin causes inflammation and reactive gliosis in the brain[2]. We have found that intracerebral injections of exogenous thrombin produce brain edema in the rat[3]. The present investigation was designed to study the role of thrombin in the formation of brain edema following intracerebral hemorrhage. To study this relationship, a specific and potent inhibitor of thrombin, hirudin, was used.

MATERIALS AND METHODS

General Preparation

Adult male Sprague Dawley rats (Charles River, Portage, MI) weighing 250-350 grams were anesthetized in a closed chamber with 5% isoflurane. Each animal was intubated with a 16 gauge angiocath. The rats were ventilated with a mixture of oxygen, nitrogen, and isoflurane. A catheter was inserted into the femoral artery and arterial blood pressure monitored continuously. The blood pressure was titrated with isoflurane to maintain a mean pressure of 100 mm Hg. Arterial blood was obtained from the femoral artery catheter for both blood gas analysis and injection into the brain. The ventilator rate, tidal volume, and inspired gas concentrations were adjusted to maintain a normal blood pH, pO_2, and pCO_2. Body temperature was kept at 37.5 °C with a heating pad.

Intracerebral Injection of Blood

The rats were positioned in a stereotactic frame. The scalp was incised longitudinally along the midline. A Zeiss operating microscope was used for the remainder of the procedure. Hemostasis was maintained with bipolar electrocautery. Using a dental drill a 2 mm burr hole was placed in the skull 3 mm lateral to the bregma. In the rats receiving an intracerebral hematoma, fresh autologous blood was withdrawn from the femoral artery catheter into a syringe. A 26 gauge needle was inserted into the right basal ganglia using stereotactic guidance at a depth of 6 mm. Blood and other fluids were infused into the brain using a Harvard pump.

Fifty microliters of unheparinized blood or saline were infused over 3 minutes. The needle was removed. Then 5 minutes were allowed for the hematoma to clot. A 20 microliter injection of thrombin inhibitor or saline was then administered through a second stereotactically placed needle over a 6 minute time period. The needle was removed and the scalp incision closed with suture. The arterial catheter was removed after ligating the femoral artery. The groin incision was closed. The inhalational anesthetic was discontinued and the animals were extubated. The rats were allowed to recover and given food and water.

Brain Water, Sodium, Potassium, and Chloride Contents

The rats were sacrificed by decapitation 24 hours after the intracerebral injection. The brains were rapidly removed. A coronal slice 5 mm from the frontal pole was cut approximately 4 mm thick. This section of brain was divided along the midline, and then the cortex was separated from the basal ganglia on each side. The blood clot was removed. The cerebellum was also detached and sliced along the midline into right and left halves. Thus, a total of 6 brain samples were produced: left and right cortex, left and right basal ganglia, and left and right cerebellum. In a portion of the animals the size of the blood clot was determined by measuring hemoglobin content spectro-photometrically (Sigma, St. Louis, MO).

The tissue samples were immediately weighed on an electronic analytical balance (Mettler AF100, Mettler Instrument Co., NJ) to the nearest 0.1 mg to obtain the wet weight (W). The tissue was then dried in a gravity oven at 95 °C for 24 hours and reweighed to obtain the dry weight (D). The water content, in grams of water per gram dry weight, was calculated as follows;

$$(W - D)/D$$

The dehydrated samples were digested in 1 ml of 1N nitric acid for a period of one week in order to release the ions into solution. A 100 microliter aliquot of this solution was diluted to 2 ml with deionized water and 3 mM $CsCl_2$ solution. The sodium and potassium contents of this solution were measured by flame photometry (IL943 TM Automatic Flame Photometer, Instrumentation Laboratory Inc., Lexington, MA). Chloride content was measured using a digital chloridometer (Model 442-5000, Haake Buchler Inc., Saddlebrook NJ). Ion content was expressed in microequivalents per gram dry weight.

Statistical Analysis

Differences in water and ion contents in the different brain regions between groups of rats were evaluated using analysis of variance. The Newman-Keuls test for significance was applied. A probability value of less than 0.05 was used to indicate a significant difference.

RESULTS

There was an increase in brain water content in both the ipsilateral ($p<0.001$) and contralateral ($p<0.001$) basal ganglia following placement of the intracerebral hematoma in untreated control animals. As shown in Fig. 1, comparison of the two groups of animals with hematomas demonstrated significantly less local accumulation of brain water in the group treated with hirudin than the saline treated controls (hirudin, 3.91 ± 0.07; saline, 4.69 ± 0.11 g/g dry weight). A similar statistically significant inhibition in edema formation was observed in the ipsilateral cortex and contralateral basal ganglia and cortex with hirudin treatment.

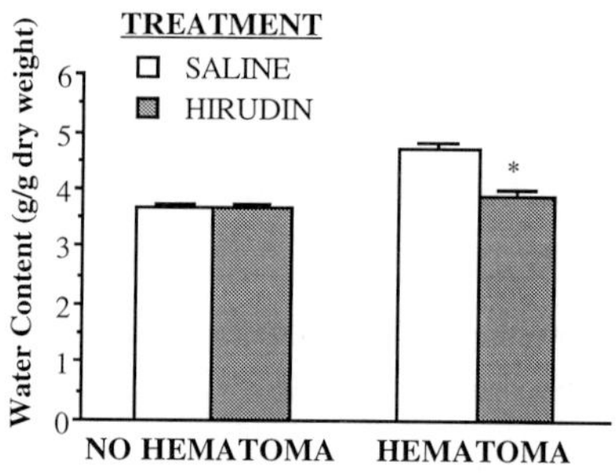

Fig. 1 Brain water content in the basal ganglia ipsilateral to the site of injection. Values are mean ± SEM. The groups without intracerebral hematomas received 50 μl injections of saline. The animals with hematomas received 50 μl injections of autologous blood from the femoral artery. Groups with and without intracerebral hematomas were treated with 20 μl of either saline or a solution of hirudin (0.5 units/μl). For each group n = 5-8; * = $p<0.001$.

Increases in brain sodium concentrations corresponded to increases in brain water content in saline treated rats with intracerebral hematomas (Fig. 2). Brain potassium content decreased with increasing edema. The changes in brain ion content in the local brain tissue surrounding the intracerebral hemorrhage were reduced in the hirudin-treated rats as compared to the group with hematomas receiving saline (sodium, $p<0.001$; potassium, $p<0.01$).

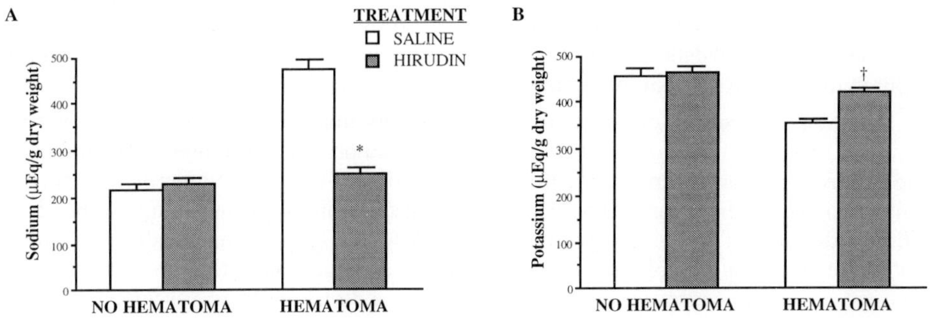

Fig. 2 Brain sodium (A) and potassium (B) contents of the basal ganglia ipsilateral to the site of injection. Values are mean ± SEM; n=6-8; * = p<0.001, † = p<0.01

The animals did not differ significantly in terms of physiological measurements including weight, blood pressure, hematocrit, and blood gases. The total hemoglobin in the intracerebral hematomas in both groups was compared in order to determine the relative volume of the clots. No difference in the hemoglobin content of the blood clots between groups was noted (saline, 4.52 ± 0.47 mg; hirudin, 4.13 ± 0.42 mg). Since the hemoglobin concentration in the blood was the same in both groups, the similar total hemoglobin content of the clots indicates that the clot mass was identical in the two groups.

DISCUSSION

Previous studies on intracerebral hemorrhage in the rat characterized the effects of blood on brain water and ion contents as well as cerebral blood flow and blood-brain barrier permeability[4]. Brain edema increases progressively in the first 24 hours along with the brain content of sodium and chloride. The edema remains elevated for several days and then begins to resolve after 4-5 days. Cerebral blood flow decreases in the tissue surrounding the clot initially. The blood flow returns to approximately baseline shortly thereafter and then slowly declines over several days. Between 4 and 12 hours the blood-brain barrier is disrupted and this increases its permeability to water and aggravates the rate of edema formation. The mediators responsible for the edema formation are unknown.

Our earlier studies showed that thrombin from an exogenous source (bovine) causes the formation of brain edema[3]. Thrombin inhibitors, such as hirudin, prevent edema formation in the presence of thrombin. Hirudin, a biological substance found in leeches, inhibits the hemostatic and receptor mediated effects of thrombin[5-9]. This protein has been used medically as an anticoagulant. Hirudin is currently being produced by recombinant DNA technology[8, 9].

This study shows that hirudin-treated animals with intracerebral hematomas accumulate less brain water than animals with hematomas which receive intracerebral injections of saline. In addition to the inhibition of edema formation hirudin also reduces the brain ion changes, including changes in sodium, potassium, and chloride. The effect does not appear to be mediated by a difference in clot mass caused by the anticoagulant properties of hirudin. Extracted clots from both groups had similar hemoglobin contents. Since hirudin is a thrombin-specific inhibitor, the effectiveness of this substance in limiting brain edema with intracerebral hematomas implicates thrombin in the pathogenesis of this form of edema.

Thrombin is a serine protease produced from its inactive zymogen, prothrombin. The predominant substrate for thrombin is the soluble plasma protein, fibrinogen. Thrombin cleaves peptide chains from fibrinogen causing the polymerization of the remaining protein to form fibrin. In addition to coagulation, thrombin has been shown to be involved in multiple other functions including induction of mitosis, chemotaxis of leukocytes, regulation of adhesion molecules, platelet aggregation, and cytokine release. Thrombin also has vasoactive properties[10-13]. In some vessels thrombin causes vasoconstriction through a direct effect on vascular smooth muscle cells in others it induces the release of vasoconstrictors like endothelin. In other vessels thrombin results in endothelium dependent vasodilation secondary to the release of endothelium derived releasing factor. An additional vascular effect of thrombin involves the modulation of endothelial cell permeability[14].

In the brain thrombin causes inflammation, scar formation, and reactive gliosis[2]. Studies have shown that thrombin binds in large quantities to the brain and spinal cord[15]. Thrombin specific receptors on platelets, endothelial cells, astrocytes, and neurons have been demonstrated[16, 17]. The brain is the only organ besides the liver which produces prothrombin. The release of prothrombin and conversion to thrombin may therefore have a role in neuromodulation. The system of inhibition of thrombin is unique to the brain. A ubiquitous thrombin inhibitor on endothelial cells, thrombomodulin, is absent in the brain[18]. Also, protease nexin 1, a thrombin inhibitor produced by astrocytes, is restricted to the extracellular matrix surrounding cerebral blood vessels.

This series of studies indicates that thrombin is involved in the pathogenesis of cerebral edema following intracerebral hemorrhage. The thrombin inhibitor, hirudin, appears to limit edema production in rats with intracerebral hematomas. Identification, however, of the precise mechanism by which thrombin causes the formation of brain edema in intracerebral hemorrhage will require further study. The possibility of clinical use of hirudin in patients with intracerebral hematomas appears promising.

ACKNOWLEDGEMENTS

This work was supported by grants from the National Institutes of Health (NS-17760 and NS-23870).

REFERENCES

1. National Center for Health Statistics (1990) Vital statistics of the United States, 1987, vol II, Mortality, part A.

2. Nishino A, Suzuki M, Ohtani H, Motohashi O, Umezawa K, Nagura H, Yoshimoto T (1993) Thrombin may contribute to the pathophysiology of central nervous system injury. J Neurotrauma 10: 167-179

3. Lee KR, Keep RF, Betz AL, Hoff JT (1994) Toxic effect of thrombin in the brain. Stroke 25: 265

4. Yang G, Betz AL, Chenevert TL, Brunberg JA, Hoff JT (1993) Experimental intracerebral hemorrhage: Relationship between brain edema, blood flow, and blood-brain barrier permeability in rats. J Neurosurg (in press)

5. Bichler J, Fritz H (1991) Hirudin, a new therapeutic tool? Ann Hematol 63: 67-76

6. Maffrand JP (1992) Direct thrombin inhibitors. Nouv Rev Fr Hematol 34: 405-419

7. Markwardt F (1988) Pharmacology of selective thrombin inhibitors. Nouv Rev Fr Hematol 30: 161-165

8. Markwardt F, Nowak G, Sturzebecher J (1991) Clinical pharmacology of recombinant hirudin. Haemostasis 21(suppl 1): 133-136

9. Talbot M (1991) Recombinant Hirudin: A New Prospect in Thrombosis. Biotechnology of plasma proteins. Curr stud hematol blood transf. 58: 1-7

10. Delin A, Olsson P, Teger-Nilsson AC (1967) Vasodilatation in the canine leg caused by intra-arterial infusion of thrombin and tissue thromboplastin. Cardiovasc Res 1: 371-378

11. Glusa E (1992) Vascular effects of thrombin. Semin Thromb Hemost 18: 296-304

12. Bacic F, Uematsu S, McCarron RM, Spatz M (1992) Secretion of immunoreactive endothelin-1 by capillary and microvascular endothelium of human brain. Neurochem Res 17: 699-702

13. White RP (1987) Comparison of the inhibitory effects of antithrombin III, macroglobulin, and thrombin in human basilar arteries: Relevance to cerebral vasospasm. J Cereb Blood Flow Metab 7: 68-73

14. DeMichele MA, Minnear FL (1992) Modulation of vascular endothelial permeability by thrombin. Semin Thromb Hemost 18: 287-295

15. Mckinney M, Snider RM, Richelson E (1983) Thrombin binding to human brain and spinal cord. Mayo Clin Proc 58: 829-831

16. Bar-Shavit R, Benezzra M, Sabbah V, Bode W, Vlodavsky I (1992) Thrombin as a multifunctional protein: induction of cell adhesion and proliferation. Am J Respir Cell Mol Biol 6: 123-130

17. Carney DH, Redin W, McCroskey L (1992) Role of high-affinity thrombin receptors in postclotting cellular effects of thrombin. Semin Thromb Hemost 18: 91-103

18. Ishii H, Salem HH, Bell CE, Laposata EA, Majerus PW (1986) Thrombomodulin, an endothelial anticoagulant protein, is absent from the brain. Blood 67: 362-365

Effect of Postischemic Transient Selective Brain Cooling on Ischemic Damage and Edema in Permanent Focal Cerebral Infarction

C.K. Park[1], C.M. Park[2], K.K. Cho[1], W.H. Sung[1], J.K. Kang[1], and C.R. Choi

Departments of [1] Neurosurgery and [2] Anesthesiology, Catholic University Medical College, Seoul, 137-040, Korea

INTRODUCTION

Recently the beneficial effects of hypothermia on ischemic or traumatic brain injury have been extensively studied in various experimental models[1,2,3,4]. In most of studies demonstrating hypothermic cerebral protection, there was concurrent lowering of body temperature. Although some of these studies have instituted moderate hypothermia, potential deleterious systemic effects of total body cooling still exist[1]. Therefore, selective brain cooling can be considered as an alternative mean[4]. However this method, the selective reduction of brain temperature while maintaining normal body temperature, has not been tried in permanent focal cerebral ischemia model yet, to our knowledge. The present study investigates the effect of moderate selective brain cooling (about 32°C of brain temperature) on ischemic brain damage and edema on permanent middle cerebral artery (MCA) occlusion in the rat.

MATERIALS AND METHODS

Eighteen adult male Sprague-Dawley rats weighing 300-400g were used in the experiments. The animals were anesthetized with a nitrous oxide-oxygen mixture (70:30%) containing 1.0 to 1.3% halothane. A mask was put on the nose and self-respiration was maintained during the time required for surgery and 30 min or 60 min of transient brain cooling. The right femoral artery was catheterized for monitoring of blood pressure and blood sampling. A small burr hole (about 3 mm in diameter) was made in the center of the left coronary suture and a micro-probe (0.5 mm in diameter) was inserted into the left frontal lobe (about 5 mm in depth) through the hole to monitor the brain temperature. All animals underwent left MCA occlusion via a subtemporal approach without removal of zygomatic arch or temporal muscle. Under high magnification of surgical microscope, the left MCA was coagulated from the olfactory tract to the most proximal portion of the MCA and cut afterward. During the surgery, mean arterial blood pressure (MABP) was recorded continuously (Model 7E Polygraph, Grass, USA). Other physiological variables such as blood gases and glucose were also measured. Brain temperature (Therm 2250-1, Ahlborn Meβ- und Regelungstechnik, Germany) and rectal temperature were monitored continuously during the surgery and brain cooling, and before sacrifice.

Three groups of animals were studied: group 1, normothermic brain temperature control (n=6): group 2, hypothermic brain temperature for 30 min (n=6): and group 3, hypothermic brain temperature for 60 min (n=6). In all groups, rectal temperature was maintained 36.5-37°C with the homeothermic system and a heating lamp. In groups 2 and 3, brain temperature was lowered to less than 34°C by active cooling 15 min following MCA occlusion. Active cooling was initiated by placing ice bags around the head and neck and applying a small electric fan onto the head, and maintained for 30 min in group 2 and 60 min in group 3. After the brain cooling treatment, the anesthesia was discontinued, the arterial catheter and the micro-probe were removed, and the head and neck were rewarmed by a heating lamp. In group 1, the animals were maintained normothermic for 75 min following MCA occlusion.

Twenty-four hours following MCA occlusion, the rats were sacrificed. Brains were removed from the calvaria immediately after sacrifice, and frozen in a cryostat (-25°C). Coronal sections (20μm thick) were cut with a cryostat and stained with hematoxylin-eosin. Infarcted area and the extent of brain swelling were readily delineated. Eight coronal sections which corresponded to planes of the preselected forebrain were selected among the stained slices, and the volume of ischemic damage was computed, as described previously[5]. To measure the volume of brain edema, the total volume of the nonischemic hemisphere in each brain was subtracted from the total volume of the ischemic one.

Significancy of the differences between the normothermic and the hypothermic groups was assessed by analysis of variance with subsequent intergroup comparison by Student's t-test with Bonferroni correction. $P<0.05$ was required for significance.

RESULTS

There were no significant differences in all physiological parameters between normothermic and hypothermic animals. The time course of the brain temperature is presented in Table 1. In the groups 2 and 3, the brain temperature was maintained between 31 and 33°C during brain cooling, while the body temperature was kept between 36.5 and 37.0°C

Table 1 Time course of brain temperature (°C) (Mean ± S.E.)

	Time (min)							
Group	-15	MCAO	15	30	45	60	75	Sacrifice
1 (normothermic)	37.0	37.1	37.0	36.9	36.9	37.0	36.8	38.1
	± 0.19	± 0.21	± 0.16	± 0.20	± 0.23	± 0.26	±0.22	± 0.26
2 (hypothermic,	37.0	36.9	33.6	32.2	32.5			38.0
30 min)	± 0.25	± 0.25	± 0.46	± 0.63	± 0.54			± 0.25
3 (hypothermic,	36.8	36.4	34.0	32.1	31.9	31.6	31.8	38.7
60 min)	± 0.23	± 0.17	± 0.02	± 0.41	± 0.36	± 0.41	± 0.64	± 0.27

Postischemic selective brain cooling for either 30 or 60 min significantly reduced the volume of infarction in the cerebral hemisphere by 14% ($P<0.05$) or by 27% ($P<0.01$) respectively. However, the volume of infarction in the caudate nucleus or the volume of brain edema, obtained by subtracting the nonischemic hemispheric volume from the ischemic hemispheric volume was not reduced by selective brain cooling (Table 2). The ratio of volumes of brain edema/infarction increased significantly in groups 2 ($P<0.05$) and 3 ($P<0.05$) compared with group 1.

Table 2 Effect of postischemic transient brain cooling on 24-hour infarction volume and ischemic brain edema (mm^3) (Mean ± S.E.)

	Infarction Volume		Edema	Edema/
Group	Hemisphere	Caudate Nu		Infarction (%)
normothermic	290.5	71.6	127.6	44
	± 9.1	± 5.7	± 7.4	± 2.5
hypothermic	249.2*	67.9	129.5	52.5*
(30 min)	± 20.1	± 4.0	± 7.7	± 2.1
hypothermic	212.8**	72.0	117.6	58.0*
(60 min)	± 24.7	± 5.3	± 9.9	± 8.2

* $P<0.05$, ** $P<0.01$ compared with normothermic group

DISCUSSION

Our results show that a transient moderate reduction of 4-6°C in brain temperature following ischemia results in attenuation of neuronal damage after permanent focal cerebral ischemia in rats. In addition, longer brain cooling further reduces ischemic brain damage. On the other hand, the striatum dose not respond favorably, and postischemic selective brain cooling appears to exacerbate ischemic brain edema to some extent.

Several theories have been proposed to explain the protection from cerebral ischemia afforded by hypothermia. It is well established that hypothermia decreases the cellular metabolic rate[6]. Hypothermia may also lower the critical threshold of cerebral blood flow (CBF), expanding the "ischemic penumbra". Recently, it has been reported in a model of permanent focal ischemia that mild hypothermia suppressed the glutamate excitotoxicity within ischemic penumbra[7]. The excessive release of glutamate particularly in the penumbra surrounding ischemic focus has been shown to contribute to the injury and death of still-viable cells[8]. Other mechanisms of this protection include reductions of intracellular acidosis[9] and edema formation[10].

According to the results of our experiments, however, the reduction of edema formation might not be a major implication for the neurporotective mechanism of selective brain cooling. The effects of hypothermia on the cerebral microcirculation have been studied both in vitro[11] and in vivo[12]. In these studies, hypothermia appeared to have a marked vasodilator effect on intracerebral arteriols, suggesting that the direct vascular effect of low temperature is to decrease vascular resistance. It is therefore also conceivable that focal hypothermia might act on the cerebral microcirculation in a way that is independent of mechanisms that occur in systemic hypothermia. Thus, selective brain cooling may result in an increase of vasodilating compounds, which can exert a protective effect against ischemic cell damage. In this setting, though, an elevation of cerebral blood flow rushing through dilated blood vessels can also contribute to permeability alterations[13]. Our finding that ischemic edema appeared to be rather exacerbated heralds a possibility that hyperemia initiated by selective brain cooling may counteract against protective effects of hypothermia.

In conclusion, in this rat model of permanent MCA occlusion, we were able to demonstrate that transient selective brain cooling reduced hemispheric infarct volume when administered 15 min after the onset of ischemia. However, ischemic edema appeared to be rather exacerbated. In its clinical application, the potential adverse effect of brain swelling on intracranial pressure should be considered.

ACKNOWLEDGMENTS

The authors thank Ms. J.A. Chun for technical assistance, and Ms. Y.J. Chung for help in preparing the manuscript.

REFERENCES

1. Kader A, Brisman MH, Maraire N, Huh J-T, Solomon RA (1992) The effect of mild hypothermia on permanent focal ischemia in the rat. Neurosurgery 31:1056-1061
2. Busto R, Dietrich WD, Globus MYT, Valdes I, Scheinberg P, Ginsberg MD (1981) Small differences in intraischemic brain temperature critically determine the extent of ischemic neuronal

injury. J Cereb Blood Flow Metab 7:729-738

3. Baker CJ, Onesti ST, Solomon RA (1992) Reduction by delayed hypothermia of cerebral infarction following middle cerebral artery occlusion in the rat: a time-course study. J Neurosurg 77:438-444
4. Kuluz JW, Gregory GA, Yu ACH, Chang Y (1992) Selective brain cooling during and after prolonged global ischemia reduces cortical damage in rats. Stroke 23:1792-1797
5. Park CK, McCulloch J, Kang JK, Choi CR (1994) Pretreatment with a competitive NMDA antagonist D-CPPene attenuates focal cerebral infarction and brain swelling in awake rats. Acta Neurochir (in press)
6. Rosomoff HL, Holaday DA (1954) Cerebral blood flow and cerebral oxygen consumption, Anesthesiology 58:527-532
7. Graf R, Matsumoto K, Risse F, Rosner G, Heiss WD (1992) Effect of mild hypothermia on glutamate consumption in cat focal ischemia. 17th International Joint Conference on Stroke and Cerebral Circulation, Phoenix, Arizona (abstr)
8. Choi DW (1990) Cerebral hypoxia: some new approaches and unanswered questions. J Neurosci 10:2493-2501
9. Norwood WI, Norwood CR, Ingwall JS, Castaneda AR, Fossel ET (1979) Hypothermic circulatory arrest. J Thorac Cardiovasc Surg 78:823-830
10. Dempsey RJ, Combs DJ, Maley MD, Cowan DE, Roy MW, Donaldson DL (1987) Moderate hypothermia reduces postischemic edema development and leukotriene production. Neurosurgery 21:177-181
11. Ogura K, Takayasu M, Dacey RG (1991) Effects of hypothermia and hyperthermia on the reactivity of rat intracerebral arterioles in vitro. J Neurosurg 75:433-439
12. Kuluz J, Smith D, Busto R, Ginsberg MD, Dietrich WD, Globus MYT (1991) Selective brain cooling increases CBF in rats. Neuroscience 17(pt 1):475
13. Ting P, Masaoka H, Kuroiwa T, Wagner H, Fenton I, Klatzo I (1986) Influence of blood-brain barrier opening to proteins on development of post-ischemic brain injury. Neurol Res 8:146-151

A Study of Microcirculation and Ultrastructure in a Sagittal Sinus Occlusion Model of a Cat

H. KUCHIWAKI, S. INAO, H. KANAIWA, K. YOSHIDA, M. YAMAMOTO, and K. SUGITA

Department of Neurosurgery, Nagoya University School of Medicine, Japan

SUMMARY

We have investigated microcirculation through a cranial window and performed ultrastuctural studies to assess treatments using a sagittal sinus occlusion model of cat (n=10). We obtained data from the control state to 120 min after occlusion. Dilatation of the venous system and partial constrictions of the arterioles were observed in early the stage after the occlusion. Blood flow decreased. This period corresponds to our previous results that a buffering circuit becomes active to decrease vascular resistance. In the later stage, subpial hemorrhages fused and edema progressed rapidly. For effective treatment, an early and transient period seems to be important after the venous occlusion.

INTRODUCTION

The patterns of venous occlusion may be divided into four groups, such as dural sinus occlusion with or without cerebral or cerebellar surface vein occlusion, the surface vein occlusion of the cerebrum or the cerebellum, and deep vein occlusion [1-5]. The diagnosis of venous occlusive diseases generally is difficult because patient conditions are similar to the diseases with other origins. Although the clinical states distribute in wide ranges from mild to severe grades, there are cases whose clinical course rapidly progress and their prognosis becomes poor [1,6]. In such cases heparin, dextran, or surgical treatment are usually suggested [1,6,7].

Pathological studies on autopsy cases [6] and experimental studies using venous occlusion models have been presented in the literature [4,5,8,9,10]. Our research group earlier reported a buffering circuit in morphological studies to explain the decrease in resistance by venous hypertension in the progress of the disease in a sagittal sinus occlusion model of a cat [11]. The present study was designed to experimentally produce a model of sagittal sinus occlusion and to analyze serial changes in vasculature, cerebral blood flow, and electron microscopic findings to assess the timing of the treatment in venous occlusive diseases.

MATERIALS AND METHODS

Eight adult cats (2.4 to 4.0 kg in body weight) were anesthetized with ketamine (40 mg/kg, i.m.), chloralose (50 mg/kg, i.v.) and urethane (200 mg/kg, i.v.). Each animal was immobilized by an i.v. injection of pancronium bromide and artificially ventilated after a tracheal cannula was inserted through a tracheotomy site. A catheter was inserted via the femoral artery into the abdominal aorta for measurement of systemic blood pressure and another via the femoral vein into the vena cava inferior. The animals were secured on a stereotactic operation table throughout the experimental period. The CO_2 concentration in an expired respiratory gas and the body temperature were continuously monitored. Thus the physiological states of the animals were kept at normal levels. A small burr was made on the superior sagittal sinus (SSS) in the occipital region. Control data were obtained 30 min after setup, when the status of each animal had been stabilized. A polyethylene catheter (1 mm dia.) whose tip was narrowed with an extension was inserted 10 mm long through the SSS in the rostral direction. A venous occlusion model was then produced by a rapid infusion of cyanoacrylate (0.05 ml). The animal was observed 120 min after an occlusion of the SSS. In this model, 1) the state of blood vessels on the brain surface was recorded via a bone fenestra of the supramarginal gyrus using a sensitive video camera (x 200); and 2) after the cats were killed, capillary specimens were obtained for electron microscopic study.

RESULTS AND DISCUSSION

The diameters of the arterioles and venules were measured in the control state. Movements of the red cells were detectable in the vein but those in the arterioles could not be found in the control. Fifteen minutes after occlusion, the arterial and venous blood flow on the brain surface decreased. Dilatation of the vunules (mean 1.33 times of the control diameter size) were observed immediately after SSS occlusion. Partial arteriolar constrictions also appear at 15 to 30 min after occlusion. Dilatation of the capillary lumen and many vesicles in the endothelium was observed electron microscopically. Within 60 minutes after the occlusion, the veins and arteries at the sites of their penetrating from or into the cortex were compressed and stenosed by small hematomas. Arterioles constricted diffusely, and the area of venous stasis increased. Blood flow became slower. At 60 min following the occlusion, extravasation was observed around large veins in which blood flow had stopped. The extent of arteriolar constriction increased with experimental time, and blood flow was intermittent. Small subpial spotty bleeding extended over a progressively larger area. At 120 min bleeding foci fused, most emissary arteries and veins showed collapse due to the hematoma, and the flow rate further decreased. Cerebral blood flow decreased even more markedly. Electron microscopy showed thinning of the endothelium and a marked increase in the perivascular space with cerebral edema.
The present results were obtained with a model of the SSS occlusion with a cortical surface vein occlusion. This model seems to be the most rapidly aggressive model among venous occlusion model [4,5]. The first stage of venous occlusion was venous dilatation and partial narrowing of arterioles in the cortical surface vasculature. Capillaries dilated and vesicles in the endothelium increased. In this period, capillaries of the cortex per unit area also increased in number [11]. This indicates the development of a transient buffering circuit to decrease high resistance in the venous circuit and allow the blood flow through the lower resistance circuit. Our results on such morphometric parameters will appear elsewhere [11].
Protection of U fiber to prevent of edema was reported also to be transiently effective [4,6]. However, this short physiological buffer effect may well be associated with down regulation of the brain metabolism soon after venous occlusion. Decreasing the increased vascular resistance and high blood viscosity, due to venous stasis and extravasation of the fluid, seems important in treating the venous occlusion this short period. At the same time it is important to protect the brain from mismatching of the decreased blood flow and the metabolism.
After 60 min, small spotted hemorrhages fused into a larger one. An increase in vascular resistance, *ie.* stasis in venous circulation, and cerebral edema, seemed to progress rapidly. In this period, brain tissue has been thought to suffer insults from ischemia and hemorrhage [9,12,13]. Surgical treatment for the mechanical obstruction is usually effective [1,2,3,6]. Characteristic findings by computed tomogram are supposed to indicate this stage[1,2,3]. This suggests that treatment is effective in the relatively early stages.
In conclusion, there is a physiological buffer capacity protecting the brain against venous occlusion. Any treatments will be effective in this period by additionally matching the brain metabolism with decreased blood flow.

REFERENCES

1. Eick JJ, Miller KD, Bell KA, Tutton RH (1981) Computed tomography of deep venous thrombosis in children. Radiology140:399-402
2. Gabrielsen TO, Seeger JF, Knake JE, Stilwill EW (1981) Radiology of cerebral vein occlusion without dural sinus occlusion. Radiology 140: 403-408
3. Erbguth F, Brenner P, Schuierer G, Druschky K-F, Neundorfer B (1991) Diagnosis and treatment of deep cerebral vein thrombosis. Neurosur Rev 14:145-148
4. Kannuki S, Cervo's-Navarro J, Matsumoto K (1989) Evolution of venous cerebral infarction and brain edema-An experimental study with sagittal sinus obstruction. Brain Nerve (Tokyo) 41:1225-1231
5. Saijou T (1992) Experimental study on cerebral venous circulatory disturbance. Okayama Igakkai Zasshi 104:871-884
6. Bonsser MG, Chiras J, Bories J, Castaigne P (1985) Cerebral venous thrombosis-Review of 38 cases. Stroke 16:199-213
7. Schmideck HH, Auer LM, Kapp JP (1985) The cerebral venous system. Neurosurgery 17:663-68
8. Miyagami M, Nakamura S, Moriyasu N (1975) Hydrodynamic of the C.S.F. under experimental occlusion of the superior sagittal sinus. Noshinkeigeka 3:739-745

9. Sato S, Toya S, Ohtani M, Kawase T (1985) The effect of sagittal sinus occlusion on blood-brain barrier permeability and cerebral blood flow in the dog. In: Inaba Y, Klatzo I, Spatz M, Brain Edema, Springer-Verlag, Berlin, Heidelberg, New York, Tokyo, pp 235-239
10. Miyamoto K, Tsujimoto S, Tominaga M, Takeshima T, Morimoto T, Tsunoda S, Sakaki T (1992) The focal brain ischemia with disturbance of venous drainage. Brain Nerve (Tokyo) 44:621-627
11. Kanaiwa H, Kuchiwaki H, Inao S, Sugita K (1994) Changes in the cerebrocortical capillary net work following venous sinus occlusion in cats. (In preparation)
12. Kurokawa Y, Hashi K, Okuyama T, Sasaki S (1989) An experimental model of cerebral venous hypertension in rats. Neurol med chir (Tokyo) 29:175-180
13. Barnett HJM, Hyland HH (1953) Non-infective intracranial venous thrombi. Brain 76:36-49

Preventing Shunt Overdrainage in Hydrocephalus: Are Anti-Siphon Devices Really Physiological?

J. Sahuquillo[1], M.A. Poca[1], M. Martinez[1], A. Rovira[2], M. Busto[2], and E. Rubio[1]

[1] Department of Neurosurgery, [2] Magnetic Resonance Imaging Unit, Vall d'Hebron University Hospital, Paseo del Vall d'Hebron s/n, 08035 Barcelona, Spain

Complications due to shunt overdrainage still have an unreasonable prevalence in high risk patients (massive ventriculomegaly, chronic adult hydrocephalus, etc.). Overdrainage is directly related to the hydrodynamic profile of shunts and is caused by the negative hydrostatic pressure generated distal to the valve when the patient assumes the erect position [1]. In the supine position, the closing pressure of the valve is the main factor that controls flow in shunts. However, when the patient assumes the erect posture, the hydrostatic pressure in the distal catheter maintains the valve continuously open even when the intraventricular pressure becomes negative [2]. Flow through the shunt in the later situation is essentially regulated by the negative pressure distal to the valve and by the resistance to outflow of the shunt (R_{shunt}). Programmable, flow-regulated or reversible occlusion valves, anti-siphon and antigravitatory devices are all designed to avoid overdrainage. The failure of programmable valves to avoid overdrainage has renewed the interest in the so-called 'anti-siphon devices' (ASD). Our purpose in this study is to evaluate 'in vivo' hydrodynamic profile and performance of a particular antisiphon, in order to study how well it reproduces the physiological changes observed in intracranial pressure (ICP) when patients assume the standing position.

CLINICAL MATERIAL AND METHODS

Nineteen adult patients with hydrocephalus of variable etiology were shunted using a differential-pressure diaphragm-based valve with an incorporated in series siphon control device (Delta valve Performance Level 1, supplied by PS Medical, USA) (DPL1). In each patient, epidural ICP was continuously monitored for at least 24 hours before shunt implantation. Postural changes in mean ICP were evaluated in supine position (**ICP_S**) and after assuming and maintaining the sitting position for at least 4 hours (**ICP_{90}**). Changes in mean ICP with changes in body position (**ICP_{grad}**) were calculated as **$ICP_S - ICP_{90}$**. In patients with communicating hydrocephalus, R_{out} and indirect PVI were calculated by the Marmarou's bolus test [3]. In every case a shunt was implanted using a right frontal ventricular approach and placing the valve in a retroauricular subcutaneous pocket with the siphon control device situated at the foramen of Monro level. To avoid variability in the induced negative hydrostatic pressure, 70 cm of distal catheter was attached to the outlet of the valve and introduced in the peritoneal cavity. ICP recording was continued after shunting and the analysis of ICP recording, postural ICP changes and hydrodynamic studies repeated 4 to 6 days later. The results of ICP_{grad} in these 19 cases were compared with normal ICP_{grad} [4] and with ICP_{grad} reported by others in patients shunted with conventional low pressure valves [5]. Our results in a group of patients shunted with a conventional low resistance cone and ball valve (opening pressure of 40 mm H2O), gave a mean ICP_{grad} of 20.3 $\pm$ 6.5 mm Hg (unpublished results) and this was also used as a control **(Fig.1)**.

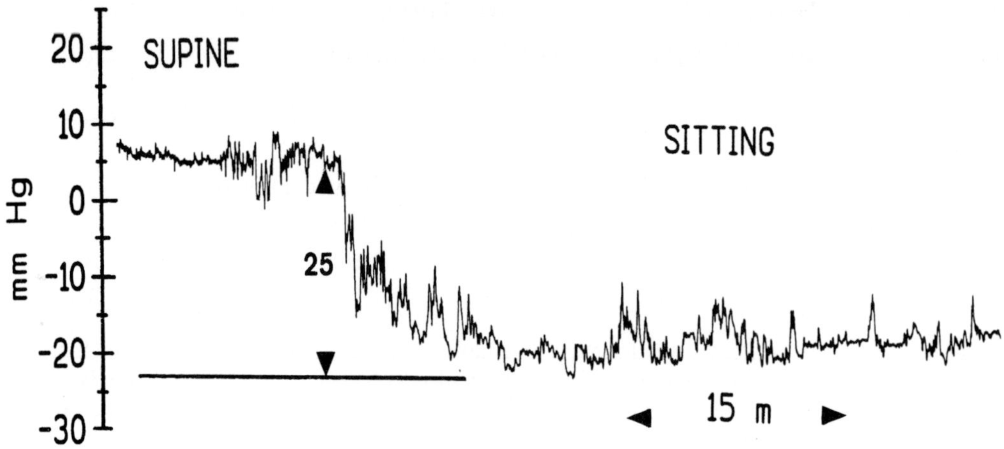

Fig.1: Post-shunt ICP recording (cone and ball low-pressure valve) in a patient with 'normal pressure hydrocephalus' syndrome. Observe the considerable ICP_{grad} of 25 mm Hg reached after about 15 minutes in the sitting position. Although, in this case, the patient did not present symptoms, overdrainage is always present in this situation.

RESULTS

Mean age for our study group was 39.2 ± 17.9 years. Of the 19 cases, 7 were male and 12 female. Mean Evans Index measured in the CT scan was 0.37 ± 0.04. Massive ventriculomegaly (Evans Index > 40) was observed in 5 cases. In five patients, the etiology of hydrocephalus was a non-tumoral aqueductal stenosis, in 6 it was related to Chiari I or II malformations, to head injury in one case and the cause was unknown in six patients. Two cases presented the so-called 'normal pressure hydrocephalus' syndrome, although in both the hydrodynamic diagnosis was of active hydrocephalus [6]. ICP before and after shunting is plotted in **Fig.1**. In 8 patients with a communicating hydrocephalus, the hydrodynamic profile showed a mean PVI of 20.6 ± 4.8 ml before shunt that increased to 60.2 ± 28.2 after shunting (P= 0.007). Mean R_{out} was 9.5 ± 4.2 mm Hg/ml/min before shunt and significantly decreased to 1.1 ± 0.8 mm Hg/ml/min after shunt. ICP_{grad} before and after shunt are summarized in **Fig.2.** Postural changes in ICP recording after shunting followed a stereotyped pattern, very different from the pattern found in shunted patients on whom antisiphon devices had not been used. After assuming the sitting position, each patient presented an immediate reduction of the ICP_S that gradually increased within the following two hours. Four hours after sitting, the median ICP_{grad} in the entire group was only slightly different from zero (3 mm Hg) and approached ICP_S in all but two patients **(Fig.3A and B)**. In each case, qualitative changes in ICP recordings were found a few minutes after assuming the sitting position. In some of them, a very irregular and abnormal chart recording was observed and in two cases, low amplitude B-waves were detected while the patients were sitting. In spite of this, mean ICP while sitting was always within the normal range and no patient presented symptoms related to low ICP. In a patient with a shunt infection and in whom the distal catheter was externalized, mean shunt drainage in supine was 0.45 ml/minute, but when a hydrostatic pressure of - 50 was added, the flow was reduced to 0.16 ml/min. Assuming an ICP of 10 mm Hg, the estimated R_{shunt} was 22 mm Hg/ml/min at 0 mm of hydrostatic pressure and increased to 292 mm Hg/ml /min when the patient was in the sitting position.

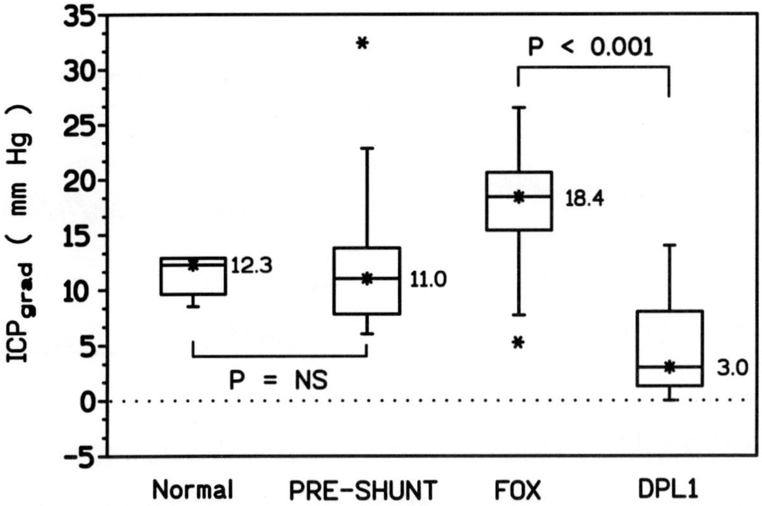

Fig.2: Boxplot summarizing postural changes before (Pre-Shunt) and after shunting (DPL1) in patients shunted with a Delta valve. Changes are compared with the normal ICP_{grad} and with the results reported by Fox et al [5]. NS= not statistically significant.

DISCUSSION

The fact that posture is one of the most important variables affecting ICP in shunted patients has been clearly demonstrated. The difference between shunted and non-shunted patients is the higher negative ICP the former can present because of the negative hydrostatic pressure transmitted to the craniospinal axis through the shunt. This negative pressure maintains the shunt open regardless of the valve's closing pressure and consequently overdrainage is produced. ASD were introduced into the neurosurgical armamentarium by Portnoy [7]. Ideally, these devices had to reproduce the physiological changes found in normal man. What ASD have to avoid is the 'excessive' ICP_{grad} that appears in shunted patients. The anti-siphon tested in our study clearly prevented overdrainage while the patient assumed the sitting position. However, ICP_{grad} reached was too small and clearly non-physiological. The ASD-induced increased in R_{shunt} to control siphoning was too high and produced, in almost every case, qualitative abnormalities in ICP recording. While a sufficient flow through the shunt exists in the supine position, an excessive reduced flow is observed when the patient assumes sitting or upright position. In one case in whom flow through the shunt was studied, a 12 times increase in R_{shunt} was observed when assuming the sitting position. Abnormal ICP chart recording in some cases, the appearance of low amplitude B-waves while sitting in others and non-physiological ICP_{grad} suggest that a modification of the shunt assembly to reduce R_{shunt} in the presence of negative hydrostatic pressure would be desirable. While these changes are not made, DPL1 valves are not recommended in those patients in whom low resistance valves are indicated ('normal pressure' hydrocephalus). In patients with hypertensive hydrocephalus and at high risk of subdural collections, this type of shunt can be a sound alternative to conventional valves. Manufacturers' shunt and ASD specifications although compliant with standard health-care regulations are clearly insufficient for the neurosurgeon. In our opinion, new devices to treat hydrocephalus, should be submitted to the discipline of clinical trials before their use in clinical practice.

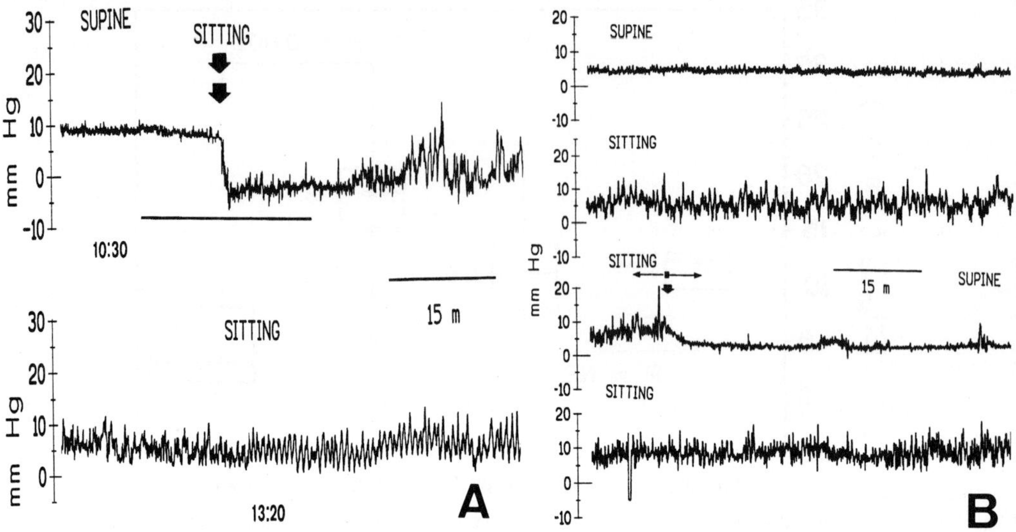

Fig.3: A) After shunt postural changes in a patient with a Chiari I malformation. In this case, a normal ICP_{grad} appears immediately after sitting (upper chart). However, the ICP_{grad} gradually disappears and qualitative abnormalities in the ICP chart are evident 30 minutes after sitting (upper chart). In this case, low amplitude B-waves are observed after 3 hours of sitting (lower chart). **B)** Shunted hydrocephalus secondary to aqueductal stenosis. Observe the normal ICP recording while supine (upper chart) and the abnormal recording two hours after sitting (second chart). In the third chart, observe the immediate normalization of the ICP recording induced while going from sitting to supine (black arrow). ICP recording becomes again abnormal immediately after sitting (lower chart).

REFERENCES

1. Tokoro, K., Chiba, Y. (1990): Optimum position of the antisiphon device. Neurosurgery 27:332.

2. Da Silva, M.C., Drake, J.M. (1990): Effect of subcutaneous implantation of anti-siphon devices on CSF shunt function. Pediatr.Neurosurg. 16:197-202.

3. Marmarou, A., Shulman, K., Rosende, R.M, (1978): A nonlinear analysis of the cerebrospinal fluid system ad intracranial pressure dynamics. J.Neurosurg. 48:332-344.

4. Loman, J., Myerson, A., Goldman, D. (1935): Effects of alterations in posture on the cerebrospinal fluid pressure. Arch.Neurol.Psychiat. 33:1279-1295.

5. Fox, J,L., McCullough, D.C., Green, R.C. (1973): Effect of cerebrospinal fluid shunts on intracranial pressure and on cerebrospinal fluid dynamics. J.Neurol.Neurosurg.Psychiatry 36:302-312.

6. Sahuquillo, J., Rubio, E., Codina, A., Molins, A., Guitart, J.M., Poca, M.A., Chasampi, A. (1991): Reappraisal of the intracranial pressure and cerebrospinal fluid dynamics in patients with the so-called "Normal Pressure Hydrocephalus" syndrome. Acta Neurochir.(Wien) 112:50-61.

7. Portnoy, H.D., Schulte, R.R., Fox, J.L., Croissant, P.D., Tripp, L. (1973): Anti-siphon and reversible occlusion valves for shunting in hydrocephalus and preventing post-shunt subdural hematomas. J.Neurosurg. 38:729-738.

The Effect of Changes in Head Position on Cerebral Hemodynamics

SHANKAR P. GOPINATH, CLAUDIA S. ROBERTSON, RAJ K. NARAYAN, and ROBERT G. GROSSMAN

Department of Neurosurgery, Baylor College of Medicine, One Baylor Plaza, Houston, TX 77030, USA

INTRODUCTION

The common causes of secondary brain damage in head injured patients include elevated intracranial pressure and hypotension, which can compromise cerebral perfusion. Elevation of the head of the bed has been the standard neurosurgical practice for management of raised intracranial pressure. However, some investigators advocate keeping the head end of the bed flat, in order to maintain maximal cerebral perfusion pressure and to prevent the occurrence of plateau waves [1,2], while others suggested 15° or 30° head elevation [3]. Our previous study did not show any significant changes in cerebral perfusion pressure or in global cerebral blood flow in most patients by elevating the head to 30° [4]. However, the most critically ill patients could not be studied at the different head positions because of the time required to do conventional measurements of cerebral blood flow. With the advent of new technologies such as near-infrared spectroscopy (NIRS), which allows estimation of trend changes in local brain tissue oxygen saturation and blood volume [5], and the thermal diffusion CBF probe, which continuously measures local cortical blood flow[6], a better understanding of the cerebral hemodynamic changes secondary to various head positions may be possible.

We used these new technologies to investigate the cerebral hemodynamic effects of head position in severely head injured patients.

MATERIALS AND METHODS

Twenty separate recordings in fifteen adult head injured patients admitted to the neurosurgical intensive care unit were obtained. The mean age of the patient was 28.4 years (range 16-50 years), and two patients were female. Twelve patients sustained closed head injury, and three had gunshot wound to the head. The primary diagnosis was acute subdural hematoma in nine patients, contusion, and intracerebral hematoma in three patients each. Postresuscitation Glasgow Coma Scale scores were 3 to 5 in ten patients, 6 to 8 in five patients.

The physiological parameters recorded continuously by a bedside computer included intracranial pressure (ICP, with the transducer zeroed at the level of the foramen of Monro), systemic mean arterial pressure (MAP), cerebral perfusion pressure (CPP), end-tidal carbon dioxide ($ETCO_2$), arterial oxygen saturation (SaO_2), continuous jugular venous oxygen saturation ($SjvO_2$) using a fiberoptic catheter, cortical cerebral blood flow (CBF) by thermal diffusion method, brain tissue oxygen saturation (SO_2), and brain tissue blood volume (BV) using near infrared spectroscopy.

The changes in the above variables were studied from: supine to 30° head elevation, supine to 60° head elevation, and supine to Trendelenberg position. In addition, changes with hyperventilation with the patient in the supine position was also recorded. While measuring the changes, the arterial pressure transducer was kept at the level of the head.

Statistical analysis was done using paired t-test. Values are expressed as percentage changes from the supine position.

RESULTS

Typical experiments are shown in fig. 1 and 2. The changes in ICP, MAP, and cortical CBF with head elevation varied from patient to patient. The most consistent changes with head position were the decrease in brain tissue BV measured with the NIRS. The decrease in BV was always greater with 60° elevation than with 30° elevation. With hyperventilation, there was the expected decrease in ICP, $SjvO_2$, and cortical CBF.

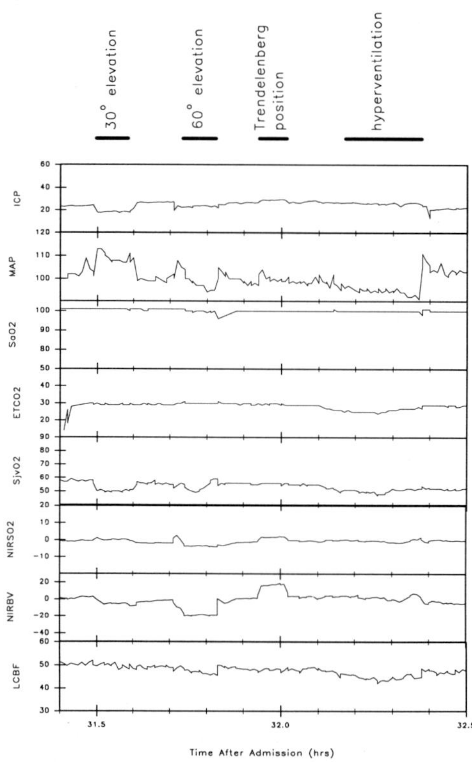

Figure 1. This patient had a significant decrease in ICP and an increase in MAP with 30° head elevation. With 60° head elevation, both ICP and MAP decreased, and cortical CBF decreased slightly.

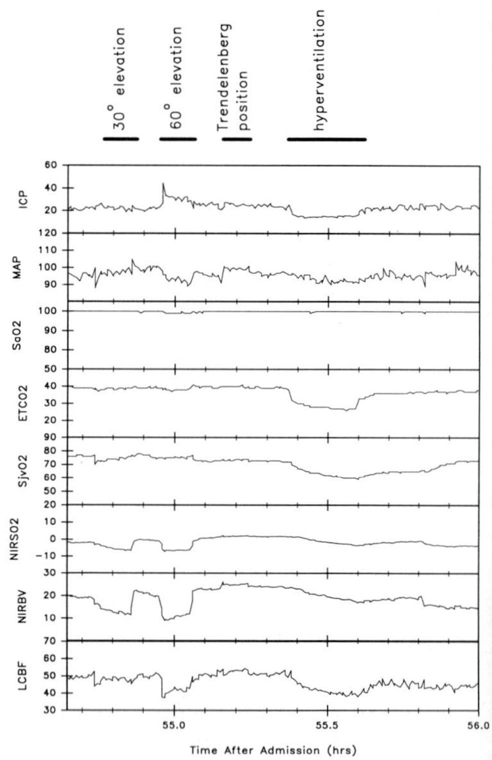

Figure 2. This patient had only a small decrease in ICP with 30° head elevation. With 60° head elevation, ICP increased and MAP decreased, resulting in a marked decrease in CPP and a decrease in cortical CBF.

The results obtained in all patients are summarized in fig. 3 (values are mean±SD, *=p<.05, paired t-test).

Head elevation from supine to 30°: The mean value for the ICP was significantly lower by 3.8 ± 2.8 without a change in mean arterial blood pressure, resulting in a 5% increase in cerebral perfusion pressure. The mean cortical cerebral blood flow increased slightly, although the change was not statistically significant. Brain tissue blood volume consistently decreased by 11%. None of the other parameters showed a statistically significant difference between head elevation at 30° and supine.

Head elevation to 60°: There was a decrease in brain tissue blood volume by 19%, almost twice the change with 30° head elevation. The changes in other variables varied from patient to patient, causing the mean changes to be not significantly different from zero (see fig. 1 and 2).

Trendelenberg position: Brain tissue blood volume increased by 5%, associated with a small increase in intracranial pressure which was not statistically significant.

Hyperventilation: Intracranial pressure and cortical cerebral blood flow consistently decreased with hyperventilation. Cerebral perfusion pressure tended to increase but the change was not significant.

Fig. 3. Summary data of all results are shown below in the graphs below. The asterisk indicates those changes that are different from zero (p<.05).

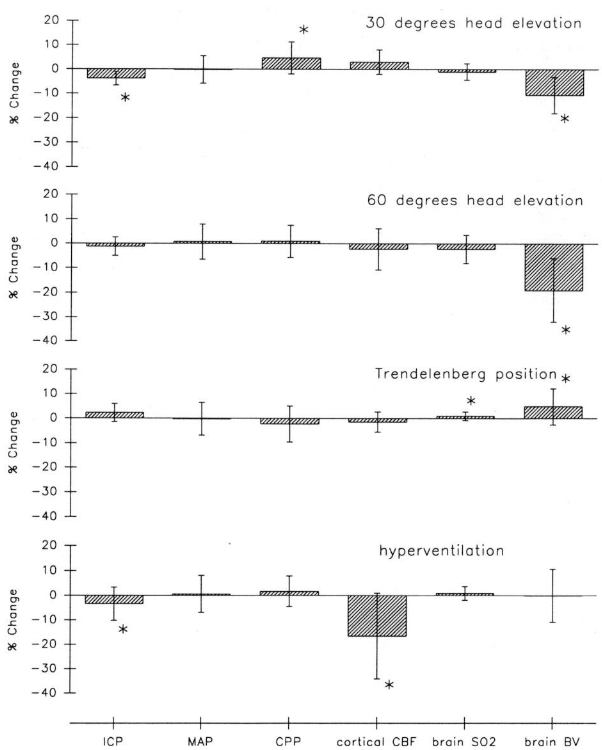

DISCUSSION

The most consistent effects of head elevation were on the changes in brain tissue blood volume obtained with the near infrared spectroscopy. Blood volume decreased with head elevation, and increased with Trendelenberg position in all patients. In contrast, the hemodynamic effects of head elevation varied with the amount of elevation, and varied from patient to patient. Head elevation to 30° consistently reduced intracranial pressure, and increased cerebral perfusion pressure. Head elevation to 60° lowered ICP in some patients and raised ICP in others. Therefore, 30° head elevation seemed to be the optimal position for most patients, but these new technologies may help individualize treatments to specific patients.

ACKNOWLEGEMENTS

This work was supported by NIH grant #PO1-NS27616.

REFERENCES

1. Rosner MJ, Coley IB (1986) Cerebral perfusion pressure, intracranial pressure, and head elevation. J Neurosurg 65:636-641
2. Rosner MJ, Daughton S (1990) Cerebral perfusion pressure management in head injury. J Trauma 30: 933-941
3. Durward QJ, Amacher AL, Del Maestro RF, Sibbald WJ (1983) Cerebral and cardiovascular responses to changes in head elevation in patients with intracranial hypertension. J Neurosurg 59:938-944
4. Feldman Z, Kanter MJ, Robertson CS, Contant CF, Hayes C, Sheinberg MA, Villareal CA, Narayan RK, Grossman RG (1992) Effect of head elevation on intracranial pressure, cerebral perfusion pressure, and cerebral blood flow in head injured patients. J Neurosurg 76:207-211
5. Smith DS, Levy W, Maris M, Chance B (1990) Reperfusion hyperoxia in brain after circulatory arrest in humans. Anesthesiology, 73:12-19
6. Carter LP, Weinand ME, Oommen KJ (1993) Cerebral blood flow (CBF) monitoring in intensive care by thermal diffusion. Acta Neurochir (Suppl) 59:43-46

Non-Physiologic Intracranial Hemodynamics in Upright Patients Shunted with Differential Pressure Valve

SOTARO HIGASHI[1], KAZUYA FUTAMI[1], HIROSHI MATSUDA[2], KAZUHIKO TOKUDA[1], SHINYA KIDA[1], and JUNKOH YAMASHITA[1]

Departments of [1] Neurosurgery and [2] Nuclear Medicine, Kanazawa University School of Medicine, 13-1 Takara-machi, Kanazawa, 920 Japan

INTRODUCTION

The introduction of shunt systems with differential-pressure (DP) valves has proven to be a definite advance in the treatment of hydrocephalus. With an ever-increasing population of shunted patients, it is apparent that the major complications of shunting are infection, shunt obstruction, and overdrainage. Continued upgrading of shunt techniques have reduced complications of infection and shunt obstruction. On the other hand, some problems relating to overdrainage still remain unsolved.

Complications due to overdrainage are directly related to significantly negative ventricular fluid pressure (VFP) in the upright position, which is caused by the hydrodynamic characteristics of valves. Many authors have investigated the effects of the head elevation on VFP in shunted patients having a deferential pressure (DP) valve.[1] However, the postural changes of cerebral blood flow (CBF), cerebral perfusion pressure (CPP), and dural sinus pressure (DSP) have been overlooked. In our opinion, there is a clear indication to clarify the effect of low VFP on intracranial hemodynamics and hydrodynamics, for the better understanding of the pathophysiology of overdrainage problems as well as for their management.

MATERIALS AND METHODS

This series included 16 shunted patients with DP valve (DP group), 13 hydrocephalic patients who had not yet received shunts (Hyd group), and 5 subjects without hydrocephalus (control). The type of shunt system used were a medium pressure DP valve (CSF-flow control valve, PS Medical Corp., Goleta, California). All of shunts were judged to be effective by the improvement in both clinical signs and ventricular size on computed tomographic scan, and in some cases by radioisotope shunt flow study.

CBF measurements were performed using technetium-99m hexamethylpropyleneamine oxime (Seletec, Amersham KK, Tokyo, Japan) (^{99m}Tc HM-PAO). Single photon emission computerized tomographic (SPECT) imaging was carried out using a three-head rotating gamma camera system (Toshiba GCA9300A). The SPECT images of the supine and the upright position were obtained using subtraction technique. Three transaxial tomographic images were selected both in the supine and upright images; the level of the basal cistern, the foramen of Monro, and the supraventricular level. For semiquantitative analysis, 10 regions of interest were drawn over the bilateral frontal, temporal, and parietal cortices in each image. Activity counts of ROIs of the upright images were compared with those of the supine images, then percent changes of regional radioactivity of the upright images to that of the supine images ($\%\Delta rCBF_{upr}$) were determined in each ROI as follows:

$$\%\Delta rCBF_{upr} = 100\ (C_{upr} - C_{sup})\ /\ C_{sup},$$

where C_{upr} and C_{sup} are the activity counts of each ROI of the upright and the supine images, respectively. Percent changes of mean CBF in the upright position ($\%\Delta mCBF_{upr}$) were taken as the average value of $\%\Delta rCBF_{upr}$.

VFP was measured from either intraventricular cannulas, chronically implanted telemetric pressure sensor, or shunt reservoir punctured by a sterile needle. Mean arterial blood pressure in the radial artery was measured with the transducer placed at the level of the foramen of Monro, giving an estimate of the mean carotid pressure (MCP). CPP was taken as the difference between MCP and VFP. DSP was measured in the jugular bulb. All pressure values were referenced to the level of the foramen of Monro and expressed as a mean value. All parameters were measured both in the supine and the upright position, and analyzed statistically.

RESULTS

Postural Changes of CBF

$\%\Delta mCBF_{upr}$ were 24.9±4.3% (mean±SE) in DP group (n = 12), 3.5±2.6% in Hyd group (n = 10), and 4.5±2.2% in control (n = 5). Significant augmentation of CBF in the upright position occurred in patients with DP valve ($p<0.01$). In contrast, there was no significant difference of $\%\Delta mCBF_{upr}$ between Hyd group and control. With regard to the difference among $\%\Delta rCBF_{upr}$ (frontal, temporal, and parietal cortices), there was no significant difference for each group (Fig. 1).

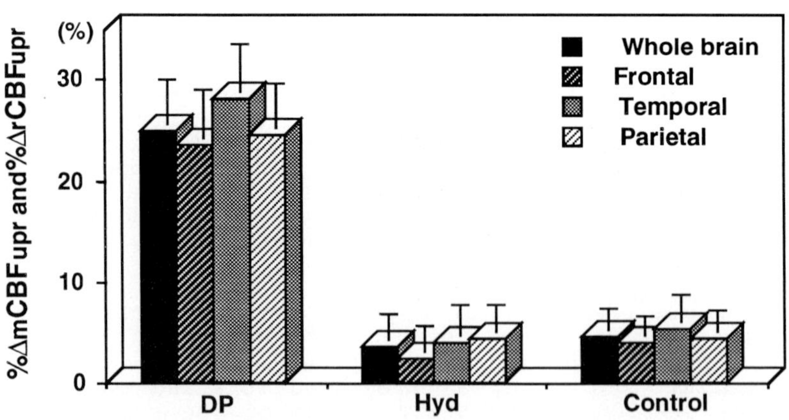

Fig. 1 $\%\Delta mCBF_{upr}$ (whole brain) and $\%\Delta rCBF_{upr}$ (frontal, temporal, and parietal cortices). In DP group, $\%\Delta mCBF_{upr}$ were significantly different from control at $p<0.01$ by unpaired t test. No statistically significant differences were detected among cortices for each group (one-way ANOVA followed by Scheffe's test). DP = differential pressure group; Hyd = hydrocephalus group. Bars and vertical lines represent mean±SE.

Fig. 2 shows the relationship between the %ΔmCBFupr and the VFP in the upright position in 12 patients with both CBF and VFP measurements available. A significant linear correlation ($r = 0.577$, $p < 0.05$) was detected between the two parameters.

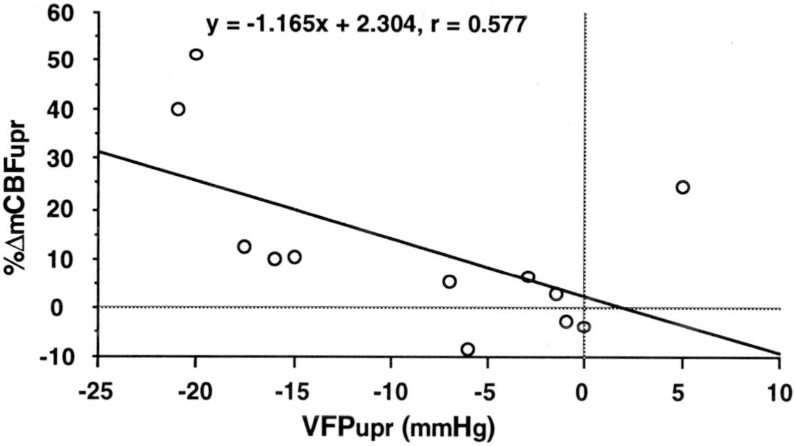

Fig. 2 Scattergram showing the relationship between the %ΔmCBFupr and VFP in the upright position (VFPupr).

Postural Changes of Pressure Parameters

Postural changes of pressure parameters are listed in Table 1. In Hyd group, there was a gradual decrement in MCP from 86.6±5.0 mmHg (supine) to 69.3±4.4 mmHg (upright) ($p<0.05$). The VFP similarly declined from 13.5±2.3 to 7.3±3.7 mmHg for the same head elevation ($p<0.05$). Since MCP declined faster than VFP, there was a net decrement in CPP from 73.1±5.0 (supine) to 62.1±5.6 mmHg (upright) ($p<0.05$). In contrast, patients with DP valves (DP group) developed significantly negative VFP of -16.7±0.8 mmHg in the upright position. This negative VFP resulted in the augmentation of CPP from 87.8±4.1 mmHg (supine) to 94.9±4.9 mmHg (upright) ($p<0.05$) and in the inversion of the pressure gradient between VFP and DSP.

Table 1 Posture-related changes of CPP, MCP, VFP and DSP

		CPP	MCP	VFP	DSP
DP group	supine	87.8±4.1	94.6±2.8	6.8±2.0	6.0
	upright	94.9±4.9	78.2±4.4	-16.8±0.8	-2.0
Hyd group	supine	73.1±5.0	86.6±5.0	13.5±2.3	6.1
	upright	62.1±5.6	69.3±4.4	7.3±3.7	-5.0

DISCUSSION

In the present study, shunted patients with DP valve consistently developed significantly negative VFP when they were upright, which is consistent with previous investigations.[1] This negative VFP is considered to attribute to augmentations of CPP during head elevation. Furthermore, significant augmentation of CBF occurred when they were upright. This CBF augmentation may be related to disturbed autoregulation of CBF to CPP. When CPP elevation occurs under intact autoregulation, vasoconstriction of the arteriole will follow to maintain CBF constant.[2] On the other hand, if autoregulation of the cerebral vessels is impaired, extraordinary increase of CBF, or relative hyperperfusion may occur. Another explanation for this CBF augmentation is overestimation of CBF due to increased cerebral blood volume (CBV). A high proportion of the radioactivity of ^{99m}Tc HM-PAO remaining in the blood is reported to be a result of the entrapment of ^{99m}Tc HM-PAO within red blood cell and plasma protein.[3] Thus, the radioactivity of whole brain may reflect not only CBF but also CBV.

The augmentation of CBF in the upright position is regarded as non-physiologic, because the concomitant negative VFP and augmentation of CPP implies an abnormal intracranial pressure environment compared with that of normal subjects. This non-physiologic intracranial environment may cause the interstitial edema and subependymal gliosis [4] induced by long-standing shunt.

In addition, the pressure gradient between VFP and DSP may not be enough to initiate CSF absorption. CSF absorption depends on the transvillus pressure gradient. [5] The flow is proportional to the pressure gradient between the subarachnoid space and the dural sinuses. The normal pressure gradient is about 3-4 mmHg. The absorption begins at a CSF pressure as low as 5 mmHg. Therefore, our results indicate that patients shunted with DP valve have less possibility of reestablishing shunt independency.

REFERENCES

1. Chapman PH, Cosman ER, Arnold MA (1990) The relationship between ventricular fluid pressure and body position in normal subjects and subjects with shunts: A telemetric study. Neurosurgery 26:181-189
2. Kontos HA, Wei EP, Navari RM, et al (1978) Responses of cerebral arteries and arteriols to acute hypotension and hypertension. Am J Physiol 234:H371-H383
3. Sharp PF, Smith FW, Gemmell HG, et al. (1986) Technetium-99m HMPAO stereoisomers as potential agents for imaging regional cerebral blood flow. J Nucl Med 27:171-177
4. Oi S, Matsumoto S (1986) Morphological findings of postshunt slit-ventricle in experimental canine hydrocephalus. Child's Nerv Syst 2:179-184
5. Gjerris F, Børgesen SE, Schmidt J, Sørensen PS (1989) Resistance to cerebrospinal fluid outflow in patients with normal pressure hydrocephalus. In: Gjerris F, Børgesen SE, Sørensen PS (eds) Outflow of cerebrospinal fluid. Munksgaad, Copenhagen, pp 329-338

Session V: Causes of Increased or Decreased ICP (2)

Chairmen: J. Ekstedt and S. Matsumoto

Dutch Normal Pressure Hydrocephalus Study
Part II. Comparison of Low and Medium Pressure Shunts

A.J.W. Boon[1], J. Th. J. Tans[1], J.A.L. Wurzer[1], D.C.J. Poortvliet[1], E.J. Delwel[2], C.J.J. Avezaat[2], D.A. de Jong[2], S.M. Egeler-Peerdeman[3], P.W. Hanlo[4], R.H.J.M. Gooskens[4], R.R.F. Kuiters[5], and J. Hermans[6]

[1] Westeinde Hospital, Postbus 432, 2501 CK The Hague, The Netherlands
University Hospitals of [2] Rotterdam, [3] Amsterdam, [4] Utrecht and [6] Leiden; [5] Leyenburg Hospital, The Hague, The Netherlands

INTRODUCTION

The selection of the shunt opening pressure for the treatment of patients with normal pressure hydrocephalus (NPH) is a matter of continuing controversy. In a retrospective study of McQuarrie better results were obtained with low than medium pressure shunts[1]. On the other hand, the patients of Larsson, who had a programmable shunt, improved at a high opening pressure without further improvement at medium and low pressures[2]. When it is thought that unfolding of the brain will only take place in the presence of a pressure gradient between brain tissue and ventricles a low pressure system is the logical choice. But when reduction of outflow resistance and brain elasticity are considered more important a medium pressure shunt might be preferred[3]. These differences of opinion call for a randomised study comparing the results of low and medium pressure shunts.

The Dutch Normal Pressure Hydrocephalus Study (DNPHS) is a multicentre trial designed to determine the positive and negative predictive value of CSF outflow resistance (Rout) regarding the results of shunting in patients with NPH. A second objective is to examine whether low or medium pressure shunts are more effective in reversing the signs and symptoms of NPH. Here we report the preliminary results of the second part of this ongoing study.

PATIENTS AND METHODS

In establishing the diagnosis of NPH all diagnostic procedures were permitted, except continuous recording of ICP and measurement of Rout. Gait disturbance was quantified by a scale consisting of 10 qualitative items of walking like the presence of wide base, small steps and shuffling as well as the number of steps and seconds required for a 10 meter walk. The range of this scale was 2 to 40. A short battery of 4 neuropsychological tests, delayed recall of 10 words after 5 minutes, digit span forwards and reverse, trail making and finger tapping, was used for evaluation of dementia, range 4 to 40. Addition of the gait and dementia scale yielded the NPH scale, range 6 to 80. Activities of daily life were classified by a modified Rankin scale, range 0 to 6.

Entry criteria for the DNPHS were: 1) A firm diagnosis of NPH made by the referring neurologist, confirmed by a trial neurologist or neurosurgeon. 2) Gait scale > 12, dementia scale > 12 and Rankin scale > 2. 3) A symmetrical communicating hydrocephalus, Evans Index > 0.30, without parenchymal lesions and without marked cortical atrophy on CT. 4) No acute or subacute symptomatic hydrocephalus or signs of raised ICP.

After entry lumbar constant flow infusion was performed and all patients received a ventriculoperitoneal Medos Hakim shunt irrespective of the value of Rout. Of the 72 evaluable patients at this interim analysis 31 were randomised to a low (opening pressure 4 cm H_2O) and 41 to a medium high pressure (opening pressure 10 cm H_2O) shunt. The unequal distribution of patients amoung the low and medium high pressure group is explained by stratification of the randomisation over the 5 participating centres. NPH and Rankin scale were determined before and 1, 3, 6, 9 and 12 months after surgery. CT scans were obtained at 0, 1, 6 and 12 months.

RESULTS

According to table 1 the randomisation process proceeded adequately. Patient characteristics that could affect the result of shunting were equally distributed amoung the low and medium high pressure group with the exception of the higher percentage of patients with idiopathic NPH in the medium high pressure group. The mean initial NPH scale was 50 $\pm$ 16.8 indicating that the average patient exhibited a substantial gait disturbance and dementia. The mean preoperative Rankin scale was 3.8 $\pm$ 1.4 designating a moderately disabled patient dependent for less then 50% of the day.

Table 1. Patients characteristics according to treatment group

	low pressure n = 31	medium high n=41
idiopathic NPH	24 (77%)	37 (90%)
symptomatic NPH	7 (23%)	4 (10%)
duration of history (years)	2.2 $\pm$ 2.7	2.3 $\pm$ 2.3
age	73.1 $\pm$ 6.4	73.1 $\pm$ 7.8
ventricular index on CT	1.18 $\pm$ 0.14	1.18 $\pm$ 0.15
baseline pressure CSF	11.2 $\pm$ 6.2	12.0 $\pm$ 4.2
follow up time (month)	9.6 $\pm$ 4.0	7.4 $\pm$ 4.4

The results of our study are summarised in table 2. Clinical improvement is expressed as the difference between the presurgery and the last postsurgery NPH and Rankin scale values. It is evident, that improvement was significantly greater in the low pressure group with a mean reduction of the NPH scale of 16.7 $\pm$ 12.7 compared to 7.5 $\pm$ 16.1 for the medium high pressure group ($p=0.01$). The Rankin scale showed the same trend with a mean difference of 1.29 for the low versus 0.68 for the medium high pressure group.

Subdural effusions were the most frequent complication occurring in no less than 44% of all patients, in 61% of the low pressure and in 32 % of the medium high pressure group. This difference was significant with a p-value of 0.02. Most effusions seemed asymptomatic or disappeared spontaneously and only 4 patients in both groups needed surgery. Looking at the influence of subdural effusions on outcome, patients within the low pressure group did better without than with effusions but the differences for the NPH as well as the Rankin scale were not significant (table 2). For the medium high pressure group the effect of subdural effusions on improvement was limited.

Table 2. Comparison of results of low and medium high pressure shunts. NPH and RANKIN scale values before and after surgery.

	HPH scale		
Shunttype	Before	After	Difference
Low	48.7 ± 18.3	31.9 ± 15.7	16.7 ± 12.7
Medium high	50.4 ± 14.8	42.9 ± 19.9	7.5 ± 16.1
p-value	0.66	0.01	0.01
Low			
no effusions	50.7 ± 16.6	31.5 ± 13.0	19.3 ± 10.8
effusions	46.7 ± 19.6	31.8 ± 17.7	14.9 ± 14.0
p-value	0.58	0.96	0.33
Medium high			
no effusions	53.4 ± 14.6	46.0 ± 18.4	7.4 ± 15.9
effusions	43.9 ± 13.7	36.1 ± 22.1	7.8 ± 17.3
p-value	0.06	0.14	0.93
		Rankin scale	
Low	3.7 ± 1.5	2.4 ± 1.5	1.3 ± 1.3
Medium high	3.9 ± 1.3	3.2 ± 1.8	0.7 ± 1.6
p-value	0.54	0.43	0.09
Low			
no effusions	3.9 ± 1.3	2.5 ± 1.4	1.4 ± 0.9
effusions	3.5 ± 1.6	2.3 ± 1.6	1.2 ± 1.4
p-value	0.45	0.69	0.67
Medium high			
no effusions	4.2 ± 1.3	3.5 ± 1.8	0.8 ± 1.6
effusions	3.2 ± 1.0	2.6 ± 1.6	0.5 ± 1.7
p-value	0.01	0.16	0.70

DISCUSSION

We chose the nonprogrammable Medos Hakim valve system for this trial, because its pressure/flow characteristics agree best with the specifications of the manufacturer and because of its long term stability and reliability[4]. In order to better assess the differences in overdrainage problems between low and medium pressure shunts we refrained from systems like PS Medical or antisiphon devices.

The very high incidence of subdural effusions can be attributed to the routine CT scan at 1 month and the strict CT criteria. Not taking into account the transient cases, our percentage of subdural effusions of 28 was comparable to the highest one reported in the literature[5].

Although our study is not yet finished convincing evidence is produced that patients with NPH do much better on a low than a medium pressure shunt. This finding is even more remarkable in view of of the significantly higher incidence of subdural effusions in the low pressure group. The results of surgery may further improve with the use of antisiphon devices or the PS Medical valve that reduce the occurence of subdural effusions. The programmable Medos Hakim shunt has the advantage that effusions can be treated by increasing the opening pressure.

REFERENCES

1. McQuarrie IG, Saint-Louis L, Scherer PB (1984) Treatment of normal pressure hydrocephalus with low versus medium pressure cerebrospinal fluid shunts. Neurosurgery 15:484-487

2. Larsson A, Jensen Ch, Bilting M, Ekholm S, Stephensen H, Wikkelso C (1992) Does the shunt opening pressure influence the effect of shunt surgery in normal pressure hydrocephalus? Acta Neurochir 117:15-22

3. Tans JThJ, Poortvliet DCJ (1988) Reduction of ventricular size after shunting for normal pressure hydrocephalus related to CSF dynamics before shunting. J Neurol Neurosurg Psychiatry 51:521-525

4. Trost HA, Heissler HE, Clausen G, Gaab MR (1991) Testing the hydrocephalus shunt valve: long term test results of various new and explanted valves. The need for a model for testing valves under physiological conditions. Eur J Pediatr Surg 1, suppl 1:38-40

5. Black PM, Ojemann RG, Tzouras A (1985) CSF shunts for dementia, incontinence and gait disturbance. Clin Neurosurg 32:632-651

Depressed Cortical Oxidative Metabolism in Chronic Hydrocephalus as Demonstrated by Cytochrome Oxidase Histochemistry

N. Tsuji[1], Y. Katayama[1], M. Fujii[1], T. Kawamata[1], T. Tsubokawa[1], and H. Nishimoto[2]

[1] Department of Neurological Surgery, Nihon University School of Medicine, Itabahi-ku, Tokyo, 173 Japan
[2] Department of Neurological Surgery, Saitama Children's Medical Center, Hasuda-shi, Saitama, 349-01 Japan

SUMMARY

In order to examine the effects of hydrocephalus on the oxidative metabolism, we evaluated changes in cytochrome oxidase (CYO) activity, a marker of mitochondrial respiration, in rats with experimental hydrocephalus. The animals were sacrificed at 4 weeks after induction of kaolin-induced hydrocephalus, and the CYO activity was determined by photometric semiquantitation using histochemical preparations. The hydrocephalus was graded into three groups by measuring the area of the coronal plane of the lateral ventricle at the level of the septal nucleus. A significant decrease in CYO activity was observed in layers II-III, IV and V in association with hydrocephalus. The decrease in CYO activity was more pronounced in animals with severer hydrocephalus. Combining these findings with the results of previous studies, it appears that the changes in cerebral metabolism occurring in chronic hydrocephalus may be characterized by a depression of oxidative metabolism and an increase in anaerobic metabolism with a maintained cerebral circulation. Such changes can be accounted for by postulating a decreased oxygen delivery due to inefficient diffusion within the brain tissue associated with hydrocephalic interstitial edema.

INTRODUCTION

Despite numerous studies, the changes in cerebral metabolism associated with neurological deficits [9] in chronic hydrocephalus remain unclear. While the cerebral blood flow (CBF) has been reported to be depressed [1,2], the observed changes are not sufficiently large to produce neuronal dysfunction or ischemic brain damage primarily. The cerebral metabolic rate of glucose (CMRglu) has been reported to be either decreased, unchanged or increased [2,3,4,5,6]. Satoh et al [2] recently measured CBF and CMRglu in the same animals, and reported that, while CBF tended to decrease, CMRglu was unchanged or even increased. The mechanism underlying such an uncoupling between flow and metabolism remains to be determined.

Little is currently known regarding the changes in oxidative metabolism. In the present study, in order to examine the effects of hydrocephalus on the oxidative metabolism, we evaluated the changes in cytochrome oxidase (CYO) activity, a marker of mitochondrial respiration, in rats with chronic hydrocephalus [7]. The biochemically determined CYO activity correlates directly with the density of histochemical staining for this enzyme. Since topographic characterization of biochemical changes was necessary, we chose to employ a histochemical technique to determine the CYO activity.

MATERIALS AND METHODS

Preparation of animals

Male Wistar rats aged 2-3 weeks (250-300 g, n=46) were used for the experiments. In one group of animals (group I, n=25), 0.1 ml of kaolin solution (200 mg/ml saline) was injected into the cisterna magna. Animals demonstrating severe weight loss or infection were excluded from the study, so that, together with rats which had died before commencing the experiments, 9 rats were excluded from the study. In an other group of animals (Group II, n=12), 0.1 ml of saline vehicle was injected into the cisterna magna. Nine other rats without any pretreatment were employed as normal controls. The animals were then placed in cages and allowed free access to water and food.

Cytochrome oxidase histochemistry

The rats were sacrificed at 4 weeks after kaolin injection. The animals were anesthetized with an overdose of pentobarbital sodium and perfused transcardially first with heparinized saline and then with 4% paraformaldehyde in phosphate buffer (0.1 M, pH 7.4). The brains were removed, postfixed in the same fixative overnight and cryoprotected with 20% sucrose in phosphate buffer. Frozen section at a thickness of 100 μm were obtained, collected in phosphate buffer and reacted for CYO.

The area of the lateral ventricle was measured planimetrically using coronal sections at the level of the septal nucleus. The hydrocephalus was graded into three groups: an increase in the measured area of <300% (grade 1), an increase in the area to 300-1000% (grade 2) and an increase in the area of >1000% (grade 3). A pair of group I and group II animals were sacrified at the same time, their brains were processed simultaneously in the same fixative and sections of the same areas obtained from the pair were reacted for CYO in the same solution.

The CYO activity in various areas was analyzed by photometric semiquantitation. The data presented here were those obtained from the somatosensory cortex. Values were obtained from 5 adjacent regions (0.3 x 0.3 mm), parallel to the cortical layers (1.5 mm in total length), at the center of each layer. The values for the group I animals were expressed as a percentage of the values obtained from the same structure of the companion sections in the group II animals.

RESULTS

A pattern of CYO activity consistent with that reported previously was noted in the group II animals (Fig. 1). Thus, higher CYO activites were seen in layers IV and VI, demonstrating a bilayer pattern. In layer IV, segmentation corresponding to a barrel-like structure was observed in the somatosensory cortex. In the animals with hydrocephalus, a discernible decrease in CYO activity was evident in the cortex (Fig. 1). A more marked decrease in CYO activity was demonstrated in the animals with hydrocephalus of higher grades. Photometric semiquantitation confirmed that these changes observed in association with hydrocephalus were statistically significant in layers II-III, IV and VI (Fig. 2).

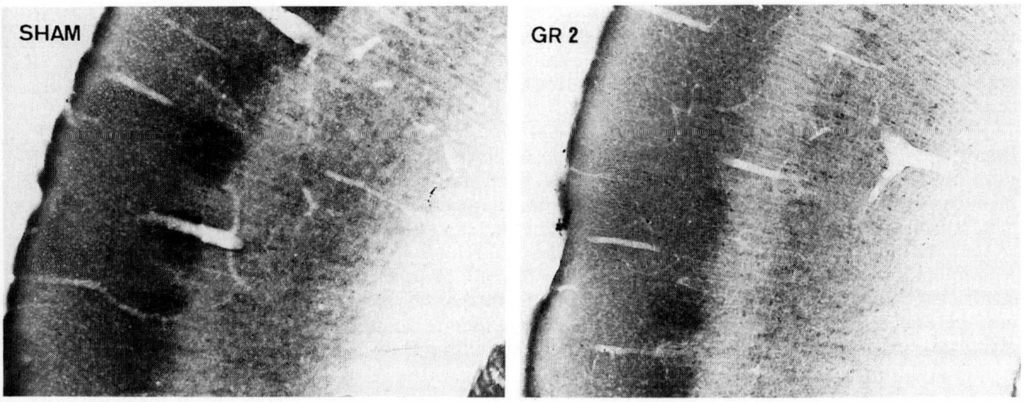

Fig. 1 Cytochrome oxidase histochemistry of the somatosensory cortex of the sham-operated rat (SHAM) and a rat with hydrocepahlus of grade 2 (GR 2). Note the decrease in CYO activity in layers II-III, IV and VI of the hydrocephalic rat.

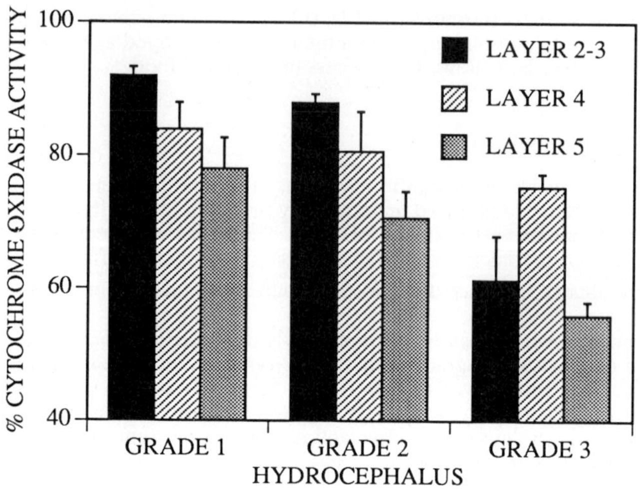

Fig. 2 Percent changes in cytochrome oxidase activity in the somatosensory cortex using photometric semiquantitation. The cytochrome oxidase activity is expressed as a percentage of the value obtained from the sham-operated animal reacted simultaneously for cytochrome oxidase. Error bars, standard deviation. n=5. P<0.05 for all columns as compared to sham-operated animals (paired t test).

DISCUSSION

Previous studies have suggested that, while CBF generally tends to decrease in chronic hydrocephalus [1,2], CMRglu does not necessarily show a concomitant decrease, and even increases in some instances [2,4]. The present data indicate that chronic hydrocephalus causes a decreased mitochondrial respiratory function in the cerebral cortex. Taking these findings together, chronic hydrocephalus appears to be associated with a depression of the oxidative metabolism and an increase in the anaerobic metabolism in the cerebral cortex.

Global impariment of the cerebral circulation due to an elevated intracranial pressure and/or mechanical distention of the brain tissue may not be the cause of such changes, since CBF is maintained far above the level that produces ischemic brain damage. Sutton et al [8] recently demonstrated that CBF is unchanged in the brain tissue associated with infusion-induced interstitial edema, if the blood flow values are corrected for dilution. We have obtained a similar results (unpublished observations). It appears unlikely, therefore, that hydrocephalic interstitial edema causes severe impairment of the cerebral circulation by itself.

Importantly, however, CMRglu has been found to be increased in the brain tissue associated with infusion-induced interstitial edema [8]. It has also been shown that lactate increases without a decrease in phosphocreatine [8]. Thus, interstitial edema appears to cause an increase in the anaerobic metabolism leaving the cerebral circulation intact. Such an event has been suggested to be induced by an inefficient diffusion of oxygen due to dilated extracellular space within the brain tissue associated with interstitial edema [8]. We have recently found that infusion-induced interstitial edema produces a significant decrease in cortical CYO activity (unpublished observations). The decrease in CYO activity may be explained by a decreased oxygen delivery, lactate accumulation arising from accelerated glycolysis or both, which have been shown to interfere with mitochondrial respiratory function [7,9].

We suggest that the metabolic changes observed in chronic hydrocephalus are at least partially attributable to a similar mechanism. Hydrocephalic interstitial edema may reduce the oxygen delivery without impairing the circulation and, thereby, enhance the CMRglu for anaerobic glycolysis and lower the CYO activity. In summary, the changes in cerebral metabolism observed in chronic hydrocephalus appear to be characterized by an increase in anaerobic metabolism without impairment of the cerebral circulation.

REFERENCES

1. Higashi K, Asahisa H, Ueda N, Kobayashi K, Hara K, Noda Y (1986) Cerebral blood flow and metabolism in experimental hydrocephalus. *Neurol Res* 8: 169-176
2. Satoh S, Shirane R, Yoshimoto T (1992) Regional CBF and regional cerebral metabolic rate of glucose in experimental hydrocephalus measured by double tracer methods of autoradiography. *Current Tr Hyd* (Tokyo) 2: 1-4
3. Miyaoka M, Ito M, Wada M, Sato K, Negishi I, Ishii S (1988) The effect of V-P shunt on local cerebral glucose utilization in HTX congenital hydrocephalic rats. *Nervous System in Children* (Tokyo) 13: 389-393 (in Japanese)
4. Richards HK, Pickard JD, Punt J (1985) Local cerebral glucose utilization in experimental chronic hydrocephalus in the rat. *Z Kinderchir* 40 (suppl) 1: 9
5. Richards HK, Bucknall RM, Jones HC, Pickard JD (1989) The uptake of [^{14}C] deoxyglucose into brain of young rats with inherited hydrocepahlus. *Exp Neurol* 103: 194-198, 1989
7. Dimlich RVW, Showers MJ, Shipley MT (1990) Densitometric analysis of cytochrome oxidase in ischemic rat brain. *Brain Res* 516: 181-191
6. Wako N (1983) Local cerebral glucose utilization on kaolin induced hydrocephalus of rats by [^{14}C] deoxyglucose method. *Brain Nerve* (Tokyo) 35: 693-701 (in Japanese)
8. Sutton LN, Greenberg J, Welsh F (1990) Blood flow and metabolism in vasogenic oedema. *Acta Neurochir* suppl 51: 397-400
9. Hillered L, Ernster L, Siesjo BK (1984) Influence of in vitro lactic acidosis and hypercapnia on respiratory activity of isolated rat brain mitochondria. *J Cereb Blood Flow Metabol* 4: 430-437
10. Tsubokawa T, Katayama Y, Kawamata T, Miyazaki S (1991) Difference in temporal patterns of impairment of hippocampal plasticity and elevation of intraventricular presure in experimental hydrocephalus. *Current Tr Hyd* (Tokyo) 1: 1-5

Ventriculostomy Infections: The MCV Experience 10 Years Late

KATHRYN L. HOLLOWAY, MARGIE RIGSBEE, and JOHN D. WARD

Division of Neurological Surgery, Medical College of Virginia, VA, USA

INTRODUCTION

In 1984 this institution published the results of a prospective epidemiologic study of ventriculostomy related infections [3]. One of the conclusions of the paper was that the incidence of ventriculostomy related infections rose after 5 days of monitoring. This led to the recommendation that catheters be prophylactically changed at 5 day intervals if prolonged monitoring was required. The literature has both supported and refuted these conclusions [1,4]. Recent studies conducted in a randomized prospective fashion on central venous catheter changes have indicated that prophylactic changes do not prevent infections and expose the patient to increased risk of complications from repeated insertion [2]. This has led us to re-examine our experience with ventriculostomy infections.

METHODS

Data on severely head injured patients with ventriculostomies were prospectively collected in two Data Banks, the Traumatic Coma Data Bank (1984-1987) and the Medical College of Virginia Neurocore Data Bank (1987-1993) and was retrospectively analyzed. Patients who had meningitis diagnosed on the day of insertion of the first ventriculostomy catheter or greater than 1 week after the removal of the final ventriculostomy catheter were excluded from analysis. Infection was defined as a positive cerebrospinal fluid (CSF) culture or white blood cells greater than 50 per cubic millimeter with greater than 50% neutrophils or a CSF glucose less than 15. For the purpose of analysis of the effect of duration on ventriculostomy infection, patients whose diagnosis of ventriculitis was made during the week after removal were considered to have become infected on the last day of monitoring.

RESULTS

There were 584 patients with 712 ventriculostomy catheters suitable for analysis. The duration of Intracranial Pressure Monitoring (ICP) monitoring via ventriculostomy ranged from less than a day to 35.8 days. The duration of an individual catheter ranged from less than a day to a maximum of 34.3 days. Sixty one patients developed ventriculitis during or immediately after the period of

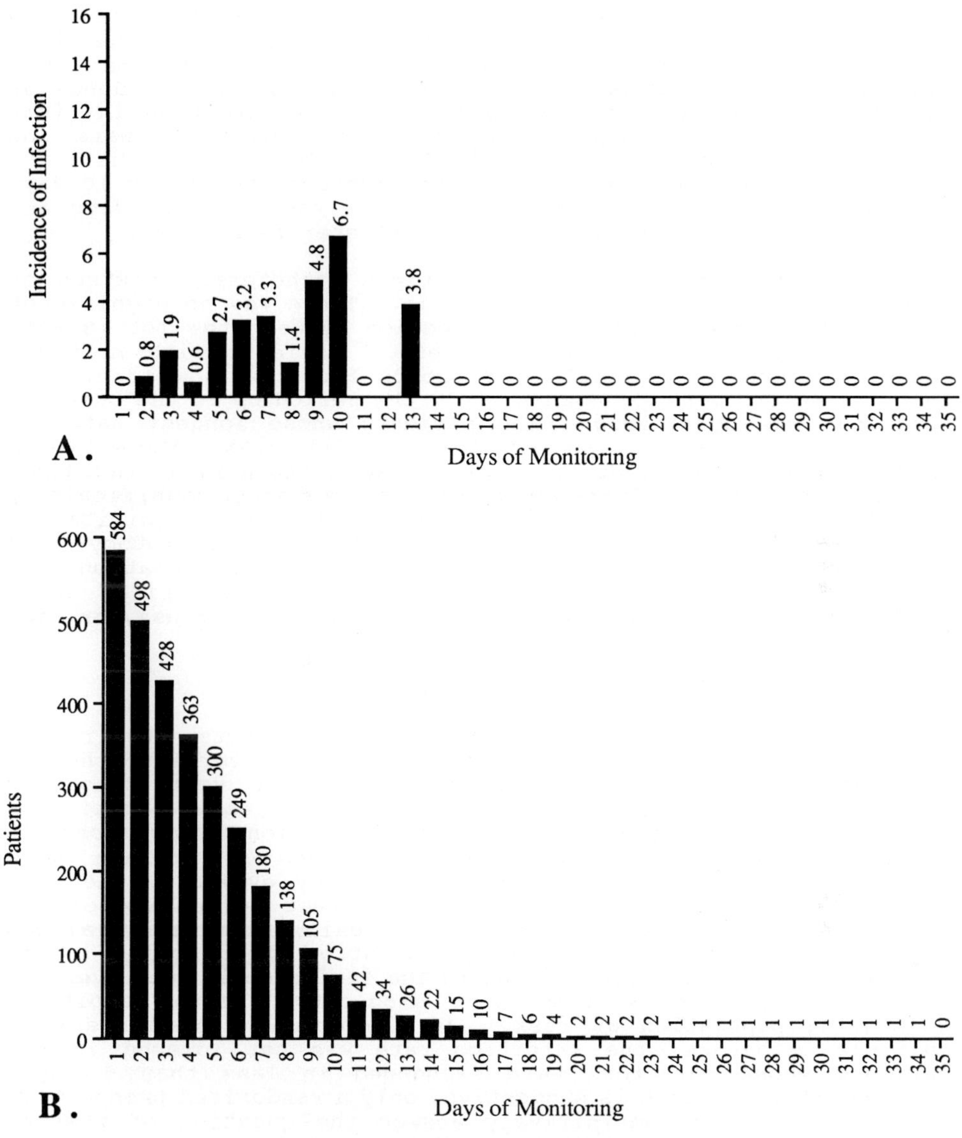

Fig. 1. Analysis of Onset of Infection in First Catheters.

A) Daily incidence of infection.

B) Daily number of patients at risk for developing infection. (# of clean first catheters) monitoring for an incidence of ventriculitis of 10.4%. The onset of infection ranged from 2-23 days after the insertion of the first ventriculostomy. Because prophylactic catheter exchanges could obscure the effect of duration of monitoring on the incidence of infection, we analyzed the daily incidence of infection in first catheters only. Subsequent catheters and infections were not included. The results are shown in Fig 1. There is a significant rise (p=.01) in the incidence of infection over the first 10 days but then the incidence falls to zero over the next few days and remains there until the last "first" catheter is removed.

There were 97 patients who had multiple catheters. Sixteen of these patients developed ventriculitis. There was no significant difference in the incidence of infection between the 1st (8.6%), 2nd (10.9%), or 3rd (5.3%) catheters. Patients with multiple catheters were divided into two groups based on how frequently their catheters were exchanged. Only the period up to the onset of infection was considered. The patients whose longest catheter duration was <5 days had an infection rate of 20.6%. The patients whose longest catheter duration was $\geq$ 5 days had a 14.3% incidence of infection. This difference was not statistically significant by a Fishers Exact Test (p=.30). Ventriculitis was significantly associated with septicemia, pneumonia and craniotomy and intraventricular blood. There was no significant association with gender, the presence of intracranial air on computerized axial tomography (CT Scan), use of steroids, Camino monitor use, or age.

DISCUSSION

Although there are some important differences between this review and our 1984 study, we believe that there are several worthwhile observations that warrant a re-examination of ventriculostomy policy. The previous study compared the average total duration of monitoring, including the time after the infection had occurred, in the infected and uninfected groups. This does not separate cause from effect. In contrast, the current study evaluates when the ventriculostomy infections developed and what percentage of the population at risk they composed. The daily examination allows greater resolution of the effect of duration on infection. With this analysis, a significant rise in the incidence is seen over the first 10 days with a subsequent drop-off to zero despite a continuing population at risk. In the group of patients with multiple catheters, the infection rate was not lowered in the patients whose catheters were exchanged in less than 5 days. Although this evidence is suggestive, only a randomized prospective clinical trial can definitively answer the question of whether prophylactic exchanging of ventriculostomy catheters is necessary or effective.

REFERENCES

1. Aucoin PJ, Kotilainen HR, Gantz, NM, Davidson R, Kellogg P, Stone B. (1986) Intracranial Pressure Monitors. Epidemiologic study of risk factors and infections. American Journal of Medicine 80:369-376.

2. Cobb DK, High KP, Sawyer RG, Sable CA, Adams RB, Lindley DA, Pruett TL, Schwenzer KJ, Farr BM. (1992) A Controlled Trial of Scheduled Replacement of Central Venous and Pulmonary Artery Catheters. New England Journal of Medicine 327:1062-1068.

3. Mayhall CG, Archer NH, Lamb VA, Spadora AC, Baggett JW, Ward JD, Narayan RK. (1984) Ventriculostomy - Related Infections. A prospective epidemiologic study. New England Journal of Medicine 310:553-559.

4. Winfield JA, Rosenthal P, Kanter RK, Casella G. (1993) Duration of Intracranial Pressure Monitoring Does Not Predict Daily Risk of Infectious Complications. Neurosurgery 33(3):424-431, 1993.

Session VI: Causes of Increased or Decreased ICP (3)

Chairmen: D.A. Hovda and T. Ohta

Development of Traumatic Brain Edema in Aged Rats

A. Unterberg, G.H. Schneider, and W.R. Lanksch

Department of Neurosurgery, Rudolf Virchow Medical Center, Free University of Berlin, 13353 Berlin, Germany

SUMMARY

Age is an important factor of mortality and morbidity following traumatic brain injury. Yet, the causes for the adverse effects of old age are still poorly understood. The aim of this study was to investigate whether old age affects posttraumatic brain edema and ICP.

In anestethized Wistar rats, a cortical freezing lesion was applied to the parietal region. 24 adult rats (4-6 months) were compared with 21 aged animals (30-40 months). 24 hours after trauma, the animals were sacrificed and hemispheric swelling, water- and electrolyte contents were determined. In subgroups, blood pressure and intracranial pressure were monitored. Moreover, the uptake of i.v. administered Evans blue as a marker of the cerebrovascular permeability was determined in the traumatized and contralateral hemisphere.

In the group of aged animals, mortality was significantly increased. Hemispheric swelling due to the cortical freezing lesion was markedly elevated. Accordingly, the increase of cerebral water content due to the lesion was more pronounced in aged rats. Intracranial pressure reached a higher level in the old age group. Moreover, there was more uptake of Evans blue in old animals. Since blood pressure was significantly decreased in the aged group, an increased vascular permeability appears to be the underlying mechanism for increased edema generation.

In conclusion, an enhanced edema formation of vasogenic origin in advanced age may be one factor of higher mortality and morbidity following brain trauma in old versus young individuals.

INTRODUCTION

Age is an important factor of morbidity and mortality as well as outcome following a traumatic brain injury, as has been shown in many experimental and clinical studies (1, 2, 4, 5, 8, 9). Yet, the causes for the adverse effects of old age are still poorly understood. Although an increased incidence age-related non-neurological complications may be one factor, the aging central nervous system appears to have an altered pathophysiological response to trauma (8). Thus it is worthwhile to study the effects of age on the generation of cerebral edema, intracranial pressure, and the response of the aging brain to mechanical stress (8). Aim of the present study was to investigate whether old age affects the development of vasogenic brain edema following a standardized cryogenic cortical lesion.

MATERIALS AND METHODS

Wistar rats with a b.w. of 420 +/- 10 g were anestetized with ketamine and xylazine. A circular craniectomy was performed over the right parietal region and a cortical freezing lesion was applied by means of a copper cylinder (diameter 5 mm), cooled with dry-ice-acetone mixture (3). The cylinder was stereotactically attached onto the intact dura for 30 seconds. Blood pressure was monitored via cannulas in the femoral or tail artery in the early peritraumatic and the late posttraumatic period. The elderly group consisted of 24 animals aged 30-40 months. This group was compared to 27 young adult rats at an age of 4-6 months. 24 hours after trauma, the animals were sacrificed and the brains were taken.

In a first series (A) the cerebral hemispheres were separated, weighed for determination of hemispheric swelling, dried and weighed again. Hemispheric swelling was determined as the difference of weight of the traumatized and contralateral hemisphere (7). Cerebral water content of

both hemispheres was obtained by dry-wet weight measurement. Sodium and potassium content were thereafter determined in dessicated brain specimen.
In a second series (B), the animals received Evans blue i.v. (2 ml/kg b.w.) and intracranial pressure (ICP) was monitored before sacrifice by ventricular puncture. The uptake of Evans blue into cerebral tissue was determined spectrophotometrically after extraction as a marker for cerebrovascular permeability (6). Finally, hemispheric swelling and cerebral water content were determined as described.

RESULTS AND DISCUSSION

All young adult rats survived the 24 hours observation period following the cortical freezing lesion, whereas 4 animals of the old age group died which corresponds to a mortality of 17% in the aged group. This difference in mortality is statistically highly significant ($p < 0.01$). Obvious reasons for the observed mortality could not be identified, in particular intracerebral hemorrhage was not found in the old rats that died.
Hemispheric swelling due to the cortical freezing lesion amounted to 10.4 +/- 0.8% in aged animals, whereas young adult animals had a swelling of 6.9 +/- 0.5% in series A ($p < 0.01$). In the second series (n = 8 each) hemipheric swelling was 8.5 +/- 0.9% young and 11.1 +/- 0,6% in old animals ($p < 0.05$; see figure 1).

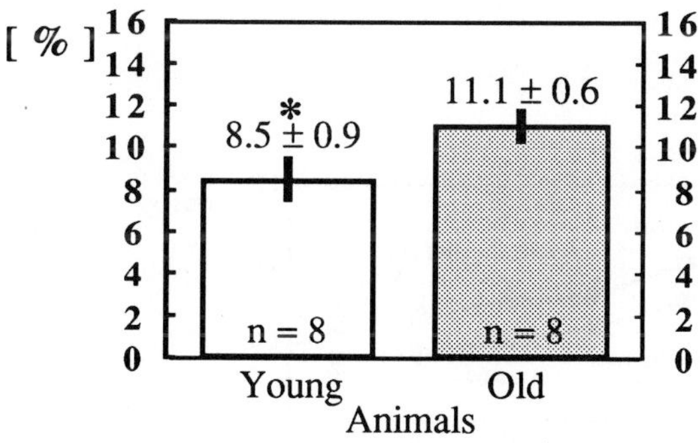

Fig. 1. Hemispheric swelling following a cryogenic lesion in young adult and aged rats. Swelling is markedly increased in the aged animals.

According to the increase in hemispheric swelling, cerebral water content was significantly more elevated following trauma in the aged group of animals. In series A the water content of the non-traumatized hemispheres was 78% and increased by 1.5% 24 hours following trauma. In old animals, the water content of the non-lesioned left hemisphere was significantly lower compared to the young group. It amounted to 76%. Following trauma, it was increased by 2% to 78%.
Following cold injury, hemispheric sodium content increased in both groups, and the potassium content declined. According to a lower water content in old animals, sodium and potassium content were also lower in the old age group.
Monitoring of mean arterial blood pressure in both groups clearly demonstrated that aged animals had a significantly decreased blood pressure compared to young animals. Thus, an increased driving force can be ruled out as the underlying mechanism for the observed increased edema formation. Based on the finding that aged animals are hypotensive, one might even argue that hypotension in old animals causes relative ischemia and the increased swelling is due to an ischemic component (1). On the other hand, it is more likely that the increased edema generation is due to an increased cerebrovascular permeability in old animals, since the Evans blue content of the traumatized hemisphere was markedly elevated in the aged group. Evans blue binds to plasmaproteins and its amount of extravasation and uptake into the tissue indicates the degree of cerebrovascular leakiness (see figure 2).

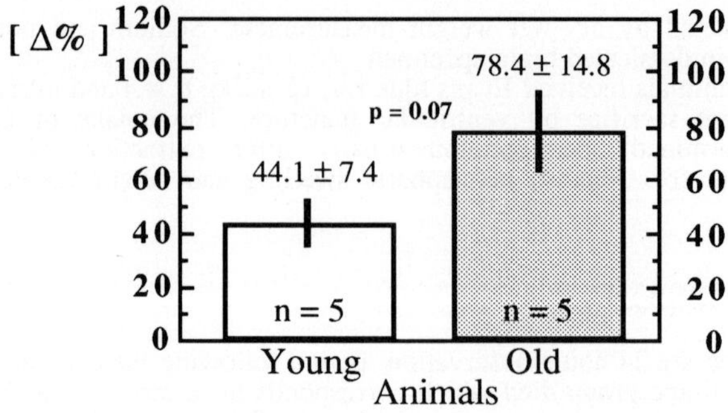

Fig. 2: Evans blue content of the traumatized hemispheres in young adult and aged animals (in percent of the non-traumatized contralateral hemispheres).

Increased edema generation in old age in associated with an increased ICP in this group as demonstrated in figure 3.
These ICP data demonstrate that the observed hemispheric swelling (of 6-12%) marginally increases intracranial pressure.

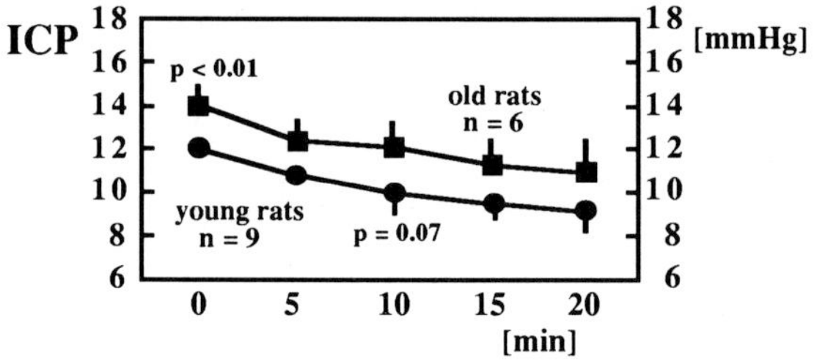

Fig. 3: Intracranial pressure shortly before sacrifice in series B. Due to the method of monitoring, i.e. ventricular puncture, ICP slowly declines to its actual value after insertion of the catheter. Obviously, ICP is marginally higher in the old aged group compared to the younger animals. ICP in non-traumatized animals is 5 +/- 1 mmHg.

In conclusion, an enhanced edema formation of vasogenic origin in advanced age might be one factor of higher mortality and morbidity following traumatic brain injury in aged individuals.

REFERENCES

1. Davis M, Mendelow AD, Perry RH, Chambers JR, James OFW (1994)
The effect of age on cerebral edema, cerebral infarction and neuroprotective potential in experimental occlusive stroke.
Acta Neurochirurgica Suppl 60: 282-284

2. Jamjom A, Nelson R. Stranjalis S, Chissel H, Kane N, Cummins B (1992)
Outcome following surgical evacuation of traumatic intracranial haematomas in the elderly.
Brit J Neurosurg 6: 37-32

3. Klatzo I, Piraux A. Laskowski EJ (1958)
The relationsship between edema, blood-brain barrier and tissue elements in local brain injury.
J Neuropath Exp Neurol 17: 548-564

4. Hamm RJ, Jenkins LW, Lyeth BG, White-Gbadebo DM, Hayes RL (1991)
The effect of age on outcome following traumatic brain injury in rats.
J Neurosurg 75: 916-921

5. Hamm RJ, White Gbadebo DM, Jenkins LW, Hayes RL (1992)
The effect of age on motor and cognitive deficits after traumatic brain injury in rats.
Neurosurgery 31: 1072-1978

6. Smith SLS, Hall ED (in preparation):
U-74006 F protects the blood-brain-barrier following head injury in the rat.

7. Unterberg A, Schmidt W, Dautermann C. Baethmann A. (1990)
The effect of various steroid treatment regimens of cold-induced brain swelling.
Acta Neurochirurgica Suppl. 51: 104-106

8 Vollmer DG, Torner JT, Eisenberg HM, Foulkes MA, Marmarou A, Marshall LF (1991)
Age and outcome following traumatic coma: why do older patients fare worse?
J Neurosurg 75: S37-S49

9. Yao H, Sadomisha S, Ooboshi H, Sato Y, Uchimara H, Fujishima M (1991)
Age-related vulnerability to cerebral ischemia in spontaneously hypertensive rats.
Stroke 22: 1414-1418

ACKNOWLEDGEMENT

The excellent technical and secretarial assistance of Ms. C. Dürre und Ms. A. Riede is highly appreciated.

Direct Intracerebral Cytokine Gene Transfer Induces Vasogenic Brain Edema: An MRI Study

JURI TJUVAJEV[1], MICHAEL KAPLITT[1], REVATHI DESAI[1], BRADLEY BETTIE[1], CORNELIA MATEI[2], JASON KOUTCHER[2], BERND GANSBACHER[3], ELI GILBOA[4], and RONALD BLASBERG[1]

[1] Department of Neurology, [2] Department of Radiology, [3] Division of Hematologic Oncology, Memorial Sloan-Kettering Cancer Center, New York, NY, USA
[4] Duke University Medical Center, NC, USA

INTRODUCTION.

Gene therapy of brain tumors is currently being vigorously explored. Direct transfer of cytokine genes into tumor cells can result in sustained local release of cytokines which is similar to that observed in the development of an immune response. Recently several groups demonstrated *in vivo* inhibition of tumor growth by genetically modifying tumor cells to produce Interleukin-2 (IL-2) [1,2]. An important aspect of cytokine gene therapy of intracerebral tumors was considered in this study, namely CNS toxicity associated with the sustained intracerebral production of cytokines. CNS toxicity associated with retroviral-mediated direct cytokine gene transfer following intracerebral implantation of vector-producer cells was evaluated in normal animals with particular emphasis on blood-brain barrier (BBB) disruption and subsequent formation of vasogenic brain edema. Changes in the brain were monitored by serial MRI, and the immune response was characterized by subtyping the infiltrating cells and reactive microglial cells.

MATERIALS AND METHODS.

Development of Vector-Producer Cell Lines. Retroviral constructs (Fig. 1) were converted to the corresponding virus using established procedures as described previously [2]. NIH3T3 murine fibroblasts were seeded in 60 mm plates. Twelve hours later, medium was removed and 3 ml of undiluted virus containing supernatants or dilutions of 1:10 to 1:10^5 of supernatants were added to the plates in presence of 8 µg/ml polybrene. Four to six hours later, supernatants were removed and standard medium was added to the plates for 24 hours and then replaced by selection medium containing 400 µg/ml of G148. Neo-resistant colonies were isolated and screened for expression of the transfected gene. All vector-producing NIH3T3 cell lines were grown in monolayers in Dulbecco's modified Eagle's (DME) medium with 10% fetal calf serum at 37°C and 5% CO_2 in a humidified incubator.

Intracerebral Inoculation. Male Fisher 344 rats weighing 250±20 g were anesthetized with a gas mixture consisting of 1.5% fluothane, 70% nitrous oxide and 30% oxygen. A 2% lidocaine gel was applied to the ears and the head was fixed in a stereotaxic device. After midline scalp incision, a burr hole was made through the skull 1 mm posterior and 3 mm lateral to the bregma. The syringe needle was then inserted 6 mm deep and the suspension of 10^5 cells in 10 µl was slowly injected. Bone wax was applied to cover the skull defect and the scalp was closed with 4.0 silk suture. After the procedure, the animals were marked and placed in standard cages.

MRI monitoring of Brain Edema. The intensity of BBB breakdown was assessed by MR imaging. MRI was performed on a General Electric CSI system with a 4.7 Tesla, 33 cm bore magnet. The rats were anesthetized as described above, placed in a special holder to stabilize the head in the midpoint of the standard imaging coil and to guarantee the reproducibility of the positioning between imaging sessions. Anesthetic gas mixture was constantly supplied to the animal throughout the imaging session via the tubing hermetically attached to the holder system. T_1-weighted post-contrast enhanced (Gd-DTPA; 0.2 mmol/kg i.v.) images were obtained [TR = 300 msec, TE = 10 msec]. Coronal slices were obtained through the area of the inoculation (3 mm thick plus 1 mm gap between slices) using a 256 x 256 matrix, 60 mm field of view. Areas of BBB disruption were detected as the contrast-enhancing regions on T_1-weighted images. The width of each hemisphere was measured and the degree of hemispheric swelling and resultant dislocation of midline structures were expressed as midline shift index (MSI; ratio of edematous to compressed hemisphere widths).

Tissue Water Content. Edematous hemisphere, and other structures of the brain were sampled, dried at 90° C in a constant temperature oven and reweighed daily until a constant dry weight was achieved (usually 3 to 4 days). Tissue water content was calculated as described elsewhere:

% Tissue Water = 100 - [(Wet weight - Dry weight)/Wet weight] x 100].

Histology and Immunofluorescence. Whole forebrains were sampled and immediately frozen in liquid freon (-78°C). Cryosections of 10 µm thickness were placed on microscopic glass slides, air-dried and fixed in cold acetone for 10 minutes. Immunofluorescent studies were performed using FITC-conjugated monoclonal antibodies (MoAB) (Serotec, Inc.): mouse monoclonal antibodies to rat CD8+ T-cells, to rat CD4+ T-cells and to macrophages, to rat OX42+ microglial cells. Histologic features of the brain tissue were assessed with light microscopy, while the cellular infiltrate was characterized using immunofluorescence under UV illumination.

RESULTS

Intracerebral Toxicity of Different Producer Cells. To analyze the direct effect of *in vivo* retroviral-mediated IL-2 and INF-γ gene transfer on normal brain, six groups of rats (5/group) were injected intracerebrally with saline or the DCA, DC-TK-IL2, DC-AD-R-IL2, N2-CMV-IL2 or DC-TK-INF vector-producer cells. There was a significant difference in the degree of BBB disruption between the experimental (DC-TK-IL2, DC-AD-R-IL2, N2-CMV-IL2, DC-TK-INF) and control (saline and DCA) groups as observed by contrast enhancement on T1 weighted MRI 7 days after inoculation **(Fig. 2)**. BBB disruption was visualized as a diffuse and moderately intense Gd-DTPA enhancement which was localized to the inoculated hemisphere. Hemispheric swelling and displacement of midline structures was most severe in the DC-TK-INF group **(Fig. 2e; and Fig. 3)**.

Among the IL-2 vector-producer groups, hemispheric swelling was greatest in the DC-TK-IL2 group **(Fig. 2d; and Fig. 3)**, and to a lesser extent in the DC-AD-R-IL2 group **(Fig. 2c; and Fig. 3)**. There was only moderate brain edema in the N2-CMV-IL2 group) **(Fig. 2b; and Fig. 3)**. In contrast, there were little or no signs of brain edema on the MR images in the DCA group **(Fig. 2a; and Fig. 3)** or saline injected controls. Interestingly, BBB disruption and hemispheric swelling decreased significantly by 12 days after inoculation of producer cells in the DC-TK-INF, DC-TK-IL2 and DC-AD-R-IL2 groups, but increased slightly in the N2-CMV-IL2 group.

Recruitment of CD4+ and CD8+ T-cells to the site of vector-producer cell inoculation and a diffuse activation of OX42+ microglial cells was observed predominantly at the site of cytokine vector-producer cell inoculation and diffusely throughout the ipsilateral hemisphere. In control groups only few OX42+ microglial cells were present.

Brain Tissue Water Content. In a separate study, the same experimental groups were produced (5 rats/group) and brain water content was measured 7 days after intracerebral inoculation of the producer cells. The degree of hemispheric brain edema, expressed as percent water content in the inoculated hemisphere, was highest in the DC-TK-INF group **(Fig. 4)**. Among the IL-2 vector-producer groups, brain edema was greatest in the DC-TK-IL2 group, but smaller in the DC-AD-R-IL2 and N2-CMV-IL2 groups. The control DCA vector-producing cell line resulted in a small amount of ipsilateral cerebral edema. No statistically significant differences in brain water content were observed in cerebellum (a remote brain structure) or in the contralateral hemisphere, although a trend is suggested **(Fig. 4)**.

A good correlation was observed between the percent water content in the inoculated hemisphere and the midline shift index (MSI) measured on MRI in correspondent groups **(Fig. 3)**. A reduction of brain edema coincided with the immunological rejection of cytokine producing fibroblasts that was observed on histology, although a small degree of swelling persisted between day 12 to day 18.

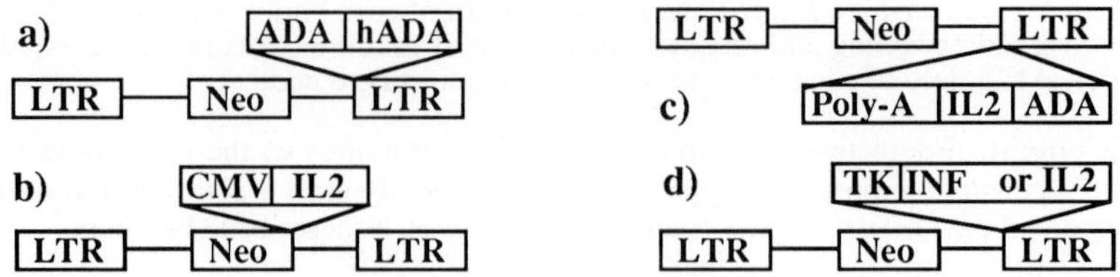

Fig. 1. Retroviral expression vectors for gene transfer.

a) DCA contains 2.1-kbp-long adenosine deaminase (ADA; EC 3.5.4.4) minigene that was inserted into the 3' LTR of the N2 retroviral vector, generating a 2.7-kbp-long chimeric LTR. **b) N2-CMV-IL2** contains a 528-bp-long DNA fragment encoding the entire coding region of a human IL-2 cDNA (without poly-A addition signal) fused to a human cytomegalovirus (CMV) promoter, cloned into the unique XhoI site of N2, downstream of the "neo" gene. **c) DC-AD-R-IL2** contains the human IL-2 cDNA fused in reverse orientation to a 832-bp-long DNA fragment of the human adenosine deaminase promoter, cloned into the Mlu I site present in the polylinker in the 3' LTR of a modified N2 vector. **d) DC-TK-IL2** and **DC-TK-INF** contain cDNA of the human IL-2 or murine interferon-γ (INF-γ), fused to a 852-bp-long DNA fragment of the Herpes simplex virus thymidine kinase (TK) promoter, cloned into the MluI site present in the polylinker in the 3' LTR of a modified N2 vector.

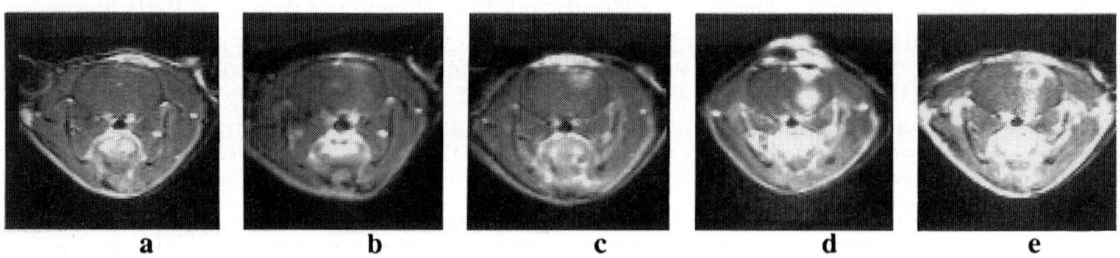

Fig. 2. T1-weighted contrast enhanced MR images of rat heads.

Representative coronal images obtained at 7 days after inoculation are presented: a) DCA control; b) N2-CMV-IL2; c) DC-AD-R-IL2; d) DC-TK-IL2; e) DC-TK-INF.

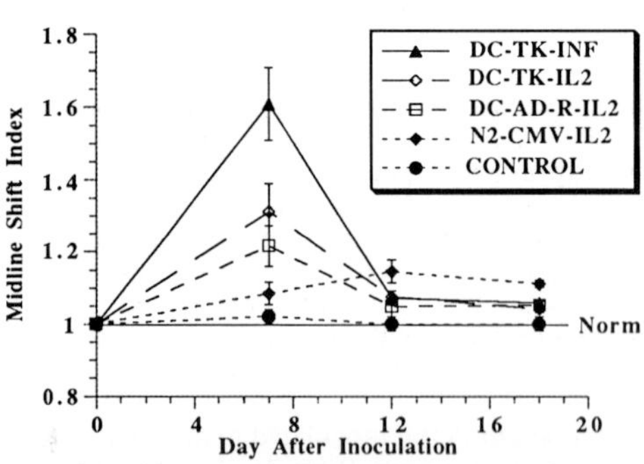

Fig. 3. Dislocation of brain midline structures. Midline shift index (MSI) changes after inoculation of vector-produces cells.

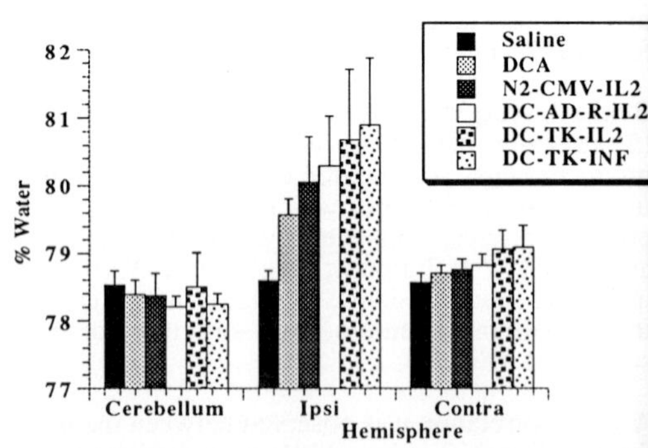

Fig. 4. Tissue water content in the brain at 7 days after inoculation with vector-producer cells.

DISCUSSION

Genetically constructed replication-deficient retroviral vectors provide the opportunity to deliver and to insert genes and promoter elements into tumor cells while sparing normal brain cells. This provides the possibility for continuous local secretion of cytokines throughout the tumor and avoids the complications associated with repeated injections of cytokines into the tumor bed.

CNS Toxicity. The greatest extent of BBB disruption and the most severe hemispheric swelling was observed following intracerebral implantation of the INF-γ-secreting DC-TK-INF vector-producer cell line. It has been shown that intracerebral injection of INF-γ causes recruitment of lymphocytes and other inflammatory cells to the injection site, including CD4+ T-cells into the perivascular space, OX42+ monocytes/macrophages and natural killer cells into brain parenchyma [3]. Other studies have shown that intracerebral injection of INF-γ causes increased MHC expression on brain cells, class I antigen on local endothelial and ependymal cells, and class II antigen on microglial ependymal and perivascular cells [3]. Intracerebral injection of IL-2 was shown to disrupt the BBB and result in the migration of inflammatory cells to the site of injection [4]. Our findings are consistent with these observations. We demonstrated disruption of the BBB and vasogenic brain edema following intracerebral inoculation of all three IL-2 vector-producing cell lines, but not in the control adenosine deaminase-producing cell line (DCA). The vasogenic brain edema was accompanied by diffuse CD4+ and CD8+ T-cell infiltration and by OX42+ microglial cells and by monocytes/ macrophages. Interestingly, the degree of vasogenic brain edema and the dislocation of the brain midline structures on MRI correlated with the levels of IL-2 production by the vector-producer cell lines. These observations raise important questions about the potential clinical applicability of intratumoral cytokine injection or cytokine gene therapy for tumors located intracranially.

CONCLUSIONS.

Our results demonstrate substantial CNS toxicity due to sustained intracerebral production of IL2 and INF-γ. The clinical application of IL-2 and INF-γ gene transfer therapy of intracerebral tumors must be approched with caution and consider the potential for the development of severe vasogenic brain edema associated with intracerebral production of these cytokines. Animal models of the sustained intracerebral production of IL2 or INF-γ could be used to further study the role of these cytokines in the development of brain edema and in the pathogenesis of other CNS diseases.

REFERENCES.

1. Porgador, A., Gansbacher. B., Bannerji, R., Tzenoval, E., Gilboa, E., Feldman, M. (1993) Anti-metastatic vaccination of tumor-bearing mice with IL-2-gene-inserted tumor cells. Int. J. Cancer, 53: p. 471-477.
2. Gansbacher, B., Zier, K., Daniels, B., Cronin, K., Bannerji, R., Gilboa, E. (1990) IL-2 gene transfer into tumor cells abrogates tumorigenicity and induces protective immunity. J. Exp. Med. 172: p. 1217.
3. Sethna, M.P., Lampson, L.A. (1991) Immune modulation within the brain: recruitment of inflammatory cells and increased major histocompatibility antigen expression following intracerebral injection of interferon-γ. J. Neuroimm. 34: p. 121-132.
4. Watts, R.G., Wright, J.L., Atkinson, L.L., Merchant, R.E. (1989) Histopathological and blood-brain barrier changes in rats induced by intracerebral injection of human recombinant interleukin 2. Neurosurg. 25: p. 202-208.

A Comparison Between Cold Injury and Contusion Injury in Relation to Cu, Zn-SOD mRNA Expression

S. Nishio, T. Fukuhara, Y. Ono, M. Kawauchi, S. Asari, and T. Ohmoto

Department of Neurological Surgery, Okayama University Medical School, Okayama, 700 Japan

SUMMARY

To examine the reaction against free radical accumulation after traumatic injury, the expression of Cu, Zn-superoxide dismutase (SOD) mRNA was analyzed in contusion injury and cold injury models. The contusion was made by a weight-drop method, and the cold injury by a standard cold injury method. Rats were decapitated six hours after the injury, and the brains were resected from three portions to examine the specific gravity and the expression of Cu, Zn-SOD mRNA by Northern blot analysis. Analysis with specific gravity, confirmed the development of brain edema in contusion and cold injury, but no difference was observed between the two groups. In the expression of SOD mRNA, however, the expression decreased in all portions in the cold injury group, but increased in the peripheral portion of the contusion group. The reason for this difference is that the extremely low temperature suppresses gene expression in the cold injury.

INTRODUCTION

Cold injury has been employed as a traumatic injury model because it causes vasogenic edema [1]. But in relation to gene expression, the issue of whether cold injury is proper as a trauma model has not been fully discussed. We compared the gene expression of Cu, Zn-SOD after contusion injury and cold injury.

MATERIALS AND METHODS

Male Sprague-Dawley rats were divided into 3 experimental groups:contusion, cold injury and control. A burr hole 5 mm in diameter was made on the right parietal portion in each rat. In the contusion group (n=8), rats underwent a traumatic insult by dropping a 20 g metallic cylinder from a height of 30 cm through a guide tube on the exposed dura of the right parietal portion. The cold injury (n=8) was produced with a metal probe cooled to -80°C with liquid nitrogen placed directly on the exposed dura of the right parietal portion. In the control group (n=7), only a burr hole was made. Six hours after the injury, all rats were decapitated. The brains were removed immediately and sectioned coronally in two slices, one including the injury portion, the other posterior to that. Samples of the cortex were taken from three portions; at the center of the injury (core), 2 mm posterior to the injury (peripheral), and the contralateral hemisphere (distal). The water content was measured with specific gravity method [2] using linear gradient columns. The columns were made of a kerosene and bromobenzene mixture, and calibrated with droplets of potassium sulfate. Specific gravity was read in the column 1 minute after immersion of the tissue samples. Cu,Zn-SOD mRNA expression (using Northern blotting) was measured in each model. RNA was quantified spectrophotometrically, assuming that 40μg RNA/ml provides an absorbance of 1.0 at 260 nm. Ten μg samples were electrophoresed in 1.1% agarose-formaldehyde gels and transferred to a nylon membrane (Hybond™-N, Amersham International, England). As a standard sample, the whole gray matter of one unoperated rat was taken. This standard sample was electrophoresed in every agarosed-formaldehyde gel to determine the relative quantification of each sample. The integrity of RNA preparations and consistency of the sample loading were verified with the loading of 5 μg total RNA by staining with ethidium bromide. The probe for hybridization was 48-mer synthetic oligonucleotide of rat Cu,Zn-SOD cDNA (base 465-512) [3]. It was end-labeled with [a-32P]ddATP using terminal transferase in a kit (3'-endlabeling kit, N4020, Amersham International). The membranes were prehybridized for 4 hours at 37°C in a buffer containing 50% deionized formamide, 1X Denhardt's solution, 4X standard saline citrate (SCC), 20 mM sodium phosphate buffer, 500 μg/ml salmon sperm DNA, 100 μg/ml yeast tRNA, 0.5% sodium dodecyl sulfate (SDS) and 5% dextran sulfate. Hybridization was carried out for 16 hours at 37°C in the same buffer. The membranes were washed twice for 30 minutes each in 1X SSC/ 0.1% SDS at room temperature and once at 50°C. The membranes were subjected to autoradiography for several days at -80°C. The intensity of the hybridization signal was analyzed densitometrically, and the ratio compared with the standard sample was calculated. Values were expressed in mean ± standard deviation. All comparisons among the three groups and the three portions were performed using analysis of variance with Scheffe's F test.

RESULTS

Table 1 Specific gravity of brain cortex in three groups

	core	peripheral	distal
control group	1.045±0.001	1.044±0.001	1.044±0.001
contusion group	1.036±0.001	1.041±0.002	1.046±0.002
cold injury group	1.038±0.002	1.042±0.002	1.045±0.002

#p<0.05, *p<0.01, **p<0.001, ***p<0.0001

The water content of both the contusion and cold injury groups was significantly higher than that of the control in the core (p<0.0001) and peripheral portions (contusion; p<0.01, cold injury; p<0.05) (Table 1). No difference was observed between the contusion and cold injury groups, which showed an almost identical degree of brain edema.

Table 2 Cu,Zn-SOD mRNA expression of the cortex in three groups

	core	peripheral	distal
control group	1.068±0.184	0.954±0.170	0.989±0.244
contusion group	1.056±0.255	1.382±0.281	1.074±0.218
cold injury group	0.279±0.047	0.293±0.110	0.229±0.084

#p<0.05, *p<0.01, ***p<0.0001

In Cu,Zn-SOD mRNA expression, a significant decrease was confirmed in all portions of the cold injury group ($p<0.0001$) (Table 2). On the contrary, a significant increase was observed in the peripheral portion of the contusion model compared with the control ($p<0.05$). No significant difference was observed in the core and distal portions compared to the control group.

DISCUSSION

It has been postulated that free radicals are produced in significant quantities in the ischemic brain, and that free radicals play a role in ischemic brain damage [4,5]. In traumatic brain damage, free radicals may play the same role as in ischemic brain injury [6]. Neurochemical analysis has increased in recent reports of experimental neurotraumatic injury that studied the formation of vasogenic edema. We investigated the expression of Cu,Zn-SOD mRNA, the increase of which has been already observed in models of ischemic injury [7,8]. Our results also show the increase of mRNA expression in the contusion injury group, but not in the cold injury group. In this experiment, however, there was a similar degree of brain edema in both the contusion and cold injury groups. These results mean that the extension of vasogenic edema is similar but the cell reactions are different after contusion injury and cold injury.

Although the accumulation of superoxide may stimulate the increase of SOD mRNA expression in ischemic injury [8], the decrease of this expression does not necessarily indicate a decrease of superoxide accumulation. In cold injury, the cells may not react against the free radical injury because of the extremely low temperature. In the contusion injury, the increase of mRNA expression was significant only in the peripheral portion, but not in the core portion, perhaps because the damaged brain cannot react against the accumulation of superoxide.

The cold injury model has been used as a closed-head injury model to investigate vasogenic brain edema [9,10,11], because the edema of cold injury is believed to be responsible for swelling after closed head injury [12]. The cold injury model is quite useful in the study of the fluid dynamics of edema [13], but that the cold injury model is essentially different from the contusion model in nuerochemical standpoint.

Based on these results, we should note the difference between contusion and cold injury when selecting an experimental model for research concerning head injury.

REFERENCES

1. Ikeda Y, Anderson JH, Long DM (1989) Oxygen-free radicals in the genesis of traumatic and peritumoral brain edema. Neurosurgery 24:213-216
2. Marmarou A, Poll W, Shulman K, Bhagavan H (1978) A simple gravimetric technique for measurement of cerebral edema. J Neurosurg 49:530-537
3. Delabar JM, Nicole A, D'Auriol L, Jacob Y, Meunier-Rotival M, Galibert F, Sinet PM, Jerome H (1987) Cloning and sequencing of a rat Cu Zn superoxide dismutase cDNA. Correlation between Cu Zn superoxide dismutase mRNA level and enzyme activity in rat and mouse tissue. Eur J Biochem 166:181-187
4. Flamm ES, Demopoulos HB, Seligman ML, Poser RG, Ransohoff J (1978) Free radicals in cerebral ischemia. Stroke 9:445-447
5. Kitagawa K, Matsumoto M, Oda T, Niinobe M, Hata R, Handa N, Fukunaga R, Isaka Y, Kimura K, Maeda H, Mikoshiba K, Kamada T (1990) Free radical generation during brief period of cerebral ischemia may trigger delayed neuronal death. Neuroscience 35:551-558
6. Kontos HA, Wei EP (1986) Superoxide production in experimental brain injury. J Nuerosurg 64:803-807
7. Matsuyama T, Michishita H, Nakamura H, Tsuchiyama M,Shimizu S, Watanabe K, Sugita M (1993) Induction of copper-zinc superoxide dismutase in gerbil hippocampus after ischemia. J Cereb Blood Flow Metab 13:135-144

8. Uyama O, Matsuyama T, Michishita H, Nakamura H, Sugita M (1992) Protective effect of human recombinant superoxide dismutase on transient ischemic injury of CA1 neurons in gerbils Stroke 23:75-81
9. Klatzo I (1967) Neuropathological aspect of brain edema. J Neuropathol Exp Neurol 26:1-14
10. Baethmann A, Maier-Hauff K, Schürer L, Lange M, Guggenbinchler C, Vogt W, Jacob K, Kempski O (1989) Release of glutamate and of free fatty acids in vasogenic brain edema. J Neurosurg 70:578-591
11. Unterberg A, Dautermann C, Baethmann A, Müller-Esterl W (1986) The kallikrein-kinin system as mediator in vasogenic brain edema. J Neurosurg 64:269-276
12. Crockard A, Kang J, Ladds G (1982) A model of focal cortical contusion in gerbils. J Neurosurg 57:203-209
13. Reulen HJ, Graham R, Spatz M, Klatzo I (1977) Role of pressure gradients and bulk flow in dynamics of vasogenic brain edema. J Neurosurg 46:24-35

The Role of Capillary Endothelial Cells and Astrocytes in the Mechanism of Volume Regulation of the Brain

Tatsuya Nagashima[1], Wu Shijing[1], Youji Tomita[1], Hidemi Nakamura[1], Akira Mizoguchi[2], Michio Yamaguchi[3], and Norihiko Tamaki[1]

Departments of [1] Neurosurgery and [2] Anatomy, [3] School of Allied Medical Sciences, Kobe University School of Medicine, 7-5-1 Kusunoki-cho, Chuo-ku, Kobe, 650 Japan

INTRODUCTION

Precise control of brain volume through adjustment of all water and electrolyte content is important for the normal function of the brain because it is confined to the semirigid and indistensible environment of the skull. Several pieces of evidence suggest that the astrocytes and capillaries play an important role in the regulation of brain water content through an ability to affect brain water and electrolyte permeability. However, a little is know about the interaction between these two cells. The purpose of this study is to establish an in vitro experimental model to analyze the interaction between brain capillary endothelial cells and astrocytes.

MATERIALS AND METHODS

(1) Cell preparations. Brain capillary endotherial cells were obtained from 10 rats cerebral cortices by the purely enzymatic isolation procedure reported by Audus and Borchard(1). The cerebral cortex were digested by two step enzymatic treatments; dispase and collagenase/dispase. And finally, the endothelial cells were purified by centrifugation over a pre-established 50% Percoll gradient. The cells were cultured by Dulbeco MEM with 13% FBS and fibroblast growth factor(FGF). The release of prostacyclin in the supernatant fluid was measured by the assay of its stable degradation product, 6-keto-PGF1α. The astrocytes were isolated from new born(1-3 days) rat brain cortices by the method reported by McCarthy(3). The cells were identified immuno-cytochemically.

(2) In vitro BBB experiment system: A monolayer of brain capillary endothelial cells were grown on a collagen membrane. Monolayer integrity was studied by ^{14}C-sucrose movement and transmembrane electrical resistance. Biochemical treatment and anoxia were applied to this membrane transport system. ^{14}C-sucrose was added in the upper chamber, then the leakage to the lower chamber was measured by liquid scintillation counter.

(3) Intracellular calcium change: Intracellular calcium concentration was measure by a confocal laser scanning microscope after labeling the cells with calcium probe Fluo-3

A/M(Fig.1). Osmotic and biochemical stimulations to the cells were studied. Confluent cultures were loaded with the calcium probe Fluo-3 A/M, then the intracellular calcium was measured. After hyperosmolar mannitol of 1.8M was applied to the endotherial cells, intracellular calcium change was monitored every 5 second. Then return of the intracellular calcium concentration was monitored for 30 minutes after the hyperosmotic treatment.

(4) Interaction between endothelial cells and astrocytes: The effect of conditioned medium on the brain capillary endothelial cells, which were exposed to anoxia, was studied by measuring the LDH release.

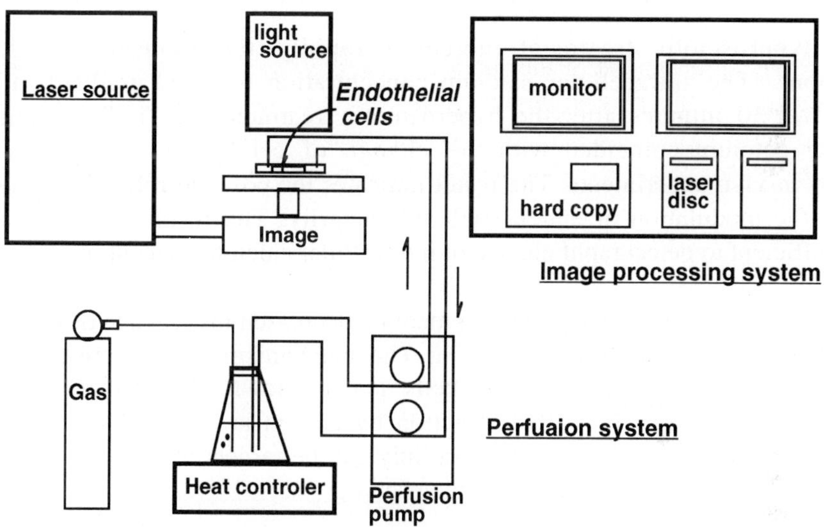

Fig.1 Confocal laser scanning microscope system. The system consists of four parts; a laser source, a laser scanning microscope, a image processing system, and a perfusion system to keep the cells in physiological condition.

RESULTS

(1) The cells retained both endothelial cell markers and some unique features typical to brain capillary endothelial cells in vivo. Their endothelial cell identity was confirmed by Factor VIII immunoperoxydase reaction and uptake of acetylated low density lipoprotein. The cells showed no evidence of GFAP. The brain capillary endothelial cell produce prostacyclin in large quantities, and this ability was unchanged by cultivation. Freshly isolated cells contain a high level of γGTP activity, which decreases with time in culture to a constant lower level. Cultured astrocyte were positively stained by

GFAP. Anoxic insult for 30 minutes caused delayed leakage of intracellular LDH that was blocked by catalase.

(2) Permeability of the endothelial cell monolayer changed rapidly after the application of hyperosmotic solution. Chemical mediators such as bradykinin, also increased it. Bradykinin is a potent vasodilator peptide that act on endothelial cells via an activation of phospholipase C, a rise in $\{Ca^{+}\}i$, and release of NO. The result demonstrated the presense of bradykinin receptor and its role as a modulator of BBB permeability. Atrial natriuretic peptide increses intracellular c-GMP concentration of the capillary endothelial cells. ANP plays an important role in the regulation of blood pressure and electrolyte metabolism. Main function of c-GMP dependent signal pathway in cerebral cepillary endothelial cells is to control transcellular ion-transport metabolism.

(3) The hyperosmotic treatment increased rapidly the intracellular calcium concentration. The intracellular calcium concentration returned gradually to the previous level 30 minutes after the hyperosmotic treatment(FIg.2). The change of intracellular calcium coincided with the change of cerebrovascular permeability observed by in vivo experiments. The result indicates the possible role of intracellular calcium in the modulation of endotherial cell integrity. The result showed that the system is sufficient to detect rapid change of intracellular calcium concentration.

(4) The presence of the astrocyte condition medium decreased the leakage of LDH from brain capillary endothelial cells by anoxia. The mechanism of protective effect of astrocyte CM on the capillary endotherial cells is not known. The blocked LDH leak by catalase indicates taht the cell destruction by anoxia is caused by oxygen free radicals. Microvascular endothelial cells not only can be targets of oxydant injury, but they also produce free radicals that injure themselves.

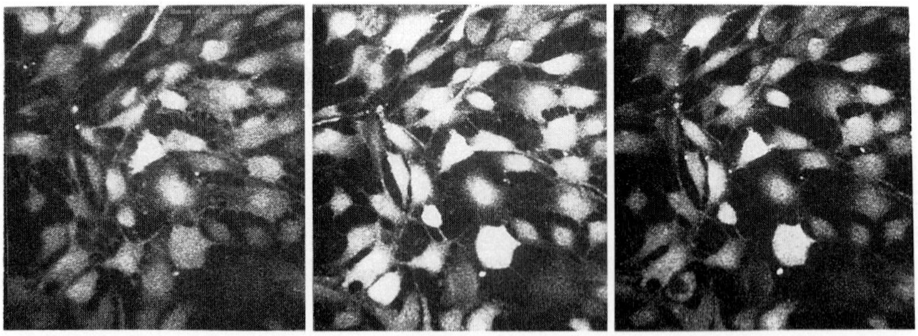

Fig.2 The change of intracellular calcium concentration before(left), 5 minutes(center) and 30 minitues(right) after the hyperosmotic treatment. The lightness of the cells indicates calcium concentration. The figure indicates the rapid increase and gradual return of the intracellular calcium concentration.

DISCUSSION

Because of semirigid nature of the cranial cavity, the intracranial volume regulation is very critical. The cytoarchitecture of the central nervous system is composed of different cell types. Each cellular component of the CNS constitutes an anatomic compartment incorporating a series of specialized biochemical functions. Many of these functions, especially interactions between brain capillary endothelial cells and astrocytes have not been well understood. The capillary endothelial cells of the brain plays an important role in homeostasis within the central nervous system by limiting the blood to brain passage of water soluble substance while facilitating transport of glucose, amino acids, etc.

Astrocytes modulate the functions of endothelial cells; increase the electrical resistance; induction of γ-GTP; modulation of hexose and amino acids transport; modulation of Na+-K+ ATPase and alkalinephosphatase activity; modulation of growth(2). Therefore, astrocytes apparently regulate the brain volume by changing the functions of capillary endothelial cells. A current interest in BBB biology address the nature of signal transduction phenomena, such as protein phosphorylation, nitric oxide release, and calcium transport, that are acutely activated within brain capillary endothelium by vasoactive agents, growth factor, or disease states. Considerable experimental attention has been focussed recently on cell culture system that reestablish functional interaction between microvascular cells in vitro to define the cellular and biochemical basis of microvessel function and blood brain barrier regulation. The results of the present study indicates that the in vitro experimental system is promising approach to study the signal transduction process.

In vitro BBB experimental system has been developed for a decade. The results of the permeability study indicated the capillary endothelium monolayer is in incomplete BBB function, however it is sufficient to study the effect of chemical mediators and anoxia. The coculture system should be established to reestablish the in vitro BBB system.

REFERENCES

1. Audus KL, Borchardt RT(1986) Characterization of an in vitro blood-brain barrier model system for drug transport and metabolism. Pharma Res 3:81-87
2. Cancilla PA, Bready J, Berliner(1993) Brain endothelial-astrocyte interactions. In Blood Brain Barrier, ed by William Pardridge, Raven Press, Ltd, New York, pp25-46
3. McCarthy KD, Vellis JD(1980) Preparation of separate astroglial and oligodendroglial cell cultures from rat cerebral cortices. J Cell Biology 85:890-902
4. Rapoport SI, Fredericks WR Ohno K, Pittigrew KD(1980) Am J Physiol 238:R421-431

Arginine Vasopressin Receptor Antagonist for Treatment of Vasogenic Brain Edema

M. Kagawa, S. Nagao, T. Ogawa, T. Kuniyoshi, Y. Honma, and H. Kuyama

Department of Neurological Surgery, Kagawa Medical School, 1750-1 Miki-cho, Kita-gun, Kagawa, Japan

SUMMARY

Recent reports indicate that centrally released arginine vasopressin (AVP) facilitates brain water permeability in normal and pathological conditions. The effects of central administration of AVP receptor antagonists on vasogenic brain edema were studied using rats. V_1 receptor antagonists of 50ng were stereotactically injected into the lateral ventricle 10 minutes prior to or 1 hour after cold brain injury. The injury resulted in significant increases in the water content of the lesion and the contralateral hemispheres. Twenty-four hours after injury, the brain water and sodium contents and plasma osmolality were measured. V_1 receptor antagonist significantly decreased the brain water and sodium contents at the adjacent cortex of the lesion without changes in serum osmolality. The V_1 receptor of AVP is thought to act on water permeability of the brain. Peptide therapy may become an additional tool for brain edema treatment.

INTRODUCTION

It is generally accepted that all membranes known to regulate water permeability are under the influence of circulating arginine vasopressin (AVP). The peptide hormone AVP is secreted and enters the cerebrospinal fluid (CSF) directly from the brain and not from the systemic circulation(4). It is reasonable to assume that brain-derived AVP should have some implication to brain water movement.

Recent studies indicated that centrally released AVP influenced water permeability of the brain in both normal(2) and pathological conditions(1,3). We undertook this study to examine the effect of intraventricular administration of V_1 receptor antagonists of AVP before and after cold injury on the brain water content.

MATERIALS AND METHODS

Sprague-Dawley rats weighing 300 to 400g were used for these experiments. After anesthesia with an intraperitoneal injection of pentobarbital sodium, a AVP V_1 receptor antagonist ([deamino-Pen^1, O-Me-Tyr^2, Arg^8]-Vasopressin) was administered into the left lateral ventricle stereotactically. A cold-injury was induced in the left hemisphere of brain by applying a cooper rod, cooled by liquid nitrogen, to the exposed bony skull for 20 seconds or 1 minute. Anesthesia was discontinued, and the animals were placed in cages and fed freely. Twenty-four hours after the injury, animals were sacrificed by decapitation. The brain was removed and divided into the injured and contralateral hemisphere immediately.

The water content in each section was determined by dry-weight method. The brain tissue

sodium and potassium were extracted with 2N nitric acid for 48 hours and analyzed using atomic absorption spectrophotometry. Before decapitation, a blood sample was taken from the femoral artery, and plasma osmolality was measured.
Animals were divided into 2 groups.
In group 1, 50 ng of V_1 receptor antagonists were given 10 minutes before 20-seconds injury and bilateral hemispheres were divided into the cortex and deep ganglia structures in 24 hours after the injury. Water, sodium and potassium contents of the two sites were evaluated.
In order to mimic clinical use, 50ng of V_1 receptor antagonist was administered 1 hour after cold injury in group 2. The animals received a 1-minute injury to promote brain edema.

RESULTS

Fifty ng of this antagonist resulted in significant decreases in water content in the cortex, but not in the deep structures (Table 1).

Table 1 Brain water contents of cortex and deep structures following administration of V_1 receptor antagonist. Asterisks indicate a value significantly different from non-treated animals. (*: P<0.05, **: P<0.01) CL:cold lesion

	water content (%)			
	cortex		deep structure	
normal (n=25)	79.32±0.04		78.32±0.05	
	lesion side	non lesion side	lesion side	non lesion side
cold lesion (n=20)	80.99±0.09	79.48±0.07	78.45±0.05	78.35±0.05
CL+V_1 50ng (n=17)	80.46±0.12*	79.28±0.05*	78.39±0.08	78.17±0.08

Changes in the tissue sodium and potassium of the cortical lesion were also significantly suppressed with V_1 receptor antagonist (Table 2). There were no significant changes in tissue sodium and potassium contents in the deep structures.

Table 2 Sodium and potassium contens of brain cortex following administration of V_1 receptor antagonist. Asterisks show a value significantly different from the values of non-treated animals. (: P<0.01) CL:cold lesion**

	Na (mmol/kg dry weight)		K (mmol/kg dry weight)	
normal (n=17)	688.7±15.8		467.5±1.8	
	lesion side	non lesion side	lesion side	non lesion side
cold lesion (n=15)	824.5±14.4	748.9±18.7	448.0±3.0	462.3±3.8
CL+V_1 50ng (n=13)	735.3±26.0**	687.8±25.5	459.9±2.7**	462.3± 2.7

With a 1-minute cold lesion, water contents of the cortex and deep structures of the lesion and non-lesion hemispheres significantly increased. Fifty ng of this antagonist administered 1 hour after the lesion also significantly suppressed increases in the water content of the bilateral cortices and had no effect on deep structures (Table 3).

Table 3 Brain water contents of cortex and deep structures with V_1 receptor antagonist which was administered 1 hour after cold lesion. Asterisks denote a value significantly different from the values of non-treated animals. (*: P<0.05, **: P<0.01) CL:cold lesion

	water content (%)			
	cortex		deep structure	
normal (n=22)	79.37±0.03		78.29±0.04	
	lesion side	non lesion side	lesion side	non lesion side
cold lesion (n=8)	81.84±0.14	79.73±0.08	78.88±0.03	78.64±0.09
CL+V_1 50ng (n=12)	81.49±0.07*	79.41±0.06**	78.74±0.06	78.55± 0.04

There were no significant changes in serum osmolality with intraventricular administration of V_1 receptor antagonists.

DISCUSSION

Centrally released arginine vasopressin is thought to be one of the substances that control brain water. In the brain, high levels of a radioiodinated V_1 receptor antagonist were found at binding sites in the choroid plexus, blood vessels, suprachiasmatic nucleus, nucleus of the solitary tract, etc.

Regarding water permeability and AVP, Raichle and Grubb(2) observed a highly significant increase in brain water permeability using $H_2{}^{15}O$ with intraventricular administration of AVP. Pharmacological doses of intraventricular AVP facilitate the production of vasogenic cold injured edema in cats(3). Significant increases in AVP in the CSF were reported in patients with intracranial hemorrhage, brain injury and ischemic stroke who have edema and intracranial hypertension(7). Thus an increase in central AVP is considered to be associated with and to facilitate brain edema. It is reasonable to assume that AVP receptor antagonists have some therapeutic significance on brain edema.

Rosenberg et al(5) reported that the increase in the brain water content induced by the infusion of AVP into bilateral caudates of normal cats was blocked by the simultaneous infusion of an AVP V_1 receptor antagonist and increased brain water and sodium contents with collagenase-induced intracerebral hemorrhage were also reduced by V_1 receptor antagonist(6). These suggest that the increase in capillary permeability is mediated by the V_1 receptor and possibility of receptor antagonist therapy for brain edema.

In our experiments, V_1 receptor antagonist were administered into the lateral ventricle because of the inability of the peptides to cross the blood-brain barrier and the blood-cerebrospinal fluid barrier. The CSF and interstitial fluid flow of the brain should serve as pathways in neuroendocrine integration(4).

Our data indicated that increases in brain water content induced by cold injury were suppressed by intraventricular administration of AVP V_1 receptor antagonist, which was compatible with the results of Rosenberg et al. The results suggest that AVP increases the water

permeability of the brain via the V_1 receptor.
Intraventricular administration of 50ng of V_1 receptor antagonist before and after cold injury showed a significant reduction of the water contents only in the cortices adjacent to the lesion. The exact reason is not clear, however, in the vicinity of the lesion, activation of AVP V_1 receptor may act as a causal factor of water movement. Central administration of V_1 receptor antagonist is thought to counter-act and reduce water permeability near the lesion site. Our results suggest that the central administration of an AVP V_1 receptor antagonist may become an effective therapeutic tool for reducing vasogenic brain edema.

REFERENCE

1. **Doczi T, Laszlo F, Szerdahelyi P, Joo F: Involvement of vasopressin in brain edema formation : Further evidence obtained from the Brattleboro diabetes inspidus rat with experimental subarachnoid hemorrhage. Neurosurgery 14:436-441, 1984**
2. **Raichle ME, Grubb RL: Regulation of brain water permeability by centrally-released vasopressin. Brain Res 143:191-194, 1978**
3. **Reeder RF, Nattie EE, North WG: Effect of vasopressin on cold-induced brain edema. J Neurosurg 64:941-945, 1986**
4. **Robinson AG, Zimmerman EA: Cerebrospinal fluid and ependymal neurophysin. J Clin Invest 52:1260-1267, 1973**
5. **Rosenberg GA, Estrada E, Kyner WT: Vasopressin-induced brain edema is mediated by V_1 receptor, in Long DM (ed): Advances in Neurology. New York: Raven press, 1990, pp 149-154**
6. **Rosenberg GA, Scremin O, Estrada E, Kyner T: Arginine vasopressin V_1 - antagonist and atrial natriuretic peptide reduce hemorrhagic brain edema in rats. Stroke 23:1767-1774, 1992**
7. **Sorensen PS, Gjerris F, Hammer M: Cerebrospinal fluid vasopressin in neurological and psychiatric disorders. J Neurol Neurosurg Psychiatry 48:50-57, 1985**

Session VII: Effects of Increased ICP (1)

Chairmen: A. Marmarou and T. Ohmoto

The Perineural Pathway of Cerebrospinal Fluid Absorption into the Cervical Lymphatic System. Morphological Findings in Rats, Cats, Dogs and Monkeys*

T. BRINKER[1], C. BÖTEL[2], H.J. ROTKÖTTER[3], G.F. WALTER[4], and M. SAMII[1]

Departments of [1] Neurosurgery Nordstadt Hospital, [2] Central Laboratory Animal Facility, [3] Anatomy and [4] Neuropathology, Hannover Medical School, Germany

SUMMARY:

The study investigates pathways for cerebrospinal fluid (CSF) outflow into the cervical lymphatic system. Dyes, fluorescent latex beads or X-ray contrast medium were infused into the cisterna magna of animals under the condition of an increase in intracranial pressure (ICP). Following a 30-minute infusion, the tracers were found in the perineural subarachnoid spaces of the cranial nerves. The dye passed the perineural arachnoidal barrier along the penetration sites of blood vessels and drained through lymph vessels of the skull base into cervical lymph nodes.

INTRODUCTION:

The fact that cerebrospsinal fluid (CSF) drains through the perineural subarachnoid space (SAS) of the cranial nerves into the connective tissue of the skull base and then into the cervical lymph system, is well known. The biological significance of this CSF outflow pathway, however, is still a matter of dispute. The present study adds some new aspects to the knowledge of the connection of CSF and lymphatic system.

MATERIAL AND METHODS:

The study was performed in anaesthetized animals. The cisterna magna was cannulated either percutaneously (cats,dogs and monkeys) or by a catheter which was introduced through a burr hole in the interparietal bone (rats). Pigment blue, india ink, 0.7 μm fluorescent latex particles or X-ray contrast medium (Isovist 300, Schering, Berlin) were infused into the cisterna magna. The rate of infusion was adjusted to each species. The infusion was performed 30 minutes in rats at a rate of 0.04 ml/min, in cats and dogs at 0.6 ml/min and in monkeys at 1ml/min. During the infusion a pressure equilibrium was attained at 40 mm Hg in rats, 50 mm Hg in dogs and cats and 80 mm Hg in monkeys. Following the infusion of dyes, the animals were killed and the eyeballs removed and fixed in 10% formalin. The eyeballs of animals, in which fluorescent latex beads had been infused, were frozen in liquid nitrogen.

RESULTS AND DISCUSSION:

CSF outflow along the optic nerve: Following the infusion of dye into the cisterna magna, transections of the orbit showed that the dye has leaked from the perineural SAS of the optic and ocular motor nerves into the retroorbital connective tissue.

---

* This study is gratefully dedicated to our teacher Prof.Dr.med.Dr.h.c.H.Dietz who founded the ICP congress in 1972 and who finished his carrier in 1993.

Transversal sections of the optic nerve showed that the dye has passed the dural sheath of the nerve along the penetration sites of blood vessels (fig. 1a). Following the infusion of the fluorescent latex beads into the cisterna magna of rats fluorescence was seen in the perineural SAS of the optic nerve. Further fluorescence was found in the center of the nerve probable in the Virchow-Robin-space around the central artery of the retina (fig. 1b).

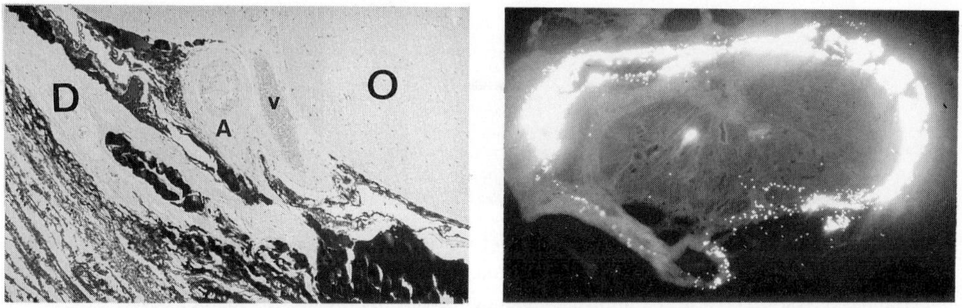

Fig. 1a (left): Cross section of the optic nerve (O) of a monkey showing the dye leaving the subarachnoid space through the dural nerve sheath (D) along a penetrating artery (A) and vein (V). Fig. 1b (right): Transversal cross section through the optic nerve of a rat after the intracisternal infusion of fluorescent latex beads. Activity is found in the perineural subarachnoid space and in the center of the nerve.

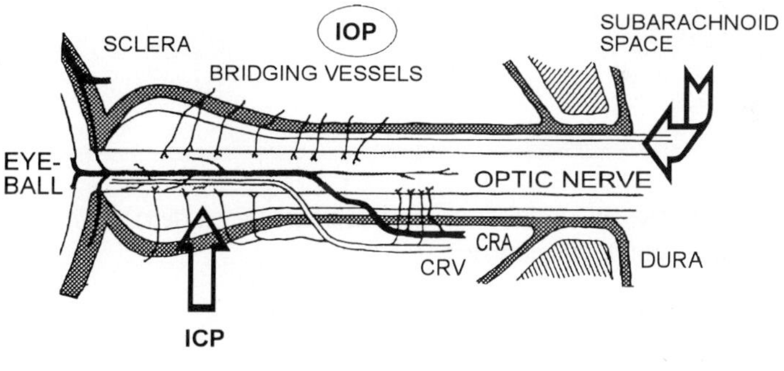

Fig. 2: Schematic drawing of the intraorbital and intracanalicular portion of the optic nerve and its sheaths. The cranial SAS communicates with the perineural SAS of the optic nerve. CSF flows through the perineural SAS and passes the dura through the penetration sites of blood vessels driven by a pressure gradient between the ICP and the intraorbital pressure (IOP).
CRA and CRV: central retinal artery and vein.

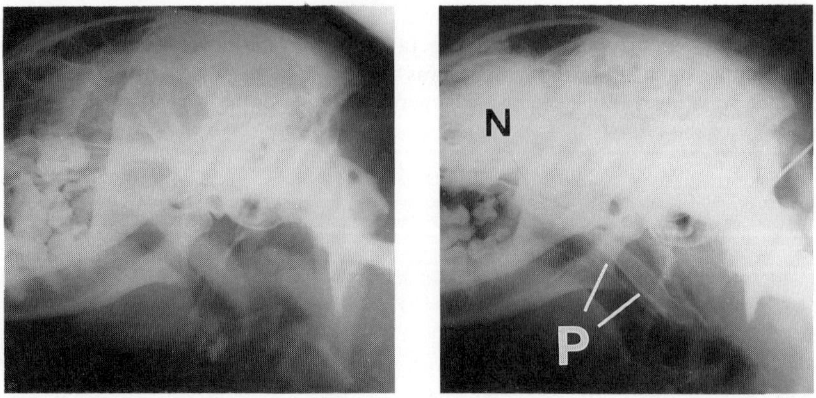

Fig.3: Lateral view of the skull of a dog before (left) and after (right) a 30-minute infusion of X-ray contrast medium into the cisterna magna. A massive leakage of the contrast medium into the the nasal region (N) and a contrast enhancement of the palate (P) can be seen.

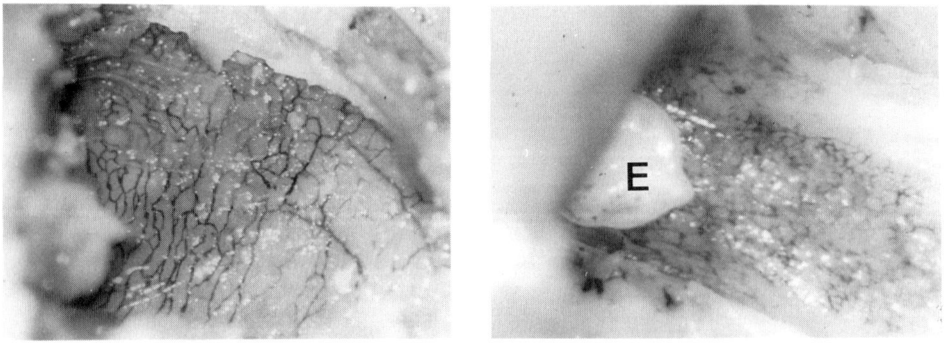

Fig.4: Networks of lymph vessels in the nasal septum of a cat (left) and in the oropharyngeal mucosa of a rat (right, E: epiglottis).

<u>CSF outflow into the lymph vessels of the skull base:</u> Following the infusion of X-ray contrast medium, an opacification of the optic nerve, a contrast enhancement of the cribriform plate and a leakage into the nasal region and the orbit were observed. In addition, a contrast enhancement of the palate was found (fig.3). Following the infusion of dyes, dense networks of lymphatic channels were found in the nasal region which were connected to lymph vessels in the oropharyngeal region. Those drained into the deep cervical lymph nodes (fig.4).

DISCUSSION:

The results of this study indicate that the perineural SAS of cranial nerves acts as a significant pathway for cerebrospinal fluid outflow into the lymphatic system. In addition to previous morphological studies [1,2] which have shown open channels at the end of the optic and olfactory nerve, it is demonstrated that CSF and even particles can pass the perineural arachnoidal barrier along the penetration sites of blood vessels.

Our light microscopic observations on the perineural dural sheath of the optic nerve are confirmed by previous ultrastructure studies showing that veins crossing the dura posses paravascular leptomeningeal protrusions which are continuous with the perineural SAS and which penetrate the dura mater. The ultrastructure of these perivascular leptomeningeal protrusions does not differ from that of the Paccionian granulations and, therefore, they have been interpreted in favor of a site of CSF outflow [3]. Paravascular leptomeningeal protrusions have yet not been shown by electron microscopy in the dural sheath of cranial nerves, but according to our results their existance is probably. These structures should form the anatomical basis for a perineural CSF outflow similar to the pressure depending bulk flow of CSF through the arachnoid villi (fig.2).

The dense networks of lymphatic channels in the skull base indicate an important biological role of the lymphatic CSF outflow pathways. The existance of those vessels has to be considered in tracer studies attempting to estimate that fraction of CSF which drains into the lymphatic system.

It is concluded that lymphatic CSF outflow pathways should be more important than suggested so far.

LITERATURE:

[1] EHRLICH, S. S., MCCOMB, J. G., HYMAN, S. & WEISS, M. H. (1986). Ultrastructure morphology of the olfactory pathway for cerebrospinal fluid drainage in the rabbit. *J Neurosurg* **64**, 466-473.

[2] EHRLICH, S. S., MCCOMB, J. G., HYMAN, S. & WEISS, M. H. (1989). Ultrastructure of the orbital pathway for cerebrospinal fluid drainage in rabbits.. *J Neurosurg* **70**, 926-931.

[3] KRISCH B, (1988). Ultrastructure of the meninges at the site of penetration of veins through the dura mater, with particular reference to Paccionian granulations. Investigations in the rat and two species of New-World monkeys. *Cell Tissue Res.* **251**, 621-631.

[4] MC COMB, J. G. (1983). Recent research into the nature of cerebrospinal fluid formation and absorption. *J.Neurosurg.* **59**, 369-383.

ACKNOWLEDGEMENTS:
This work is supported in part by the Deutsche Forschungsgemeinschaft (Grant No. Br 1416/1-1).

Morphological Aspects of Interstitial Fluid Drainage from the Rat Brain

S. Kida[1], Y. Okamoto[1], S. Higashi[1], K. Futami[1], T. Yamashima[1], J. Yamashita[1], and R.O. Weller[2]

[1] Department of Neurosurgery, Kanazawa University School of Medicine, Kanazawa, Japan
[2] Department of Neuropathology, School of Medicine, University of Southampton, Southampton, UK

SUMMARY

There is firm physiological evidence for the lymphatic drainage of interstitial fluid from the brain of experimental animals. Studies using tracers have demonstrated that a significant fraction of fluid in the brain drains into deep cervical lymph nodes within a short time. To define morphological aspects of such pathways, 2 µl of Indian ink were injected into the rat caudoputamen over a period of 60 min using an infusion pump. The distribution of the ink as it spread from the site of injection was documented by 2 mm thick slices of brain and skull base, and by decalcified paraffin sections. Interstitial fluid of the ink spread diffusely through the white matter and appeared to drain into the ventricular cerebrospinal fluid. In gray matter, Indian ink passed along perivascular spaces to the surface of the brain and into the subarachnoid cerebrospinal fluid. Indian ink particles were accumulated in the paravascular compartments around subarachnoid blood vessels which followed the course of branches of the middle cerebral artery to the circle of Willis and thence, along the nasal-olfactory arteries toward the cribriform plate. Carbon particles in the subarachnoid space beneath the olfactory bulbs entered discrete channels which passed through the arachnoid and holes in the cribriform plate then, connected directly with lymphatics in the nasal submucosa. This study demonstrates the direct drainage of interstitial and cerebrospinal fluid through anatomically defined pathways into deep cervical lymph nodes. Such pathways are compatible with the observed rapidity of the bulk flow drainage of fluid in the rat brain.

INTRODUCTION

Drainage of cerebrospinal fluid (CSF) and interstitial fluid from the brain into deep cervical lymph nodes has been well documented in a number of mammalian species for over a century[1]. Physiological studies using a variety of tracers have demonstrated that a significant fraction (14-47%) of CSF drains into deep cervical lymph nodes [2]. However, the exact anatomical connections between the subarachnoid space and the nasal lymphatics are still obscure.

Erlich et al. [3] proposed that macromolecules pass from the subarachnoid space into olfactory perineural spaces in the rabbit and then diffuse to nasal lymphatics through submucosal connective tissue. Yamazumi et al. [4], on the other hand, demonstrated that Indian ink injected into the cisterna magna in the rabbit reached the cervical lymph nodes within 1 min. Yamazumi's observations suggest that there may be a more direct pathway for the drainage of CSF than by diffusion through the nasal mucosa.

In the present study, we test the hypothesis that there is a direct connection between the cranial subarachnoid space and nasal lymphatics which would facilitate the observed rapid and high flow lymphatic drainage of interstitial fluid and CSF from the brain. The aim of the present study, therefore, is to review the distribution of tracers (Indian ink) injected into the rat brain.

MATERIALS AND METHODS

A total of 30 male Wistar rats weighing 200 g were used in this study. The animals were anesthetized with a mixture of nitrous oxide/oxygen (70%:30%) containing 1.5% halothane. Animals were placed in a stereotactic frame and a burr hole was made at 2.5 mm lateral to the bregma, this site was calculated for injection into the caudoputamen. The arachnoid mater was perforated and CSF was allowed to flow out for 5 min. A 30 gauge needle was inserted vertically through the burr hole to a depth of 3 mm and 2 µl of Indian ink suspension (Rotring, Germany; 20-50 nm particle size) were injected over a period of 60 min using an infusion pump (Harverd, USA). The needle was then withdrawn, the burr hole closed with bone wax, and the skin sutured.

Except for 10 animals killed within 30 min after injection, animals were subsequently anesthetized and killed by intracardiac perfusion with 10% buffered formalin at 6 h (10 animals) or 24 h (10 animals) following the injection.

The head and neck regions were removed *en bloc* at the cervico-thoracic junction and the skin was stripped. These specimens were further fixed by immersion in 10% buffered formalin for 3 days and decalcified by immersion in 5% nitric acid for 3 days. Each specimen of skull base and brain was cut coronally into 2 mm slices. Half the specimens of skull and brain from each time point were dehydrated and embedded in paraffin wax. Sections (5 µm) were cut in coronal and stained with hematoxylin and eosin. The rest of the specimens were dehydrated in alcohol, cleared in cedar wood oil and examined by transillumination with a stereoscopic microscope.

RESULTS

Within 30 min of the injection of Indian ink into the caudoputamen, the peripheral regions of the deep cervical lymph nodes on both sides turned black in all animals examined. Light microscopy confirmed that carbon particles were present in the marginal sinuses of the deep cervical lymph nodes.

The distinct subarachnoid pathways of drainage for the tracer were seen on the surface of the rat brain. Indian ink passed in broad channels besides branches of the middle cerebral artery towards the base of the brain. Some pooling of the ink occurred near the circle of Willis, just lateral to the optic chiasm but a thin line of ink extended forwards towards the undersurface of the olfactory bulbs and there is well-marked paravascular blackening along the nasal-olfactory artery. Examination of the skull base revealed Indian ink accumulation above the cribriform plate. This demonstrates a highly selective, directional flow of Indian ink from the base of the brain (Fig. 1).

In 2 mm slices of brain and skull cleared in cedar wood oil, Indian ink could be seen distributed along the base of the brain. The only pathway by which Indian ink was observed leaving the subarachnoid space in these specimens was through the nasal mucosa. In three-dimensional views with the stereoscopic microscope, many thin channels were outlined by Indian ink, originating at the cribriform plate and spreading through the nasal mucosa. Carbon particles were also seen in the subarachnoid space of the optic nerve but extended no further than the orbital end of the optic nerve; no lymphatic drainage of carbon from this area was seen. No carbon particles were found along any other cranial nerves; in particular, no carbon particles were associated with the fifth or eighth cranial nerves once they had left the subarachnoid space.

Light microscopic study revealed the perivascular spread of Indian ink in the gray matter of the caudoputamen and the cortex. Particles of ink were detected mainly around arteries and veins but small amounts were also seen around capillaries. In the white matter, the ink had spread diffusely between nerve fibers and had extended into the lateral ventricles. In low power views of the cribriform plate and the nasal mucosa, ink was seen widely distributed in channels in the submucosa. At higher power, tortuous channels containing Indian ink were identified passing from the subarachnoid space, through the cribriform plate, often, but not always, alongside olfactory nerves and into the nasal submucosa. These thin-walled channels are most likely to be lymphatics as in the occasional poorly perfused animal, blood was seen in the blood vessels in the submucosa but none was seen in the carbon-containing vessels.

DISCUSSION

From the results of the present study and those of previous studies [5,6,7,8,9,10], it is now possible to suggest an anatomical pathway for the drainage of interstitial fluid from the brain to lymph nodes under physiological and pathological conditions.

Tracers injected into the gray matter of the rat brain pass along perivascular pathways which are in direct continuity with perivascular compartments of meningeal arteries[5]. It is probable that fluid and tracers pass through the meningeal coatong of vessels into compartments of the subarachnoid space that form paravascular pathways of nasal-olfactory artery to the cribriform plate. Tracers, such as Indian ink, then pass in channels, through the cribriform plate into nasal lymphatics and to deep cervical lymph nodes.

Previous studies in experimental animals[11] have emphasized the possible routes of lymphatic drainage from the subarachnoid space surrounding the optic nerve. Such studies suggest that soluble markers and small particles such as ferritin enter cervical lymph nodes via this route. Although there is no evidence that carbon particles escaped from the subarachnoid space into the lymphatics by this route, passage of smaller molecules and particles by the optic route cannot be excluded.

Our finding that direct channels connect the subarachnoid space to nasal lymphatics correlates well with the observed physiological and immunological characteristics of lymphatic drainage from the brain in the number of experimental animal species[2]. The well-developed direct channels found in the rat would serve a high flow, lymphatic drainage from the rat brain.

Furthermore, lymphocytes and macrophages may also drain from the brain by this route, as it has been reported that lymphocytes, macrophages and erythrocytes injected into the central nervous system accumulate in deep cervical lymph nodes. In pathological brains, macrophages and lymphocytes typically accumulate in perivascular spaces[1]. It seems, therefore, that both the perivascular space in the brain and paravascular compartments in the subarachnoid space might be equivalent to lymphatics in other organs of the body.

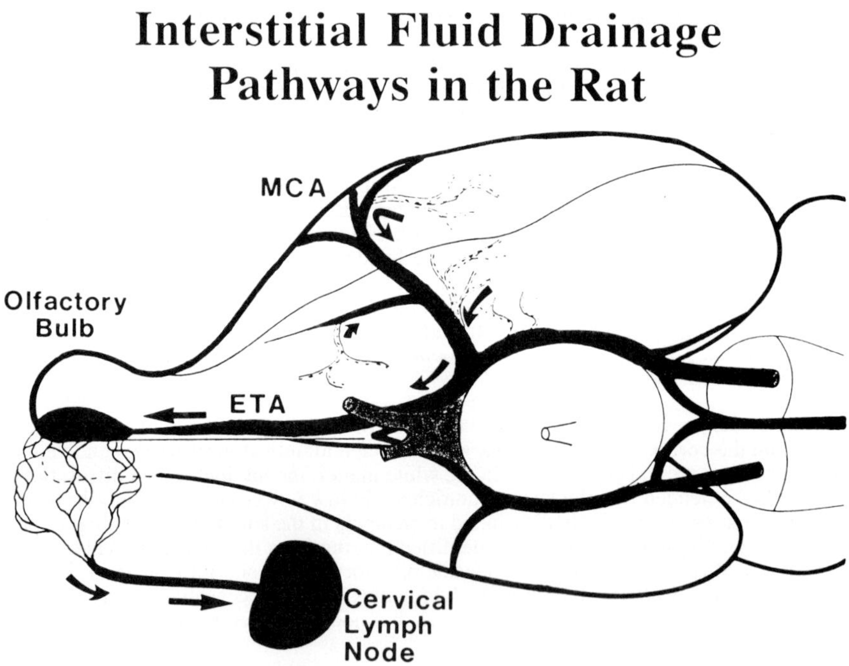

Fig. 1 Interstitial fluid drainage pathways from the rat brain to cervical lymph nodes. Interstitial fluid in the gray matter passes along perivascular spaces which are in direct continuity with paravascular compartments of subarachnoid arteries. The fluid goes along branches of the middle cerebral arteries to the circle of Willis. The fluid further passes along paravascular pathways of the nasal-olfactory (or ethomoidal) artery on the undersurface of the olfactory bulb. Through direct channels via the cribriform plate, the fluid finally drains into nasal lymphatics and deep cervical lymph nodes.

REFERENCES

1 Weller RO, Kida S, Zhang ET (1992) Pathways of fluid drainage from the brain: Morphological aspects and immunological significance in rat and man. Brain Pathol 2:277-284
2. Cserr HF, Harling-Berg CJ, Knopf PM (1992) Drainage of brain extracellular fluid into blood and deep cervical lymph and its immunological significance. Brain Pathol 2: 269-276
3. Erlich SS, McComb JG, Hymann S, Weiss MH (1986) Ultrastructural morphology of the olfactory pathway for cerebrospinal fluid drainage in the rabbit. J Neurosurg 64: 466-473
4. Yamazumi H (1989) Infiltration of Indian ink from subarachnoid space to nasal mucosa along olfactory nerves in rabbit. Nippon Jibiinkoka Gakkai Kaiho 92:608-616
5. Zhang ET, Inman CBE, Weller RO (1990) Interrelationships of the pia mater and perivascular (Virchow-Robin) spaces in the human cerebrum. J Anat 170: 111-123
6. Zhang ET, Richards HK, Kida S, Weller RO (1992) Directional and compartmentalized drainage of interstitial fluid and cerebrospinal fluid from the rat brain. Acta Neuropathol 83: 233-239
7. Kida S, Steart PV, Zhang ET, Weller RO (1993) Perivascular cells act as scavengers in the cerebral perivascular spaces and remain distinct from pericytes, microglia and macrophages. Acta Neuropathol 85: 646-652
8. Kida S, Weller RO (1993) Morphological basis for fluid transport in and around ependymal, arachnoidal and glial cells. In: Raimondi AJ (ed) Principles of pediatric neurosurgery: Intracranial cystic lesions. Springer-Verlag, New York, pp37-52
9. Kida S, Pantazis A, Weller RO (1993) CSF drains directly from the subarachnoid space into nasal lymphatics in the rat: Anatomy, histology and immunological significance. Neuropathol Appl Neurobiol 19: 480-488
10. Kida S, Ellison DW, Steart PV, Iannotti F, Weller RO (1994) Perivascular edema fluid pathway in astrocytic tumors. Acta Neurochir 60: 384-386
11. Erlich SS, McComb JG, Hymann S, Weiss MH (1989) Ultrastructure of the orbital pathway for cerebrospinal fluid drainage in rabbits. J Neurosurg 70: 926-931

Quantitative Analysis of CSF Dynamics in Patients with Benign Intracranial Hypertension

S.S. Gasparian[1], A.Y. Razumovsky[2], A.R. Shakchnovitch[1], A.A. Tumanova[1], and N.A. Vladimirova[1]

[1] Burdenko Neurosurgical Institute, Moscow, Russia
[2] Johns Hopkins Medical Institutions, Baltimore, USA

SUMMARY

The syndrome of BIH is manifested by papilloedema, raised intracranial pressure with normal or low range of protein concentration in cerebrospinal fluid, absence of neurological deficits and ventriculomegaly on computerized tomography [1,2]
The evolution of BIH leads to visual deficits up to blindness. 75 adult patients were investigated by standard neurological examination, CT and CPIT. We found elevation of P csf in 99% of patients, raised R in 82% of patients, elevation of El in 61% of patients. Pis in 8 patients was slightly increased in one case and was normal range in others. The production of CSF was normal.
The correlation analysis between clinical findings, CT data and parameters of CSF dynamics showed the relations, which confirmed the important role of raised R , El and PVO in evolution of clinical signs of BIH syndrome.

INTRODUCTION

The clinical manifestation of BIH syndrome may be caused by disturbances of CSF or venous outflow [1,2]. Our previous investions found the elevation of Pcsf,R and El in patients with syndrome of BIH, but it possible correlations between clinical criterias, CT data and quantitative parameters of CSF dynamics were not estimated.
The aim of our study was to determine changes in characteristics of CSF dynamics and to analies possible correlations between them and clinical signs in patients with syndrome of BIH.

MATERIAL AND METHODS

The study was carried out in 75 adult patients (61 women and 14 men, aged 17-66 years). They were examined using standard neurological method with computerized tomography and CPIT [3,4] in order to determine Pcsf, R, El, Pis, F, PVO, VI, PO (by quantitative papillometric method), POD, VF. Correlation analysis between these characteristics was performed.

1 Abbreviations. BIH-benign intracranial hypertension; Pcsf-cerebrospinal fluid pressure; R-outflow resistance; El-elastance of the brain; CPIT-constant pressure infusion test.

RESULTS

As a result of our study we found the following changes: raised Pcsf, which was increased in 75% of patients (average 23,7 mmHg range 18-30 mmHg), in 13 patients Pcsf was more than 30 mm Hg and in one case 49,5 mmHg.

R was increased in 82% of patients (average 27,6 mmHg/ml/min-1 range 12,9-116 mmHg/ml/min-1). In 3 patients R was more than 100 mmHg/ml/min-1; 12 patients had normal R. El was increased in 46 patients (average 1,03 ml-1 range 0,6-1,82 ml-1). In 29 cases we found normal El. Pis was determined in 8 cases and in 7 of them this parameter was normal and in one case Pis =14 mmHg. F was in normal range (0,2-0,6 ml-1).

Correlation analysis between clinical characteristics, CT data and parameters of CSF dynamics showed the following:

Pcsf and PO : $r=0,4$ $p<0,01$; Pcsf and POD: $r=0,3$ $p<0,02$;
R and POD : $r=0,3$ $p<0,02$; R and VI : $r=-0,2$ $p<0,05$;
El and PVO : $r=0,2$ $p<0,02$; VF and PO : $r=0,2$ $p<0,05$.

DISCUSSION

The obtained data may be inetrpreted as a confirmation of the wide possibilities of compensative capacity of cerebrospinal system in evolution of severe intracranial hypertension.

Increased R as a result of inflammatory and adhesive processes in arachnoid cover leads to disturbances of CSF and venous outflow. It causes increased cerebral blood volume and not rarely associates with periventricular oedema, that leads to raised El and decreased ventricular size. We suppose, that raised El may be caused not only by disturbances of CSF outflow, but more lightly by disorders of venous outflow at the level of arachnoid cover,bridging veins and the venous circulation of the brain.

These changes lead to decrease of compensative capacity of cerebrospinal system and clinical manifestation of the syndrome of BIH with increased Pcsf and papilloedema, that will be resulted in decreased VF.

We support the hypothesis about important role of CSF disorders, venous outflow failures in genesis of the BIH syndrome. But the role of endocrinological disorders and possible hyperproduction of CSF is not very clear (we have measured F only for 8 patient).

We are sure, that it will be possible to answer these questions in future to improve the results of conservative therapy and shunting operations in patients with the syndrome of BIH.

REFERENCES

2 Abbreviations. CPIT-constant pressure infusion test; Pis-intrasinus pressure; F-rate of production; PVO-periventricular oedema; VI-bicaudate ventricular index for anterior horns; PO-degree of papilloedema; POD-duration of papilloedema; VF-degree of visual function.

1.Janny P.,Chazal J.,ColnetG.,DevoizeJ.L.,Baretto L.L.(1981) L'hypertension intracranienne benigne. Etude clinique, physiopathologique et nosographique. Neurochirurgie,27:79-88.
2 Johnston I.,Paterson A.,Besser M.(1981) The treatment of benign intracranial hypertension: a review of 134 cases. Surg.Neurol.16:218-224.
3. Portnoy H.D.,Croysant P.D.(1976) A practical method for measuring hydrodynamics of cerebrospinal fluid. Surgical Neurology v 5,5,273-277.
4. Szevzykovsky E.,Shakchnovich A.R.,Konovalov A.N.,Tomas D.G.,Korsak-Sliwka, Dubova S.B.,Kunicky A.,Sliwka S, Milovanova L.S.(1983) Using of computer estimation for intensive care of the patients in neurosurgical clinic. Voprosy neurochirurgii 3, 7-16 (in russian).

Session VIII: Effects of Increased ICP (2)

Chairmen: R.M. Bullock and H. Kanaya

Waveform Analysis of Blood Pressure, Intracranial Pressure and Transcranial Doppler Signals and Their Relationship to Cerebral Perfusion Pressure in Head Injured Patients

F.C. Wong, I.R. Piper, and J.D. Miller

Department of Clinical Neurosciences, University of Edinburgh, Western General Hospital, Edinburgh, UK

INTRODUCTION

The use of non-invasive methods of monitoring like transcranial doppler sonography (TCD) has definite advantages in head injured patients. Previous work in our department had demonstrated that cerebral perfusion pressure (CPP) has a defined relationship to the pulsatility index (PI) of the middle cerebral artery (MCA) flow velocity waveform (1). This paper examines the potential uses of an on-line computerised analysis system of the intracranial pressure (ICP), blood pressure (BP) and TCD waveforms. The main aim was to define in patients the threshold for the treatment of reduced CPP and hence reduce the incidence of secondary insults in the injured brain.

MATERIALS AND METHODS

Patients admitted to the intensive care unit with head injuries severe enough to require ICP monitoring and assisted ventilation were studied. Multiple physiological parameters were monitored continuously including BP, ICP, and in some patients, jugular venous oxygen saturation (Sjo2). TCD monitoring was carried out continuously by fixing the doppler probe to the patient's temporal region using a velcro headband. Simultaneous sampling of corresponding pulses of BP, ICP and TCD signals with signal averaging were carried out and their derived parameters from waveform analysis displayed on computer in real time. Patients were monitored for several hours if required, under various physiological conditions and therapeutic manoeuvres for reduced CPP. The relationship between CPP and PI and other derived parameters were examined.

RESULTS

Waveform analysis data were obtained from fourteen patients monitored during spontaneous and treatment induced periods of changing CPP. There were a total of twenty recording episodes which generated about 3100 data points.

It was possible to demonstrate a relationship between CPP and PI and between CPP and the other waveform analysis derived parameters for eg. the fundamental transfer function from BP to ICP (Xfra). Using a sequential analysis of variance, a breakpoint near 63 mmHg of CPP could be demonstrated for the grouped data when PI was plotted against CPP (fig.1). However, this form of continuous on-line analysis could also demonstrate the breakpoint value to differ between patients and to change within the same patient on different days by at least 10mmHg of CPP. A breakpoint could be demonstrated only when a sufficient range of CPP was encountered during the monitoring periods.

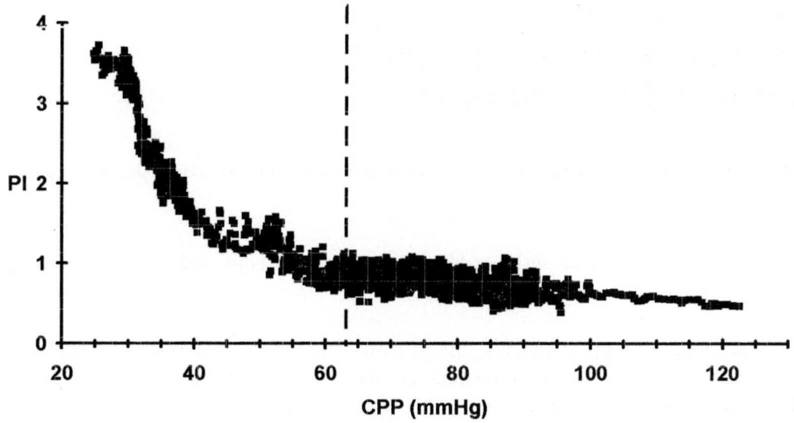

Fig.1 Graph of pulsatility index (PI) plotted against cerebral perfusion pressure (CPP) for the total grouped data. The CPP breakpoint value (dotted line) was estimated to be at around 63 mmHg by sequential analysis of variance.

In the individual patient, plotting the Xfra against CPP could also demonstrate the breakpoint at a similar CPP value when compared to the breakpoint value of PI plotted against CPP. There was good correlation between the PI and transfer function data in 17 out of the 20 recording episodes. Limited data from jugular venous oxygen saturation monitoring supports the presumption that these CPP breakpoint values may represent the lower limit of autoregulation in these head injured patients.

DISCUSSION

We have demonstrated that CPP breakpoint values can be determined by other waveform parameters besides the PI of the MCA flow velocity waveform. Simultaneous monitoring of BP, ICP and TCD signals can help to determine the minimum values above which patients' CPP should be maintained. Such a continuous monitoring system can "tailor" the CPP management thresholds to the individual patient.

REFERENCE

1. Chan KH, Miller JD, Dearden NM, Andrews PAJ, Midgley S (1992) The effect of changes in cerebral perfusion pressure upon middle cerebral artery flow velocity and jugular bulb venous oxygen saturation after severe brain injury. J Neurosurg 77:55-61,

Can TCD Pulsatility Indices Be Used for a Non-Invasive Assessment of Cerebral Perfusion Pressure in Head Injured Patients?

M. Czosnyka, P. Kirkpatrick, E. Guazzo, P. Smielewski, H. Whitehouse, and J.D. Pickard

MRC Cambridge Centre for Brain Repair and Academic Neurosurgical Unit, Addenbrooke's Hospital, Cambridge, UK

Pulse waveform of Transcranial Doppler (TCD) blood flow velocity depends on the magnitude of arterial blood pressure pulsations and the hydrodynamic conditions affecting blood flow: the geometry of cerebrovascular bed, vascular resistance, elasticity of compliant walls, viscosity of blood and many other factors. Among various indices describing pulse waveform of blood velocity the so called Gosling's Pulsatility Index (PI= peak-to-peak pulse amplitude divided by mean flow velocity) is one of the most frequently used. The authors are well aware that PI cannot be regarded as a function of cerebrovascular resistance (CVR). This can be demonstrated by the adverse effect of hypercapnia, when CVR and PI decrease and systemic hypotension when CVR decreases but PI increases.
Our aim was to study the correlation between TCD pulsatility indices and measured CPP to assess the accuracy of possible non-invasive estimation of CPP using TCD waveform analysis. This methodology was presented for the first time by Aaslid [1] but still awaits clinical validation.

MATERIAL AND METHOD

We studied 42 severely head injured patients with a mean Glasgow Coma Scale of 6 on admission. They were all sedated and ventilated and had ICP and systemic arterial blood pressure (ABP) monitored continuously. The blood flow velocity in the middle cerebral artery was recorded daily for periods of 15 to 120 mins. A hundred and ninety-three computer recordings (3800 minutes) of ICP, ABP and FV waveforms were analysed. Signals were sampled and subjected to spectral analysis to calculate the amplitudes of the fundamental (ICPa, ABPa and FVa relatively) and higher harmonics of pulse waveforms.
The following indices of TCD pulsatility were considered:
a. Gosling's Pulsatility Index (PI)
b. Spectral Pulsatility Index: PIs = FVa/FVmean,
c. Standardised Pulsatility Index: SPI= PIs/ABPa.
Calculation of the SPI allows change in TCD pulsatility that are not a result of changes in pulse wave of ABP to be detected. (correlation between ABPa and FVa was strong, $r=0.601$; $p<0.00001$).
One-minute average values were taken to evaluate the relationships between selected indices and cerebral perfusion pressure (CPP=ABP-ICP) using ANOVA or analysis of regression (Statgraphics +, Manugistics, USA)

RESULTS AND DISCUSSION

The relationship between mean FV and CPP was of bi-phasic character. For CPPs above 55 mmHg FV was not correlated to CPP ($r=-0.0289$, $p<0.35$). Below this threshold FV decreased when CPP was decreasing ($r=0.377$; $p<0.00001$). This was mainly due to decreaseing diastolic FV ($r=0.601$; $p<0.000001$). Systolic FV was stable even for low CPPs ($r=0.0012$; $p<0.451$). Increasing divergence between flow velocity systolic and diastolic caused an increase in FVa with CPP decerasing.

This steady increase was noticed even for relatively high CPPs (above 60 mmHg, r=-0.323; p<0.00001). As a result of the gradual increase in FV amplitude (or peak-to-peak pulse) and decreases in FV, PI and PIs were steadily increasing with decreasing CPP (r around -0.60; p<0.001). Because the amplitude of ABP was decreasing significantly with CPP (r=0.648; p<0.0001), SPI was more convergent increasing when CPP was falling (r=-0.702; p<0.00001)- see Fig.1.

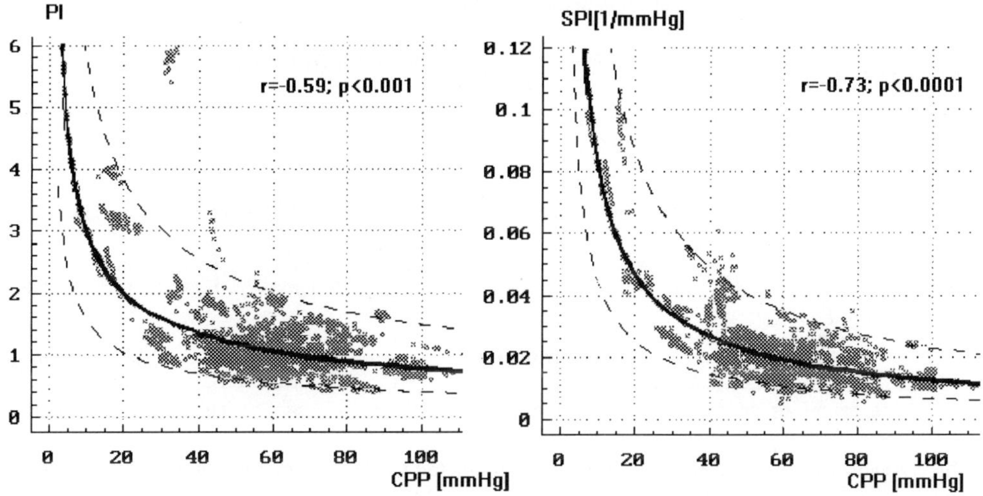

Fig.1 Relationship between Gosling's Pulsatility Index (PI) and Standardised Pulsatility Index (SPI) and CPP in 42 head injured patients. Correlation coefficients were highest for the inverse model (y=1/(ax+b)) for both variables.

Good correlation between SPI and CPP in a heterogeneous group of head injured patients facilitated the use of this parameter for non invasive estimation of CPP. ANOVA showed a good convergence of mean estimated (CPPe= 1/SPI) and real CPP (p <0.00001) - see Fig.2. However, the regression analysis demonstrated that predictive power of CPPe was still small. The correlation coefficient between predicted and measured CPP was not sufficiently high for accurate predictions: r=0.601; p<0.001 with the wide 95% confidence limit for predictors (+/- 30 mmHg). Analysis of variance of CPP versus CPPe showed two distinct relationships: For low CPP (below 40 mmHg) the correlation coefficient between CPP and CPPe was r=0.77, with a 90% confidence limit for predictors less than 12 mmHg. For very low CPP (below 30 mmHg) the correlation coefficient increased to 0.936 with a 90% confidence limit for predictors of only 5 mmHg. For CPPs above 50 mmHg the confidence limit for predictors increased to above 20 mmHg. On average, CPPe was lower than real CPP (p<0.001), with a mean difference of 7 mmHg and standard deviation of 17 mmHg. Measurement of CPPe requires the direct monitoring of arterial blood pressure and computer analysis of ABP and FV waveforms. It would be convenient to replace direct ABP by cuff measurement of systolic/diastolic pressure and Gosling's PI. The modified formulae would be: CPPg= ABPsystolic-diastolic / PI. The correlation between CPPg and CPPe was quite high (r=0.792, p<0.0001). CPPg was statistically lower than CPPe. Correlation coefficient between CPPg and CPP was not worse than for CPPe (r=0.601; p<0.0001). However, CPPg did not indicate better predictive power than CPPe.

However, even with the limited accuracy the non-invasive CPP assessment may be still useful in specific conditions:

A. The correlation coefficient between CPPe and real CPP increases to $r=0.882$; $p<0.001$, if the spectral pulsatility index is higher than 0.9. Similarly correlation between CPPg and CPP is $r=0.87$; $p<0.0001$ if PI exceeds 1.5. Therefore the practical application of a non-invasive assessment of CPP would be: If after TCD examination PI is higher than 1.5, real CPP is higher than the peak-to-peak ABP divided by PI. Therefore, CPPg is helpful in limiting the possible range of CPP.
B. CPPe or CPPg are useful for deteotion of dynamic changes in CPP. In 23 recordings, when CPP was varying by more than +/- 10 mmHg, CPPe was correlated to real CPP better than $r=0.9$, $p<0.0001$. This dynamic correlation is demonstrated in Fig.3

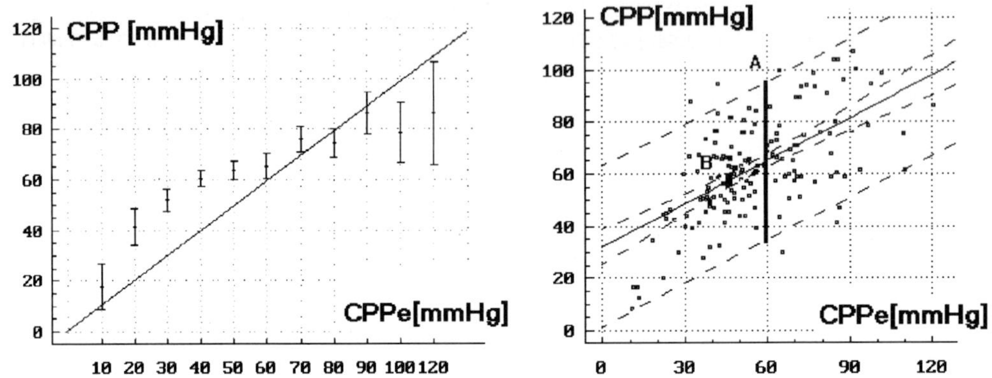

Fig.2 Analysis of variance of real CPP versus predicted CPPe (left graph) shows that relationship is not ideally linear. For CPPs below 60 mmHg the CPPe underestimates the real CPP. Analysis of regression (right graph) demonstrates that 95% confidence limits for means is less than 10 mmHg (section B) for the middle range of CPPs. However 95% confidence limits for predictors (section A) is about +/- 30 mmHg, demonstrating a poor predictive power of CPPe.

Fig.3 Example of continuous recording of ICP, CPP and TCD flow velocity during plateau wave of ICP in head injury. Both predictors of CPP: CPPe and CPPg were well correlated to real CPP ($r=0.96$; $p<0.00001$). X axis-time in minutes.

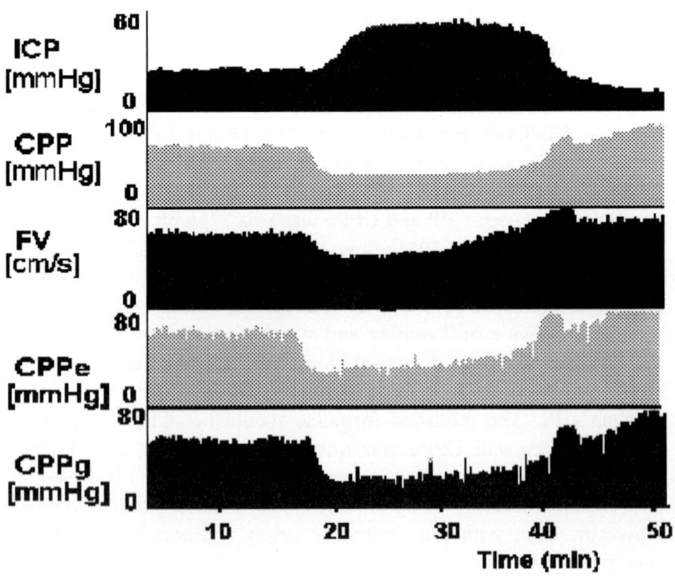

C. Estimated CPP correlates to outcome. Patients were divided according to Glasgow Outcome Score to three groups: I- good and moderate outcome (n=20), II -severe disability (n=11) and III- persistent vegetative state or dead (n=11). Significant difference in correlation coefficients between CPP and CPPe was found (I: r= 0.242, p<0.01; II: r=0.66, p<0.0001; III: r=0.791, p<0.0001). Therefore, the good convergence of CPPe to real CPP may be considered as a predictor of poor outcome. This finding was not surprising, because all pulsatility indices were found (see Table) to increase with worse outcome.

Table. Mean values of TCD pulsatility indices in different outcome groups (I-good and moderate, II- severe disability, III- PVS and dead). * and ** denote statistically significant difference between different groups (p<0.05).

	Group I	Group II	Group III
PI	1.18	1.35	1.78*
PIs	0.51	0.64*	0.93**
SPI [1/mmHg]	0.019	0.020	0. 026 *

CONCLUSION

In conclusion, the method of non-invasive assessment of CPP by TCD pulsatility indices is not accurate. However, in cases of increased PI (>1.5) the estimated CPP may be taken as a measure of real cerebral perfusion pressure. The method seems to be sufficiently accurate to detect dynamic changes in CPP. Good correlation between estimated and real CPP is a bad prognostic for outcome.

REFERENCES

1. Aaslid R, Lundar T, Lindegaard KF, Nornes H (1986) Estimation of Cerebral Perfusion Pressure from Arterial Blood Pressure and Transcranial Doppler Recordings. In: Miller JD, Teasdale GM, Rowan JO, Galbraith SL, Mendelow AD (eds) Intracranial Pressure VI. Springer-Verlag Berlin Heidelberg, pp 226-229

Intracranial Blood Flow Velocity After Minor Head Injury in Children: A Transcranial Doppler Ultrasound Study

S.C.P. NG, K.H. CHAN, K.N. HUNG, Y.W. FAN, and C.F. FUNG

Division of Neurosurgery, Department of Surgery, The University of Hong Kong, Queen Mary Hospital, Hong Kong

INTRODUCTION

Transcranial Doppler ultrasonography (TCD) enables noninvasive and repetitive measurement of blood flow velocity of the major basal intracranial arteries. Since flow velocity is proportional to the ratio of cerebral blood flow (CBF) to the cross-sectional area of blood vessel examined, changes in flow velocity may occur in association with alterations in CBF or vessel diameter. TCD can therefore provide a means of monitoring changes in the cerebral circulation. Blood flow velocity changes had been well documented after severe, moderate and minor head injury in adult [2]. Whether changes also occur after head injury in children is unknown. The aim of this study is to define the relationships between blood flow velocity and age, and time after head injury in children.

PATIENTS AND METHODS

From March 1993 to February 1994, 106 patients (74 males and 32 females; mean age 6.1 years, range: 1 month to 15 years) with minor head injury defined as admission Glasgow Coma Score of 13 to 15 points were included in the study. All patients had computerised tomography scanning to define the brain pathology.

Blood flow velocity of at least both middle cerebral arteries (MCA) was determined as soon as possible after admission according to the method described by Aaslid [1]. TCD examination was performed daily during hospitalisation and at two weeks after discharge using the same window and depth for each patient. The highest time-averaged mean flow velocity was chosen for recording.

TCD examinations were performed on 25 normal control (16 males and 9 females; mean age 7.3 years, range: 4 months to 15 years) without past history of brain pathology to establish the normal values of blood flow velocity in children. Increased blood flow velocity was defined as velocity above 120cm/second.

Previous study showed that the incidence of intracranial complications occurring after head injury varied according to the developmental skull changes in children, patients could be divided into four age ranges: (I) <2 years, (II) 2-6 years, (III) 7-10 years and (IV) 11-15 years of age [4]. We first analysed our data in all patients and then according to this classification. Statistical analyses were by t-test, significance was taken at 5% level.

RESULTS

There was no significant side to side difference in right and left MCA velocity in normal control and in our patients at different time periods, the average of the two velocities was used for analysis.

In all 106 patients, there was no significant change in MCA velocity from normal at different time period during hospitalisation and at two weeks after discharge. When analysis was performed in relation to developmental skull changes and the 106 patients were subdivided into 4 age groups, the following results were obtained:

Group I (n=25): admission velocity, 90.0 (83.7, 96.3)cm/s (mean (95% confidence limits)) was not significantly different from the normal value, 89.5 (81.6, 93.6)cm/s of the group (Fig.1). Velocity 97.57 (90.0, 105.1)cm/s increased and was significantly higher than normal by day 1 and reached a maximum of 99.88 (94.7, 105.0)cm/s by day 2. Velocity then returned to normal afterwards. Increased velocity above 120cm/s was noted in three patients and they all had bilateral velocity elevation.

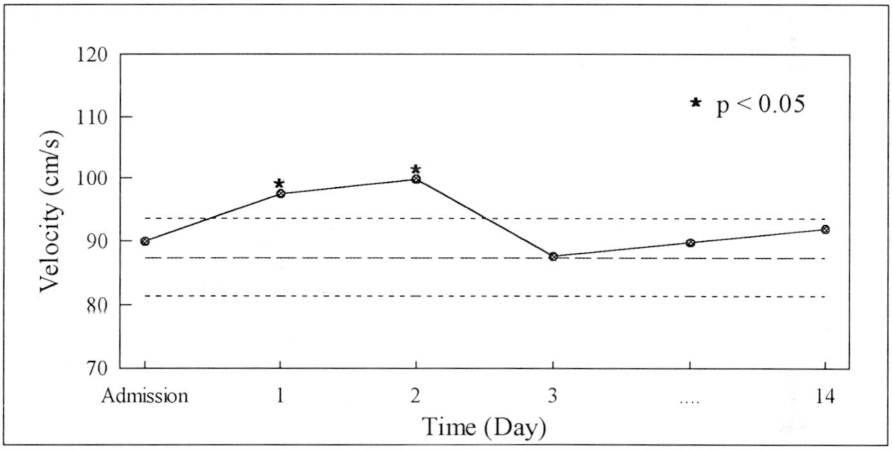

Fig. 1 Plot of velocity against time in group I patients (dotted lines represent the mean and 95% confidence limits of normal value of the group)

Group II (n=34): velocity on admission, 97.3 (91.6, 102.8)cm/s and on day 1, 98.12 (92.5, 103.8)cm/s were significantly below normal 109.1 (99.5, 118.7)cm/s of the group. Velocity returned back to normal afterwards.

Group III (n=27): admission velocity, 92.9 (86.7, 99.0)cm/s was significantly below normal of 104.1 (94.5, 113.7)cm/s. Velocity remained normal at other time period during hospitalisation and at discharge.

Group IV (n=20): admission velocity, 78.05 (73.1, 83.0)cm/s was not significantly different from normal, 82.9 (77.3, 88.6)cm/s (Fig. 2). Velocity on day 1, 91.1 (86.3, 95.9)cm/s was significantly

Two patients had velocity increase above 120cm/s. They all had unilateral MCA velocity elevation. One patient with unilateral MCA velocity increase had persistent hemiparesis of the side of the body contralateral to the site of velocity elevation.

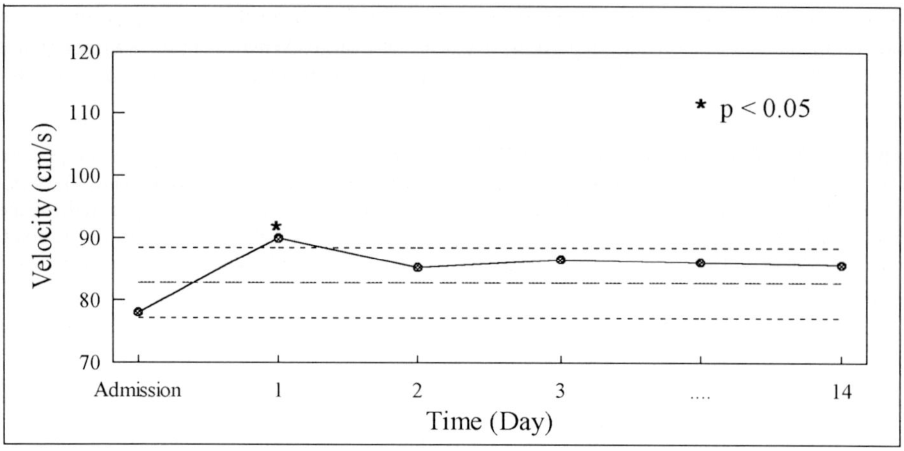

Fig. 2 Plot of velocity against time in group IV patients (dotted lines represent the mean and 95% confidence limits of normal value of the group)

In our patients with unilateral velocity increase, there was a notch noted at diastole, which was absent in those patients with bilateral MCA velocity elevation (Fig. 3).

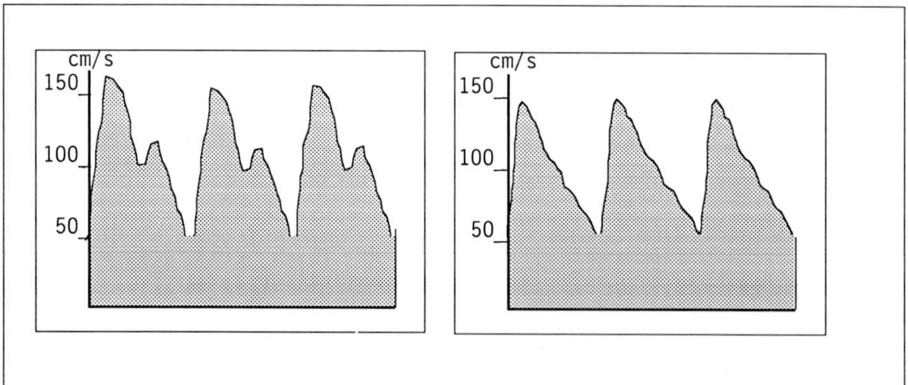

(i) Unilateral velocity increase (ii) Bilateral velocity increase

Fig. 3 (i) Diagram showing unilateral velocity increase doppler waveform with a notch at diastole. (ii) Diagram showing bilateral velocity increase doppler

DISCUSSION

Our results showed that the paediatric population was not a homogenous group after they sustained head injury. Velocity changes observed in the different age groups suggested that alterations in cerebral circulation occurred even after minor head injury in children. This is in accord with observations in adult [2]. Chan et al found that after head injury in adult, velocity decreased in severe, moderate and minor head injury. The most significant decrease was noted in the severe injury group. Decreased velocity on admission in our patients was observed only in group II and III (3-10 years). This may be a result of differences in pathology in the various groups.

High flow velocity may be due to the occurrence of post-traumatic increase of CBF (cerebral hyperaemia) or narrowing (vasospasm) of the major cerebral arteries [3]. These changes probably played a major role in the peaking of flow velocity observed in group I and IV patients. Previous study has shown that bilateral MCA velocity increase and absence of a notch at diastole in the velocity waveform were found in hyperaemic patients, whereas, cases with possible vasospasm had unilateral MCA velocity elevation and a notch at diastole in the doppler waveform [3]. These similar observations together with the neurological deficit developed which was relevant to the side with increased velocity suggested that unilateral velocity increase may represent vasospasm and bilateral velocity elevation may indicate hyperaemia.

REFERENCES

1. Aaslid R, Markwalder TM, Nornes H (1982) Noninvasive transcranial doppler ultrasound recording of flow velocity in basal cerebral arteries. J Neurosurg 57:769-774.

2. Chan KH, Miller JD, Dearden NM (1992) Intracranial blood flow velocity after head injury: relationship to severity of injury, time, neurological status and outcome. J Neurol Neurosurg Psychiatry 55:787-791.

3. Chan KH, Dearden NM, Miller JD, Midgley S, Piper IR (1992) Transcranial doppler waveform differences in hyperemic and nonhyperemic patients after severe head injury. Surg Neurol 38:443-446.

4. Mann KS, Chan KH, Yue CP (1986) Skull fractures in children: their assessment in relation to developmental skull changes and acute intracranial hematomas. Child's Nerv Syst 2:258-261.

Electrocortical Activity Recovery After Prolonged Experimental Brain Tamponade

C. Anile[1], A. Mangiola[1], R. Gaspari[2], F. Della Corte[2], D. Catapano[1], F.F. Angileri[1], P. Santini[1], and G. Maira[3]

Institutes of [1] Neurosurgery and [2] Anesthesiology, Catholic University, Rome, Italy
[3] University of Perugia, Italy

INTRODUCTION

Electrophysiological and metabolic cerebral recovery after prolonged global brain ischemia, produced by cardiac arrest or vascular occlusion at different levels, has been well documented in several experimental models on different animal species, primates included [1]. Furthermore, evidence does exist in monkeys that post-ischemic morphological alterations observed after 1 hour of complete brain ischemia can be reversed, in the majority of the anatomical cerebral areas explored, if adequate reperfusion follows [2]. In the same report the authors concluded that "the majority of the neurons of monkey brain survive complete cerebrocirculatory arrest of 1 hour for at least 1 day".

Brain tamponade represents a dramatic event of cerebrocirculatory arrest caused by abnormally increased intracranial pressure (ICP) due to different causes, traumatic, hemorrhagic, tumoral, etc.. Few papers have reported the possibility of a successful reversibility of such a condition lasting for some minutes. To our knowledge, no successful reversibility has been documented in cases of longer lasting intracranial circulatory arrest [3]. For this reason the brain tamponade has been considered until now as an irreversible intracranial hemodynamic alteration leading unavoidably, in a very short time, to a condition of brain death.

In this paper we report the results of an investigation aimed at exploring the possibility of an electrocortical functional recovery after a prolonged transitory global brain ischemia in an experimental model reproducing a reversible brain tamponade phenomenon.

MATERIALS AND METHODS

Following our previous studies, an experimental reversible condition of intracranial hypertension was produced by infusing saline into a lateral ventricle until ICP approached arterial blood pressure (ABP). In this new experimental series nine domestic pigs (all female) weighing between 20 and 25 kg were used. The animals were tranquilized with 5 mg/kg ketamine, paralyzed with 0.4 mg/kg/hr pancuronium bromide and mechanically ventilated with a gas mixture of 0.5 - 1% halothane, 50% N_2O, the rest oxygen. The respiration of the animals was adjusted to yield a $PaCO_2$ of about 35 mmHg and a PaO_2 of more than 100 mmHg. No artificial system to kept a constant body temperature was utilized. General anesthesia was discontinued when the brain tamponade condition was reached and resumed only after the electrocortical recovery .

ICP was measured through the same 18G epidural needle utilized for the infusion; ABP through a 16G catheter inserted into the right common carotid artery in the neck. Cerebral blood flow (CBF) variations were analyzed by evaluating CBF velocities measured by utilizing two ultrasound 8 and 4 MHz continuous wave probes located intracranially at the sagittal sinus and at the left internal carotid artery level through two adequately tailored skull windows positioned respectively in the posterior part of the middle vertex and in the left temporal bone. The anatomy of the intracranial cerebral arterial and venous system in pig is quite similar to that found in man; the sagittal sinus, in particular, is devoted to drain exclusively from cortical and bridging veins to systemic circulation [4]. Furthermore, the characteristic feature of this structure, delimited by rigid walls, permits us to regard the measurement of the blood flow velocity variations, recorded by doppler technique at this site, as a reliable evaluation

of the global CBF variations.
The integrity of the skull was reconstitued with dental acrylic cement.
Electrocortical activity was recorded by 4 screw electrodes located on the skull in symmetrical bilateral fronto-parietal position at distance of about 4 cm; electrocardiac activity by spindle electrodes at the extremities.
All signals were continuously recorded both on chart and on magnetic tape for delayed automatical data processing and storage utilizing self-developed software based on the Fourier frequency analysis. The electrocortical activity was evaluated qualitatively by looking at the chart recording and quantitatively by calculating the sum of the amplitudes of the different frequencies of the power spectrum (total power spectrum).
Saline was infused at a progressively increasing rate, starting from 12 ml/hr, until a condition of brain tamponade was reached as documented by the observation of a reverberating blood flow velocity wave pattern both at internal carotid artery and sinus level with a mean value of zero. This condition was maintained for 15' in 4 animals, 30' in 3 and 60' in the last two. At the end of the infusion the experimental observation was prolonged until an electrocortical activity was again clearly evident.
Statistical analysis was carried out by utilizing the linear correlation method.

RESULTS

In all animals the cerebral perfusion pressure (CPP = mean ABP - mean ICP) decrease produced by the intraventricular saline infusion was associated to a relative stability of the electrocortical activity until values of less than 40 mmHg were reached; then it abruptly reduced and disappeared at CPP value of about 20 mmHg when a typical recording of "electrocortical silence" became evident (Fig. 1).

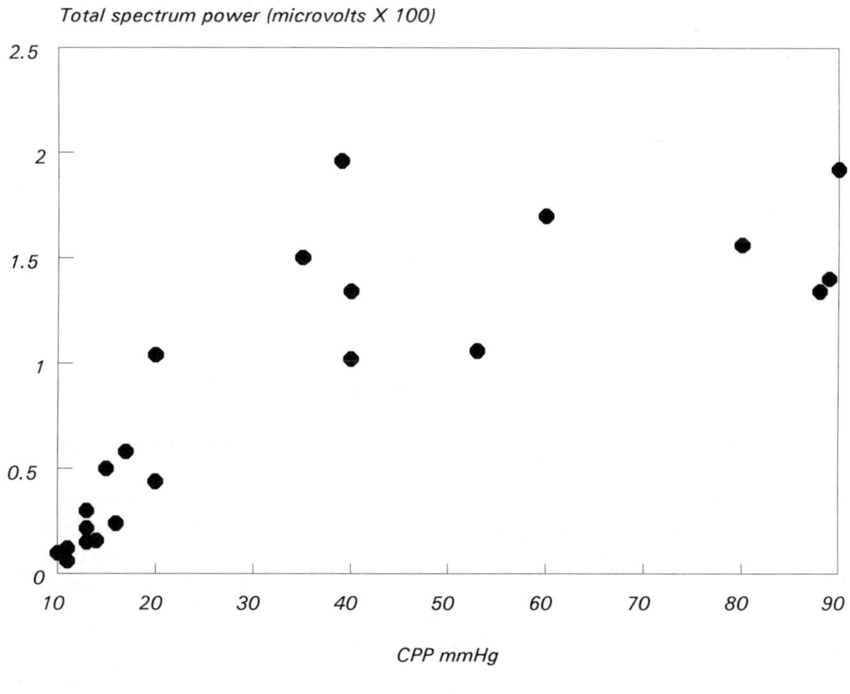

Fig. 1: An example of elctrocortical activity variation during CPP decrease induced by saline infusion
A few seconds later the typical reverberating wave patterns appeared both at sinus and internal carotid

level indicating the zero CBF value. Shortly after the disappearance of the electrocortical activity bilateral mydriasis and corneal areflexia occurred.
At the end of the infusion, arterial and venous CBF velocity immediately restored following the CPP increase; an electrocortical activity became again evident in all the animals after CBF restoration in a time linearly correlated with the duration of the brain tamponade condition. The first signs of the electrocortical activity recovery were represented by bursts of low voltage waves separated by isoelectric periods of diminishing length. Progressively the intervals between the bursts shortened and the voltage increased until continuous background activity was again observed about 50' after CBF restoration in those animals with a 15' duration of brain tamponade; in the other ones the time of experimental observation before sacrifice was, probably, too short to permit a complete recovery. However, in both groups of animals, the entity in the electrocortical activity recovery was linearly correlated with the lapse of time after CBF restoration (Fig. 2).

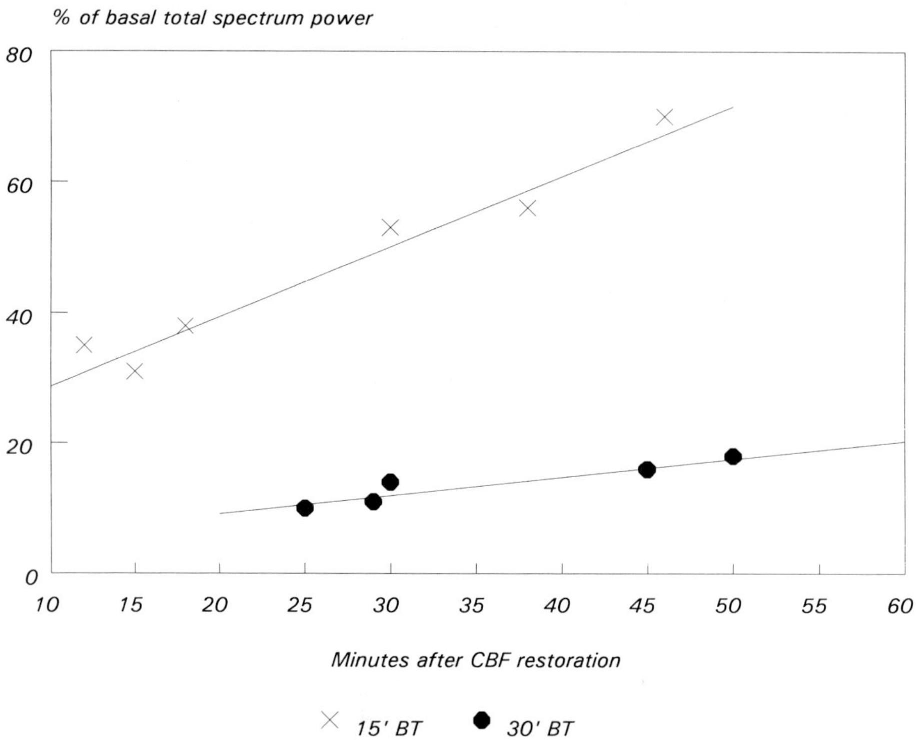

Fig. 2: Electrocortical activity recovery after 15' - 30' of brain tamponade (BT)

As expected the slope of these correlations indicated that the shorter the duration of the brain tamponade condition and the faster the recovery of the electrocortical activity. No such correlation was observed in the two animals with a 60' brain tamponade duration probably because the observation time had been interrupted too soon. It should be mentioned, however, that even in these animals an initial electrocortical activity recovery was evident 40' and 60' after CBF restoration. Furthermore, in all the animals the pupils regained normal size and normal light responsiveness and corneal reflex reappeared.

DISCUSSION

Reversibility of intracranial circulatory arrest in man is controversial. Only few reports support this possibility [3]. In our as in other experimental models, however, not only CBF, but also electrocortical activity, recovered even after 1h of complete global brain ischemia. Our results present some similarities but also some discrepancies compared to the previous cited reports. The time of recovery in the experimental models in which a condition of brain global ischemia was produced by vascular occlusion is generally longer than in our and other model of intracranial hypertension, probably because this latter experimental preparation induces less systemic circulatory effects so favouring an optimal brain reperfusion. The time of recovery observed after 30' of brain tamponade in our model is in agreement with that reported by Ichord et al. [5] in a similar experimental model; however in 6 out of 16 animals (8 piglets and 8 pigs) no EEG recovery was observed. No finding about the rate of recovery was indicated.

Even if the linear correlations among brain tamponade duration, delay and rate in the electrocortical recovery suggest a time-related reduction in the capability of the neurons to restore their functional activity, nevertheless, they do not indicate a clear-cut limit beyond which the recovery becomes impossible. De la Torre et al. reported in 1991 [6] neuroelectric and metabolic activity recovery even after 75' of global brain ischemia in rats. On the other hand, Hossmann et al. [1] reported that in their model of 1 hour global brain ischemia in monkeys "despite progressive EEG recovery, animals exhibited no signs of consciousness during the observation period" up to 24 hours.

This finding may indicate irreversible brain damage or the necessity of a longer period to restore a more complex function than the electrocortical activity, such as consciousness requires.

In conclusion, even if the transposition of this experimental data to the human pathology may be considered unsuitable, nevertheless, all the findings here reported not only indicate that the intracranial circulatory arrest may not be the equivalent of an irreversible lethal condition such as "brain death" [3], but also refute the reliability of a functional criterion, such as the absence of an electrocortical activity, in the diagnosis of this condition.

REFERENCES

1. Hossmann K-A, Grosse Ophoff B (1986) Recovery of monkey brain after prolonged ischemia. I.Electrophysiology and brain electrolytes. JCBFM 6:15-21.
2. Bodsch W, Barbier A, Oemhichen M, Grosse Ophoff B, Hossmann K-A (1986) Recovery of monkey brain after prolonged ischemia. II. Protein synthesis and morphological alterations. JCBFM 6:22-33.
3. Steinmetz H, Hassler W (1988) Reversible intracranial circulatory arrest in acute subarachnoid haemorrhage (letter). JNNP 51:1355-6.
4. Fries G, Wallenfang T, Hennen J, Velthaus M, Heimann A, Schild H, Perneczky A, Kempski O (1992) Occlusion of the pig superior sagittal sinus, bridging and cortical veins: multistep evolution of sinus-vein thrombosis. J Neurosurg 77:127-133.
5. Ichord RN, Kirsch JR, Helfaer MA, Haun S, Traystman RJ (1991) Age-related differences in recovery of blood flow and metabolism after cerebral ischemia in swine. Stroke 22:626-634.
6. de la Torre JC, Fortin T, Saunders J, Butler K, Richard M (1991) Return of ATP/PCr and EEG phosphate energy metabolism after 75 minutes of global brain ischemia. Brain Res 542:71-76.

Acknowledgements: we are grateful to Mrs. Anna Capuano for her precious technical collaboration.

Session IX: Biophysics (1)

Chairmen: A. Marmarou and S. Ishii

PVI-Timed Wake Up in Head-Injured Patients

R.L. Bernays[1], Th. Bischoff[1], R. Stocker[2], and H.-G. Imhof[1]

[1] Department of Neurosurgery, [2] Division of Trauma Surgery, University Hospital Zürich, CH-8091 Zürich, Switzerland

Introduction:

The necessity of sedation after head injury is clear and established, but the timing of wake up is unclear. The timing of wake up in the head injured patient's course of treatment is critical because stopping sedation and weaning from mechanical ventilation is often associated with elevation of intracranial pressure (ICP) and deterioration of cerebral perfusion pressure (CPP)[1,2]. In order to co-ordinate respiratory care with protection of the brain against secondary cerebral insults, we applied the pressure-volume-index (PVI) as defined by Marmarou [3,4] as a predictor of outcome on wake up. Outcome was defined as ICP remaining below 15 mm Hg, or rising above 15 mm Hg, which required resedation and continued mechanical ventilation. We compared this method of predicting outcome on wake up with the method we used until 1993. Before 1993 we did not calculate PVI and began wake up if ICP remained below 15 mm Hg for 24 hours.

In head injured patients PVI ($PVI = \Delta V/\log\{Pp/Po\}$) is a valuable parameter for defining brain tightness or cerebral compliance [5], which according to several authors represents the compressibility of the brains vascular system [6,7]. PVI has been proved in clinical practice to be a valuable decision-making-tool for further diagnosis and therapy [8,9] as well as an indicator for an impending rise of ICP [10,11] and prognosis of neurologic outcome [12]. Some authors have criticized PVI-calculations [13,14,15] stating that they are difficult to perform, time-consuming, susceptible to artifacts and without correlation to pulsatile ICP changes [16].

We have improved PVI calculations by introducing a new, easy to use computer-based protocol which produces reliable and stable PVI values during 30 minutes bedside testing.

Materials and Methods:

Head injured patients with an initial GCS ≤ 8 and/or CT abnormalities were intubated and transferred to ICU after surgery. Multimodality monitoring routinely was employed, including ICP monitoring, arterial and jugular venous bulb oxygen saturation, arterial pressure, as well as CPP, SEP and EEG monitoring. ICP was monitored either with a subdural Wilkinson-cup-catheter or with an intraventricular catheter. Patients were treated with a standard protocol including intravenous muscle relaxants and sedatives, mechanical ventilation, osmotherapy, CSF drainage for ICP > 15 mm Hg and barbiturates.

Until 1993 wake up was initiated after the ICP remained below 15 mm Hg for 24 hours. These patients are allocated to the "*ICP-based group*". In 1993 we started to apply the PVI-based-protocol: a PVI value ≥ 18 ml was interpreted as a value which allowed initiating wake up. These patients are allocated to the "*PVI-based group*".

ICP-based group:

The data of 52 patients with severe head injury admitted to the ICU in 1992 were retrospectively analyzed. 8 patients in this group had to be excluded because of incompleteness of data and 8 patients died before wake up could be initiated. The remaining 36 patients had a median age of 35 with an initial median GCS of 6. All patients had ICP monitoring, 11 with an intraventricular catheter, 25 with a subdural catheter.

PVI-BASED GROUP:

The PVI-based group included 10 patients with a median age of 33 with an initial median GCS of 6. In this group only intraventricular catheters have been used. Because PVI determination requires an intraventricular catheter patients without intraventricular catheters were not included in the PVI-based group.

Table 1: Distribution of age, sex, initial GCS, duration of sedation and type of ICP catheter used in the two groups.

	ICP-based group	**PVI-based group**
Median, mean and range of age	35, 39, 16 - 68	33, 33, 18-55
Ratio: female:male	11:25	1:9
Init. median GCS	6	6
Median, range of duration of sedation	8.5. 1-27	15, 2-34
Number of patients	36	10
Number of ventricle. catheters	11	10
Number of subdural catheters	25	0

PVI MEASUREMENT PROTOCOL:

As referred to by several authors [13,14] and according to our early experience there can be considerable variability between sequential PVI values, partially due to baseline floating, e.g. B-waves. In a majority of recorded pressure curves under ICU conditions it is insufficient only to consider cardiac and respiratory cycles to choose Po and Pp (Po = median preinjection/withdrawal ICP, Pp = median postinjection/withdrawal ICP value), see Fig.1. Using Marmarou's standard equation stated above we developed a computer-based protocol for sampling PVIs, which improved the technique for determining PVI significantly.

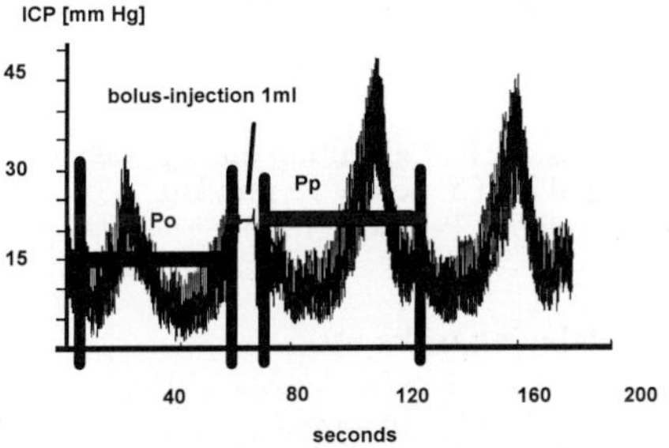

Fig. 1 Illustrating median Po and median Pp determination in time windows, considering the slowest underlying wave-period.

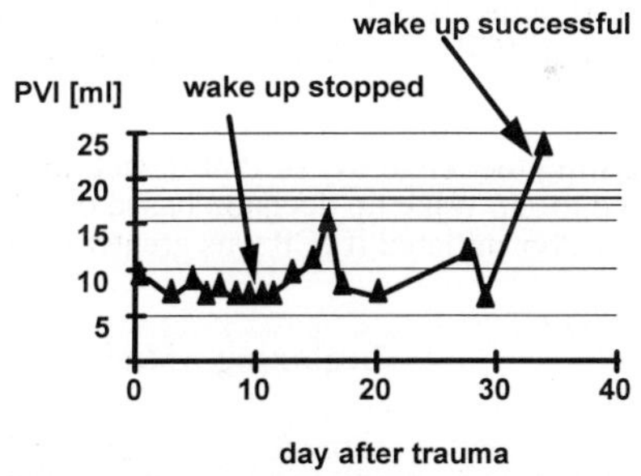

Fig. 2 Illustrating the course of PVI in a patient where wake up at a PVI < 18 ml had to be stopped and later at PVI ≥ 18 ml was successful.

PVI calculations were started within the first 24 hours after insertion of a ventricular catheter and were repeated at 24 hour intervals. Preceding a PVI-study, ICP was recorded at slow speeds during 5 minutes in order to get an estimate of recording quality and possible baseline floating.
For patients with ICP below 15 mm Hg, 0.5 - 3 ml Ringer's solution at room temperature was injected at 1 ml/sec into the lateral cerebral ventricle. For patients with ICP above 15 mm Hg 0.5 - 3 ml CSF was drained at 0.5 ml/sec. Usually 5 (no baseline floating) to 15 (considerable baseline floating) PVI calculations, bolus-injections and CSF-drainage's of defined volumes alternately, were done per study. One study was done per day. Using a mouse driven computer cursor, two time windows were selected before and after injection/withdrawal, see Fig.1. From these Po and Pp were determined and PVI calculated. Depending on the amount of baseline floating this PVI calculation was repeated 5 -15 times.

A median PVI then was calculated and recorded as the PVI for that day. A PVI-study took approximately 30 minutes per patient.

HARDWARE AND SOFTWARE USED FOR RECORDINGS:

A commercially available A/D (analogue/digital) data acquisition board (8-channel, 12-bit resolution, 100 kilosample/sec, Keithley MetraByte) with data acquisition and analysis software (Easyest LX, Keithley Asyst) had been installed in a 486-PC. This equipment enabled us to program automated recording-protocols and bed-side PVI calculations of the recorded data. All recordings and calculations could be visualized on the PC screen and be printed out.

RESULTS:

ICP-BASED GROUP:

In all the patients (intraventricular and subdural catheters), the prediction concerning timing of wake up was correct 22 times for 22 patients (61%) so that ICP remained below 15 mm Hg and resedation was not required. The prediction for wake up was incorrect 18 times for 14 patients. Thus 39% of patients in this group underwent multiple wake ups.
As mentioned above there were 11 patients with intraventricular catheters and 25 patients with subdural catheters in the ICP-based group. 6 patients (55%) with intraventricular catheters did not show any rise of ICP during wake up, 3 patients (27%) required 2 wake up attempts and 2 patients (18%) required 3 wake up attempts. Of the 25 patients with subdural catheters 16 patients (64%) showed no ICP problems during initial wake up, 7 patients (28%) needed 2 and 2 patients (8%) needed 3 wake up attempts.
The median times from onset of treatment of ICP to initiation of wake up were as follows: all patients 8.5 days, patients with intraventricular catheters 13 days (mean = 12.5 days), patients with subdural catheters 5 days (mean = 7.4 days).

PVI-BASED GROUP:

Wake up was initiated 4 times in patients with PVI values < 18 ml and these patients were subsequently resedated, for example see Fig. 2. Wake up was initiated 10 times in patients with PVI values ≥ 18 ml. In each of these 10 patients ICP remained below 15 mm Hg during wake up. The median times from onset of treatment of ICP to initiation of wake up were 15 days.

Table 2: Illustrating the reliability of PVI-detection of patients at risk for ICP elevation during wake up. In the ICP-based group wake up decision based on a 24 hour's period of ICP below 15 mm Hg.
* Wake up was never initiated if ICP was greater than 15 mm Hg in the ICP-based group.

	beginning wake up		**delaying wake up**	
	correct predictions	incorrect predictions	correct predictions	incorrect predictions
ICP-based group	22 (55%)	18 (45%)	-*	-*
PVI-based group	10 (100%)	0	4 (100%)	0

DISCUSSION:

The number of investigated patients is rather small, nevertheless there is a striking distinction between the results of the two treatment protocols. PVI calculations are able to detect the patients likely to develop elevated ICP during the weaning phase. Indeed, several patients with PVI < 18 ml underwent unsuccessful wake up attempts due to elevated ICP. PVI calculations also detected patients who would tolerate wake up.

In the PVI-based group the duration of sedation was considerably longer than in the ICP based group. It may be concluded that the success at wake up was on the basis of a longer time of sedation. Nevertheless, underlying this is the realization that cerebral compliance, which is measured by PVI, improves over time. Unterberg et al. [17] found a secondary rise of ICP commencing between day 3 and 10 after trauma in 28% of their investigated head injured patients. This finding corresponds with the long sedation period observed in a subgroup of our patients.
An other reason accounting for the difference of duration of sedation is a selection bias. At our institution more severely injured patients receive an intraventricular catheter instead of a subdural catheter. During the time that the patients were selected for PVI determinations less severely injured patients were monitored by subdural catheters. Comparing only the cases with intraventricular catheters in the ICP-based group with the PVI-based group the difference of duration of sedation becomes minimal: 15 days (median) in the PVI-based group and 13 (median) days in the ICP-based group.

Further experience and a higher number of investigated patients will be necessary to confirm the reliability and show the range of confidence of this computer based PVI-assessment system for timing wake up in head-injured patients and preventing secondary cerebral insults during this critical phase.

REFERENCES:

1. Jaskulka R, Weinstabl C, Schedl R (1993) [The course of intracranial pressure during respirator weaning after severe craniocerebral trauma]. Unfallchirurg 96:138-141
2. Williams G, Roberts PA, Smith S, Stevens FA, Tompkins P, Arancibia , C. , Pollay M (1991) The effect of apnea on brain compliance and intracranial pressure. Neurosurgery 29 (2):242-246
3. Marmarou A, Shulman K, LaMorgese J (1975) Compartmental analysis of compliance and outflow resistance of the cerebrospinal fluid system. J Neurosurg 43:523-534
4. Marmarou A, Shulman K, Rosende RM (1978) A nonlinear analysis of the cerebrospinal fluid system and intracranial pressure dynamics. J Neurosurg 48:332-344
5. Bouma GJ, Muizelaar JP, Bandoh K, Marmarou A (1992) Blood pressure and intracranial pressure-volume dynamics in severe head injury: relationship with cerebral blood flow. J Neurosurg 77 (1):15-9
6. Muizelaar JP, Marmarou A, DeSalles AA, Ward JD, Zimmerman RS, Li Z, Choi SC, Young HF (1989) Cerebral blood flow and metabolism in severely head-injured children. Part 1: Relationship with GCS score, outcome, ICP, and PVI. J Neurosurg 71:63-71
7. Marmarou A, Maset AL, Ward JD, Choi S, Brooks D, Lutz HA, Moulton RJ, Muizelaar JP, DeSalles A, Young HF (1987) Contribution of CSF and vascular factors to elevation of ICP in severely head-injured patients. J Neurosurg 66:883-890
8. Shapiro K, Marmarou A (1982) Clinical applications of the pressure-volume index in treatment of pediatric head injuries. J Neurosurg 56 (6):819-25
9. Wachi A, Sato K, Inao S, Maset AL, Marmarou A (1990) Pvi in analyzing pressure volume relationship--effect of a bolus mannitol administration. No To Shinkei 42 (7):661-7
10. Maset AL, Marmarou A, Ward JD, Choi S, Lutz HA, Brooks D, Moulton , R J, DeSalles A, Muizelaar JP, Turner H, et al. (1987) Pressure-volume index in head injury. J Neurosurg 67 (6):832-840
11. Muizelaar JP, Ward JD, Marmarou A, Newlon PG, Wachi A (1989) Cerebral blood flow and metabolism in severely head-injured children. Part 2: Autoregulation. J Neurosurg 71:72-76
12. Stocchetti N, Mattioli C, Mainini P, Furlan A, Paparella A, Zuccoli , P. (1993) (clinical use of cerebral elastance and intracranial dynamics measurements). Minerva Anestesiol 59 (1-2):1-9
13. Tans JT, Poortvliet DC (1983) Intracranial volume-pressure relationship in man. part 2: clinical significance of the pressure-volume index. J Neurosurg 59 (5):810-6
14. Christensen L, Borgesen SE (1989) Single pulse pressure wave analysis by fast fourier transformation. Neurol Res 11 (4):197-200
15. Friden HG, Ekstedt J (1983) Volume/pressure relationship of the cerebrospinal space in humans. Neurosurgery 13 (4):351-66
16. Kosteljanetz M (1986) Acute head injury: pressure-volume relations and cerebrospinal fluid dynamics. Neurosurgery 18 (1):17-24
17. Unterberg A, Kiening K, Schmiedek P, Lanksch W (1993) Long-Term Observation of Intracranial Pressure after Severe Head Injury. The Phenomenon of Secondary Rise of Intracranial Pressure. Neurosurgery 32:17-24

Periventricular Glial Proliferation and Intracranial Compliance in Experimental Hydrocephalus

F. Takei[1], R. Tsugane[1], Y. Hashimoto[1], H. Takasawa[2], S. Oi[2], and O. Sato[2]

[1] Department of Neurosurgery, Tokai University Oiso Hospital, Nakagun, Kanagawa, 259-01 Japan
[2] Department of Neurosurgery, Tokai University, School of Medicine, Isehara, Kanagawa, 259-11 Japan

INTRODUCTION

From clinical experience in performing the ventricular tap of long-standing hydrocephalic cases, we sometimes feel a high resistance when the needle just before penetrates the ventricular wall. This phenomenon seems to reflect a glial bundle formation in the periventricular tissue and lead to lower intracranial compliance. However, there is no counterevidence of this clinical imagination. This study aims to analyze the influence of periventricular morphological alterations upon the intracranial compliance and ventricular dilatation in hydrocephalus.

MATERIALS AND METHODS

We evaluated intracranial pressure dynamics and morphological alterations using six feline kaolin-induced hydrocephalus models, 4-8 weeks after kaolin induction into the cisterna magna, and 4 non-treated normal cats as a control.

Intracranial Pressure Dynamic Analysis

To identify the intracranial pressure dynamic property of the periventricular tissue (PVT) in normal and hydrocephalic condition, we analyze following three parameters such as intraventricular pressure (IVP) as ICP, pressure volume index (PVI: bolus technique) as an indicator for intracranial compliance and penetrating pressure of the brain parenchyma (PPB) as an indicator for local tissue rigidity.
In measuring PPB, a fiberoptic (camino) pressure transducer was used and this pressure was recorded on the strip chart while the transducer was introduced into the brain parenchyma from the cortical surface to lateral ventricle using an infusion pump with a constant rate.

Morphological Analysis

In normal and hydrocephalic animals, the periventricular region 1 (R1) and region 2 (R2) along the ventricular tap tract by pressure transducer was analyzed by means of light and transmission electron microscope. R1 was the region of an initial inner quarter from ventricular surface and R2 was second inner quarter from the surface of lateral ventricle.

Assessment of Parameters Observed

Pattern of PPB in R1 and R2 recorded on the strip chart was assessed by delta P (pressure difference between maximum and minimum pressure: mmHg) and peak pressure. These two parameters and PVI were compared with corresponding regions observed morphologically.

RESULTS

All animal received kaolin suspension obtained ventricular dilatation.
ICP of non-treated normal and hydrocephalic animal were 9.78 +/- 0.83mmHg, 9.05 +/- 0.60mmHg; PVI was 0.76 +/- 0.22ml, 2.11 +/- 0.42ml respectively (Table 1). PVI in hydrocephalics increased significantly after initiation of hydrocephalus ($P<0.05$) even ICP remained within same range ($P>0.05$).

Table 1. Comparison of ICP and PVI in normal and hydrocephalic condition

	Normal	**Hydrocephalus**	
ICP	9.78 +/- 0.83	9.05 +/- 0.60	(mmHg)
PVI	0.76 +/- 0.22	2.11 +/- 0.42*	(ml)

*: P< 0.05 (mean +/- S.D.)

Penetrating pressure of brain parenchyma in hydrocephalics corresponding to the region of PVT (R1 and R2) significantly increased while PPB in other outer regions in normal group slowly increased. On the other hand, PPB in control animals did not show any significant increase when the transducer penetrated over the region of R1 and R2. Delta P and peak pressure of PPB were 31.5 +/-

20.4mmHg, 72.8 +/- 33.0mmHg (R1), 36.5 +/-25.5mmHg, 52.0 +/- 18.7mmHg (R2) in hydrocephalic animal and 6.8 +/- 9.4mmHg, 32.5 +/- 20.6mmHg (R1), 10.8 +/- 10.6mmHg, 41.5 +/- 18.7mmHg (R2) in normal group respectively (Table 2).
In morphological observation in hydrocephalics, dense layer of glial proliferation observed in R1 while morphological changes in R2 were similar to normal group (Fig.1) and this was as same as previously reported elsewhere[1].

Table 2. Regional difference in measured PPB (delta P and peak pressure) in normal and hydrocephalic condition

		Normal delta P (peak pressure)	**Hydrocephalus** delta P (peak pressure)
PPB (mmHg)	**R1**	6.8 +/- 9.4 (32.5 +/- 20.6)	31.5 +/- 20.4 (72.8 +/- 33.0)
	R2	10.8 +/- 10.6 (41.5 +/-18.7)	36.5 +/- 25.5 (52.0 +/- 18.7)

(mean +/- S.D.)

DISCUSSION AND CONCLUSIONS

In our preliminary observation, increased penetrating pressure in the region of periventricular tissue seems to correspond with its periventricular glial proliferation and other pathological alteration observed in hydrocephalus. However a high PPB that obtained over the PVT in hydrocephalus, intracranial compliance, assessed with PVI by bolus technique, did not indicate such result. This result suggested that intracranial compliance did not simply correlate with periventricular morphological alterations both in normal and hydrocephalic condition and the resistance on performing ventricular tap does not truly reflect the intracranial compliance.
In hydrocephalus, mechanism of ventricular dilatation is still unclear and various factors[2,3,4,5] besides intracranial compliance should also involve in its entity.
Therefore we emphasized that, considering distensibility of ventricular system in hydrocephalus, development of increased PPB implying high tissue resistance and glial proliferations observed on PVT may act as a self-limiting factor for ventricular dilatation. Furthermore, regarding the unsolved mechanism of termination of ventricular enlargement in arrested hydrocephalus, the results obtained in this study may answer to such a long-standing debatable questions.

REFERENCES

1. Takei F, Shapiro K, Hirano A, Kohn I (1987) Influence of the rate of ventricular enlargement on the ultrastructual morphology of the white matter in experimental hydrocephalus. Neurosurg 21: 645-650
2. Bering E.A., Jr. (1962) Circulation of the cerebrospinal fluid. Demonstration of the choroid plexus as the generator of the force for flow of fluid and ventricula enlargement. J Neurosurg 19: 405-413
3. Shapiro K, Kohn I, Takei F, Zee C (1987) Progressive ventricular enlargement in cats in the absence of transmantle pressure gradients. J Neurosurg 67: 88-92
4. Takei F, Ito K, Sato O (1991) The role of altered brain properties in ventricular dilatation. In: Matsumoto, Tamaki N (eds) Hydrocephalus : pathogenesis and treatment. Springer, Tokyo, pp 279-291
5. Shapiro K, Takei F, Fried A, Kohn I (1985) Experimental hydrocephalus: The role of biomechanical changes in ventricular enlargement in cats. J Neurosurg 63: 82-87

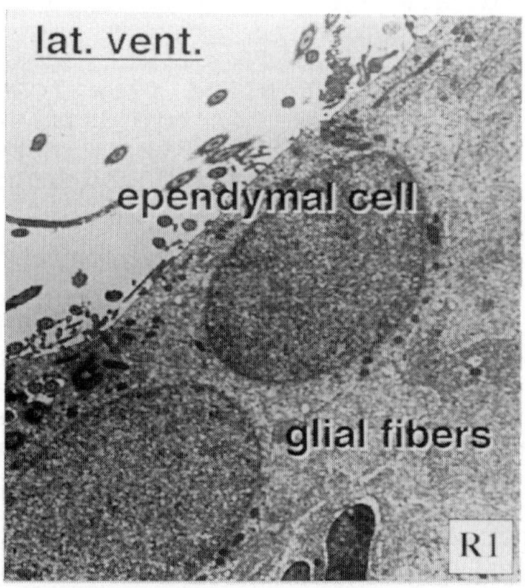

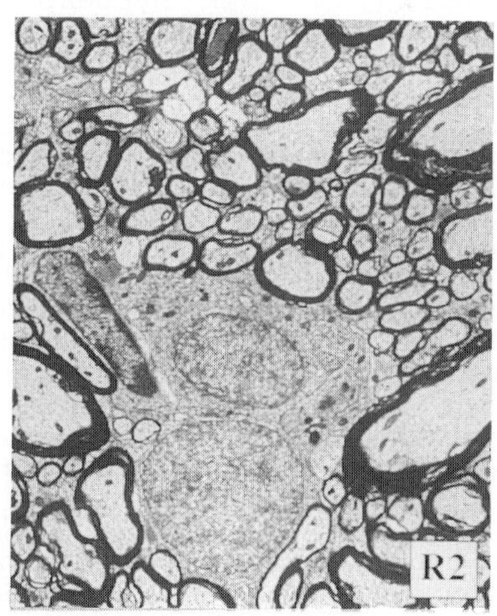

Fig.1 These electron photomicrographs show the histological alterations in hydrocephalic animal. R1 (left) : stretched ependymal cell is seen. A number of the cilia and microvilli are decreased. The glial fibers are rich in volume in the subependymal region. (x 5500) b) R2 (right) : Appearance of cellular components is similar to the normal condition (x 4500).

Intracranial Volume-Pressure Relationship During Desflurane Anesthesia in Dogs; Comparison with Isoflurane and Thiopental/Halothane

A.A. Artru

Department of Anesthesiology, RN-10, University of Washington School of Medicine, Seattle, WA, USA

INTRODUCTION

Previous studies with desflurane reported that in dogs ICP was higher after 30 min at 1.0 MAC desflurane (15 ± 3 cmH_2O, mean ± SEM) than after 30 min at 1.0 MAC halothane (10 ± 1 cmH_2O), enflurane (8 ± 1 cmH_2O) or isoflurane (4 ± 2 cmH_2O); and ICP during 0.5 or 1.0 MAC desflurane did not decrease with hypocapnia but did decrease with hypocapnia during 1.0 MAC halothane, enflurane or isoflurane. In patients with supratentorial mass lesions, ICP increased progressively during 45 min hypocapnia and 1.0 MAC desflurane, but not during 45 min hypocapnia and 1.0 MAC isoflurane.

Because desflurane-induced increase of cerebral blood flow (CBF) is similar to that with other inhalational anesthetics, but desflurane-induced increase of ICP is greater, it seems unlikely that increased cerebral blood volume (CBV) accounts for desflurane-induced increase of ICP unless the CBV/CBF ratio is significantly higher with desflurane than with the other inhalational anesthetics.

A second cause of increased ICP is increased brain tissue water content and, consequently, increased brain tissue volume. In a previous study from this laboratory brain tissue water content following desflurane anesthesia in dogs was not significantly different from previously reported normal values. Thus it seems unlikely that increased brain tissue volume explains the desflurane-induced increase of ICP.

A third cause of increased ICP is increased cerebrospinal fluid (CSF) formation rate (V_f) or increased resistance to reabsorption of CSF (Ra) and, consequently, increased CSF volume. A previous study from this laboratory reported that desflurane increased V_f during hypocapnia and increased CSF pressure but not during hypocapnia and normal CSF pressure or during normocapnia. Desflurane also caused no significant change in R_a. Thus, a desflurane-induced increase of CSF volume may explain previous reports that ICP does not decrease with hypocapnia during desflurane anesthesia and that ICP increases progressively during hypocapnia in patients with supratentorial mass lesions. However, that mechanism does not explain a desflurane-induced increase of ICP during normocapnia.

A fourth cause for increase of ICP is an alteration of the intracranial volume-pressure relationship such that there is (a) an exaggerated CSF pressure increase when CSF volume increases and/or (b) a decreased capacity for CSF pressure to return to baseline following a CSF pressure increase (impaired CSF pressure normalization). The effects of desflurane on the intracranial volume-pressure relationship have not previously been reported. Accordingly, the present study was designed to determine the effects of desflurane on the two above mentioned phases of the CSF pressure response to increase of CSF volume: the CSF pressure increase due to increase of CSF volume, and the capacity of CSF pressure to return to baseline values following a CSF pressure increase.

METHODS

In 12 dogs receiving desflurane (groups 1 and 2) the four experimental conditions were: 0.5 MAC desflurane at normal CSF pressure, 1.0 MAC desflurane at normal CSF pressure, 0.5 MAC desflurane at elevated CSF pressure, and 1.0 MAC desflurane at elevated CSF pressure. The six dogs in group 1 were examined at normocapnia (P_aCO_2 35-40 mmHg) and the six dogs in group 2 were examined at hypocapnia (P_aCO_2 18-22 mmHg). In 6 dogs receiving isoflurane (group 3) the four experimental conditions were: normocapnia at normal CSF pressure, hypocapnia at normal CSF pressure, normocapnia at increased CSF pressure, and hypocapnia at increased CSF pressure. In 6 dogs in group 4 (thiopental/halothane controls) the four experimental periods were at each of four time periods comparable to those in groups 1-3. In all 24 dogs in the present study, 0.5 ml infusions of mock CSF at each experimental condition caused an abrupt increase of ventricular and cisternal CSF pressure, followed by a slower, biphasic return of CSF pressure towards pre-infusion values. The CSF pressure increase due to increase of CSF volume was determined during approximately the first 20 s after mock CSF infusion, and the capacity of CSF pressure to return to baseline volumes was determined during approximately the 20 s-3 min interval following mock CSF infusion. At 3 min after volume infusion, 0.5 ml was withdrawn from the cisterna magna to restore CSF volume to its pre-infusion value.

CSF Pressure Increase due to Increase of CSF Volume
The values determined from each CSF pressure response were CSF pressure prior to volume infusion (Po) and peak CSF pressure following volume infusion (Pp). From these, three previously described and frequently cited measures of the intracranial volume-pressure relationship were calculated: intracranial compliance (C), the volume pressure response (VPR, a measure of intracranial elastance) and the pressure volume index (PVI, a measure relating change of intracranial volume [ΔV] and log ICP). C was calculated as the ratio of ΔV to change of CSF pressure (ΔP). C values were expressed as ml/cmH_2O. VPR was calculated as the ratio of ΔP to ΔV. VPR values were expressed as cmH_2O/ml. PVI was calculated as $\Delta V/[\log P_p/P_o]$. Calculated PVI values were expressed as ml. Marmarou and colleagues, who described PVI, also described an estimate of C (C_e) based on the values obtained with PVI. Utilizing their equation, C_e was calculated as $[0.4343\ (PVI)]/P_o$. Calculated C_e values were expressed as ml/cmH_2O.

Capacity of CSF Pressure to Return to Baseline Values Following a CSF Pressure Increase
Values relating to CSF pressure normalization were determined from the CSF pressure curve during the time period following the peak increase of CSF pressure due to mock CSF infusion. These values previously were reported as measures of the capacity of the CSF and surrounding tissues to return CSF pressure toward preinfusion values. Two of the characteristics of the CSF pressure response to volume infusion occurring at normal CSF pressure were the first phase slope of decrease of CSF pressure from P_p (S_1), and the second phase slope of decrease (S_2). S_1 and S_2 were expressed as cmH_2O/min. A third characteristic of the CSF pressure response was the duration of S_1 (DS_1), expressed in seconds. A fourth characteristic of the CSF pressure response was the CSF pressure change equaling the difference

between P_o and the CSF pressure at which extrapolation of S_2 intersected the slope of CSF pressure increase from P_o (ΔP_s). ΔP_s was expressed as cmH_2O/ml. Under conditions of elevated CSF pressure the slope of the decrease of CSF pressure from P_p did not occur in two distinct phases, so the average slope (S_{1-2}) was calculated, and ΔP_s and DS_1 were not calculated.

Statistical comparisons within groups were made using repeated-measures analysis of variance, and comparisons between groups were made using multiple analysis of variance. Where the calculated F value exceeded the critical value for the 0.05 probability level, the Student-Newman-Keuls' test was used to determine which differences were significant at $P < 0.05$. Values are tabulated as mean ± SD.

RESULTS

During desflurane or isoflurane anesthesia (groups 1-3) and in the control group (group 4), P_O and the responses to volume infusion were not significantly affected by the order of presentation of the experimental conditions. In addition, in all four groups P_o, P_p, VPR and PVI increased and C and C_e decreased when CSF pressure was increased to >30 cmH_2O as compared to when CSF pressure was at baseline values.

During normal CSF pressure and normocapnia or hypocapnia, desflurane decreased C_e (0.06±0.02 ml/cmH_2O) as compared to control values (0.09±0.01 ml/cmH_2O) but did not consistently alter other measures of the CSF pressure response to increase of CSF volume. Both 0.5 and 1.0 MAC desflurane decreased C_e. During normal CSF pressure and normocapnia, desflurane increased S_2 (1.5±0.5 cmH_2O/min). Desflurane did not significantly change any of the other measures of the capacity of CSF pressure to return to baseline values following a CSF pressure increase during normal CSF pressure and normocapnia or during any other experimental condition.

During normal CSF pressure and normocapnia or hypocapnia, isoflurane decreased C_e (0.04±0.01 ml/cmH_2O) as compared to controls but did not consistently alter other measures of the CSF pressure response to increase of CSF volume. C_e with 0.5 MAC isoflurane was not significantly different from C_e with 0.5 MAC desflurane. During hypocapnia and increased CSF pressure 0.5 MAC isoflurane increased VPR (71±15 cmH_2O/ml). During normal CSF pressure and normocapnia or hypocapnia, isoflurane decreased S_1 (20±6 and 19±9 cmH_2O/min) and increased ΔP_s (21±6 and 20±8 cmH_2O/min) as compared to controls. Under conditions of increased CSF pressure, isoflurane did not consistently alter other measures of the CSF pressure response or any of the measures of CSF pressure normalization.

During normocapnia and normal or increased CSF pressure, both measures of the CSF pressure response and measures of CSF pressure normalization in the control group (group 4) were not significantly different from values taken from two previous studies under similar experimental conditions.

DISCUSSION

Decrease of C_e during both desflurane or isoflurane and normocapnia at normal CSF pressure suggests that desflurane and isoflurane may decrease intracranial compliance. That C_e was similarly decreased with 0.5 MAC or 1.0 MAC desflurane and 0.5 MAC isoflurane indicates that altering the concentration of desflurane within the 3.5-7.0%

range does not significantly alter its effect on C_e. Continued decrease of C_e with hypocapnia suggests that hypocapnia does not reverse desflurane- or isoflurane-induced decrease of intracranial compliance. However, these results are not consistent with the C data from the present study which indicated no significant change in intracranial compliance with 0.5 or 1.0 MAC desflurane or 0.5 MAC isoflurane as compared to controls. Because C_e is derived from PVI and previously was reported to provide results that are sometimes inconsistent with C and VPR, C may be more reliable than C_e as a measure of intracranial compliance. The decrease of C_e seen with desflurane and isoflurane also is not consistent with the VPR data which indicated no significant change in intracranial elastance. Decrease of C_e with desflurane or isoflurane at normal CSF pressure but not at increased CSF pressure suggests that the decrease of intracranial compliance caused by increasing CSF pressure to >30 cmH_2O exerts such a great influence on C_e that the effects of desflurane or isoflurane are no longer demonstrable.

Isoflurane decreased S1 and increased ΔP_s, whereas desflurane caused no consistent change in S_1, S_2, S_{1-2}, DS_1, or ΔP_s. These results indicate that at normal CSF pressure and with normo- or hypocapnia, isoflurane but not desflurane impairs the capacity of CSF pressure to return to baseline values following a CSF pressure increase. While the processes responsible for the above mentioned characteristics of the CSF pressure relaxation curve are uncertain, S_1 presumably reflects rapidly occurring CSF pressure buffering events such as compression of cerebral veins from which blood may be rapidly conducted (such as sigmoid veins) and translocation of CSF through large diameter, high conductance pathways. S_2 presumably reflects more slowly occurring and "recruitment" of CSF pressure buffering responses such as compression of cerebral veins from which blood is not rapidly conducted (such as parenchymal veins), translocation of CSF through smaller diameter pathways, displacement of brain tissue, and reabsorption of CSF. At increased CSF pressure much of the first-occurring CSF pressure buffering capacity, i.e., the processes responsible for S_1, are probably exhausted accounting for the monophasic rather than biphasic character of the CSF pressure curve as CSF pressure decreases following CSF volume infusion. DS1 presumably reflects the reserve represented by or the capacity within the processes responsible for S_1, while ΔP_s presumably is determined by both the capacity within S1 and the steepness of the slope of S_1. In the present study isoflurane appears to have slowed the rapid CSF pressure buffering processes (as indicated by decreased S_1 in group 3) but not to have limited the capacity of those processes (as indicated by unchanged DS_1 in group 3) so that during isoflurane, CSF pressure at end S_1 did not decrease as much as with desflurane or in the controls (as indicated by increased ΔP_s in group 3). With 0.5 or 1.0 MAC desflurane at either normo- or hypocapnia there was no impairment of the capacity of CSF pressure to return to baseline values following a CSF pressure increase as compared to controls.

Time Pattern of ICP After Bolus Injection as an Indicator of Intracranial Disturbances

N. Stocchetti[1], S. Rossi[1], P. Ceccarelli[1], M. Ursino[2], and D. Mancia[3]

[1] First Department of Anesthesia and Intensive Care, Hospital of Parma, Italy
[2] Department of Electronics and Automatics, University of Ancona, Italy
[3] Department of Neurology, University of Parma, Italy

Introduction

Bedside evaluation of intracranial pressure-volume characteristics has been reported in head injured patients [1,2]. After injection of fluid, pressure increases, allowing calculation of Pressure Volume Index (PVI); the rate of reduction in ICP after the peak has been suggested as an indicator of resistance to CSF outflow [1]. In some cases after the initial peak, ICP behaves differently, with further increase starting 8-10 seconds after bolus injection and lasting for minutes. We have indicated this pattern as paradoxical response (PR). This phenomenon is investigated in a group of comatose head injured patients in order to 1) quantify the frequency of PR and 2) to assess the association of this pattern with relevant clinical variables.

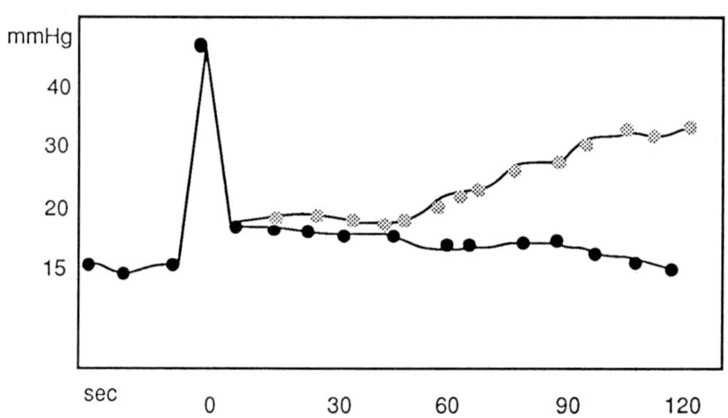

Fig.1: ICP recording during PVI testing. In black the expected response after bolus injection, in gray the Paradoxical Response

Methods

34 head injured patients, 4 female, with a mean age of 33 years (14-64) were studied. Median motor GCS on admission was 3; CT Scan diagnoses on admission were: epidural hematoma (1 case), subdural hematoma (11), contusions (12) and diffuse damage (8). The basal cisterns were normal in 19 patients, compressed in 8 and absent in 7 cases. ICP was recorded through ventricular catheters; analog data regarding ICP and Mean Arterial Pressure (MAP) was processed by an Analog-Digital Converter (Mac Lab Word Precision Instruments, New Haven - Connecticut USA) and sent to a computer for storage and analysis. Pressure-volume studies were done using the bolus technique, injecting and withdrawing 1-3 ml of saline six times for each study; studies were repeated every 12 hours. Only bolus injection studies were considered for analysis. The occurrence of B-waves, defined as repetitive oscillations in ICP at frequencies of 0.5- 2 waves per minute [3], before each test was recorded.
After injection the ICP immediately following the bolus and values at different times (30, 60, 90 and 120 seconds) were measured. Estimated intracranial volume change (EIVC) was calculated at 1 and 2

minutes after injection for studies showing PR. Calculation was based on the following equation, modified from Marmarou [4]:

$$EIVC = PVI * \log (ICP \text{ at time 1 or 2}/ICP \text{ Peak}).$$

This equation allows calculation of the volume changes at 1 and 2 minutes after the test, excluding changes produced by the bolus itself.

A stepwise regression showed that the degree of PR after 90 seconds was the best predictor of the ICP in the following 12 hours: in order to simplify the analysis only this value was considered for comparison among the different groups.

The severity of PR was assessed by calculating the percentage of tests in which ICP 90 seconds after injection was greater than ICP immediately following the bolus addition. Patients showing PR in up to 20% of tests were classified as Grade 0, patients with a PR present in 21 to 50% of tests as Grade 1 and cases with PR in more than 50% of tests as Grade 2.

The highest ICP lasting more than 5 minutes was recorded every 12 hours and was indicated as maximal ICP.

Outcome was asessed six months after trauma using a modified version of the Glasgow Outcome Score [5].

Differences among percentages were assessed by using a Fisher exact test and among means by using a one-way ANOVA.

Results

Mean ICP was 21.95 mmHg (sd 7.94), mean ICP maximal was 37.04 mmHg (sd 14.66) and mean PVI was 24.79 ml (sd 10.64).

A total of 461 pressure-volume tests was examined in 34 patients.

Sixty seconds after the injection ICP was above the peak level in 184 studies, at the peak level in 176 and only in 101 tests the ICP value decreased toward the baseline value. Two minutes after injection the ICP value was still higher than the peak in 171 tests. The mean EIVC was 1.48 ml at 1 minute (range 0.51-3.22 ml sd) and 0.97 ml (range 0.49-3.11 sd) at two minutes.

The occurrence of B-waves was detected in 181 tests; it was present in 76 tests showing PR and it was not associated with the severity of PR itself.

Twelve patients were classified as Grade 0, 16 as Grade 1 and 6 as Grade 2. Main data regarding the clinical presentation and outcome for the different groups are reported in the following table (Table 1).

Table 1

	n°pt	Median motor GCS	Average PVI (*)	Average ICP (*)	Average ICP maximal (*)	Compressed or absent cisterns (*)	Good outcome (*)	Poor outcome (*)
Grade 0	12	3	27.05 ml (sd 9.84)	17.23 mmHg (sd 2.69)	27.14 mmHg (sd 4.8)	4	10	2
Grade 1	16	3	24.91 ml (sd 6.51)	24.88 mmHg (sd 12.61)	36.82 mmHg (sd 14.47)	7	9	7
Grade 2	6	4	21.95 ml (sd 7.84)	28.28 mmHg (sd 11.04)	57.55 mmHg (sd 12.01)	4	3	3

Legend: the first column shows the number of patients of each group, Average PVI is the mean of PVI of all patients of each group, Average ICP is the mean value of ICP recorded for all patients of each group; Average ICP maximal is the mean of the highest ICP lasting more than 5 minutes recorded in the same group of patients. Good outcome includes good recovery and moderate disability while poor outcome indicates severe disability. When significant differences ($p<0.05$ or lower) are detected, they are indicated by (*).

Discussion

PR is a rather frequent finding in this group of head injured patients since it was detected in 40% of PVI tests. Twenty-two patients in 34 showed PR in more than 20% of their pressure-volume tests. This paradoxical response was associated with a greater increase both in mean ICP and in the maximal ICP. It was also associated with lower values of PVI, suggesting reduced intracranial compliance, and with a

greater incidence of compressed or absent basal cisternes. This data indicates that a more severe disturbance of the intracranial system is present when PR is identified. Patients classified as Grade 1 and 2 had a significantly worse outcome.
Mean EIVC at one minute was 1.48 ml. Since no more fluid is added to the intracranial system from the outside at that time, and changes in PVI are not suitable, the ICP rise that we have labelled PR indicates that changes in intracranial content are due to modifications of one or more intracranial components.
This behavior of ICP is elicited by the bolus injection, since it is not associated with the occurrence of B-waves preceding the test.
The short time of onset of PR suggests that the most probable cause of PR itself is a modification in vascular components; in fact CSF recirculation takes longer than the few seconds measured in these cases and modifications of cerebral tissue are not probable. Assuming that vascular factors are implied in determining PR, the net increase in intracranial volume may be explained both by a decrease in cerebrovascular resistances and/or by an increase of resistance to venous outflow.
Due to the associaton of this phenomenon with important clinical variables, we suggest that after bolus injection the trend of ICP should be considered as a significant sign of instability of the intracranial system.

References

1) Marmarou A, Maset AL, Ward JD, et al. (1987). Contribution of CSF and vascular factors to elevation of ICP in severely head-injured patients. J Neurosurg 66:883-890.
2) Kosteljanetz M (1986) Acute Head Injury. Pressure-Volume Relation and Cerebrospinal Fluid Dynamics. Neurosurgery 18:17-23.
3) Marmarou A, Wachi A. (1987). Blood volume responsivity to ICP change in head injured patients. Intracranial Pressure VII Eds.: Hoff JT and Betz AL, Springer-Verlag Berlin Heilderberg , pp 688-689.
4) Newell DW et al. (1992). The relationship of blood flow velocity fluctuations to intracranial pressure B waves. J. Neurosurgery 76: 415-421.
5) Jennet B, Bond M (1975). Assessment of outcome after severe brain damage. Lancet 1:480-484.

Regional Tissue Compliance of Edematous Brain in Water Intoxication Edema—Comparison to Vasogenic Edema

T. Kuroiwa[1], M. Ueki[1], I. Taniguchi[2], H. Ichiki[1], and R. Okeda[1]

[1] Department of Neuropathology, [2] Department of Neurophysiology, Medical Research Institute, Tokyo Medical and Dental University, Bunkyo-ku, Tokyo, 113 Japan

SUMMARY

The purpose of present study was to elucidate the biomechanical characteristics of edematous brain tissue in water intoxication by measuring regional tissue compliance and water content and to compare with those in vasogenic edema. Water intoxication was induced in cats by drip infusion of ADH and distilled water for 6 h, and the animals were sacrificed under deep anesthesia by an injected overdose of potassium chloride. Vasogenic edema was induced in cats by cold lesion made on the left ectosylvian gyrus, and the animals were sacrificed at 4 h after lesioning. In both groups, the brain was cut in coronal plane and prepared for determination of regional tissue compliance (indentation method) and water content (gravimetry) at various locations of the coronal plane and for histological study. BBB permeability was assessed by i.v.injection of Evans Blue. In water intoxication group, blood osmolarity reduced from 316 to 278 mOsm. Water content significantly increased to 80.5% in the gray matter (78.5% in the control) and 69.1% in the white matter (65.8% in the control). Regional tissue compliance in the corresponding sites were 102.4% and 127.2% of the control value, respectively. In cold lesion edema, water content increased to 82.7% in the edematous white matter (65.3% in the control). Regional tissue compliance in the corresponding site increased to 402% of the control value. Present study showed that (1) accumulation of edema fluid induced by water intoxication is more pronounced in the white matter than gray matter, (2) the change in tissue compliance induced by water intoxication is not significant and much milder than the change observed in vasogenic edema induced by cold lesion.

INTRODUCTION

Brain Edema - a common complication of various intracranial disorders such as cerebral ischemia, tumor and trauma - is a major risk factor for fatal cerebral herniation. It also causes demyelination, ischemia and the other secondary brain injuries. Biomechanical changes of edematous tissue is an important factor in the process of these edema-mediated tissue injuries. Therefore basic knowledge on the biomechanical characteristics of edematous as well as normal brain tissue is indispensable for studying the pathophysiology.

In this study , we measured regional difference in the tissue water content and tissue compliance in brain edema induced by water intoxication and cold lesion. We observed that the edema fluid accumulates more in the white matter than gray matter[1] in water intoxication and the change in tissue compliance induced by water intoxication is significantly milder than the change in vasogenic edema induced by cold lesion.

MATERIALS AND METHODS

Adult mongrel cats (N=13) weighing 2.5- 4 kg were used in the following experiments. The anesthesia was induced by intramuscular injection of ketameine (30mg/kg) and maintained by additional injections during surgical preparation. Catheters were inserted into the femoral artery and vein for monitoring of arterial blood pressure (ABP) , and injection of tracers and drugs. Water intoxication was induced by drip infusion of ADH and distilled water for 6 h[1]. Blood osmolarity was intermittently measured to control the level about 40 mOsm lower than the control value. The animal was sacrificed by an injected overdose of potassium chloride. Vasogenic edema was induced by cold lesion made on the left ectosylvian gyrus[2], and the animal was sacrificed at 4 h after lesioning. In both groups, the brains were cut in coronal plane and prepared for the following studies. Regional tissue compliance was measured by using indentation method[2]. The water content of brain tissue was measured by gravimetry [2] at various locations of the coronal plane. Water content value was calculated from the specific gravity value according to the equations reported by Marmarou A et. al[3]. The tissue sections used for compliance measurement were immersion fixed, embedded in paraffin and prepared for histological study. BBB permeability was assessed by i.v.injection of Evans Blue (2 cc/kg, 2% saline solution).

RESULTS AND DISCUSSION

Systemic ABP and blood gases were maintained within the physiological ranges. Very mild and diffuse EB extravasation in the cerebrum was observed in one animal in water intoxication group. Intense EB extravasation was observed in the subcortical white matter under the lesioned cortex and adjacent semioval center in cold lesion group.

Fig. 1. Light micrograph of the white matter in the control (left), water intoxication edema (middle) and cold lesion edema (right). Note the dissociation of neuronal fibers in the edematous white matter (HE staining, x52).

Light microscopical examination showed marked dissociation of neuronal fibers and dilatation of extracellular space in the edematous white matter in cold lesion group. In water intoxication group, very mild dissociation was observed in the white matter. No noticeable change was observed in the gray matter in either group (Fig. 1).

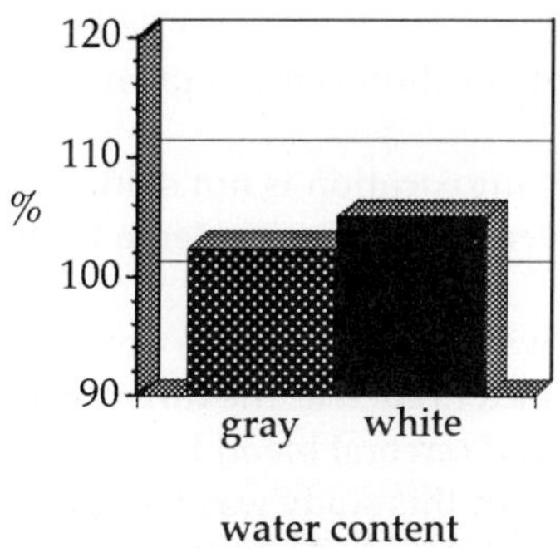

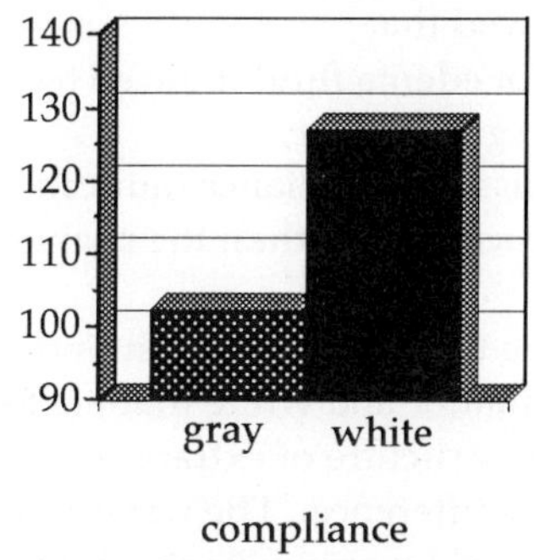

Fig. 2 % Increase of regional tissue water content (left) and compliance (right) in water intoxication edema

In water intoxication group, mean blood osmolarity reduced from 316 to 278 mOsm. The water content increased from 78.5±0.82% (mean±SD) to 80.5±0.56% in the gray matter and from 65.8±0.25% to 69.1±0.75% in the white matter (102.4 % and 105.1 % of the control value, respectively). The *p* values by unpaired Student *t*-test were 0.004 and 0.0006, respectively. Regional tissue compliance increased from 0.000141±0.000091 cm^2/dyn to 0.000144±0.000042 cm^2/dyn in the gray matter and from 0.00018±0.000081 cm^2/dyn to 0.00023±0.000062 cm^2/dyn in the white matter (102.4 % of the control value in the gray matter and 127.2 % of the control value in the white matter). The increase in either group was not significant (p=0.95 in the gray matter and p=0.34 in the white matter, Fig. 2).

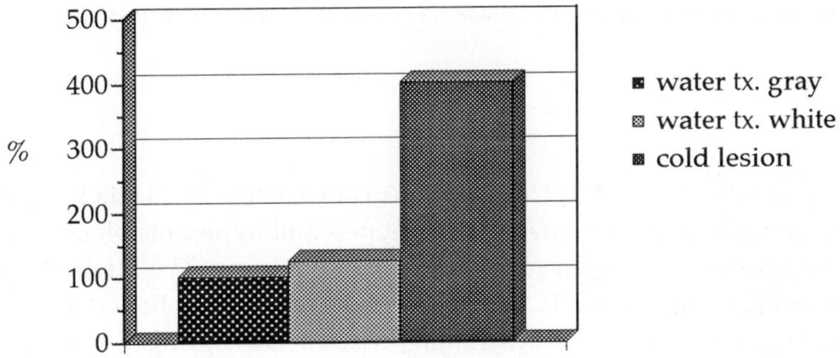

Fig. 3 % Increase of regional tissue compliance in water intoxication edema (left; gray matter, middle; white matter) and cold lesion edema (right)

In cold lesion group, the water content of edematous white matter increased from 65.3±3.5% to 82.7±5.2% ($p \leq 0.00001$, 126.6 % of the control value). Regional tissue compliance in this group increased from 0.00010±0.000026 cm^2/dyn to 0.000403±0.000274 cm^2/dyn (p=0.00019, 402.1 % of the control value).

Present study showed that ;
(1) accumulation of edema fluid induced by water intoxication is more pronounced in the white matter than gray matter,
(2) the change in tissue compliance induced by water intoxication is not statistically significant and much milder than the change observed in vasogenic edema induced by cold lesion.
The increase in the tissue water content induced by water intoxication is not uniform between the gray matter and white matter. Several factors such as the differences in the intracellular space, structure of extracellular matrix and cerebral blood flow are probably responsible for the difference. The water intoxication in this study was designed as a model for water intoxication occasionally observed in the neurosurgical and ICU practices. Further study is needed to examine if the observed dissociation exists in different level and duration of water intoxication.
As we have presented in the ICP symposium in 1991[2], we observed a significant increase in regional tissue compliance in vasogenic edema induced by cold lesion. However, we were not able to detect any significant increase in regional tissue compliance in water intoxication edema either in the gray matter or white matter. It is probably due to the milder edema in water intoxication. Another factor contributing to the difference is probably different localization of edema fluid. In vasogenic edema - in which edema fluid distributes mainly in the extracellular space -, water accumulation causes marked increase in the tissue compliance. However, in water intoxication edema - in which edema fluid distributes to all compartments of brain tissue to equilibrate the osmotic difference among them - water accumulation causes minimal increase in tissue compliance. This speculation fits to our recent observation on cerebral ischemia, in which intracellular accumulation of edema fluid (ischemic edema) causes decrease in regional tissue compliance[4].

REFERENCES

1. Ueki M, Kuroiwa T, Okeda R (1991) Ueki M, T, Kuroiwa, Chen Q, Okeda R (1992) Analysis of regional brain water content under hyper- and hypotonic blood osmolallity. Abstract for 10th World Congress of Anesthesiologist in Hague, The Netherland.
2. Kuroiwa T, Taniguchi I and Okeda R. (1991) Regional tissue compliance of edematous brain after cryogenic injury in cats. Intracranial Pressure VIII Springer-Verlag pp 127-129
3. Marmarou A, Tanaka K, Schulman K (1982) An improved gravimetric measure of cerebral edema. J Neurosurg 56: 246-253
4. Kuroiwa T, Ueki M, Suemasu H, Taniguchi I, Okeda R (1994) Biomechanical characteristics of brain edema. Acta Neurochir [Suppl] 60: 158-161

Quantitative Hysteresis Area Rate as an Indicator for Changes in Intracranial Components

M. MAEDA[1], K. NAKAJIMA[1], Y. SAKAI[2], M. MIYAZAKI[1], and S. SUZUKI[3]

[1] Department of Neurosurgery and Casuality Center, Juntendo University Izunagaoka Hospital, Izunagaoka-cho, Tagata-gun, Shizuoka, 410-22 Japan
[2] Department of Engineering, Chuo University, Bunkyo-ku, Tokyo, 112 Japan
[3] Numazu College of Technology, Numazu, Shizuoka, 410 Japan

[INTRODUCTION]

Synchronization of changes in the intracranial pressure pulse wave (ICPPW) with the cardiac best was first reported in the 1950s [1]. Intracranial components may also influence the ICPPW [2,3]. Conventional analyses of the ICPPW have focused on the peaks [4,5,6] and amplitude [2] of the wave. System analysis attempts to obtain a transfer function for the intracranial cavity, in order to analyze the intracranial physical environment [7,8]. The system analysis approach tries to characterize the ICPPW by the response to a known input signal, the systemic arterial pulse wave (SAPW). We previously proposed a quantitative hysteresis area ratio (Rh%) based on the observation that the time delay between the SAPW and ICPPW demonstrates hysteretic damping [9]. The present study investigated how Rh% changes under pathophysiological conditions, such as hypercapnia, cerebral vasoconstriction due to hyperventilation, and increased ICP.

[MATERIALS AND METHODS]

Eighteen cats were used for the experiments under chloralose anesthesia. The animals were immobilized by pancuronium bromide and artificially ventilated. Both femoral arteries and veins were dissected and cannulated with polyethylene catheters pushed into the thoracic part of the aorta and the superior vena cava for blood sampling and pressure recording, respectively. End-tidal CO_2 concentration was continuously monitored. The lateral ventricle was punctured with a needle for ICP recording. The ICPPW was also continuously monitored by a Camino fiber optic transducer inserted into the white matter of the occipital lobe. The Rh% was calculated as follows: A Cartesian plot of the SAPW (X-axis) and the ICPPW (Y-axis) traces a closed loop locus in a counterclockwise direction (Fig 1A).

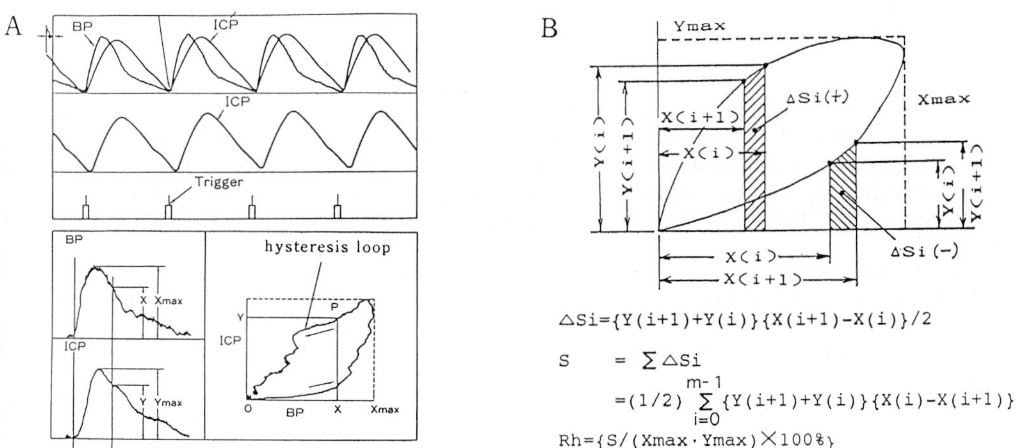

$$\Delta Si=\{Y(i+1)+Y(i)\}\{X(i+1)-X(i)\}/2$$

$$S = \sum \Delta Si = (1/2)\sum_{i=0}^{m-1}\{Y(i+1)+Y(i)\}\{X(i)-X(i+1)\}$$

$$Rh=\{S/(Xmax \cdot Ymax)\times 100\%\}$$

Fig.1 Calculation procedure for hysteresis area rate (Rh%)

Rh% was defined as the ratio of the hysteresis loop area to the rectangular area which circumscribed the hysteresis loop. Analogue information of SAPW and ICPPW with sampling time 2 msec was digitized into values X(i) and Y(i) on the Cartesian coordinates, and the area of the trapezoid ($\triangle Si$) integrated.
Then, Rh% = $\{S/(X_{max} \cdot Y_{max})\} \times 100$ (Fig 1B).
Analysis of the Rh% was carried out during hypercapnia (5% CO_2 and 95% O_2), intravenous injection of acetazolamide (Diamox) (15 mg/kg), hyperventilation, acute brain compression and decompression by epidural balloon inflation and deflation, and intraventricular infusion (IVI) of saline.

[RESULTS]

Hypercapnia was induced by ventilation with 5% CO_2 and 95% O_2. An example of the changes in the hysteresis loop from the early phase of hypercapnia to equilibrium is shown in Fig 3A. There was progressive rounding of the ICPPW (Fig 2A) and the hysteresis loop (Fig 2B), and Rh% remarkably increased to 53% (Fig 2B,C).

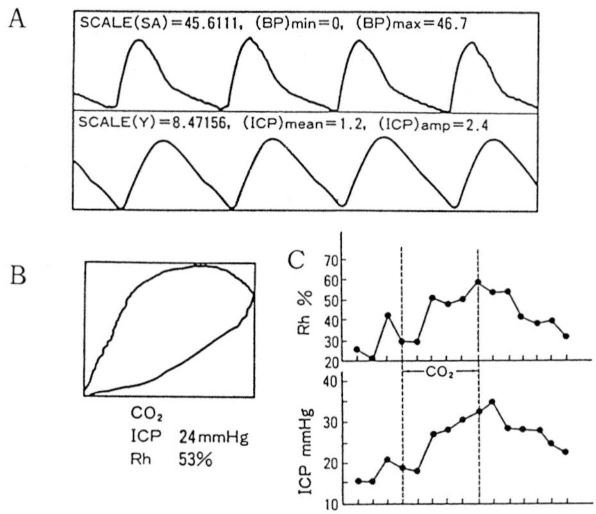

Fig.2 Changes in SAPP, ICPPW, Hysteresis loop and Rh(%) during CO_2 inhalation.
A: systemic arterial pulse wave (upper trace) and intracranial pressure pulse wave(lower trace)
B:hysteresis loop, C:Rh(%) and ICP during hypercapnia

In an another animal, Rh% progressively increased from 24.1% to 39.7% and 57.5%, then returned to 29.3% after cessation of CO_2 inhalation (Fig 3A). Plotting of the ICP and Rh% during hypercapnia showed that the onset of increased ICP was slightly preceded by an increase in Rh%. Intravenous injection of acetazolamide, which acts as a cerebral vasodilator, also provoked a slight increase in Rh%.
The changes in Rh% during IVI was much smaller than those during hypercapnia at the same mean levels of ICP.
Cats were hyperventilated with room air. An example of the changes in the hysteresis loop under hyperventilation is shown in Fig 3A. Rh% decreased to 15.6% during hyperventilation and returned to 24.1~33.9% after return to normoventilation. Plotting of the mean ICP and Rh% measured during hyperventilation showed that a decrease in Rh% preceded or was synchronized with the decrease in ICP (Fig 3B).

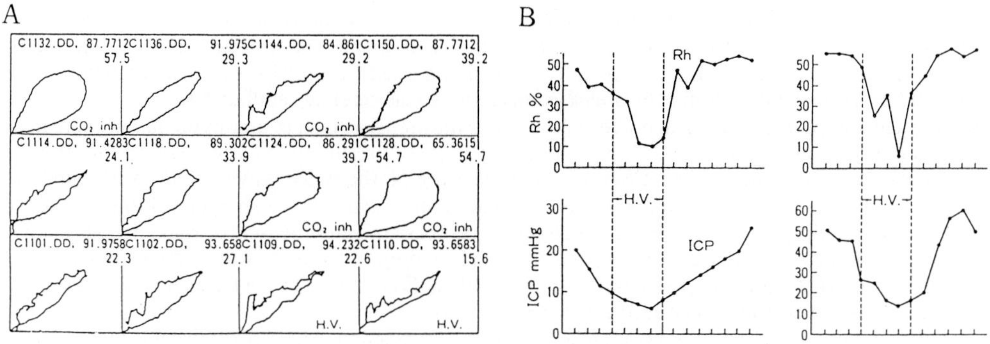

Fig.3 Changes in hysteresis loop during hyperventilation and CO2 inhalation (A), and decrease of Rh(%) and ICP during hyperventilation (B)

Progressive increase in ICP induced an increase in Rh%. When acute brain compression and decompression was repeatedly induced by balloon inflation-deflation, concomitant changes in Rh% were elicited with variations in ICP (Fig 4A,B). Following the second inflation and deflation, the ICP returned to the previous level. However, the Rh% remained higher as shown by the open triangles of Fig 4A.

We recorded ICPPW and SAPW in patients who developed clinical vasospasm following aneurysmal subarachnoid hemorrhage. At the onset of clinical vasospasm, a slight decrease in Rh% was observed within the normal limits of ICP.

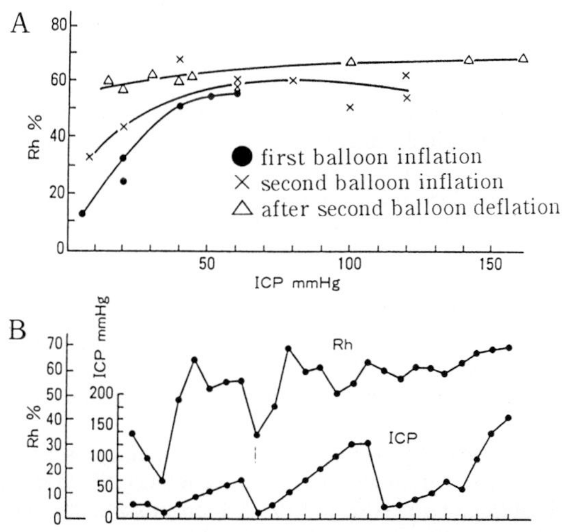

Fig.4 Changes in Rh(%) and ICP during acute brain compression and decompression

[DISCUSSION]

The ICPPW is similar to the arterial pulse, but the exact origin of the wave has not been determined [4,10]. Bering [1] believed that the cerebrospinal fluid pulse wave (CSFPW) emanated from the choroid plexus, while Dunber et al. [10] suggested the feeding vessels. Portnoy et al. [11] reported that the CSFPW is derived from the transmission of an arterial pulse into the cerebral veins, and the pulsations within the thin-walled vein are then transmitted to the CSF. Nagai et al. [12] used a newly devised epidural transducer to study how the pulse wave form changed when blood pressure was elevated or reduced by a hypertensive or hypotensive agent. They suggested that the cerebrovascular tone contributes to the form of the pulse wave under increased ICP.

Hamer et al. [4] studied the CSFPW in dogs under normovolemic hypotension or hypertension, concludin that both systemic blood pressure and cerebrovascular reactivity are major determinants for the shape an pressure amplitude of the ICPPW. Cerebral vasodilatation caused cerebral vascular damping of the arteri pulse and the arterial pressure may be directly transmitted to the cerebral capillary bed.

Portnoy and Chopp [3] investigated CSFPW analysis during hypercapnia and hypoxia. Hypercapnia an hypoxia produced an increase in CSF pulse pressure ($\triangle P_{CSF}$) resulting in an increase in the amplitude c the fundamental frequency of the CSFPW with rounding of the pulse wave. They suggested that th increase in $\triangle P_{CSF}$ is related to cerebral arteriolar vasodilation and not to a sharper volume-pressure curv and that the rounding of the CSFPW is related to a decrease in cerebrovascular tone. In our study, CC inhalation produced an increase in pulse pressure with rounding of the pulse wave and an increase in Rh% The changes in Rh% during hypercapnia were greater than those during IVI at the same mean levels of ICI In contrast, hyperventilation produced a decrease in Rh%.

Our study showed that acute brain compression and decompression caused a remarkable increase in Rh% It is well known that cerebrovascular tonicity is seriously damaged by mechanical or metabolic facto caused by acute increase in ICP. Our results suggest that the Rh% is primarily dependent on th cerebrovascular tone in the intracranial vasculature. The increase in Rh% caused by acetazolamide injectic or the decrease in Rh% in patients with cerebral vasospasm corresponds with cerebrovascular dilatation c constriction, respectively. Continuous monitoring of the Rh% may be an useful indicator for pathologic changes in intracranial components, especially cerebrovascular tone.

[ACKNOWLEDGEMENTS]

This work was supported in part by a grant awarded to prof. Minoru MAEDA (NO.06671420) from th Japanese Ministry of Education, Science and Culture.

[REFERENCE]

1. Bering EA Jr (1955) Choroid plexus and arterial pulsation of cerebrospinal fluid. Demonstration of choroid plexus as a cerebrospinal fluid pump. Arch Neurol Psychiatry 73 : 165-172
2. Avezaad CJJ, Van Eijndhoven JHM, Wyper DJ (1979) cerebrospinal fluid pulse pressure and intracranial volume pressure relationship. J Neurol Neurosurg Psychiatry 42 : 687-700
3. Portnoy HD, Chopp M (1981) Cerebrospinal fluid pulse wave form analysis during hypercapnia and hypoxia. Neurosurgery 9 : 14-27
4. Hamer J, Alverti E, Hoyer S, Wiedemann K (1977) Influence of systemic and cerebral vascular factors on the cerebrospinal fluid pulse wave. J Neurosurg 46 : 36-45
5. Hirai O, Handa H, Ishikawa M (1984) Epidural pulse wave form as an indicator of intracranial pressure dynamics. Surg Neurol 21 : 67-74
6. Nitta M (1982) The effect of increased intracranial pressure on pulse wave. Neurol Med Chir 22 : 193-200 (Jpn)
7. Chopp M, Portnoy HD (1980) System analysis of intracranial pressure. Comparison with volume-pressure test and CSF-pulse amplitude analysis. J Neurosurg 53 : 516-527
8. Kasuga Y, Nagai H, Hasegawa Y, Nitta M (1987) Transmission characteristics of pulse waves in the intracranial cavity of dogs. J Neurosurg 66 : 907-914
9. Maeda M, Nakajima K, Sakai Y, Miyazaki M, Suzuki S (1993) Analysis of a quantitative hysteresis area rate as an indicator for pathological changes in intracranial components. Progress in Research on ICP : 13-19
10. Dunber HS, Guthrie TC, Karpell B (1966) A study of the cerebrospinal fluid pulse wave. Arch Neurol 14 : 624-630
11. Portnoy HD, Chopp M, Branch C, Shannon MB (1982) Cerebrospinal fluid pulse wave form as on indicator of cerebral autoregulation. J Neurosurg 56 : 666-678
12. Nagai H, Kamiya I, Ikeyama J (1980) A newly devised transducer for epidural pressure measuremen and its clinical use. In : Shulman K, Marmarou A, Miller JD (eds) Intracranial Pressure Ⅳ. Springer, Berlin Heiderberg New York : 417-418

Session X:
Biophysics (2)

Chairmen: A. Unterberg and H. Nagai

Statistical Analysis of ICP and Frequential Analysis of Slow Waves During the Course of Subarachnoid Haemorrhage Following Arterial Aneurysm Rupture: Effects of Vasospasm

J.-J. Lemaire[1], B. Irthum[1], J. Chazal[1], and J.-Y. Boire[2]

[1] Service of Neurosurgery, University Hospital, Clermont-Ferrand, France
[2] Laboratory of Biomathematics, Statistics and Medical Computing, Faculty of Medicine, Clermont-Ferrand, France

SUMMARY

Twenty patients (pts) suffering from subarachnoid haemorrhage following arterial aneurysm rupture were studied: 10 male, 10 female; mean age 53.4 ranging from 25 to 70; 1 pt grade I WFNS, 5 pts II, 1 pt III, 7 pts IV, and 6 pts V. All pts had a nimodipine treatment during the study. ICP monitoring was realised during a temporary external ventricular drainage performed to treat an acute CSF flow disturbance. The frequency and the duration of the daily recordings were guided by clinical conditions. ICP data analysis have consisted in : 1°) a descriptive statistical study with calculation of the mean pressure (MeP) and its standard deviation (SDm), the modal pressure (MoP) and the left and right standard deviations and their sum (SDsum); 2°) a study in the frequential domain which provided the power spectrum of which we have noted the frequency (F, Hz) of the most important spike of power (P, arbitrary unit: a.u.), and this for the frequency bands of B waves (BW, from $8 * 10^{-3}$ Hz to $50 * 10^{-3}$ Hz) and infra B waves (IB, below $8 * 10^{-3}$ Hz): FBW and PBW, FIB and PIB, respectively. We have defined a daily analysis period: after the drainage closing, we have looked for a stable ICP level with the highest value of the whole of the daily recording. We have differentiated ICP recordings, associated (V+, n=20) or not (V-, n=28) with an angiographic vasospasm phase, and these realised during a sedation period (sed+, n=25) or not (sed-, n=23). We found: 1°) increasing exponential relations between the Glasgow Coma Scale score and SDsum (sed-, $P<0.01$), GCS score and PBW (sed-, $P<0.01$), GCS score and PIB (sed+, $P<0.05$); 2°) a reduction of high PBW values ($100*10^{-3}$ a.u.$<$PBW$\leq 1000*10^{-3}$ a.u.) for the V+ group (χ^2 test, $P<0.01$). The pathophysiological considerations are discussed.

INTRODUCTION

Previous clinical studies showed patterns of slow ICP fluctuations [1] [2] during the course of subarachnoid haemorrhage following arterial aneurysm rupture. ICP slow waves (A, B, C) were analysed less in these circumstances [3] and a relationship has been demonstrated between the cerebral dysfunction status and patterns of slow pressure waves.

We decided to evaluate the informative value of these ICP slow waves notably when there was an angiographic vasospasm. In this aim we used the descriptive statistical analysis of ICP and a study in the frequential domain of the slow waves. Because of technical constraints we were limited to the so called B and A waves.

MATERIALS

Twenty patients (pts) were studied: 10 male and 10 female with a mean age of 53.4 ranging from 25 to 70. The majority of them were in severe initial clinical conditions: 1 pt grade I WFNS, 5 pts II, 1 pt III, 7 pts IV, and 6 pts V. They all had an acute CSF flow disturbance which indicated a temporary external ventricular drainage and permitted a discontinuous ICP monitoring (P10EZ* transducer, Gould Medical, U.S.A.; CM 130* monitor, PPG Hellige, France). CSF flow disturbance was evoked if we noted a widening of ventricular size (Bifrontal Index [4] increase on successive CT scans) or a massive subarachnoid and/or ventricular haemorrhage associated with a rapid consciousness impairment.

To record the ICP signal we used a device sampling at 166.6 * 10^{-3} Hz (PICSOFT*, Sophysa, France) [5], connected downstream from the monitor. Because of spontaneous ICP variations and/or necessity of CSF drainage, we were obliged to define an analysis period inferior to an hour per recording-day (numbered in relation to the date of the aneurysm rupture): after a drainage closing we looked for a stable ICP level, and we selected the highest ICP level value obtained from the whole of the daily recording (e.g. fig 3). The duration and the frequency of the daily recordings were laid down by clinical conditions. Forty eight recording periods were analysed (Fig 1).

A recording was considered as associated with a vasospasm phase if it was realised: 1°) Any day inside a period during the course of which an angiogram showed a spasm (positive angiogram): periods were determined according to classical notions of vasospasm risk, early from D0 to D4, common from D5 to D10 and from D11 to D15, late from D16 to D21, and ultra-late beyond D21; 2°) the day after a positive angiogram carried out at the upper boundary of one of the periods defined above; 3°) between two positive angiograms. Beyond D15, if no spasm was proved before, and if there were good clinical and CTscan conditions, no angiogram was performed, and we considered that there was no vasospasm. Angiograms never showed diffuse vasospasm.

Twenty recordings were realised during a vasospasm phase (V+), and twenty-eight out of a vasospasm phase (V-) (Fig 1).

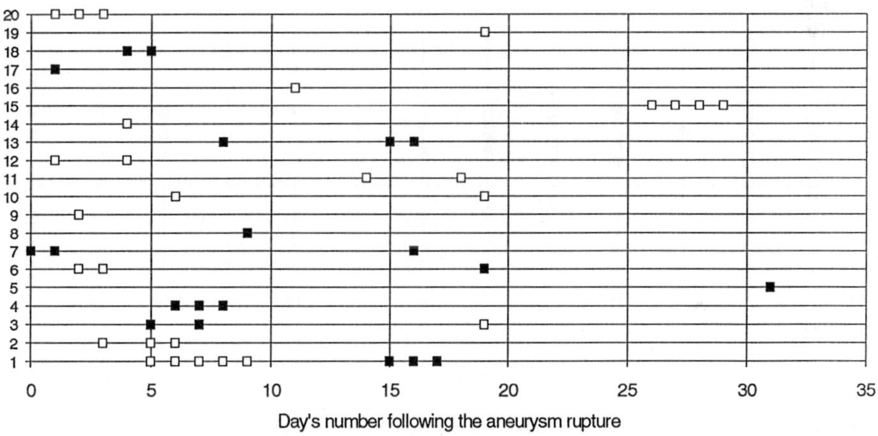

Fig 1 Time distribution of the recordings (n=48) carried out during (n=20, solid square) or out of (n=28, empty square) a vasospasm phase. Patient's references are figured on y axe (20 patients).

Comatose patients were, if necessary, sedated (sed) with benzodiazepine and morphinic. All patients had a nimodipine treatment from their admission to D21, or beyond, if there was an ultra-late vasospasm.

METHOD

°) ICP Curve Analysis

We were limited for the duration of the analysed periods to 25 and 51 min because of frequential analysis technical constraints. Each selected recording was examined with the two durations which overlapped.

Descriptive statistical parameters: The mean pressure (MeP) and its standard deviation (SDm), the modal pressure (MoP) and the left and right standard deviations (SDl, SDr) [6], were calculated.

Frequential analysis: According to a method previously described [7], we used a fast Fourier transform which provided the power spectrum, and we noted the frequency (F, Hz) of the most important spike of power (P, arbitrary unit: a.u.). This was done only (because of the Shannon theorem) for the frequency bands of B waves (BW, from 8 * 10^{-3} Hz to 50 * 10^{-3} Hz) and infra B waves (IB, below 8 * 10^{-3} Hz) which included the A waves: FBW and PBW, FIB and PIB, respectively.

2°) Global Data Analysis

We have separated the 25 and 51 min durations. Clinical data (Glasgow Coma Scale score, temperature), patient sedation (25 recordings with sed, sed+; 23 without sed, sed-) and angiographic spasm were correlated with the ICP data.

RESULTS

1°) Relationships between Clinical Status and ICP Data

We found an increasing exponential relation between SDsum (SDr+SDl) versus GCS score ($r=0.5649$; $P<0.01$) which corresponded essentially to the sed- group (sed+ group $r=0.2059$; $P>0.05$) (Fig 2a).
We found an increasing exponential relation between PBW and GCS score for the sed- group ($r=0.747$; $P<0.01$) (Fig 2b), also between PIB and GCS score for the sed+ group ($r=0.4273$; $P<0.05$).
These results were found for both 25 and 51 min durations.

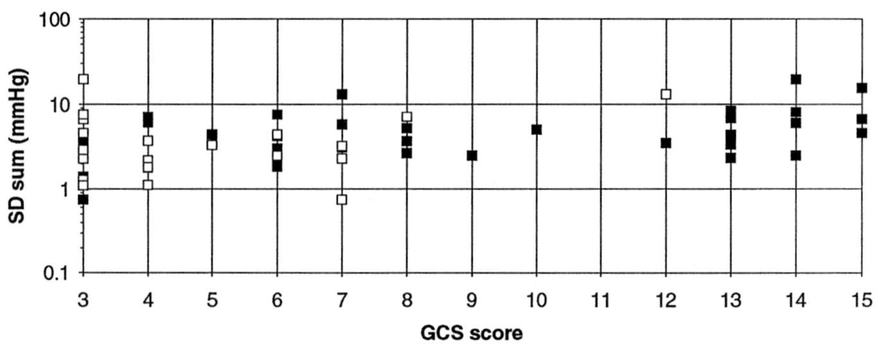

(a)

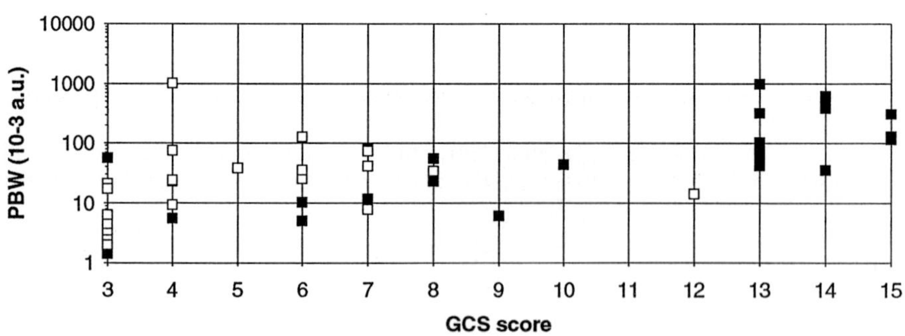

(b)

Fig 2 Relationships between SD sum (a) or PBW (b), and GCS score: cases with sedation (n=25, empty square), cases without sedation (n=23, solid square).

2°) Relationship between ICP Data and Vasospasm

The distribution of PBW was different for V+ and V- groups (χ^2 test, P<0.01) with a reduction of high PBW values ($100*10^{-3}$ a.u. < PBW ≤ $1000*10^{-3}$ a.u.) in the V+ group (Fig . 3 and 4). This result was found only for the 25min-period analysis.

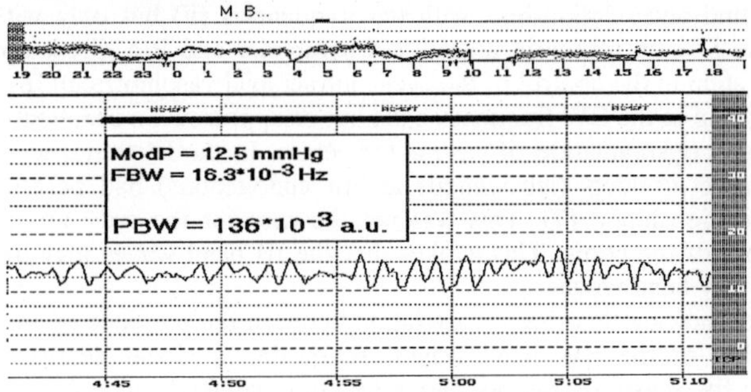

(a)

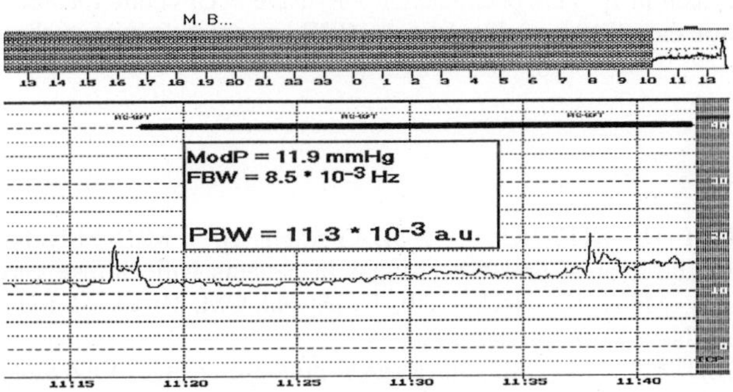

(b)

Fig 3 Example of reduction of PBW and vasospasm. Patient of 54 years old, female, WFNS II on admission D0, anterior communicating cerebral artery aneurysm, endovascular embolization D1 (coils), external ventricular drainage D4, death D25 (polyvisceral failure). (a) D8 no vasospasm , (b) D17 vasospasm.

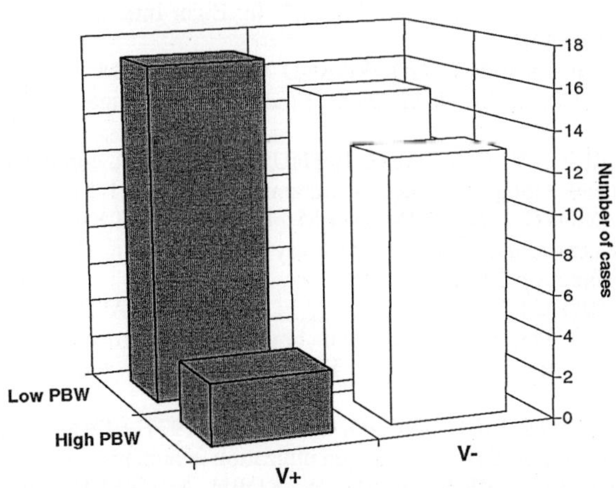

Fig 4 Distribution of the high ($100*10^{-3}$ a.u.< PBW ≤ $1000*10^{-3}$ a.u.) and low (PBW ≤ $100*10^{-3}$ a.u.) PBW values, function of the association with a vasospasm phase (V+) or not (V-). Analysis of the 25min-periods.

DISCUSSION

Our results seem to show that not ICP values but slow ICP waves are closely dependant on the status of awakeness. We didn't find any relationships with the frequencies (F) but only with the pressure wave amplitude, of which the SDsum represent an indirect parameter and P a direct one. This suggests the implication of the brain stem in the control of the cyclic intracranial vasomotricity [8] [9]. This phenomena was clear for the sed- group in the BW frequency band but disappeared if a sedation was induced probably because of the therapeutic dysregulation of vasomotor centre. In the IB frequency band, because of the slow frequencies, pressure artefacts (iatrogenous and/or endogenous) had parasited the analysis thus masking the possible relationship(s) [7]. This was not the case for the sed+ group for which PIB was correlated with the depth of the coma. This evokes that the IB band waves may be less sensitive to the sedative drugs than the BW band waves.

The results also seem to indicate that there is a relation between the presence of angiographic vasospasm and the power reduction of the BW band waves, suggesting a global decrease of the arterial bed vasomotricity, of which the spasm represents only a focused manifestation, catalysed by the presence of local chemical factors. This power reduction might be due to the decrease of the cerebral blood flow (CBF) during the vasospasm [10]. This phenomenon may have been counterbalanced by a CBF increase with nimodipine [11], but the effects of this drug on CBF are controversial in these pathophysiological circumstances [12].

REFERENCES

1. HAYASHI M, FUJII H, KITANO T, KOBAYASHI H, MUNEMOTOS S, HANDA Y, YAMAMOTO S (1979) Intracranial pressure changes in patients with diffuse cerebral vasospasm. In: Shulman K, Marmarou A, Miller JD, Becker DP, Hochwald GM, Brock M (eds) ICP IV. Springer-Verlag. Berlin, Heidelbrg, New York, pp 215-219.

2. VOLBY B, ENEVOLDSEN E.M (1982) Intracranial pressure changes following aneurysm rupture. J Neurosurg 56: 186-196.

3. HAYASHI M, MARUKAWA S, FUJII H, KITANO T, KOBAYASHI H, YAMAMOTO S (1977) Intracranial hypertension in patients with ruptured intracranial aneurysm. J Neurosurg 46: 584-590.

4. HAHN FJ, RIM K (1976) Frontal ventricular dimensions on normal C.T. Am. J. Roentgenol. 126: 593-596.

5. LEMAIRE J-J, CHAZAL J, IRTHUM B, FAISANDIER Y, COLNET G, JANNY P (1991) ICP recording and spectral analysis : the software Picsoft*. In: Eight International Symposium on Intracranial Pressure, Rotterdam, Abstr.34.

6. JANNY P, JOUAN J-P, JANNY L, GOURGAND M, GUEIT U-M (1972) A statistical approach to long-term monitoring of ICP. In: Brock M, Dietz H (eds) ICP I. Springer. Berlin, Heidelberg, New York, pp 59-64.

7. LEMAIRE J-J, BOIRE J-Y, CHAZAL J, IRTHUM B (1994) A computer software for frequential analysis of slow ICP waves. Comput Methods Programs Biomed 42 : 1-14.

8. HIGASHI S YAMAMOTO S HASHIMOTO M FUJII H ITO H KOGURE Y TOKUDA K (1989) The role of vasomotor centre and adrenergic pathway in B-waves. In: Hoff JT, Betz AL (eds) ICP VII. Springer. Berlin, Heidelberg, pp 220-224.

9. HASHIMOTO M, HIGASHI S, KOGURE Y, FUJII H, YAMASHIMA T, TOKUDA K, ITO H, YAMAMOTO S (1989) Pressure waves and brain stem microcirculatory disturbance following experimental subarachnoid haemorrhage. In: Hoff JT, Betz AL (eds) ICP VII. Springer. Berlin, Heidelberg, pp 748-753.

10. GRUBB RL, RAICHLE M, EICHLING JO, GADO MH (1977) Effects of subarachnoid haemorrhage on cerebral blood volume, blood flow, and oxygen utilization in humans. J Neurosurg 46 : 446-453.

11. GAAB MR, HAUBITZ I, BRAWANSKI A, KORN A, CZECH TH (1985) Acute effects of nimodipine on the cerebral blood flow and intracranial pressure. Neurochirurgia 28: 93-99.

12. NEIL-DWYER G, MEE E, DORRANCE D, LOWE D (1987) Early intervention with nimodipine in subarachnoid haemorrhage. Europ Heart J 8 (suppl K) : 41-47.

Pressure Volume Index as a Function of Head Elevation

RANDOLPH BISHOP[1], J. BISHOP[2], and MICHAEL J. ROSNER[1]

[1]Division of Neurosurgery, University of Alabama at Birmingham, Birmingham, AL, USA
[2]Division of Anesthesiology, University of Alabama at Birmingham, Birmingham, AL, USA

INTRODUCTION

Pressure volume index (PVI) can be a useful tool in determining the "stiffness" of the neuraxis, although a better term is "volume tolerance" as defined by Schrader et al [1]. The PVI is calculated from the ICP response to the addition of a known volume into the ventricular system.

We tested the hypothesis that the volume tolerance of the brain as measured by the pressure volume index would decrease as the head was elevated from zero to 45 degrees. The rationale for this hypothesis was based upon the linear relationship of PVI and cerebral perfusion pressure (CPP) above the lower limits of autoregulation [2]. Rosner and Coley [3] have demonstrated the decrease in CPP with increasing head elevation. Therefore, we predicted that PVI would decrease with increasing head elevation.

METHODS

The PVI was measured in 15 adult neurosurgical intensive care patients at head elevations of zero, 15, 30, and 45 degrees. Serial determinations of systemic arterial blood pressure (SABP) at the head and heart, CPP (SABP - ICP), central venous pressure (CVP), and intracranial pressure (ICP) were made at each elevation. The pCO_2 was held constant throughout each experiment.

The pressure volume index was obtained by injecting one cc of normal saline into the lateral ventricle over one second and recording the change in ICP and CPP. The following relationship was then used:

$$PVI = 1/Log\ (P_P / P_O)$$

P_P = Post-injection pressure
P_O = Pre-injection pressure

Three determinations of PVI were made at each level (zero, 15, 30 and 45 degrees) of head elevation, and the mean of the three measures calculated for each of the head positions.

RESULTS

PVI decreased in all patients as a function of increasing head elevation ($PVI_0 = 33.1 \pm 18.1$, $PVI_{45} = 13.57 \pm 5.4$, $p = 0.002$). ICP decreased by -3.9 ± 5.6 mmHg ($p = .018$) as did CPP (-13.9 ± 20.7 mmHg, $p = .021$) with increasing head elevation.

DISCUSSION

This study examined the relationships between ICP, CPP, and PVI under constant end-tidal CO_2 during incremental head elevation from zero to 45 degrees. PVI was found to decrease as the head was elevated from zero to 45 degrees (decreasing by 19.5 ± 19.2). One possible mechanism for the decrease in the PVI seen with head elevation is an increase in CBV. This proposed increase in CBV can be explained by examining the vasodilatory cascade model [4]. As the head position is elevated, CPP decreases [2,3,4]. This decrement in CPP causes a decrease in CBF which initiates vasodilation. The increased CBV as a result of vasodilation is reflected by the decreased PVI with head elevation. Thus, head elevation in the brain injured patient actually results in decreased perfusion, decreased volume tolerance, and increased cerebral blood volume.

As previously demonstrated, ICP and CPP were found to be highest in the flat position (ICP = 36 ± 25.8 mmHg, CPP = 79.9 ± 34.3 mmHg) and progressively fall as the head was elevated to 45 degrees (ICP = 32.3 ± 24.0 mmHg, CPP = 66.1 ± 32.0 mmHg). The degree of decrease of the CPP exceeded that of the ICP (ICP = 3.87 ± 5.6 mmHg, CPP = 13.9 ± 20.7 mmHg).

Controversy exists concerning head position in the treatment of intracranial hypertension. Traditional therapy has advocated a raised head position because of the observed effect on ICP and the assumption that head elevation decreases cerebral blood volume (CBV) by facilitating venous drainage. Recent studies examining CPP, ICP, and outcome in patients treated in the flat position suggest ICP is less important than CPP in the brain injured patient [3].

The decrease in ICP with head elevation has traditionally been felt to be the result of increasing venous drainage with a secondary decrease in CBV. This study suggests that CBV may actually be increased with head elevation. This apparent contradiction can be explained as follows: The ICP is a summation of the tissue, blood, and cerebrospinal fluid pressures within the cranium. The tissue component of the ICP is elastic and may lower ICP, as the brain "pulls" away from the skull's inner table, although the blood component may actually be greater.

CONCLUSIONS

1. Pressure-volume index varies inversely with head elevation in the brain injured patient operating within the limits of autoregulation.

2. These data contradict the assumption that the decrease in ICP seen with head elevation is the result of a reduction in cerebral blood volume. Rather, cerebral blood volume most likely increases with increasing head elevation in the brain injured patient.

3. In terms of pressure-volume index and cerebral perfusion pressure, a flat head position is superior to a raised head position in the management of the brain injured patient. The patient is more "volume tolerant" when flat.

REFERENCES

1. Schrader H, Lofgren J, Zwetnow NM: Influence of blood pressure on tolerance to an intracranial expanding mass. Acta Neuro Scand 71;114-126, 1985.

2. Gray WJ, Rosner MJ: Pressure-volume index as a function of cerebral perfusion pressure. J Neurosurg 67:369-376, 1987.

3. Rosner MJ, Coley IB: Cerebral perfusion pressure, intracranial pressure, and head elevation. J Neurosurg 65:636-641, 1986.

4. Rosner MJ, Daughton S: Cerebral perfusion pressure management in head injury. J Trauma 30:933-941, 1990.

Changes in Pulse Waveform of Cerebral Venous Pressure During Acute Intracranial Hypertension

YUKIHIKO UEDA[2], HAJIME NAGAI[1], MITSUHITO MASE[1], and KEN KAMIYA[1]

[1] Department of Neurosurgery, Nagoya City University Medical School, Mizuho-ku, Nagoya, Aichi, 467 Japan
[2] Department of Neurosurgery, The National Tousei Hospital, Shimizu-cho, Suntou-gun, Shizuoka, 411 Japan

INTRODUCTION

Some research has revealed that pulse waveform of intracranial pressure (ICP-PWF) is formed by pulsation of arteries in the cerebrospinal cavity [1]. On the other hand some research has suggested that ICP-PWF is generated by the venous system, because ICP-PWF was similar to the pulse waveform of the cerebral vein [2], and also because there is similarity between the ICP-PWF and the pulse waveform of superior sagittal sinus pressure from the viewpoint of systems analysis, suggesting that ICP-PWF transmits to the intracranial cavity through the cerebral venous system, of which the venous walls are thin [3]. Some investigators, however, believed that ICP-PWF was produced mainly by the arterial pulse wave with the influence of the venous pulse wave [4]. Though the origin of ICP-PWF in physiological ICP has been investigated, little is known about ICP-PWF at high ICP, especially in comparison with the pulse waveform of the cerebral venous system. Authors performed the following experiment to clarify the extent to which ICP-PWF is influenced by the pulse waveform of the cerebral venous system, i.e., the cortical venous pressure-pulse waveform (CoVP-PWF) and the superior sagittal sinus pressure-pulse waveform (SSSP-PWF), under the condition of intracranial hypertension.

MATERIALS AND METHODS

Eleven adult mongrel dogs weighing about 10kg were under general anesthesia with ketamine hydrochloride, and were mechanically ventilated, given alcuronium chloride intravenously. Blood gas was checked frequently and maintained in the physiological level throughout the experiment (mean±s.d., pH: 7.376±0.034, $PaCO_2$: 33.05±1.69 mmHg, PaO_2: >100 mmHg). ICP was measured epidurally (Epidural Pressure: EDP) by an epidural pressure sensor (Tokai Rika Denki Manufactory, TICP-1, Japan). Common carotid arterial pressure (CAP), cerebral cortical venous pressure (CoVP), and superior sagittal sinus pressure (SSSP) were measured through hard polyethylene tubes connected with pressure transducers (Statham Co. Ltd; P-23D for measuring CAP, P-50 for CoVP and SSSP). Polyethylene tubes with outer diameters approximately 0.9 mm for CAP and 0.8 mm for CoVP and SSSP were catheterized directly in the vessels after having been tapered so as not to interfere with the intraluminal blood flow. The length of the polyethylene tubes was designed with a shortness of 15 cm to prevent damping effect for pressure value and pulse waveform. All of the damage to the bone was repaired with bone cement and the catheters were heparinized. The cisterna magna was punctured percutaneously with a needle, which was connected with a drip infusion system of saline. ICP was increased stepwise by about 10 mmHg from the initial pressure up to 40 mmHg by slow injection of saline into the cisterna magna. While recording the pressure, artificial respiration was stopped and the endotracheal tube was opened to the atmosphere for 2 to 3 seconds to exclude the influence of respiration and the change of intrathoracic pressure on the pulse waveforms. Data obtained in the tape recorder were put into the minicomputer after A/D converting as the data per heart beat. By computerized treatment, pressure value, pulse pressure (PP), and bottom-peak interval (time-lag from the lowest pressure to the highest pressure in one waveform) were obtained in each pulse. Statistical analysis was performed by simple regression,

Student's paired or unpaired *t* test.

RESULTS

Heart rate and pulse pressure of carotid arterial pressure were stable during the course of ICP elevation, but carotid arterial pressure was slightly elevated when ICP was high ($y=0.51x+118$; $r^2=0.056$; $n=114$; $p<0.02$).

Change in Cortical Venous Pressure (CoVP) and Superior Sagittal Sinus Pressure (SSSP) according to Increase of ICP (Epidural Pressure; EDP)

CoVP increased linearly as EDP increased up to 40 mmHg (Fig.1). A detailed observation disclosed that CoVP was higher than EDP at physiological ICP and that the difference between those two pressures decreased according to the increase of ICP. SSSP was at the same level as EDP in the physiological ICP and increased linearly according to the increase of EDP, while SSSP was lower than EDP at high ICP. Thus, the pressure difference between CoVP and SSSP increased progressively according to the increase of ICP.(Fig.1)

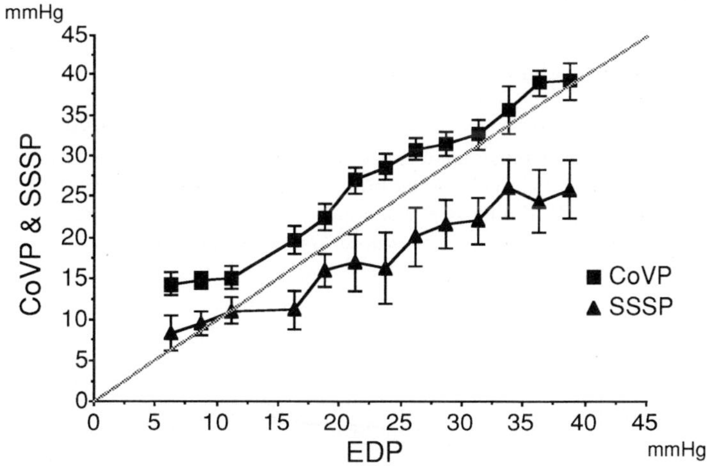

Fig.1 Change in cortical venous pressure (CoVP) and superior sagittal sinus pressure (SSSP) according to increase of ICP (epidural pressure; EDP).
CoVP: $y=0.85x+7.13$; $r^2=0.789$; $n=98$; $p<0.001$, and SSSP: $y=0.58x+4.25$; $r^2=0.376$; $n=109$; $p<0.001$. Mean±SEM (n=11).

Change in Pulse Pressure (PP) of ICP and Cerebral Venous Pressure according to Increase of ICP

Like EDP-PP, CoVP-PP and SSSP-PP increased almost linearly as ICP was elevated.(Fig.2) But the magnitude of the increase in CoVP-PP was smaller than that in EDP-PP and the difference between CoVP-PP and EDP-PP became larger as EDP was increased. The magnitude of the increase in SSSP-PP according to increase of EDP was smaller even than that in CoVP-PP.

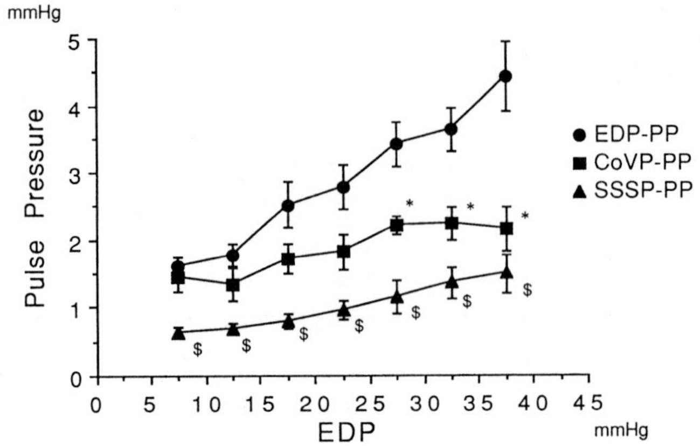

Fig.2 Change in pulse pressure (PP) of EDP, CoVP and SSSP according to increase of ICP.
EDP-PP: $y=0.099x+0.705$; $r^2=0.484$; n=109; $p<0.001$, CoVP-PP: $y=0.035x+1.017$; $r^2=0.329$; n=45; $p<0.001$, and SSSP-PP: $y=0.033x+0.301$; $r^2=0.257$; n=109; $p<0.001$. The */$ symbols refer to the comparison of single data points of the corresponding data of EDP-PP (*p<0.05 and $p<0.001). Mean±SEM (n=11).

Change in Bottom-Peak Interval of Pulse Waveform according to Increase of ICP

Change in the bottom-peak interval of the pulse waveform of EDP, CoVP, SSSP or carotid arterial pressure according to the increase of intracranial pressure is shown in Fig.3. The bottom peak interval of EDP was slightly longer than that of carotid arterial pressure but shorter than those of CoVP and SSSP. The bottom-peak interval of EDP at high ICP was longer than that at normal ICP (141±5 msec.and 118±5 msec., respectively, $p<0.02$). But there was no difference in the bottom-peak interval of CoVP, SSSP or carotid arterial pressure when ICP was between normal and high.

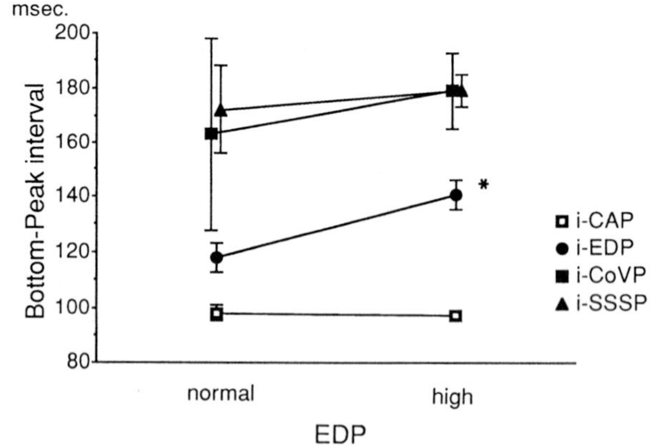

Fig.3 Change in bottom-peak interval of pulse waveform of carotid arterial pressure (i-CAP), EDP (i-EDP), CoVP (i-CoVP) and SSSP (i-SSSP) according to ICP increase.
Normal ICP is less than 15 mmHg. High ICP is more than 15 mmHg and up to 40 mmHg. *p<0.02 different from the value at normal ICP. Mean±SEM (n=11).

DISCUSSION

Increase of CoVP-PP was not as prominent as that of EDP-PP even though value of EDP and CoVP were nearly equal during ICP elevation (Fig.1&2), indicating that pulsation in the cerebral cortical vein was suppressed when ICP was high. SSSP-PP was remarkably smaller than CoVP-PP (Fig.2).

The time-lag from the bottom to the peak of ICP-PWF (bottom-peak interval) was slightly longer than that of carotid arterial pressure -PWF and shorter than that of CoVP-PWF or SSSP-PWF at normal ICP (Fig.3). According to the increase of ICP, the bottom-peak interval of ICP-PWF was elongated whereas that of carotid arterial pressure -PWF, CoVP-PWF or SSSP-PWF did not show any significant change (Fig.3). The result in this experiment might support one of the following assumptions; that is, when ICP is increased, a time-lag will be produced during transmission of the pulse in the intracranial cavity [5], or one of the peaks of ICP-PWF will be more prominent than others [6].

Our results showed that both of pulse pressure of CoVP-PWF and SSSP-PWF were smaller than that of ICP-PWF when ICP was increased, and that the bottom-peak interval of CoVP-PWF or SSSP-PWF did not show any significant delay at high ICP whereas the bottom-peak interval of ICP-PWF did, indicating that ICP-PWF is not much influenced by the cerebral venous system at high ICP. The authors assume that CoVP-PWF might be passively produced by transmission of ICP-PWF through the venous wall of the cortical vein, where CoVP-PWF might be dampened.

REFERENCES

1. Dunbar HS, Guthrie TC, Karpell B (1966) A study of the cerebrospinal fluid pulse wave. Arch Neurol 14: 624-630
2. Hamit HF, Beall AC Jr., De Bakey ME (1965) Haemodynamic influences upon brain and cerebrospinal fluid pulsations and pressure. J Trauma 5:174-184
3. Portnoy HD, Chopp M, Branch C, Shannon MB (1982) Cerebrospinal fluid pulse waveform as an indicator of cerebral autoregulation. J Neurosurg 56: 666-678
4. Kasuga Y, Nagai H, Hasegawa Y, Nitta M (1987) Transmission characteristics of pulse waves in the intracranial cavity of dogs. J Neurosurg 66: 907-914
5. Nitta M, Kasuga Y, Hasegawa H, Nagai H (1983) Conduction time of the pulse through the brain with increased intracranial pressure. In: Ishii S, Nagai H and Brock M (eds) Intracranial Pressure V. Springer-Verlag, Berlin Heidelberg New York Tokyo, pp211-215
6. Shigemori M, Tokutomi T, Kawaba T, Nakashima H, Kuramoto S (1986) Analysis of epidural pressure pulse wave(EDP-PW) and common carotid blood velocity (CBFV) in acute intracranial hypertension. Neurol Res 8: 105-108

Analysis of Intracranial Pressure Pulse Wave in Experimental Hydrocephalus

T. Matsumoto[1], H. Nagai[2], T. Fukushima[3], and M. Mase[2]

[1] Department of Neurosurgery, Meitetsu Hospital, Nishi-ku, Nagoya, Aichi, 451 Japan
[2] Department of Neurosurgery, Nagoya City University Medical School, Mizuho-ku, Nagoya, Aichi, 467 Japan
[3] Department of Neurosurgery, Nagoya East General Hospital, Chikusa-ku, Nagoya, Aichi, 464 Japan

INTRODUCTION

We have some information regarding the relationship between the pulse pressure(PP) of the intracranial pressure pulse wave(ICP pulse wave) and ventricle dilatation [1].Some data suggest that high PP is the cause of hydrocephalus [2.3], and other authors have reported that high PP results from decreased intracranial compliance[4]. In order to clarify these points, the amplitude of PP and pressure-volume response(PVR: as an indicator of intracranial compliance) were measured in bilateral ventricle using Hochwald's hydrocephalic model (right-left difference in ventricle size is clearly due to hemicraniectomy)[5].

MATERIALS AND METHODS

Hydrocephalus was developed by means of an intracisternal injection of a kaolin powder solution using adult mongrel dogs. The ventricle dilatation was confirmed by MRI 4-31 days after kaolin injection. The ICP was measured with two Camino fiberoptic ICP monitoring systems placed intraventricularly. The mean ICP was calculated from the diastolic pressure plus one third of the pulse pressure. The PP of the ICP pulse wave was measured from the bottom to the highest peak of the pulse wave. PVR was obtained from the ventricles on both sides following rapid injection of saline(0.5ml/s) into each ventricle. Each parameter was evaluated under pathologic conditions induced by the following procedures. Group A, the control group, had kaolin-induced hydrocephalus without craniectomy. In group B animals kaolin induction of hydrocephalus was followed by right craniectomy. Group C had kaolin-induced hydrocephalus with right craniectomy and dural resection. Group D had kaolin-induced hydrocephalus with right side craniectomy, dura resection and temporal muscle resection.

RESULTS

Fig.1 shows the MR images obtained in each group. The same degree of symmetrical ventricle dilatation was identified in all groups except group D. Group D alone demonstrated differences in ventricular size(larger on the craniectomy side than on the non-craniectomy side).

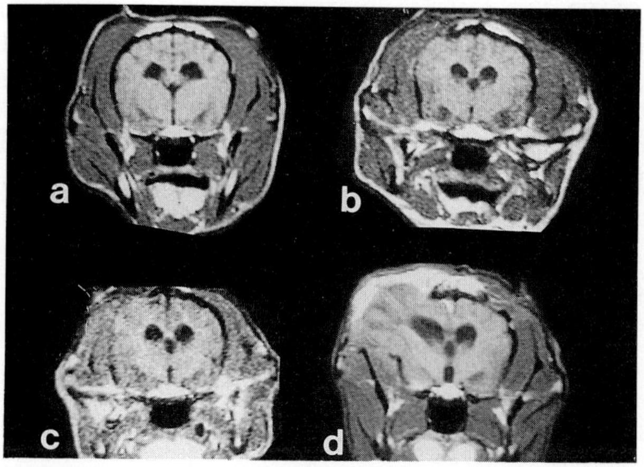

Fig.1 MRI(T1-weighted, , coronal section) of animals with kaolin-induced hydrocephalus. Groups A (control, no craniectomy), B (craniectomy), C (craniectomy + dural resection) and D(craniectomy + dural resection + temporal muscle resection). Group D shows laterality of ventricles.

All parameters which affect the ICP pulse wave, remained stable throughout the experiment (Table 1). Also, there was no appreciable difference in mean ICP between any two of the groups.

Table1. Summary of four groups. Intracranial pressure(ICP), pulse pressure(PP), pressure-volume response(PVR), systemic arterial pressure(SAP), arterial pulse pressure(dSAP), heart rate (HR) and ventricle size. Groups as in Fig.1. *gradual decrease of PP and PVR, ** right-left difference in ventricle size.

Animal number	*ICP mmHg*	*PP* mmHg*	*PVR* mmHg*	*SAP mmHg*	*dSAP mmHg*	*HR*	*Vent. Size mm*
GA(No.1) (rt)	12.5	1.7	47.2	123.3	70.0	181	10.9
(lt)	11.1	1.6	44.8				10.6
GB(No.2) (rt)	16.5	1.4	31.0	118.3	55.0	144	11.2
(lt)	20.2	1.3	29.0				10.6
GC(No.3) (rt)	11.4	0.6	9.2	148.3	55.0	188	10.9
(lt)	13.3	0.7	9.2				10.0
(No.4) (rt)	13.8	0.8	12.0	143.8	55.0	220	9.1
(lt)	9.3	0.8	12.6				9.1
GD(No.5) (rt)	1.6	0.6		100	75.0	150	10.9**
(lt)	4.1	0.4					4.5**
(No.6) (rt)	11.7	0.4	2.8	100	75.0	150	20.0**
(lt)	7.9	0.5	3.2				10.9**
Mean(SD) (rt)	11.3	0.92	20.4	122.3	64.2	181	12.2
	(5.1)	(0.52)	(18.3)	(20.7)	(10.2)	(39.2)	(3.9)
(lt)	11.0	0.88	19.9				9.3
	(5.5)	(0.48)	(16.9)				(2.4)

The amplitude of the PP decreased stepwise from group A to group D, while there was no difference in PP amplitude between right and left ventricles in any group. Even in the larger ventricle in group D, the amplitude of PP was the same as that of the left ventricle, and much smaller than that in other groups. Like the amplitude of PP, PVR also showed a stepwise decrease from group A to group D, without any right-left difference. Again, even on the larger ventricle side in group D, the PVR was the same as that of the left ventricle and much smaller than that of other groups [Fig.2].

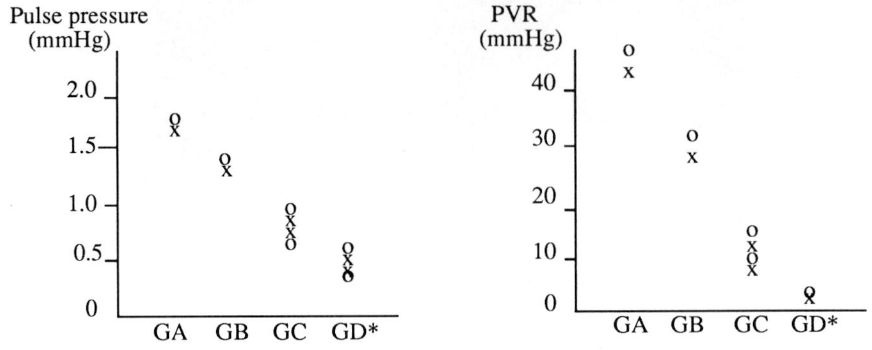

Fig.2 Absolute values of pulse pressure (left) and volume pressure response (right) in each group. Groups as in Fig. 1.
* Ventricle was greater on right than on left.

DISCUSSION

The size of the ventricle is in a dynamic equilibrium between forces that tend to expand them(for instance, CSF production and resistance to the out flow of CSF) and forces that constrict them(CSF absorption and compliance of container). Hydrocephalus results when some pathological process unbalances this dynamic equilibrium. However except this general pathogenesis, several investigations have adressed other mechanisms by which the ventricle size becomes large. One of the theory is the water hummer effect on the ICP pulse wave. Di Rocco [2,3] produced an experimental hydrocephalic model in which hydrocephalus was induced in lambs by an artificial increase of the amplitude of the ICP pulse wave without concomitant changes of the mean ICP. We also measured the amplitude of ICP pulse wave in experimental and clinical hydrocephalus [1,4]. Our results also showed that with approximately the same ICP level, the PP was higher in some kinds of hydrocephalus. However we have reported that, in many cases, the high PP had resulted from decreased intracranial compliance, the results of this study also showed that even in the larger ventricle the amplitude of PP was the same as that in the ventricle on the other side, and much smaller than in other groups. In addition the amplitudes of PP and PVR are highly correlated. This suggests that, in this model, PP can be a good parameter of intracranial compliance, but not the driving force of the ventricle dilatation.

CONCLUSION

The results of our research suggest that:
1) There was no relation between ventricle dilatation and the amplitude of PP. This means that the increased amplitude of PP was not the cause of the ventricle dilatation in this model. 2) There was a high degree of correlation between the amplitude of PP and the PVR. This means that PP can be a good parameter of intracranial compliance in this model.

REFERENCES

1. Nagai H, Kamiya K, Ohno M, Matsumoto T (1983) Importance of the pulse amplitude in ventriculomegaly. In: Ishii S (ed) Hydrocephalus. Excerpta Medica, Amsterdam, pp 126-134
2. Di Rocco C, Pettorossi VE, Caldarelli R (1977) Experimental hydrocephalus following mechanical increment of intraventricular pulse pressure. Experimentia 33:1470-1472
3. Di Rocco C, Pettorossi VE, Caldarelli R (1978) Communicating hydrocephalus induced by mechanically increased amplitude of the intraventricular cerebrospinal fluid pressure. Exp Neurol 59:40-52
4. Matsumoto T, Nagai H, Kasuga K, Kamiya K (1986) Changes in intracranial pressure(ICP) pulse wave following hydrocephalus. Acta Neurochir 82: 50-56
5. Hochwald GM, Epstein F. Malahan C (1972) The role of the skull and dura in experimental feline hydrocephalus. Dev Med Child Neurol 14[Supp 27]: 65-69

Prognostic Significance of the ICP Pulse Waveform Analysis After Severe Head Injury

M. CZOSNYKA, E. GUAZZO, P. KIRKPATRICK, H. WHITEHOUSE, Z. CZOSNYKA, P. SMIELEWSKI, and J.D. PICKARD

MRC Cambridge Centre for Brain Repair and Academic Neurosurgical Unit, Addenbrooke's Hospital, P.O. Box 167, Cambridge CB2 2QQ, UK

The exponential shape of the pressure-volume relationship cannot be regarded as the only factor influencing the magnitude of ICP pulse wave. Four simultaneous mechanisms should be considered:

(i) gradient of the pressure-volume curve, being the measure of the brain elasticity which increases with mean ICP ;

(ii) pulsatile inflow of arterial blood increasing with falling CPP;

(iii) delay between arterial inflow and venous outflow profiles, varying with ICP;

(iv) delay between arterial blood inflow and CSF outflow through the foramen magnum to the spinal subarachnoid space.

Mechanism (i) can be investigated using well established pressure-volume studies. Factor (ii) needs continuous monitoring of blood flow velocity in basal cerebral arteries. The third mechanism has not been fully investigated: the parallel recording of blood flow profiles in basal cerebral arteries and straight sinus, reported by Aaslid et al. [1] may help in answering this question. To study the fourth factor, the highly specialized dynamic magnetic resonance imaging technique is needed.

Therefore, it is difficult to investigate all these factors in parallel in clinical practice. Our methodology is much simpler: The relationship between ICP pulse amplitude and mean ICP has been studied in a heterogenous group of 56 head injured patients. High statistical convergence of data suggested that its shape reflects a general relationship describing cerebrospinal pressure-volume compensation. Additional questions regarded whether the outcome of head injured patients correlated with the shape of the amplitude-pressure curve?

MATERIAL AND METHODS

ICP was monitored continuously in 56 head injured ventilated patients with a mean Glasgow Coma Score 6 (range 3-13) with only 5 patients having a GCS > 8 after resuscitation.

ICP was monitored using a fibre-optic transducer (Camino Direct Pressure Monitor, Camino Laboratories, US), inserted in an intradural location (35 cases) or a subdural catheter connected via a standard manometer line to the pressure transducer (21 cases).

Systemic arterial blood pressure and ICP waveforms were read digitally by a bed-side computer. The fundamental harmonic of ICP pulse amplitude and the mean ICP over one minute periods were calculated using FFT algorithm [2]. Heart rate variability analysis was used to filter out measurement artifacts. The moving correlation coefficient between the fundamental harmonic of ICP pulse wave and the mean ICP (RAP: R-symbol of correlation between A-amplitude and P-pressure) was evaluated within consecutive one minute periods. RAP describes the time-dependent changes in correlation between amplitude and the mean ICP.

RESULTS AND DISCUSSION

On statistical analysis (ANOVA, more than 130 000 minute-averages of the pooled data were analysed) of the whole group first harmonic of the ICP pulse amplitude increased as ICP rose to 36 mmHg and then began to decrease (see Fig.1a). This upper breakpoint was not related to specific changes in the pulse amplitude of the arterial blood pressure: the ratio between the first harmonic of ICP and ABP pulse amplitudes showed the same breakpoints (see Fig 1b). For the ICP lower than 36 mmHg RAP was higher than 0.5 ($p<0.0001$) while for the higher ICP it decreased and became negative ($RAP<0$; $p<0.01$) when ICP raised above 55 mmHg. Finally , relationship between ICP pulse amplitude and mean CPP exhibited a character dual to AMP/ICP curve. AMP started to rise with CPP decreasing below 85 mmHg and reached the maximaum at 40-35 mmHg (Fig 1 c and d).

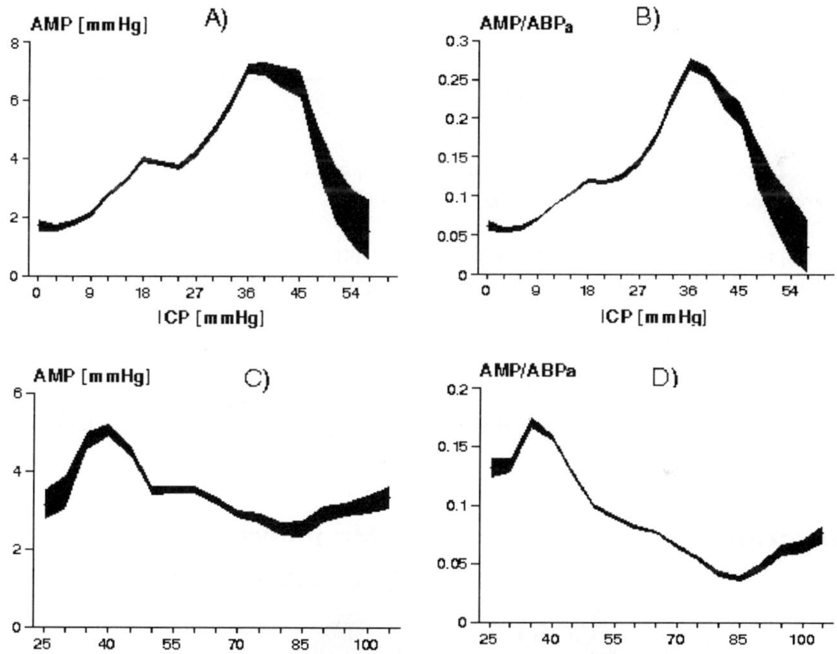

Fig.1 . 95% confidence area for averaged pulse amplitude of ICP (A and C) and ratio of pulse amplitudes of ICP and ABP (AMP/ABPa) (B and D) versus mean ICP (A,B) and CPP(C,D).

Mathematical model of cerebrospinal [3] space offers a theoretical explanation of the observed breakpoints. Pulse wave of intracranial pressure is derived from the arterial pulse , transmitted through elastic walls of cerebral arteries to compliant CSF containers [4]. Thus , the transmission coefficient can be expressed as ratio of compartmental compliances Ca (arterial) and Ci (CSF container):

$$Transmission = \frac{Ca}{Ca + Ci}$$

Model simulation shows that Ca increases with decreasing CPP until maximal vasodilation and then starts to decrease gradually because of passive decrease of the arterioral radius [5]. Ci decreases uniformly with increasing ICP. The relationship between simulated Transmission and pulse amplitude of ICP versus CPP is plotted in Fig.2.

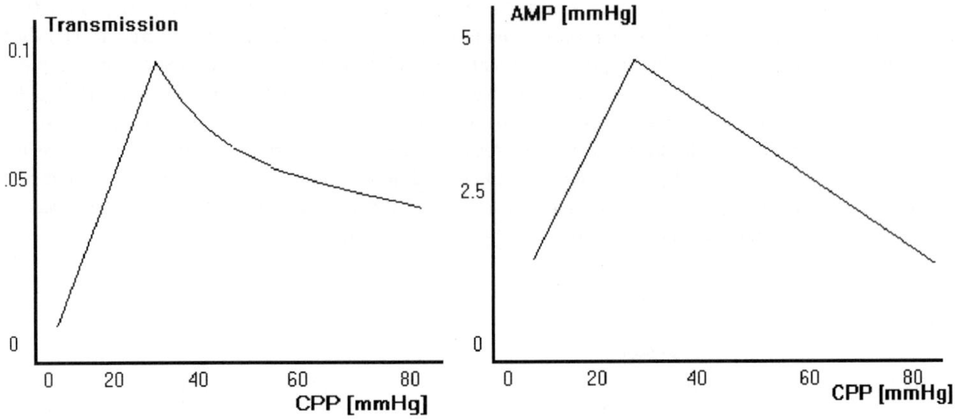

Fig2. Simulated Transmission Coefficient (left) and pulse amplitude of ICP versus CPP. Lower breakpoints of both curves mark the lower limit of maximal vasodilatation.

All patients had their outcome assessed using the Glasgow Outcome Scale between 4 and 19 months (mean 12) after injury. They were grouped as follows and the AMP/ICP and AMP/CPP relationships for each group was analysed:
(i) **GOS 1 or 2** - good or moderate disability (n=30)
(ii) **GOS 3** - severe disability (n=13)
(iii) **GOS 4 or 5** - PVS or dead (n=13)
Pulse amplitude of AMP of ICP was plotted against mean ICP and CPP in these three different outcome groups (see Fig.3).

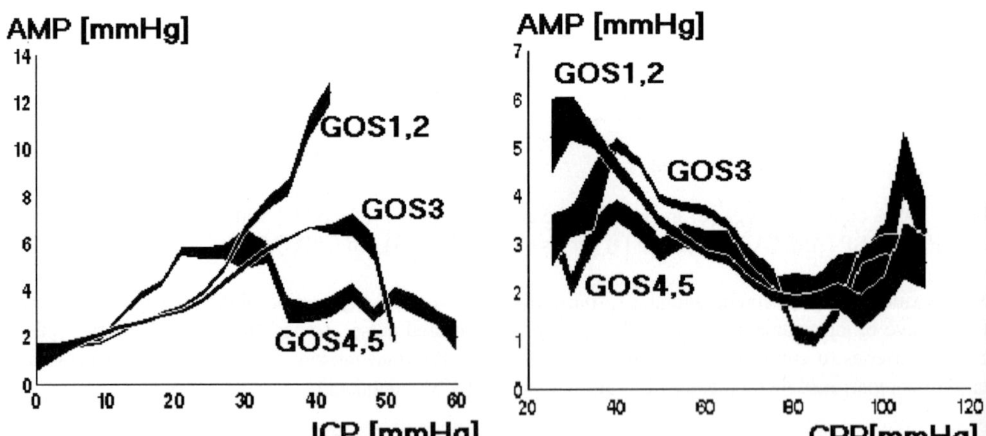

Fig.3. ANOVA relationships between pulse amplitude of ICP (y) and mean ICP (left plot) or mean CPP (right plot) plotted in three different outcome groups.

Upper an lower breakpoints of AMP/ICP and AMP/CPP differ in three different outcome groups (see Table). The upper breakpoint of AMP/ICP curve decreases with a worse outcome. The lower breakpoint of AMP/CPP curve was around 40 mmHg for unfavourable outcome patients, no breakpoint was seen in the favourable outcome group. It is interesting that the upper breakpoint of AMP/ICP curve gives a better statistical convergence in heterogenous group of head injured patients than lower breakpoint of AMP/CPP.

Table. Upper and lower breakpoints of AMP/ICP and AMP/CPP relationships in three outcome groups.
* denotes values significantly different in rows

	GOS 1,2	GOS3	GOS4,5
AMP/ICP	non-detectable	47 mmHg*	30 mmHg
AMP/CPP	non-detectable	40 mmHg	40 mmHg

As the upper breakpoint of the AMP/ICP curve can be interpreted as an index of terminally elevated ICP, affecting cerebral circulation, the moving correlation coefficient RAP can be used to detect the episodes of the terminal hypertension in time. If ICP is elevated above 20 mmHg correlation between AMP and ICP should be high , unless cerebrovascular reserve is exhausted.
RAP is less than 0.5 when for only 14% of time when ICP is elevated above 20 mmHg in group GOS 1, 2. This percentage is significantly higher in group GOS 3 (31%) and GOS 4,5 (75%, with $p<0.001$).
Therefore, clinically useful conclusion may be, that in states of intracranial hypertension , the poor correlation between pulse amplitude and mean ICP, detected using RAP is an indicator of unfavourable outcome [6].

REFERENCES

1. Aaslid R, Newell DW, Stoss R, Sorteberg W, Lindegaard KF (1991) Assessment of cerebral autoregulation dynamics from simultaneous arterial and venous transcranial Doppler recordings in humans. Stroke, 22: 148-1154
2. Czosnyka M, Batorski L, Laniewski P, Maksymowicz W, Koszewski W, Zaworski W (1990) A computer system for the identification of the cerebrospinal compensatory model. Acta Neurochirurgica, 105: 112-116
3. Czosnyka M, Harris NG, Pickard JD: CO2 cerebrovascular reactivity as a function of perfusion pressure- a modelling study .Acta Neurochirurgica 121:159-165,1993
4. Piper I, Miller JD, Dearden M (1990) System analysis of cerebrovascular pressure transmission : an observational study in head injured patients. J Neurosurg 73:871-880
5. Kontos H, Wei EP, Navari RM, Levasseur JE, Rosenblum WI, Patterson JL (1978) Response of Cerebral arteries and arterioles to acute hypotension and hypertension. Am J of Physiology H371-H383
6. Czosnyka M. Price JD , Williamson M (1994): Monitoring of cerebrospinal dynamics using continuous analysis of intracranial pressure and cerebral perfusion pressure in head injury, Acta Neurochirurgica (Wien) 126: 113-119

Regional Cortical Blood Flow in Appearance of Pressure Wave—A Clinical Study in Patients with B Waves

T. Onitsuka, Y. Takeda, T. Miki, J. Haraoka, and H. Ito

Department of Neurosurgery, Tokyo Medical College, 6-7-1 Nishi-shinjuku, Shinjuku-ku, Tokyo, 160 Japan

INTRODUCTION

Cerebral perfusion pressure (CPP) is defined as a disparity between blood pressure (BP) and intracranial pressure (ICP) , and in normal situations the cerebral blood flow (CBF) is considered to maintain a given value unless there is no significant change in CPP . although these relation breaks down in association with a rise in ICP . although it is considered that CPP and CBF may decrease in the appearance of A waves , actual conditions of CPP and CBF in the appearance of B waves seemed to be obscure . in this study , using a laser doppler microcirculation flowmetry, we measured regional cerebral cortical blood flow (cCBF) in the appearance of B waves and assessed the changes .

MARERIALS AND METHODS

We investigated the four adult cases of brain tumors with rised ICP . these patients showed hydrocephalus except for one case . cCBF was measured using laser doppler microcirculation flowmetry (TSI , BPM 403 A) . The probe was implanted on the surface of the frontal lobe keeping away from large vessels . The averaging time was set to 0.2 seconds . Ventricular fluid pressure or epidural pressure was monitored by pressure transducer (Statham , P50 , Gaeltec , ICT/b) . Systemic arterial pressure was monitored by pressure transducer from radial artery (Statham , P50) . All of them and CPP which was calculated by the value of ICP and BP using DC amplifier (Nihon Kohden , AD-601G) , were putted in data recorder (Sony , KS-609) and continuously monitored from 24 to 48 hours and analyzed later . BP , ICP , CPP and cCBF were analyzed in average values , one-third value of their amplitude in addition to their minimum values .

RESULTS AND DISCUSSION

Case 1 . This is the data from a 60-year-old male of metastatic brain tumor . During the B waves , Parameters showed increase from 77 to 105 mmHg in BP , from 12 to 38 mmHg in ICP , and scarce increase from 65 to 67 mmHg in CPP . cCBF changed from 17 to 27 ml/100g/min (Fig. 1) .
Case 2 . This is a 71-year-old male of meningeal carcinomatosis . Parameters showed increase from 75 to 100 mmHg in BP , from 12 to 26 mmHg in ICP , and moderate increase from 63 to 74 mmHg in CPP . cCBF changed from 17 to 32 ml/100g/min .
Case 3 . This is a 67-year-old female of tentorial meningioma . parameters showed increase from 73 to 104 mmHg in BP , from 9 to 16 mmHg in ICP , from 64 to 88 mmHg in CPP . cCBF changed from 6.6 to 12 ml/100g/min .
Case 4 . This is a 40-year-old male of cerebellar hemangioblastoma . parameters showed increase from 78 to 117 mmHg in BP , from 20 to 47 mmHg in ICP , and moderate increase from 58 to 70 mmHg in CPP . cCBF remarkably increased from 59 to 120 ml/100g/min .

Fig. 1 The data of case 1 , a 60-year old male of metastatic brain tumor .

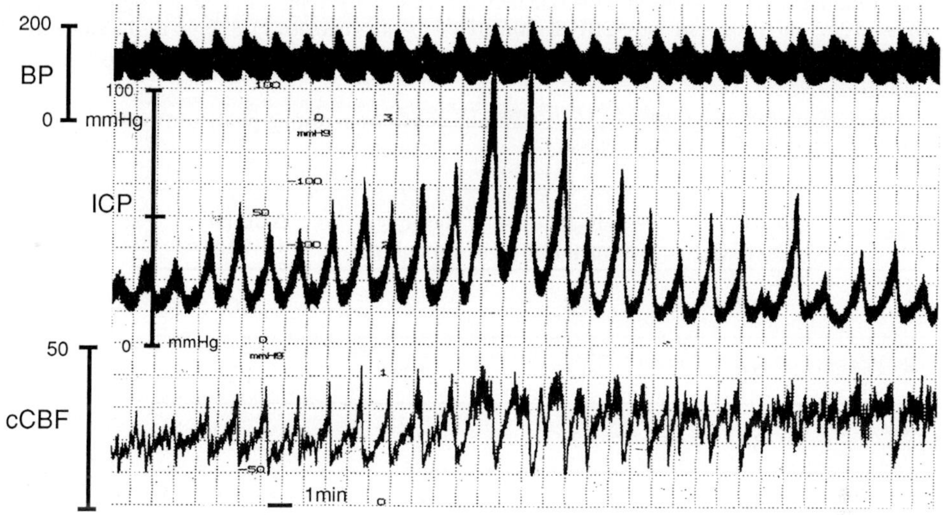

We calculated the average value of values of the above four cases . In resting phase of B waves , monitor showed 75.8 mmHg in BP , 13.3 mmHg in ICP , 62.5 mmHg in CPP and 24.9 ml/100g/min in cCBF . In the appearance of B waves , ICP increased to 31.8 mmHg , BP also increased 107 mmHg , and CPP moderately increased to 74.8 mmHg . cCBF showed remarkable increase in value 47.8 ml/100g/min (Table 1) .

Table 1 Values of blood pressure (BP) , intracranial pressure (ICP) , cerebral perfusion pressure (CPP) and regional cortical cerebral blood flow (cCBF) in resting phase and B waves .

Case	Resting phase				B waves			
	BP (mmHg)	ICP (mmHg)	CPP (mmHg)	cCBF (ml/100g/min)	BP (mmHg)	ICP (mmHg)	CPP (mmHg)	cCBF (ml/100g/min)
1	77	12	65	17	105	38	67	27
2	75	12	63	17	100	26	74	32
3	73	9	64	6.6	104	16	88	12
4	78	20	58	59	117	47	70	120
Mean	75.8 ±2.22	13.3 ±4.72	62.5 ±3.11	24.9 ±23.3	107 ±7.33	31.8 ±13.6	74.8 ±9.29	47.8 ±48.9

we calculated the change of the value of those parameters from resting phase to B waves . ΔCPP showed 12.3 mmHg and CPP showed moderate increase 19.6 % up to the value in resting pressure , ΔcCBF showed 25.7 ml/100g/min and cCBF demonstrated drastic increase 91.8 % up to the value in resting pressure (Table 2) .

Table 2 The change of the value of BP , ICP , CPP and cCBF from resting phase to B waves , and increasing rate of those parameters .

Case	ΔBP (mmHg)	ΔICP (mmHg)	ΔCPP (mmHg)	ΔcCBF (ml/100g/min)
1	28	26	2	10
2	25	14	11	15
3	31	7	24	5.4
4	39	27	12	61
Mean	30.8±6.02	18.5±9.68	12.3±9.03	25.7±22.9
Increasing Rate (%)	40.6	140	19.6	91.8

The respective parameters changed in the following patterns in the appearance of B waves . ICP gradually increased in B wave ascending phase . BP scarcely increased in the early ascending phase and rapidly increased in the late ascending phase . this resulted in CPP decrease in the early ascending phase and increased in the late ascending phase . Although , it's increase and decrease showed within normal range of CPP . In the descending phase , ICP showed rapid decrease , but BP showed comparatively gradual decrease . The changing pattern of cCBF was similar of ICP in the case 1 , 2 , 3, and was similar to that of BP in the case 4 .

These findings definitely indicated that cCBF demonstrated rhythmic change , a significant increase during the B waves , while , CPP remained in it's normal range .

Uede , et al. , reported that , in the normal brain condition , CBF is maintained at a certain level by autoregulation if CPP changes within the range of 40 to 150 mmHg . In the four cases studied , CPP changed in the appearance of the B waves within this range but cCBF dynamically changed . these findings suggested that cCBF may change in the manner out of regulation by CPP , and may be affected by some other factors during the appearance and disappearance of B waves .

Table 3 The changing patterns of BP , ICP , CPP and cCBF in B waves .

		Early ascending Phase	Late ascending Phase	Descending Phase
BP		scarcely increased	rapidly increased	gradually decreased
ICP		gradually increased		rapidly decreased
CPP		within normal limited (decreased)	within normal limited (increased)	within normal limited (decreased)
cCBF	Case 1,2,3	gradually increased		rapidly decreased
	Case 4	scarcely increased	rapidly increased	gradually decreased

REFERENCES

1. DAVID W. NEWELL (1992) The relationship of blood flow velocity fluctuation to intracranial pressure B waves. J Neurosurg 76 : 415-421
2. B. A. Meyerson (1991) Bedside monitoring of regional cortical blood flof in comatose patients using laser doppler floemetry. Neurosurgery 29 : 750-755
3. Uede T (1988) Intacranialpressure and Intracranial hemodynamics. Clinical Neuroscience 6 : 1073-1074

Barodynamic Analysis of Intracranial Pressure Change After Intraventricular Hemorrhage—An Experimental Study

F. Takei[1], R. Tsugane[1], Y. Hashimoto[1], H. Takasawa[2], S. Oi[2], and O. Sato[2]

[1] Department of Neurosurgery, Tokai University Oiso Hospital, Nakagun, Kanagawa, 259-01 Japan
[2] Department of Neurosurgery, Tokai University School of Medicine, Isehara, Kanagawa, 259-11 Japan

INTRODUCTION

Intraventricular hemorrhage (IVH) is one of the defeated factors in clinical prognosis in patients with cerebrovascular disease. However, accompanying with the development of modern technology, especially the case with asymptomatic IVH is ordinary treated conservatively and its prognosis is better than expected. In such situation, intracranial pressure dynamics may involve the patients' prognosis in its clinical entity. The purpose of this study is to evaluate intracranial pressure dynamic change due to IVH together with other parameters including CSF hydrodynamics and morphological alterations.

MATERIALS AND METHODS

Eight IVH models that are induced by fresh autologous blood injection into the lateral ventricle, and 4 non-treated normal cats as a control group were studied. At the time of blood injection, contralateral intraventricular pressure (IVP) was monitored to avoid the periependymal tissue damage that was caused by excessive increments of ICP. Pressure volume index (PVI) by bolus technique calculated as intracranial pressure dynamic evaluation. The obtained ICP and PVI in the chronic phase (post IVH: 6-8 weeks after initiation of IVH) were compared with the initial states (pre IVH). In this analysis, series of PVI measurements were made in both pre and post IVH conditions at two different levels of ICP (one was ICP below 20 mmHg as a baseline condition, the other was beyond 20 mmHg as an elevated ICP condition). The elevated ICP condition was produced by fluid induction into the cisterna magna.

In post-IVH, the histological alteration of periependymal tissue of lateral ventricle was observed by means of light and transmission electron microscope as a morphological evaluation. The pattern of HRP distribution in the region of periventricular tissue was evaluated as the sequela of CSF dynamic change due to IVH by HRP perfusion technique from lateral ventricle to cisterna magna.

RESULTS

Clinical Profiles of IVH model

The mortality rate due to manipulation of intraventricular blood injection in IVH model was 88% and none of the survived animals (N=7) showed clinical deterioration during observation period. In seven survivors, six of animals showed normal ventricle in size and one showed ventricular dilatation. This hydrocephalic animal was excluded because the process of ventriculomegaly itself might affect to observed histological alteration and CSF dynamics.

Intracranial Pressure Dynamic Change

Mean baseline and elevated ICP were 10.0+/-2.4 mmHg, 24.0+/-2.7 mmHg in pre-IVH and 10.2 +/-2.3 mmHg, 24.6+/-2.7 mmHg in post-IVH condition respectively. There was no statistically significance between the values obtained in each condition observed (Table 1).
Mean of PVI calculated at baseline and elevated ICP level was 0.84+/ 0.1 ml, 0.82+/-0.1 ml in pre-IVH and 0.90+/-0.2 ml, 0.75+/-0.1 ml in post-IVH condition respectively. Statistically different between these PVIs values was noted in post-IVH (*P<0.05) while no such difference was observed in pre-IVH condition (Table 1). Average of individual correlation coefficient of linear regression between PVI and ICP obtained at baseline and elevated ICP condition was 0.31, 0.26 in pre-IVH (P>0.05) and 0.24, 0.77 in post-IVH (**P<0.05) respectively (Table 1 and Fig.1).

Table 1. Intracranial pressure dynamic change in pre and post IVH condition

	Pre-IVH		Post-IVH	
	baseline ICP (< 20mmHg)	elevated ICP (> 20mmHg)	baseline ICP (< 20mmHg)	elevated ICP (> 20mmHg)
IVP (mmHg)	10.0 +/- 2.4	24.0 +/- 2.7	10.2 +/- 3.2	24.6 +/- 2.7
PVI (ml)	0.84 +/- 0.1	0.82 +/- 0.1	0.90 +/- 0.2	0.75 +/- 0.1 *
Average of Cor.Coef.	0.31	0.26	0.24	0.77 **

IVH : intraventricular hemorrhage IVP : intraventricular pressure mean +/- S.D
PVI : pressure volume index Cor.Coef : correlation coefficient */** : P< 0.05

Histological Alterations

Various periependymal tissue damages observed even the condition which ICP did not increase or the ventricle did not dilate. Distribution of the cilia and microvilli at the apical surface of the ependyma cell was diminished. Increased glial fibers and some degenerated intracellular organelles were observed frequently in the ependyma and other glial cells that were located in the region of subependymal tissue. A number of mitochondria were somewhat increased (Fig. 2a, b).

CSF Hydrodynamic Change

Distribution pattern of HRP was not similar to normal group showing Fig. 2c

DISCUSSION AND CONCLUSIONS

Most of asymptomatic IVH are now treated conservatively owning to the advances of therapeutic modalities. In such situation, Asai has reported the influence of intraventricular blood to the CSF hydrodynamics[1,2]. Thompsom[3] and Murakami[4] documented histological alterations due to IVH in experimental animals. According to other reports regarding IVH and our results, IVH seems to cause various changes in the intracranial pressure dynamics, morphology and CSF dynamics in the region of periependymal tissue even when ICP was the normal and the clinical deterioration was not obvious.

It was concluded that 1) IVH resulted in periventricular tissue damage and disturbed transependymal CSF circulation without dynamic insult to the region observed. 2) IVH induced an undermining damage in intracranial pressure dynamics and may be the cause of overt intracranial dynamic distress when ICP was elevated. 3) Clinical profiles due to IVH itself did not correlate with changes both in intracranial pressure dynamics and the transependymal CSF circulation occurring as long as ICP remained within normal range. 4) Special attention must be paid to ICP evaluation after an IVH episode regardless of the clinical symptoms to prevent undesirable cerebral disaster.

REFERENCES

1. Asai T (1977) The effect of the intraventricular blood component on both the production and absorption rate of the cerebrospinal fluid in dog (part-I). Neurol Med Chir 17: 487-492
2. Asai T (1977) The effect of the intraventricular blood component on both the production and absorption rate of the cerebrospinal fluid in dog (part-II). Neurol Med

Chir 17: 493-498
3. Thompson RK, Manganiello LOJ, Nichols P (1947) Intracranial hemorrhage. Some experimental and clinical observations. South Med J 40: 990-996
4. Murakami T (1981) Experimental study of prognosis-aggravating factors in the acute stage of intraventricular hemorrhage. Nichidai-isi 40: 1361-1374

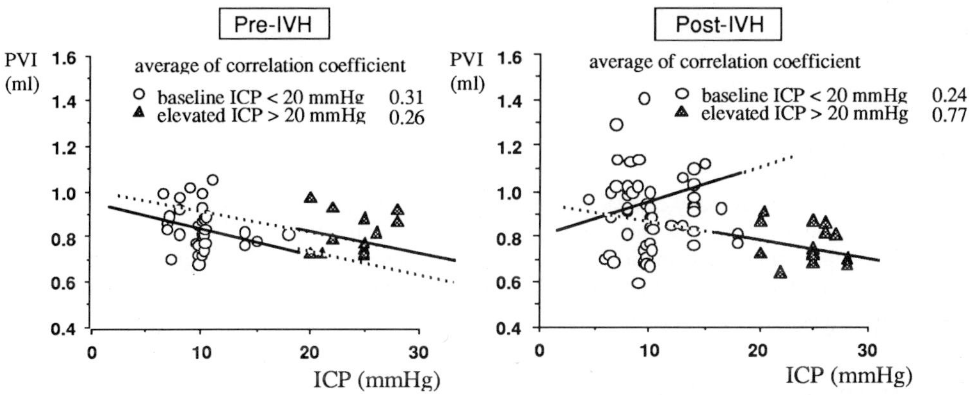

Fig.1. Relationship between PVI and ICP in pre-IVH (left) and post-IVH (right) condition. PVI decrease according to ICP elevation after IVH (right) episode while PVI in pre-IVH (left) does not correspond with increment of ICP.

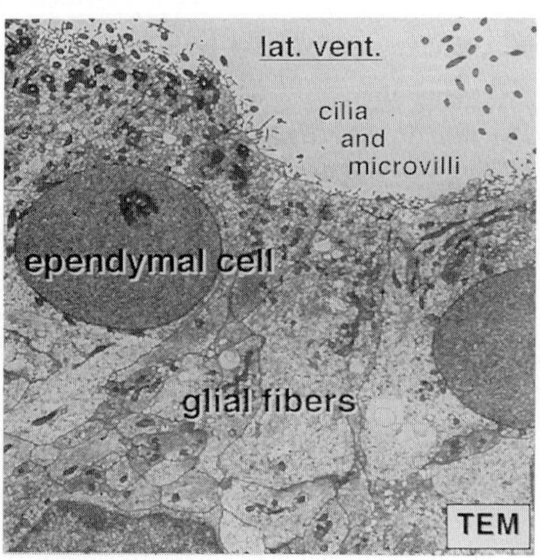

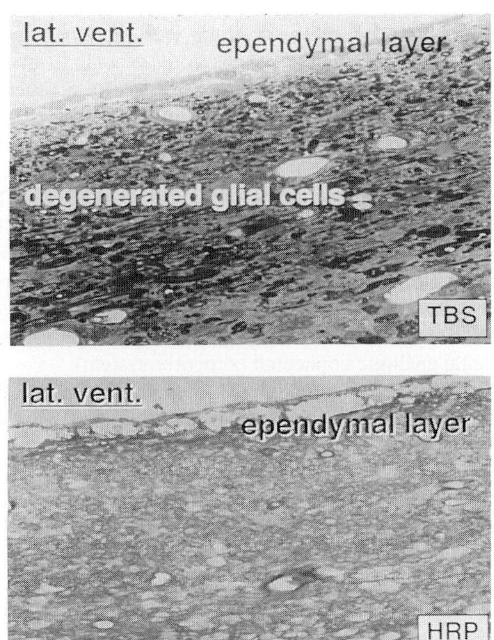

Fig.2. Histological alterations after IVH. a) The cilia and microvilli are diminished and glial fibers are increased in number. (transmission electron microscope (TEM) x 3000). b) Degenerated glial cells are abundant in the region of periependymal layer. (toluidine blue stain (TBS) x 25). c) HRP is densely migrated into the periependymal layer. (x 20).

Early ICP Monitoring: Relevant Essay for Prognosis in Severe Head Injury, Pilot Study in 30 Patients

L. Cristofori, R. Foroni, R. Gambin, C. Vivenza, S. Turazzi, and A. Bricolo

Department of Neurosurgery, University of Verona City Hospital, Verona, Italy

INTRODUCTION

One of the mean effort of many clinical studies in severe head injured patients is to point out robust outcome predictors for prognosis and assessment of the value of therapy [1,2].
Furthemore , application of numerical methods to determine the prognostic significant of clinical factors, is to weigh those associated with a poor prognosis [3,4,5]. This lead improve to understanding of pathophysiology and cure of head injuried.

CLINICAL MATERIAL AND METHODS

To verify the two hypothesis of this study, predictor value of the early ICP monitoring on global observation and the power of early ICP as descriptor for explaining outcome, we included only patients with continued ICP monitoring throught at least 48 hours and started within 6 hours post injury.
To obtain an homogeneus group with the aim to restrict as more as possible the variables linked to other definited predictors we selected planning a prospective study 30 head injuried patients affered to our Department from november 1991 to october 1993. Were included patients with GCS 4-8, furthermore were excluded patients in pediatric age (less than 16 years) and older than 50 years. Another exclusion criteria was bylateral not reacting pupils. To avoid overlapping with secondary ischemic brain damage patients with persistent systemic hypotension or hypoxia before arrival, were not included. Patients with normal CT scan (Diffuse Injury I) on admission were also excluded.
All patients were treated by the same medical and ICU nursing staff. Elevations of ICP greater than 20 mm Hg were treated according to applied sequence of Therapy Intensive Level (TIL) as descripted in Traumatic Coma Data Bank [6]. Device choosen was always Camino fiberoptic (24 subdural - intraparenchymal and 6 ventricular bolts). Continous recording of blood pression (BP), cerebral perfusion pression (CPP) and ICP were obtained connected patients to the data collection system (digital analogic connected computer system).
For all patients were defined 13 descriptors (ICP, CPP, BP, GCS, TIL, pupils, age) based on medium values obtained during global monitoring; for ICP, BP, CPP we defined 24 hours, 48 hours and global observation as separated descriptors.
A Cluster procedure was used to select a subset of potential candidate and possible interrelations. A priori none of single descriptors was overstimated. In addition we performed ICP data analysis following the usual signal approch (FFT, Spectrum Analysis, ARMA). Furthermore, medium values of ICP data of all patients (global of extended observation versus 24 hours, versus 48 hours) were analysed with 2 way ANOVA [7,8,9,10,11].
Six months outcome was evaluated with Glasgow Outcome Scale (GOS).

RESULTS

We collected data over 30 patients with mean age of 31,6 years and median of 29; 27 males and 3 females. GCS, motor score and GOS are shown in Table I.

Table I. GCS, motor score and GOS over 30 patients.

N° pts	GCS	N° pts	Motor Score	N° pts	GOS
4	8	2	5	10	Good
2	7	13	4	3	Moderate
12	6	4	3	7	Severe
3	5	9	2	-	Vegetative
9	4	2	1	10	Death

On entry 27 (90%) patients had both reactive pupils while one was not reacting over 3. CT findings showed Diffuse Injury (DI) in 17 patients: DI I in 6 patients, DI with edema in 10, DI with shift in 1. The focal lesions were evacuated mass lesion in 10 and not evacuated in 3.
Mean ICP and CPP values are shown in Table II and Fig. 1a, 1b.

Table II. ICP and CPP results in 30 patients.

	ICP 24 hrs	ICP 48 hrs	ICP global	CPP 24hrs	CPP 48 hrs	CPP global
Maximum	48	44	46	103	98	100
Minimum	3	4,5	5,6	57	49	49
Mean	15,5	16,3	18,7	87	84,2	81,6
Stand. Dev.	10,7	9,7	10,7	11,2	12,3	14,3

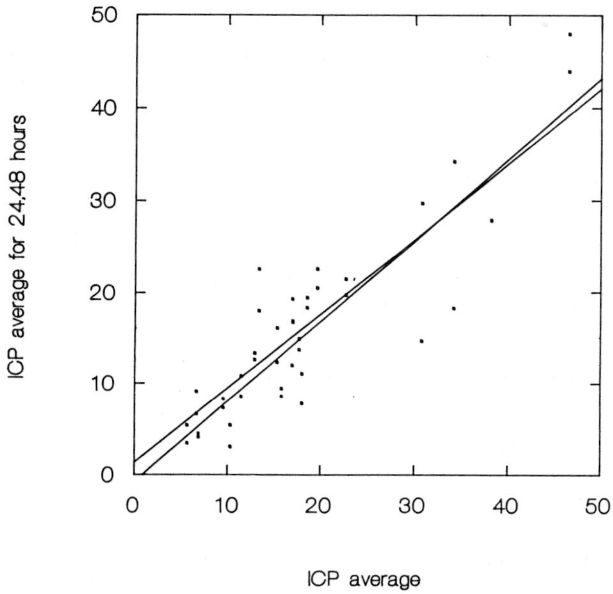

Fig. 1a

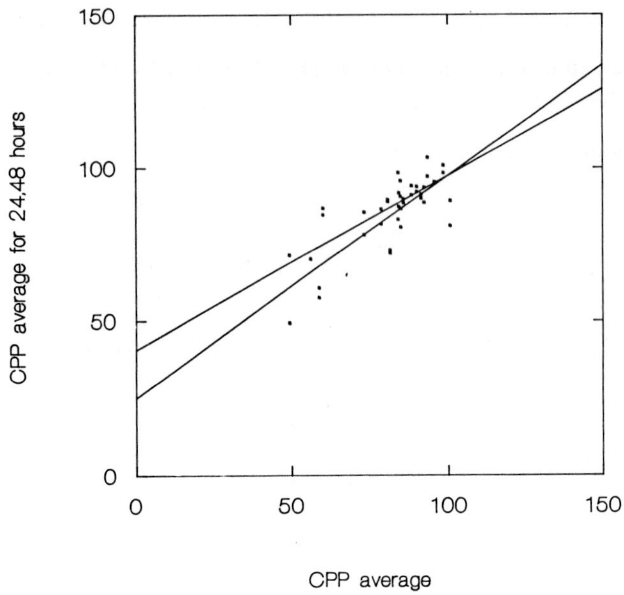

Fig. 1b

Fig. 1a, 1b. Linear regression analysis of ICP and CPP at 24, 48 hours versus global ICP and CPP (r = . 8 for ICP; r = .85 for CPP)

The F-Fischer test of two way ANOVA over 30 patients, was not significative in the differences between the three medium ICP and CPP values (24, 48 hours and global extent of observations).
Using Cluster analysis, Spearman test and autocorrelation matrix were found high correlations between outcome and ICP, CPP, TIL. Motor score, age and BP showed a lower correlation (Table III)

Table III. Autocorrelation coefficients between the multiple predictors. The interrelations tend to be stronger if the coefficients tend to be closer to 1; on the contrary the interrelations are weaker if the coefficients tend to be closer to 0; MS = motor score

	GOS	ICP	CPP	BP	TIL	AGE	MS
GOS	1						
ICP	.82	1					
CPP	.73	.84	1				
BP	.36	.2	.23	1			
TIL	.78	.84	.73	.4	1		
AGE	.28	.48	.36	.16	.34	1	
MS	.32	.2	.23	.14	.32	.07	1

DISCUSSION

From our knowledge, in the literature reports seldom is underlined the delay between the time of head injury and the start of ICP monitoring. The relevance of our study is concerning about to restrict and to evaluate in an homogeneous group only patients in whom ICP (within 6 hours from injury) surely describes the post injury acute damage. The criteria of group homogeneity, described in the previous

clinical materials, try to point out early ICP as predictor apart the others already well defined predictors. [2,3,4,5]
The early ICP monitoring is strongly predictive of global trend; our results about ICP predictive value confirm the study of Pitts and coworkers [12] on a larger number of patients, but in this previous study the patients selection criteria were not closed and signal approaches were not considerated.
Statystical analysis with Cluster and correlation matrix highlight as ICP values at 24, 48 and global monitoring are robust outcome predictors while motor score, TIL and CPP are the others, less significative, outcome predictor factors. Finally BP and age were less significative parameters (homogeneity in age and no hypotension).
Correlation between outcome and TIL was, as expected, equally strongly significant and statystical analysis showed a close association between TIL and ICP. Predictor values for CPP and BP as single factors on outcome is questionable and source of criticisms [2,13]; we observed that in our group, 9 patients received high dose barbiturate. Although is unquestioned the benefit effect of barbiturate in lowering ICP [14,15], the real degree of influence on BP and CPP is still uncleared and the question cannot be answered by this pilot study.
These preliminary results should be confirmed with a larger number of patients.

Acknowledgements. We wish to thank the ICU nursing staff for their invaluable cooperation.

REFERENCES

1. Marshall LF, Gautille T, Klauber MR, Eisenberg HM, Jane JA, Luerssen TG, Marmarou A, Foulkes MA (1991) The outcome of severe closed head injury. J Neurosurg 75:28-36.
2. Marmarou A, Anderson RL, Ward JD, Choi CS, Young HF, Eisenberg HM, Foukles MA, Marshall LF, Jane AJ (1991) Impact of ICP instability and Hypotension on outcome in patients with severe head trauma. J. Neurosurg. 75 (Suppl.):559-566.
3. Becker DP, Miller JD, Ward JD (1977) The outcome from severe head injury with early diagnosis and intensive management. J. Neurosurg 47:491-502
4. Eisenberger HM, Cayard C, Papanicolaou A (1983) The effects of three potentially preventable complications on outcome after severe closed head injury. In: Ishii S, Nagai H, Brock M (eds) Intracranial Pressure V Berlin: Springer-Verlag, pp. 549-553.
5. McGraw CP, Howard G., O'Connor C (1983) Outcome associated with management based on ICP monitoring. In: Ishii S., Nagai H., Brock M., (eds) Intracranial Pressure V. Berlin: Springer-Verlag, pp. 558-561.
6. Marmarou A, Anderson RL, Ward JD, Choi CS, Young HF, Eisenberg HM, Foukles MA, Marshall LF, Jane AJ (1991) NINDS Traumatic Coma Data Bank: Intracranial pressure monitoring methodology. J Neurosurg 75 (Suppl.): 521-527
7. BMDP. Statistical software manual. Vol. 1. University of California Press, pp. 259-289.
8. Montgomery A (1991) Designe and analysis of Experiments. Willey eds, pp. 350-367.
9. Young F. (1984) Recursive estimation and time series analysis. Springer-Verlag, pp. 58-75.
10. Anderson P (1957) An introduction to multivariate statystical analysis. Willey eds, pp. 80-85.
11. Kilders A (1978) Modern Spectrum Analysis. IEEE Press, pp. 112-120.
12. Pitts LH, Kaktis JV, Juster R (1980) ICP and outcome in patients with severe head injury. In: Shulman K, Marmarou A, Miller JD (eds) Intracranial Pressure IV. Berlin: Springer-Verlag, pp. 5-9.
13. Miller JD, Becker DP, Ward ID (1981) Significance of intracranical hypertension in severe head injury. J Neurosurg 47: 503-516.
14. Eisenberg MH, Frankowski FR, Contant CF, Marshall FL, Walker DM (1988) High-dose barbiturate control of elevated intracranial pressure in patients with severe head injury. J Neurosurg 69:15-23.
15. Bricolo A., Glick R. (1981) Barbiturate effects on acute experimental intracranial hypertension. J Neurosurg 55: 397-406.

Session XI: Treatment for Abnormal ICP (1)

Chairmen: A. Baethmann and N. Kodama

CPP Management I: Results

MICHAEL J. ROSNER and SHEILA D. ROSNER

Division of Neurosurgery, University of Alabama at Birmingham, Birmingham, AL, USA

INTRODUCTION

Cerebral ischemia dominates traumatic brain injury as the single most important event determining outcome [1,2]. The ultimate basis for the iatrogenic maintenance of CPP is the prevention and extension of ischemic injury. The primary role of CPP maintenance is the preservation of cerebral blood flow (CBF); regardless of spasm, abnormalities of autoregulation, or vessel obstruction, it is this pressure gradient (CPP) which will be most important in maintaining CBF and the most amenable to manipulation by the physician.

Mortality and morbidity have been improved with CPP based regimes. Rosner & Daughton reported a small series of GCS ≤ 7 patients with an overall mortality of 25% and improved morbidity [3]. We have continued to refine these techniques with treatment directed at CPP maintenance.

METHODS

158 patients, GCS ≤ 7 were managed using vascular volume expansion, CSF drainage via ventriculostomy, systemic vasopressors (phenylephrine, norepinephrine) and normocapnia to maintain a minimal CPP ≥ 70 mmHg. Detailed outcomes and follow-up data bases have been kept. No barbiturates nor hypothermia were used.

RESULTS

CPP averaged 85 ± 15 torr, ICP averaged 25 ± 12 torr and SABP 109 ± 14 torr. CSF drainage averaged 123 ± 120 cc/day; intake (5580 ± 3745 cc) was carefully titrated to output (5042 ± 3745 cc/day) and mannitol averaged 48 ± 118 gm/day. The ratio of favorable (good and moderate disability) to poor outcomes (severe, vegetative, or dead) was calculated for each GCS category and compared with the same ratio from the Traumatic Coma Data Bank (Traumatic Coma Data Bank).

CPP management improved the ratio of favorable : unfavorable outcomes when compared to TCDB results many fold: GCS = 3 by 5.9 ($p < .001$); GCS = 4 by 5.2 ($p < .001$); GCS = 5 by 2.4 ($p = .03$), and GCS = 6 by 4.4 fold ($p < .001$). GCS = 7 were not statistically different from the TCDB results (Pearson Chi square and Fisher Exact Test).

DISCUSSION

Cerebral perfusion pressure is the stimulus to which the autoregulatory response of the vasculature occurs [4]. The absolute arterial pressure has historically been the parameter varied in "tests" of autoregulation [5-7]. As a result, conclusions about the "intactness" of cerebral pressure autoregulation were often based upon undefined and abnormally low CPP.

Table 1: CPP vs. Traumatic Coma Data Bank Outcome vs. Glasgow Coma Scale

	GCS3		GCS4		GCS5		GCS6		GCS7		TOTAL	
	Fav	Unfav	Fav	Unfav	Fav	Unfav	Fav	Unfav	Fav	Unfav	Fav	Unfav
CPP	8	15	14	16	17	17	36	8	18	8	93	64
TCDB	7	90	16	95	24	58	57	56	102	46	206	345
***p=**	0.004		0.001		0.05		<.001		0.82		p<.001	

*Fisher Exact Test

Traumatic and other brain injury shifts the cerebral autoregulatory curve to the right. I.e., the injured brain will require a higher than normal CPP before relatively "normal" levels of CBF are attained [8,9]. This "lower limit " of autoregulation is not only higher than normal, it is depressed as well at a time when the cerebral tissue is highly vulnerable to ischemic insults [10]. The cerebral vascular resistance is higher generally and the critical closing pressure is also much higher [11,12]. Decrements in cerebral perfusion pressure, acting as an autoregulatory stimulus, are capable of precipitating plateau or Lundberg "A" waves which are associated with cerebral ischemia [13]. "B" waves, while shorter lived than "A" waves are qualitatively identical and also represent suboptimal and variable CPP [14]. By stabilizing CPP at or above the threshold level for "A" and "B" wave occurrence, they can be effectively eliminated. However, this threshold may be 85 mmHg or even higher [3,8]. These CPP levels appear extreme but for the reasons above are required. They must be obtained with significant systemic arterial hypertension which, as a result of early studies which only examined SABP and not CPP, concluded that arterial hypertension was harmful. However, Schrader et al have demonstrated that systemic hypertension is protective in the face of intracranial hypertension and mass lesion [15] and this is consistent with emerging clinical studies as well [3,16].

Because of the intense inter-relationships which exists between the autoregulatory response and other therapeutic modalities such as barbiturates and mannitol, CPP effects play an important, permissive role in their application. Barbiturate therapy is most effective when CPP is high, though these drugs may lower the CPP threshold needed. Mannitol requires an "adequate" CPP for its effects on ICP to be realized and in part works by increasing CPP as well as through viscosity effects [17,18].

Cerebral perfusion pressure is a parameter intimately linked with intracranial pressure and of the two, is most determinant of cerebral hemodynamic responses and effects. It can safely be manipulated to reduce frequency of CSF pressure waves with attendant ischemia: CPP is a viable and effective end point in the treatment of the intracranial hypertension associated with Traumatic Brain Injury.

CONCLUSION

CPP management yields favorable clinical results up to six-fold better than traditional techniques directed at ICP. When causes of mortality are examined, it appears that traumatic brain injury death rates can be reduced by another 33-50% by refinements in CPP management alone. Beyond this future morbidity/mortality reduction will require use of additional therapeutic modalities.

REFERENCES

1. Bouma GJ, Muizelaar JP, Choi SC, et al: Cerebral circulation and metabolism after severe traumatic brain injury: the elusive role of ischemia. J Neurosurg 75:685-693, 1991

2. Obrist WA, Langfitt TW, Jaggi JL, et al: Cerebral blood flow and metabolism in comatose patients with head injury. Relationship to intracranial hypertension. J Neurosurg 61:241-253, 1984

3. Rosner MJ, Daughton S: Cerebral perfusion pressure management in head injury. J trauma 30:933-941, 1990

4. Rosner MJ: Intracranial Pressure: A critical examination of its physiology and pathophysiology, in B.Andrews (ed): Neurosurgical Intensive Care.. New York, McGraw-Hill:57-112, 1993

5. Langfitt TW: Increased intracranial pressure. Clin Neurosurg 16:436-471, 1969

6. Langfitt TW, Tannenbaum HM, Kassell NF: The etiology of acute brain swelling following experimental head injury. J Neurosurg 24:47-56, 1966

7. Langfitt TW, Weinstein JD, Kassell NF: Cerebral vasomotor paralysis produced by intracranial hypertension. Neurology 15:622-641, 1965

8. El-Adawy Y, Rosner MJ: Cerebral Perfusion Pressure, Autoregulation and the PVI Reflection Point: Pathological ICP, in Hoff, JT, et al (eds): Intracranial Pressure VII. Springer-Verlag:829-833, 1988

9. Gray J, Rosner MJ: Pressure volume index Part II: The effects of low cerebral perfusion pressure and autoregulation. J Neurosurgery 67:369-376, 1987

10. Jenkins LW, Moszynski K, Lyeth BG, et al: Increased vulnerability of the mildly traumatized rat brain to cerebral ischemia: the use of controlled secondary ischemia as a research tool to identify common or different mechanisms contributing to mechanical and ischemic brain injury. Brain Res 477:211-224, 1989

11. Dewey RC, Pieper HP, Hunter WE: Experimental cerebral hemodynamics. Vasomotor tone, critical closing pressure, and vascular bed resistance. J Neurosurg 41:597-606, 1974

12. Fein JM, Lipow K, Marmarou A: Cortical artery pressure in normotensive and hypertensive aneurysm patients. J Neurosurg 59:51-56, 1983

13. Rosner MJ, Becker DP: The origin and evolution of plateau waves: Experimental observations and a theoretical model. J Neurosurgery 60:312-324, 1984

14. Rosner MJ: Cyclic CSF pressure waves causally relate to systemic arterial blood pressure, in Avezaat CJJ, van Eijndhoven JHM, Maas AIR, et al Intracranial Pressure VIII. Berlin, Springer-Verlag:414-417, 1993

15. Schrader H, Lofgren J, Zwetnow NM: Influence of blood pressure on tolerance to an intracranial expanding mass. Acta Neuro Scand 71:114-126, 1985

16. McGraw CP: A cerebral perfusion pressure greater than 80 mm Hg is more beneficial, in Hoff JT, Betz AL (eds): Intracranial Pressure, VII. Berlin, Springer-Verlag:839-841, 1989

17. Muizelaar JP, Bouma GJ, Levasseur JE, et al: Effect of hematocrit variations on cerebral blood flow and basilar artery diameter in vivo. Am J Physiol 262:H949-H954, 1992

18. Rosner MJ, Coley I: Cerebral perfusion pressure: A hemodynamic mechanism of mannitol and the post mannitol hemogram. Neurosurgery 21:147-156, 1987

CPP Management II: Optimization of CPP or Vasoparalysis Does Not Exist in the Living Brain

MICHAEL J. ROSNER and SHEILA D. ROSNER

Division of Neurosurgery, University of Alabama at Birmingham, Birmingham, AL, USA

INTRODUCTION

The foundation for the theoretical and practical development for cerebral perfusion pressure (CPP) management techniques is the continuing reactivity of the cerebral vasculature [1-5]. We asked: (1) Could we objectively determine an optimal CPP from the ICP-CPP relationships for not only the group, but the individual patient? And (2) Was there any patient where ICP varied directly with CPP (i.e., were we hurting patients by iatrogenically increasing CPP)?

METHODS

158 patients GCS ≤ 7, suffering traumatic brain injury were managed using previously described techniques. CPP was actively increased using vasopressors, euvolemia, the flat position and without hyperventilation. 105 physiological and other variables were recorded daily including the highest, mean, and lowest SABP, ICP, and CPP. We analyzed the relationship between CPP and ICP for both the group and individuals, for the average of ten days, by single treatment days, and in a subset of patients by hour.

RESULTS

[Outcomes have been reported in Part I.]. No patient demonstrated a direct relationship between CPP and ICP. For the group as a whole, a quadratic function based upon the mean daily ICP and CPP ($ICP = 0.006\ CPP^2 - 1.35\ CPP + 95$, $p < .001$ for all coefficients, $r = .499$, $r^2 = .25$) suggested a <u>decreasing</u> ICP up to a CPP of 112 mmHg ($ICP' = 0$) where a very gradual increase would then occur (Figure 1). The same general relationship held on a daily basis but the CPP at which the ICP increased began at 112 mmHg (day = 1), became maximal at 130 mmHg (day 3 and 5) and then declined to 94 mmHg by day 7.

When analyzed by hourly ICP and CPP means, the relationship showed a gradually <u>increasing</u> ICP <u>up</u> to CPP = 48 mmHg ($ICP' = 0$) where $ICP = -.002\ CPP^2 + .19\ CPP + 19$, $p < .001$) where it then declined. For <u>individuals</u> the CPP above which the ICP declined varied from 43 mmHg to 127.5 mmHg with a mean of 72 mmHg.

1. ICP does <u>not</u> vary directly with CPP.
2. For the group, ICP declines as average CPP increases up to about 112 mmHg.
3. This CPP level varies with time after injury and may reach 130 mmHg or greater.
4. Individuals demonstrated an increasing ICP as CPP increased to above threshold values whence ICP declined; this point varied individually from 43 to 130 mmHg but averaged 72 mmHg.

DISCUSSION

The concept of "vasoparalysis" occurring after traumatic brain injury implies that increasing systemic blood pressure will be harmful by potentiating cerebral hyperemia, cerebral edema, and ICP [6,7]. However, cerebral ischemia is the fundamental cause of subsequent neurologic demise [8] and not high cerebral blood flow (CBF). If CBF is to be maintained, a minimal level of cerebral perfusion pressure will be required.

The importance of these findings, i.e., the decrementing of ICP as CPP is brought to higher levels argues that "vasoparalysis" does not exist as a generalized phenomena in the injured brain. Rather, the ability of the cerebrovasculature to respond remains intact but blunted and supranormal levels of CPP are required. The effect of achieving these levels is to decrease ICP by both vasoconstriction and reduction of cerebral edema through improved tissue perfusion.

CONCLUSION

These data suggest neurovascular reactivity is intact after severe trauma, varies with time (nadir about day 3-5) and ICP follows an expected course of increasing with CPP from very low CPP until a threshold is reached, where upon ICP decreases as a function of high CPP acting to stimulate vasoconstriction. This threshold varies individually and the quadratic relationship can be used to identify it quantitatively to help guide individual management.

Figure 1.

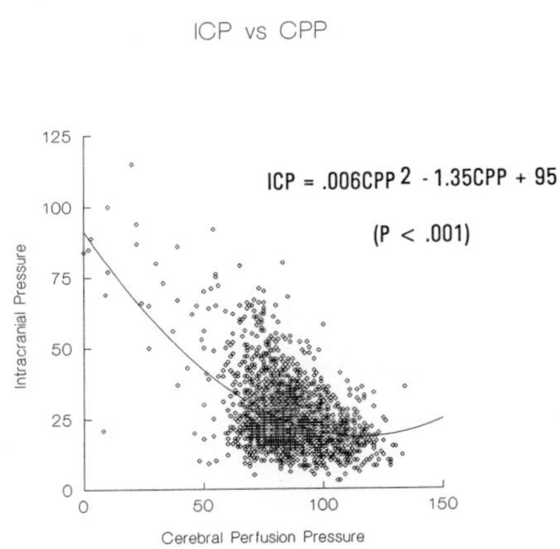

REFERENCES

1. Rosner MJ: Intracranial Pressure: A critical examination of its physiology and pathophysiology. In B. Andrews (ed.): Neurosurgical Intensive Care. McGraw-Hill, New York, 57-112, 1993.

2. Rosner MJ, Daughton S: Cerebral perfusion pressure management in head injury. J Trauma, 30:933-941, 1990.

3. El-Adawy Y, Rosner MJ: Cerebral Perfusion Pressure, Autoregulation, and the PVI Reflection Point: Pathological ICP, in Hoff, JT, et al (eds): Intracranial Pressure VII. Springer-Verlag: 829-833, 1988.

4. Gray J, Rosner MJ: Pressure Volume Index Part II: The effects of low cerebral perfusion pressure and autoregulation. J Neurosurg 67:369-376, 1987.

5. Rosner MJ: Cerebral perfusion pressure: The link between intracranial pressure and systemic circulation, in Wood, JH (ed.): Cerebral Blood Flow: Physiologic and Clinical Aspects. New York, McGraw-Hill, 425-448, 1987.

6. Langfitt TW, Weinstein JD, Kassell NF: Cerebral vasomotor paralysis produced by intracranial hypertension. Neurology 15: 622-641, 1965

7. Marshall WJS, Jackson JLF, Langfitt TW, et al: Brain swelling caused by trauma and arterial hypertension: Hemodynamic aspects. Arch Neurol 21:545-553, 1969.

8. Obrist WA, Langfitt TW, Jaggi JL, et al: Cerebral blood flow and metabolism in comatose patients with head injury. Relationship to intracranial hypertension. J Neurosurg 61:241-253, 1984.

Influence of Small-Volume Resuscitation on Formation of Brain Edema in Rabbits with Hemorrhagic Shock and Brain Injury

R. HÄRTL[1], L. SCHÜRER[2], C. DAUTERMANN[2], S. BERGER[3], F. RÖHRICH[2], K. MESSMER[1], and A. BAETHMANN[1]

[1] Institute for Surgical Research, [2] Department of Neurosurgery, Klinikum Großhadern, Ludwigs-Maximilians-University, 81336 Munich, Germany
[3] Department of Pediatric Surgery, Johannes-Gutenberg-University, 55131 Mainz, Germany

SUMMARY

The efficacy of small volumes of hypertonic/hyperoncotic solution (HHS), e.g. 7.2% NaCl / 10% dextran 60 is practically unmatched in reestablishment of the cardiovascular function in severe hemorrhagic shock under emergency conditions. Previous studies of this laboratory have indicated absence of adverse side effects of this treatment on cerebral blood flow or the cerebral O_2-supply in the presence of a focal brain lesion. The current investigations were carried out to elucidate, whether or not HHS enhances posttraumatic brain edema in animals with hemorrhagic hypotension and acute brain injury opening the blood-brain barrier. HHS was found to afford recovery albeit transiently of systemic blood pressure, and to decrease hematocrit from hemodilution. Serum-Na^+-levels were intermittently increased by 30 - 50 mM/l, subsequently followed by almost complete normalization. The focal lesion of the brain led to a significant decrease in specific gravity (SG), indicating accumulation of water in grey and white matter adjacent to the focal brain lesion. SG of grey matter was close to normal in animals with shock and HHS while reduced in animals with trauma without HHS. SG changes were similar in affected white matter, with the decrease being most pronounced in animals with trauma only, while SG changes in other groups with and without trauma following treatment with HHS were less severe. The data indicate altogether that HHS does not enhance brain edema in animals with hemorrhagic shock in the presence of a focal brain lesion. To the contrary, HHS seems to afford inhibition of edema formation early after trauma. Reservations against the treatment of patients with shock and head injury with HHS are not justified.

INTRODUCTION

Findings obtained by the US Traumatic Coma Data Bank Study indicate that mortality is doubled in severe head injury in the presence of hemorrhagic shock (14), highlighting the significance of prompt and effective shock treatment on the scene (18). So far, no treatment modality of severe hemorrhagic shock is available, which as rapidly normalizes cardiovascular function as small volume resuscitation with HHS. Effectiveness and safety of this regimen to restore cardiovascular competence and to improve the microcirculation is well documented (9). These attributes render resuscitation with HHS superior for the treatment of severely head injured patients in shock. These considerations notwithstanding, experience of side effects is limited in the presence of a traumatic brain lesion, particularly with regard to posttraumatic brain edema (3, 4, 7, 15, 16, 17, 21, 22). The present experiments were carried out using 7.2 % NaCl/10% dextran 60 (HHS) to obtain further information on this aspect.

METHODS

Preparation: 30 New Zealand rabbits of 2.6-3.5 kg body weight were utilized as experimental animals. Anaesthesia was induced by repetitive doses of thiopental (total 25-35 mg/kg b.w.) and continued by infusion of alpha-chloralose. Animals were tracheotomized and paralyzed for artificial ventilation. Arterial CO_2 was maintained at 35 mm Hg. A catheter was introduced into a femoral artery for monitoring of arterial blood pressure and for blood sampling to assess blood gases and others. The animals head was immobilized in a sphinx position by a stereotactic holder.
Cold injury: A trephination was made over the left cerebral hemisphere for induction of a cold lesion of the brain according to KLATZO (1967) with employment of a stainless steel cylinder (6 mm Ø; -68°C; duration: 1 min). Hemorrhagic shock was induced by withdrawal of one third of the circulating blood volume until MAP fell to 40 mm Hg for 30 minutes.
Resuscitation: A bolus of 4 ml/kg of 7.2% NaCl/10% dextran 60 (HHS; Hyperdex®, Schiwa GmbH, Glandorf, FRG) was infused through an ear vein within 2 min. No further infusions followed.

Specific gravity: At termination of the experiment animals were rapidly sacrificed by KCl. For measurement of specific gravity (SG) the brain was carefully removed and frozen at -70°C. A Percoll® (Pharmacia Fine Chemicals, Uppsala, Sweden) density gradient as described by TENGVAR et al. (1983) and introduced for tissue density measurement by PERTOFT and AKERSTRÖM et al. (1, 13) was prepared. The brains were dissected into 4 coronary slices. Samples of grey and white matter of ca. 4 mm^3 were punched from defined areas, defrosted in a humidified chamber and immersed at the surface of the Percoll column. One minute later the position of the floating sample was read in arbitrary units given at the glass cylinder. SG was calculated by employment of a calibration curve obtained with standard beads (12).

Experimental protocol: Animals were randomly divided into six groups. At conclusion of the preparation, baseline values of MAP, hematocrit (Hct), colloidosmotic pressure (COP), and serum Na^+ were established. In group I (sham; n=6) measurements continued for 240 minutes. Group II (HHS only; n=6) was infused with 4 ml/kg b.w. at 60 min (t=60 min) followed by observation for another 180 min. Group III (trauma only; n=6) underwent brain injury at t=0 min without subsequent treatment. In group IV (HHS & shock; n=6) hemorrhagic shock was induced at 30 min after beginning of the experiment (t=30) with infusion of HHS 30 min. later (t=60). In group V (trauma & HHS; n=6) brain injury (t=0) was followed by HHS infusion at 60 min later. In group VI (trauma & shock & HHS; n=6) brain injury was combined with hemorrhagic hypotension followed by infusion with HHS.

Statistics: SG of corresponding brain hemispheres of different groups was analyzed by the Kruskal-Wallis test in the computer version of Theodorsson-Norheim (20). Comparisons between both brain hemispheres were made according to Conover. $p<0.05$ was required for rejection of the null hypothesis.

RESULTS

Table I Specific gravity (g/cm^3; mean ± SEM) of grey and white matter of the left (traumatized) and right cerebral hemisphere. SG measurements are based on 150 - 200 specimens in grey matter, while on 50 - 75 specimens in white matter.

Grey matter	Left / lesioned		Right / control	
	Mean	SEM	Mean	SEM
Group I	1,03904	0,001	1,03921	0,0011
Group II	1,03996	0,0019	1,04176	0,00332
Group III	1,03665	0,00115	1,03804	0,0007
Group IV	1,04162	0,00172	1,041	0,00132
Group V	1,03818	0,00237	1,03962	0,00177
Group VI	1,03993	0,0022	1,0413	0,00101

White matter	Left / lesioned		Right / control	
	Mean	SEM	Mean	SEM
Group I	1,03448	0,00158	1,03553	0,00158
Group II	1,03635	0,00164	1,03711	0,00176
Group III	1,03217	0,00088	1,03442	0,00112
Group IV	1,03684	0,00111	1,03708	0,00098
Group V	1,03552	0,00161	1,03647	0,00101
Group VI	1,03633	0,00146	1,03844	0,00146

Systemic parameters: MAP was 89 ± 2 mm Hg in the early control phase in sham animals, remaining largely unchanged during the experiment. Neither HHS nor induction of the cold lesion affected MAP significantly. In groups IV and VI (hemorrhagic shock) ca. 20 ml /kg blood were withdrawn to lower MAP to 40 mm Hg. Infusion of HHS led to short recovery of MAP to 72 ± 3, or 67 ± 2 mm Hg in these groups, respectively. In groups II, IV, V and VI HHS infusion caused a decrease of Hct by ca. 10 % from hemodilution. Hct was similar in groups IV and VI with hemorrhage. COP ranged from 15 to 17 mm Hg in all groups under control conditions. Hypovolemia decreased COP to 11 - 12 mm Hg, while HHS afforded transient recovery. Serum Na^+-levels were in the range of 138 - 150 mM/l, which was unaffected by the cold lesion or hemorrhage. HHS, however, was transiently raising serum-Na^+ by 30 - 50 mM/l, followed by near normalization within 120 min.

Specific gravity: Brain edema is associated with a decrease in specific gravity of affected tissue. Mean SG per hemisphere (± SEM) is given in table I. In white matter 50 - 75 specimens were studied per experimental group, in grey matter 150 - 200 specimens

Grey matter: SG of grey matter was 1.03904 g/cm^3 in sham animals in the left, while 1.03921 g/cm^3 in the right hemisphere. Significant differences in grey matter between the left and right hemispheres were found only in group III (trauma only). SG of grey matter of the exposed hemisphere was highest in group IV (shock + HHS), while lowest in group III (trauma only), with both SG values being significantly different from controls. Grey matter of the right, non-lesioned hemisphere had a similar pattern. The lowest SG value was found in group III indicating more edema, while high SG levels in groups II, IV or VI which, however, were all significantly different from SG in group I.

White matter: The focal brain lesion led in white matter to a particularly pronounced decrease in SG, involving all groups except group IV (shock + HHS). Maximum edema was found in group III, while SG changes were less pronounced in groups II, IV, V and VI, which again were significantly different from that in white matter of the control group.

DISCUSSION

Mechanisms underlying recovery of the cardiovascular function from shock by hypertonic saline are quite well understood (11). Accordingly, the osmotic gradient between the intra- and extravascular space is rapidly attracting water accross the vascular border including from endothelial cells as well as from the extracellular space of the parenchyma and beyond. Nevertheless, only limited data is available on the effects of this treatment in the CNS with an open blood-brain barrier (3, 4, 7, 15, 16, 17, 21, 22). Reduction of ICP is well understood by hypertonic fluid attributable to the dehydration of brain tissue with an intact blood-brain barrier (BBB) (2, 17). A compromised BBB in patients with head injury, however, not only may limit effectiveness of HHS, but could also support development of brain edema by this treatment (5, 10). Enhancement of edema could be brought about by extravasation of the colloid (dextran) into brain parenchyma as a basis of fluid retention (6). The current experiments were made to shed further light on this aspect, paying special attention to brain edema formation from a focal cerebral lesion.

The results do not support that HHS early after administration enhances brain edema, if the blood-brain barrier is open, while edema was maximal in animals (trauma only) which did not receive treatment. Administration of HHS in animals with trauma was associated with a significantly reduced water content (i.e. high SG) in white matter of the exposed hemisphere. The present findings seem to be at variance with that of other laboratories (3, 17, 21, 22) who reported that hypertonic solutions (without colloids) attenuate brain edema only in tissue areas with an intact BBB. Based on these and our present findings we assume that it is the combination of cristalloids with hyperoncotic colloids which is rendering small volume resuscitation superior to cristalloids alone.

In conclusion, administration of HHS in animals with hemorrhagic shock and a focal brain lesion does not increase vasogenic brain edema. Just to the contrary, animals with treatment had a lower water content in both, the traumatized as well as contralateral brain hemispheres early after fluid administration. Due to the powerful properties of HHS to restore cardiovascular function in hemorrhagic shock, this treatment appears to be particularly beneficial in polytraumatized patients and severe head injury to prevent development of secondary brain damage from cerebral ischemia.

REFERENCES

1. Akerström G, Pertoft H, Grimelius L, and Johansson H: Density determinations of human parathyroid glands by density gradients. Acta Pathol Microbiol Scand (a) 2:91-6, 1979
2. Battistella F and Wisner D: Cerebral dehydration following hypertonic saline resuscitation. Circ Shock 37:16, 1992
3. Battistella FC and Wisner DH: Combined hemorrhagic shock and head injury: effects of hypertonic saline (7.5 %) resuscitation. J Trauma 31:182-8, 1991
4. Berger S, Schürer L, Dautermann C, Härtl R, Murr R, Röhrich F and Baethmann A: Hypertonic solutions in treatment of intracranial pressure. Zentralbl Chir 118:237-43, 1993
5. Gröger U and Marmarou A: Importance of protein content in the edema fluid for the resolution of brain edema. Adv Neurol 52:215-8, 1990
6. Gunnar WP, Merlotti GJ, Barrett J and Jonasson O: Resuscitation from hemorrhagic shock. Alterations of the intracranial pressure after normal saline, 3 % saline, and dextran-40. Ann Surg 204:686-92, 1986
7. Härtl R, Schürer L, Dautermann C, Röhrich F, Berger S, Murr R, Messmer K and Baethmann A: Effect of hypertonic-hyperoncotic solutions (HHS) on increased ICP after a focal brain lesion and inflation of an intracranial balloon. in: Avezaat CJJ et al. (eds). Intracranial pressure VIII, Springer, pp 612-614, 1993
8. Klatzo I: Presidential address. Neuropathological aspects of brain edema. J Neuropathol Exp- Neurol 26:1-14, 1967
9. Kreimeier U, Frey L and Messmer K: Small-volume-resuscitation. Curr Op Anaesth 6:400-408, 1993
10. Kuroiwa T, Chan R, Juhler M, Goping G, Campbell G and Klatzo I: Role of extracellular proteins in the dynamics of vasogenic brain edema. Acta Neuropathol 66:3-11,1985
11. Mazzoni MC, Borgström P, Arfors KE and Intaglietta M: Dynamic fluid redistribution in hyperosmotic resuscitation of hypovolemic hemorrhage. Am J Physiol 255:H629-37, 1988
12. Nelson SR, Mantz ML and Maxwell JA: Use of specific gravity in the measurement of cerebral edema. J Appl Physiol 30:268-71,1971
13. Pertoft H, Laurent TC, Laas T and Kagedal L: Density gradients prepared from colloidal silica particles coated by polyvinylpyrrolidone (Percoll). Anal Biochem 88:271-82, 1978
14. Piek J, Chesnut RM, Marshall LF, van Berkum-Clark M, Klauber MR, Blunt BA, Eisenberg HM, Jane JA, Marmarou A and Foulkes MA: Extracranial complications of severe head injury. J Neurosurg 77:901-7, 1992
15. Prough DS, Johnson JC, Poole G Jr., Stullken EH, Johnston W Jr. and Royster R: Effects on intracranial pressure of resuscitation from hemorrhagic shock with hypertonic saline versus lactated Ringer´s solution. Crit Care Med 13:407-11,1985
16. Schürer L, Dautermann C, Härtl R, Murr R, Berger S, Röhrich F, Messmer K and Baethmann A: Treatment of hemorrhagic hypotension with hypertonic/hyperoncotic solutions: effects on regional cerebral blood flow and brain surface oxygen tension. Eur Surg Res 24:1-12, 1992
17. Shackford SR, Zhuang J and Schmoker J: Intravenous fluid tonicity: effect on intracranial pressure, cerebral blood flow, and cerebral oxygen delivery in focal brain injury. J Neurosurg 76:91-8, 1992
18. Siegel JH, Gens DR, Mamantov T, Geisler FH, Goodarzi S and Mac Kenzie EJ: Effect of associated injuries and blood volume replacement on death, rehabilitation needs, and disability in blunt traumatic brain injury. Crit Care Med 19:1252-65, 1991
19. Tengvar C, Hultström D and Olsson Y: An improved Percoll density gradient for measurements of experimental brain edema. Addition of sucrose to an isotonic gradient in an attempt to balance osmotic conditions during density determinations. Acta Neuropathol 61:201-6, 1983
20. Theodorsson-Nordheim E: Kruskal-Wallis test: BASIC computer program to perform nonparametric analysis of variance and multiple comparisons on ranks of several independent samples. Comput Methods Programs Biomed 23:57-62, 1986
21. Wisner DH, Schuster L and Quinn C: Hypertonic saline resuscitation of head injury: effects on cerebral water content. J Trauma 30:75-8, 1990
22. Zornow MH, Scheller MS and Shackford SR: Effects of a hypertonic lactated Ringer´s solution on intracranial pressure and cerebral water content in a model of traumatic brain injury. J Trauma 29:484-8, 1989

Controlled External Lumbar Drainage for Treatment of Severe Intracranial Hypertension

F. Artru[1], C. Mottolese[2], D. Peillon[1], C.M. Mottolese[1], and C. Jourdan[1]

[1] Department of Anesthesia, [2] Department of Neurosurgery, Neurological Hospital, Lyon, France

INTRODUCTION

Lumbar drainage is commonly employed to treat post-operative CSF fistulae or to drain CSF spaces after subarachnoidal hemorrhage. However, several cases of transtentorial herniation have been reported [1, 2] and attributed to overdrainage and creation of a pressure gradient between the supratentorial and lumbar compartments. More recently, the procedure has been reported to be useful in controlling refractory intracranial hypertension in children with severe diffuse head injury [3]. In the present series, we tried to avoid the risk of cerebral herniation in restricting lumbar drainage to patients retaining a free communications between intracranial and extracranial CSF spaces, as judged from visible basal cisterns on C-T scan. Moreover, to limit the pressure gradient, a counter-pressure was practised by keeping the drainage system above the patient's head.

MATERIALS AND METHODS

The series comprised 13 patients (age : 49 ± 13 yrs) who were comatose from head injury (n=5) or intracerebral hemorrhage (n=8). GCS before intubation was 6.6 ± 1.9. Mean ICP over a 24 h period exceeded 30 mmHg. Management included controlled ventilation and a combination of therapies, the intensity of which was evaluated according to a special scale (fig. 2). On C-T scan, basal cistern appeared compressed in 12/13 patients but remained visible with an effacement score [4] not exceeding 9/14. Lateral ventricules were generally small, sometimes normal-sized but never dilated.

A lumbar F5 catheter was inserted through a 14 G Tuohy needle (Cordis® lumbar catheter accessory kit) and connected to an external drainage system (Cordis® external drainage set). The drainage height was set 30 cm above the tragus. No effort was done to limit the CSF output. Cell count, glucose level and culture of the CSF was daily performed and all catheters were cultivated after removal. ICP was continuously monitored with a Camino sensor along with arterial blood pressure and CPP. Daily mean values of ICP and CPP were calculated.

RESULTS

CSF drainage data

Lumbar catheters were placed 7.8 ± 4.2 days after onset of the coma. The duration of drainage was 6.7 ± 5.1 days. Mean daily output amounted to 147 ± 122 ml. Two catheters became obstructed and had to be replaced and another was accidently pulled out. After removal of his catheter, one patient developped a Staphylococcus Epidermidis meningitis which was rapidly controlled with antibiotics. In 2 other patients, catheter culture was positive with the same germ.

Effect on ICP and CPP

On the first post-insertion day, the lumbar drainage caused a reduction of daily mean ICP from 33 ± 3 mmH to 19 ± 9 mmHg. This reduction remained significant during 3 days (fig. 1). Patients could be divided in categories : in 9 patients, the drainage was immediately and permanently effective on ICP level. Such a cas is illustrated on figure 3. These patients were moderately or severely disabled after six months except fc one who died from sepsis. In one patient with a very low daily CSF output (16 ml), the drainage totally faile to influence the ICP level and death from sepsis occured one week later. In 3 other patients, ICP lev remained low for respectively 2, 5 and 10 days. Afterwards, ICP rose again, despite persistance of a larg CSF output. Pupils became non-reactive to light. Two patients progressed to cerebral death. The third benefite of an external ventricular drainage, recovered his pupils reactivity and subsequently awoke from coma.

Effect on basal cistern volume

During the drainage, basal cistern effacement judged on a 14 points scale increased significantly compare to pre-insertion values (from 6.3 ± 2.7 to 12.4 ± 2.0 ; $p<0.005$). Cisterns even completely disappeared in patients. Within the first week after cessation of drainage, basal cisterns were again well visible with tl effacement score decreasing to 4.2 ± 2.8 ; $p<0.0005$.

Effect on the therapy level intensity

For the whole series, the therapy intensity decreased significantly during the first 3 days from a pre-insertic level of 4.5 ± 2.2 to 2.4 ± 1.4 and remained significantly lower for the first 3 days. (fig. 2)

DISCUSSION

The initial effectiveness of lumbar drainage in reducing high ICP can be related to the persistance on C- scan of visible CSF spaces at the cranial basis. To explain the secondary reascension of ICP in 3 patien with the later occurence of herniation signs, one has to assume that a free communication was no long present at that time. Overdrainage and consecutive collapsus of CSF communication channels probab promoted the creation of a craniospinal pressure gradient and the caudal displacement of brain structure Analysis of these cases did not point to any specific sign preceeding the occurence of herniation except tl reascension of ICP above 30 mmHg. The day pupils became nonreactive, daily CSF output figures were n decreased and were actually among the highest of the series (330-345-265 ml) suggesting a direct role overdrainage in the determination of transtentorial herniation. Basal cisterns were collapsed but the san held true for other patients who did not deteriorate.

From these series, we conclude that, in order to avoid possible deleterious effect of lumbar drainage, thr precautions should be added to the protocole :
- drainage should be not only pressure-controlled but also volume-controlled in elevating the drainage syste at levels sufficiently high to keep the early CSF output under 5 ml
- if after a few days and despite a productive drainage, ICP rise again above 30 mmHg or if the differenti between ICP and lumbar pressure exceeds 10 mmHg [5] , the procedure should be promptly discontinue

Lumbar drainage thus appears a useful alternative or adjunct to the usual management of seve intracranial hypertension. The procedure should be however indicated in selected cases and obey a str monitoring protocole.

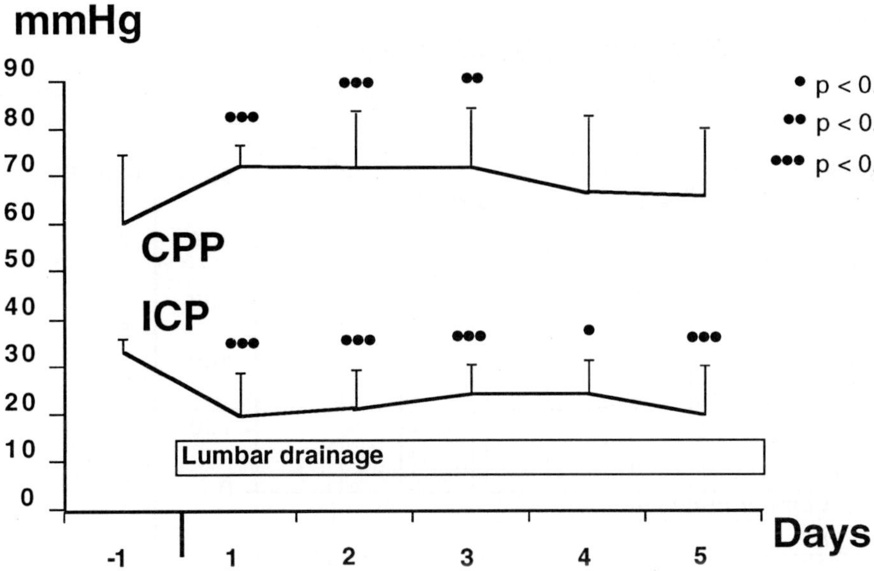

Fig. 1 : Effect of lumbar drainage on daily mean ICP and CPP.

Therapy	Score
Mannitol	
< 1g/kg/d	1
≥ 1g/kg/d	2
Thiopental	
< 30 mg/l	1
< 30 mg/l + ¥OH bolus	2
> 30 mg/l ± lidocaine	3
negative water balance	1
THAM	1
Dopamine	1

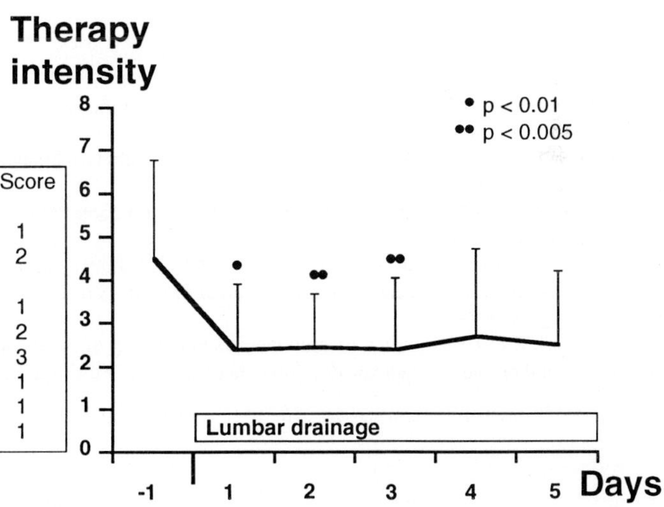

Fig. 2 : Effect of lumbar drainage on daily mean therapy intensity level score. Weights of the different treatments are listed on the left.

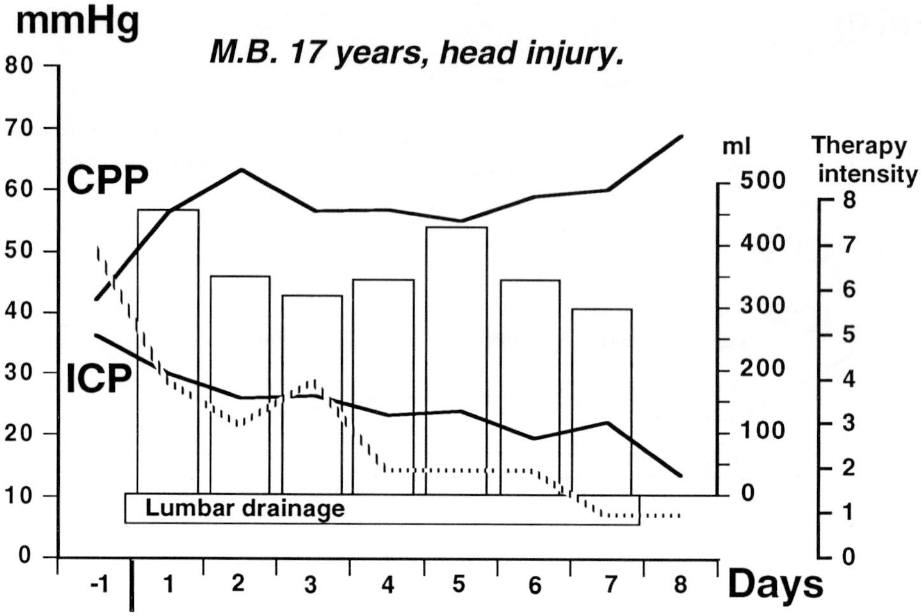

Fig. 3 : Decrease in ICP, increase in CPP and reduction of the therapy intensity level score during a seven days lumbar drainage in a head injury patient.

REFERENCES

1. Snow RB, Kuhel W, Martin SB (1991) Prolonged lumbar spinal drainage after the resection of tumors of the skul base: a cautionary note. Neurosurg. 28(6) : 880-883.
2. Roland PS, Marple BF, Meyerhoff WL, Mickey B (1992) Complications of lumbar spinal fluid drainage. Otolaryngol Head Neck Surg 107:564-569.
3. Baldwin HZ, Rekate HL (1991-92) Preliminary experience with controlled external lumbar drainage in diffuse pediatric head injury. Pediatr Neurosurg 17:115-120.
4. Artru F, Jourdan C, Convert J, Duquesnel J, Deleuze R (1990) An effacement score for basal cisterns to predict ICP level and outcome after severe head injury. Intracranial Pressure VII, Eds:J.Hoff and A.Betz, Springer-Verlag Berlin-Heidelberg, pp 603-605.
5. Kaufman GE, Clark K (1970) Continuous simultaneous monitoring of intraventricular and cervical subarachnoid cerebrospinal fluid pressure to indicate development of cerebral or tonsillar herniation. J Neurosurg 33:145-150

Impact of Moderate Hypothermia on Therapies for Intracranial Pressure Control in Severe Traumatic Brain Injury

T. Hirayama[1], Y. Katayama[1], T. Kano[1], N. Hayashi[2], and T. Tsubokawa[1]

[1] Department of Neurological Surgery, [2] Division of Emergency and Critical Care Medicine, Nihon University School of Medicine, Itabashi-ku, Tokyo, 173 Japan

SUMMARY

We report here the effects of hypothermia on intracranial pressure (ICP) and the intensity level of therapies for its control observed in a randomized study of moderate hypothermia (32-33°C for 48 hours) in 22 patients with severe traumatic brain injury (Glasgow Coma Scale score ≤7). No significant differences in absolute values of ICP were demonstrated at any time between the normothermia (n=10) and hypothermia (n=12) groups. However, hypothermia appeared to have lowered ICP for some extent since ICP levels during hypothermia was significantly lower than ICP levels following termination of hypothermia (P<0.01). No such changes were observed in normothermia group. Mannitol dosage used for ICP control was significantly lower during hypothermia as compared with the normothermia group (P<0.05). While SjO_2 and $PaCO_2$ values demonstrated significant positive correlations in the normothermia group (P<0.05), no such correlation was observed during hypothermia. These findings suggest that hypothermia may increase therapeutic efficiency of hyperventilation due partly to less marked impact on the balance between cerebral circulation and metabolic demand, and reduces the intensity level of therapy for ICP control using mannitol.

INTRODUCTION

Clifton et al. [1] recently reported results for a randomized trial of moderate hypothermia (32-33°C) in 46 patients with severe traumatic brain injury (Glasgow Coma Scale (GCS) scores ≤7). They observed strong indications of an improved outcome with minimal toxicity in the hypothermia group. Cooling was begun within 6 hours post-trauma and continued for 48 hours. Such a level of hypothermia has been well established to represent the optimal range for avoiding toxicity and serious complications [2].

We have also performed a randomized trial of moderate hypothermia in patients with severe traumatic brain injury (GCS scores ≤7), employing a similar protocol to that reported by Clifton et al. [1]. We report the results at this stage, since several lines of evidence have suggested that hypothermia reduces the intracranial pressure (ICP) or increases the efficiency of therapies for ICP control. ICP can be controlled by various means other than hypothermia, so that comparisons of absolute values of ICP between normothermia and hypothermia groups may not reveal a difference [1]. We therefore evaluated the intensity level of therapies [8] for ICP control. The present study was performed a the one-year period from 1992 [5].

MATERIALS AND METHODS

A total of 22 patients aged 18-81 years with closed head injury and post-resuscitation GCS scores of ≤7 were included in the study. All of the patients were transported directly to our service within 2 hours posttrauma. The initial patient management consisted of rapid intubation and ventilatory support. Computerized tomography (CT) scans were performed at the Emergency Center and craniotomies for hematomas were carried out immediately. ICP was monitored with a fiberoptic catheter (Camino Co.) introduced via, a frontal burr hole. An arterial catheter and Swan-Ganz catheter were routinely inserted. A ...e fiberoptic catheter system (4Fr. Opticath and Oximetrix III Systems) was used for continuous measurement of the jugular bulb oxygen saturation (SjO_2) [3,6,9,10]. The catheter was placed in the dominant side based on the findings of CT scans and previous angiography. The arterial blood oxygen saturation was monitored from withdrawn arterial blood as well as by pulse oximetry at the finger, and was maintained at ≥92 percent. Morphine (10-20 mg/hour) was infused for sedation, and pancuronium bromide (4 mg) was given hourly to control ventilation. When the ICP was not greater than 20 mmHg, ventilation was adjusted to maintain a PaO_2 of ≥100 mmHg and $PaCO_2$ of ≥35 mmHg. An increased ICP was managed first by hyperventilation using an SjO_2 of 55 percent to determine the lowest level of $PaCO_2$. Mannitol was infused at a rate of 12.5 grams IV q 5min PRN when the ICP exceeded 20 mmHg, until a serum osmolarity of > 315 mosm was reached. Ten patients were treated under standard management at 37-38°C (normothermia group). Twelve patients were treated at 32-33°C (hypothermia group) beginning within 6 hours post-trauma employing cooling blankets (Blanketrol II, Cincinnati Sub-Zero Co.). These patients were re-warmed by 1°C every 4 hours beginning at 48 hours after a temperature of 32-33°C had been reached. These protocol of patient management and procedures for hypothermia were broadly identical to those reported by Clifton et al. [1]. Physiologic and laboratory data were averaged for each 24 hour block. The intensity level of therapies for ICP control was evaluated from the $PaCO_2$ values and the mannitol dosage averaged also for each 24-hour time block. The outcome was assessed from by the Glasgow Outcome Scale (GOS) at 3 months post-trauma.

RESULTS

The age, GCS, pupillary reactivity, time of emergency department admission soon after admission primary diagnosis and initial ICP levels were similar in both groups. Among the physiologic data (Table 1), heart rate was significantly lower in the hypothermia group during both the first and second 24-hou blocks (P<0.01, unpaired t-test). The mean arterial blood pressure was slightly lower in the hypothermi group, but the difference was not statistically significant. Laboratory data (Table 1) demonstrated decrease in serum potassium in the hypothermia group, although the values were not significantly different a compared to those in the normothermia group due to replacement therapy.

Table 1. The comparison of physiologic data in both groups

Chracteristic / Time (hrs)	Normothermia		Hypothermia		t-test
	mean	SE	mean	SE	
mean arterial pressure					
0-24	93.90	2.37	93.25	3.98	NS
24-48	93.70	4.14	86.50	3.83	NS
48-72	94.90	3.83	91.83	4.21	NS
intracranial pressure					
0-24	18.10	5.86	11.00	2.77	NS
24-48	21.8	4.99	12.33	2.42	NS
48-72	26.4	5.49	19.67	3.45	NS
heart rate					
0-24	100.60	5.32	70.25	3.32	p<0.01
24-48	97.20	4.09	65.59	2.66	p<0.01
48-72	97.40	3.70	86.50	3.15	p<0.05
potassium					
0-24	3.86	0.22	3.15	0.25	NS
24-48	3.83	0.19	3.86	0.32	NS
48-72	3.92	0.29	3.82	0.13	NS

NS = no significance

No significant differences in absolute values of ICP were noted between the normothermia an hypothermia groups during either the first and second 24-hour blocks, or the subsequent 24-hour block which hypothermia was terminated (Table 1). However, there were indications that the ICP levels we lowered by the hypothermia during the first and second 24-hour blocks, while such an effect disappeare during the subsequent 24-hour block in association with the termination of hypothermia. Thus, the IC levels during the first and second 24-hour blocks were significantly lower than those during th subsequent 24-hour block in the hypothermia group. No such changes in ICP were detected in th normothermia group.

There was a difference in intensity level of therapy for ICP control: the mannitol dosage used during th first and second 24-hour blocks was significantly lower in the hypothermia group (P<0.01, unpaired t-te Fig. 1). The mean $PaCO_2$ values during either the first or second 24-hour blocks were not significan different between the normothermia and hypothermia groups. It was found that, while the SjO_2 and PaC(values demonstrated significant positive correlations in the normothermia group during the first 24-ho block (P<0.05, Spearman rank correlation; Fig. 2), no such correlation was evident in the hypothermia group (Fig. 2).

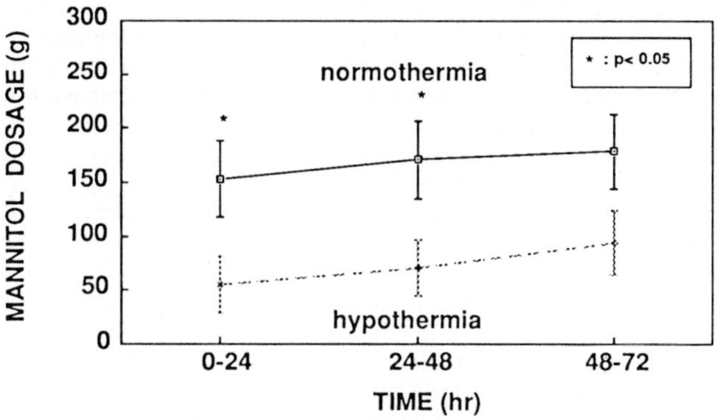

Fig. 1. The mannitol dosage used during the first and second 24-hour blocks was significantly lower in the hypothermia group (P<0.01, unpaired t-test).

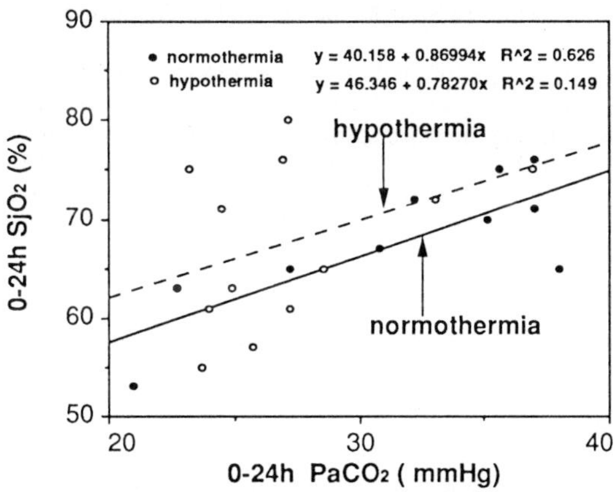

Fig. 2 The SjO2 and PaCO2 values demonstrated significant positive correlations in the normothermia group during the first 24-hour block (P<0.05, Spearman rank correlation). No such correlation was evident in the hypothermia group .

The mortality rate was 50 percent in the normothermia group and 33.3 percent in the hypothermia group. In the normothermia group, 30 percent of patients were in a state of good recovery or moderate disability and 70 percent were either severely disabled, vegetative or dead at 3 months posttrauma. In contrast, 66.7 percent of patients were in a state of good recovery or moderate disability and 33.3 percent were either severely disabled, vegetative or dead in the hypothermia group. While all of these measures of outcome were consistently better in the hypothermia group, the differences did not reach a statistically significant level.

DISCUSSION

The results of the present study on various aspects of moderate hypothermia were consistent with the previous observations reported by Clifton et al. [1]. It is now clear that moderate hypothermia can be employed with minimal toxicity. Definite conclusions regarding improvement of outcome due to hypothermia must, however, await further investigations with larger numbers of patients. The present study failed to demonstrate a significant difference in absolute values of ICP between the normothermia and hypothermia groups. Since ICP levels can be controlled by therapies other than hypothermia, absolute values of ICP may not reveal such an effect by themselves, especially in patients with a mildly elevated

ICP. The lower intensity level of therapies for ICP control using mannitol also indicates that moderate hypothermia may exert a favorable effect on an elevated ICP.
These findings suggest that hypothermia can either reduce ICP by itself or increase the efficiency of other therapies for ICP control. In the normothermia group, SjO_2 decreased as the $PaCO_2$ values were reduced by hyperventilation. This effect could be a consequence of cerebrovascular constriction which reduces the cerebral circulation to below the level which meets the cerebral metabolic demand for oxygen. In contrast, such a decrease in SjO_2 was not clearly observed during the earlier post-traumatic period with hypothermia. Since CO_2 reactivity of the cerebral vasculature was obviously preserved during moderate hypothermia, absence of SjO_2 responses in the hypothermia group may suggest that a decrease in $PaCO_2$ during hypothermia has a lesser impact on the balance between the cerebral circulation and metabolic demand.

Evidence has been accumulated to suggest that cerebral metabolic demand increases during the early period after traumatic brain injury in rodents [4,7,12]. It has also been found that the cerebral circulation is relatively impaired as compared to the metabolic demand during the early period in patients with severe traumatic brain injury [3,10]. A decrease in $PaCO_2$ through hyperventilation may be hazardous under such circumstances, which can be manifested as a decrease in SjO_2 to the critical level. It is possible that hypothermia may attenuate the adverse effects of a decrease in $PaCO_2$, presumably through reducing the cerebral metabolic demand during the early period after traumatic brain injury. Future studies should clarify the detailed response characteristics of SjO_2 to changes in $PaCO_2$ during hypothermia.

An increase in ICP was observed in association with the termination of hypothermia in the present study. It appears that 48 hours of hypothermia may not be sufficiently long to counteract the acute post-traumatic pathological process which may continue for more than 72 hours. In experimental animals, toxicity arising from moderate hypothermia occurs as the duration of hypothermia is increased [11]. Future studies should also determine the optimal duration of hypothermia for the management of severe traumatic brain injury.

REFERENCES

1. Clifton GL, Allen S, Barrodale P, Plenger P, Berry J, Koch S, Fletcher J and Hayes RL (1993) A phase II study of moderate hypothermia in severe brain injury. J.Neurotrauma 10(3): 263-271
2. Clifton GL, Allen S, Berry J and Koch SM (1992) Systemic hypothermia in treatment of brain injury. J. Neurotrauma 9 suppl 2: 487-495.
3. Hirayama T, Kinoshita K, Katayama Y and Tsubokawa T (1993) Relative ischemic condition during ultraacute phase in patients with traumatic diffuse brain injury. Neurotraumatology (Tokyo), 16:93-99 (in Japanese).
4. Katayama Y, Becker DP, Tamura T and Hovda DA (1990) Massive increases in extracellular potassium and the indiscriminate release of glutamate following concussive brain injury. J. Neurosurg 73: 889-900.
5. Katayama Y, Hirayama T and Tsubokawa T (1993) Therapeutic hypothermia in patients with severe traumatic brain injury. Neurotraumatology (Tokyo) 16: 133 (in Japanese).
6. Katayama Y, Tsubokawa T, Hirayama T and Himi K (1994) Continuous monitoring of the jugular bulb oxygen saturation as a measure of the shunt flow of cerebral arteriovenous malformations. J. Neurosurg 80:826-833.
7. Kawamata T, Katayama Y, Hovda DA, Yoshino A and Becker DP (1992) Administration of excitatory amino acid antagonists via microdialysis attenuates the increase in glucose utilization seen following concussive brain injury. J. Cereb. Blood Flow Metab 12: 12-24.
8. Marmarou A, Anderson RL, Ward JD, Choi SC, Young HF, Eisenberg HM, Foulkes MA, Marshall LF and Jane JA (1991) NINDS traumatic coma data bank: Intracranial pressure monitoring methodlogy J. Neurosurg 75 suppl: 21.
9. Robertson CS, Grossman RG and Goodman JC (1987) The predictive value of cerebral anaerobic metabolism with cerebral infarction after head injury. J. Neurosurg 67:361-368.
10. Sheinberg M, Kanter MJ, Robertson CS, Contant CF, Narayan RK and Grossman RG (1992) Continuous monitoring of jugular venous oxygen saturation in head-injured patients. J.Neurosurg 76:212-217.
11. Steen PA, Soule EH and Michenfelder JD (1979) Detrimental effect of prolonged hypothermia in cat and monkeys with and without regional cerebral ischemia. Stroke 10: 522-529.
12. Yoshino A, Katayama Y, Kawamata T and Becker DP (1992) Hippocampal CA3 lesion prevents the post-concussive metabolic derangement in CA1. J. Cereb.Blood Flow Metab 12: 996-1006.

Session XII: Treatment for Abnormal ICP (2)

Chairmen: L. Symon and J. Yamashita

Experience with the Glutamate Antagonist CGS19755 in Severe Human Head Injury: Evidence for ICP Lowering Effect

R. BULLOCK[2], G.M. TEASDALE[1], A. KOTAKE[3], L. STEWART[1], and A. WAGSTAFF[1]

[1] Department of Neurosurgery and Neuroanesthesia, University of Glasgow, Scotland, UK
[2] Department of Neurosurgery, Medical College of Virginia, Richmond, VA, USA
[3] Ciba-Geigy, Summit, NJ, USA

INTRODUCTION:

Glutamate antagonists are currently the focus of intense interest as neuroprotective compounds for both severe head injury and stroke. This is because these compounds have shown a greater magnitude of neuroprotective efficacy in laboratory studies than any other agents so far tested.[1] This effect has been most consistently seen in models of focal ischemia (middle cerebral artery occlusion [2], but efficacy has also been seen in global ischemia models, and in trauma models such as fluid percussion injury [3] and subdural hematoma in the rat.[4]

Prolonged high level glutamate release has now been shown in human traumatic brain injury (TBI), particularly when focal injuries or raised intracranial pressure are present.[5] The competitive NMDA glutamate antagonist, CGS19755, has a high margin of efficacy in laboratory ischemia and TBI models, and it has been shown to be safe in humans. We have accordingly performed an open-label, dose escalation, safety and efficacy study with this compound in thirty-one patients with severe TBI, who were selected because of the need for intracranial pressure monitoring, based upon their CT scan appearances. In this paper, we report the effect of the compound upon hemodynamic parameters and ICP.

PATIENTS AND METHODS:

Over a 40 month period, we have selected 31 severe TBI patients for the study, based upon the following enrollment criteria:

1) Age between 16 and 65 years,
2) Glasgow Coma Score range between 4 and 9 (not obeying commands),
3) Stable hemodynamic status - MABP > 70 mmHg,
4) CT scan appearances of focal mass lesion or brain swelling,
5) At least one pupil reacting to light, and
6) Absence of major concomitant systemic injuries or pre-existing significant medical condition.
7) Recent rapid deterioration in neurologic status, with CT evidence of injury, (within 3 days of injury)

Administration of CGS19755:

The dose escalation regime used is shown in Table 1. The drug was given as two intravenous bolus doses twenty-four hours apart. CGS19755 was made up to 10ml in normal saline and administered via a peripheral vein.

TABLE 1
DOSE ESCALATION FOR CGS19755 IN SEVERE HEAD INJURY

Dose (mg/kg)	Number of Patients
1	2
1.5	2
2	5
3	8
4	3
5	5
6	6
	31

TABLE 2
CLINICAL FEATURES IN 31 SEVERELY HEAD INJURED PATIENTS TREATED WITH CGS19755

Mean age (range)	31yrs (16-65 yrs)
Sex	26 male
Admission GCS (range)	(4-12)
3-8	20 patients
9-12	10 patients
12-15	1 patient
Surgically evacuated hematomas/contusions	19
Diffuse brain swelling	12

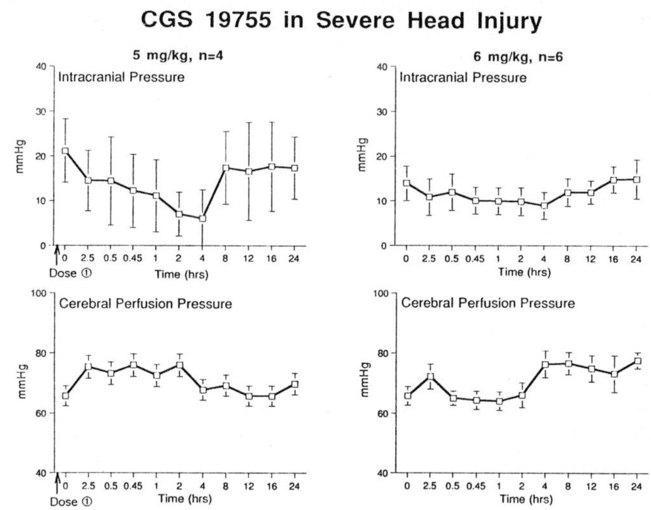

Figure 1: Effect of CGS 19755 at two doses, upon ICP and CPP

Monitoring:

In all patients, the following parameters were monitored for two hours prior to, and twenty-four hours after drug administration: Mean arterial blood pressure (MABP), ICP and cerebral perfusion pressure (CPP), jugular vein saturation ($SJVO_2$), middle cerebral artery Doppler velocity, and neurological status. Outcome was also measured at three and 6 months, using the Glasgow Outcome Scale.

RESULTS:

The characteristics of the thirty-one patients enrolled, are shown in Table 2. These were typical for severely head injured patients from our institution. However, patients with uncontrollable raised intracranial pressure (>30mm Hg) within 4 hours after admission, were excluded from this study.

Effect of CGS19755 on Hemodynamic Parameters and ICP:

CGS19755 had no effect on blood pressure or pulse rate, until the 6mg/kg dose level was reached. Mean arterial blood pressure become slightly lower after the 6mg/kg dose. (Figure 1) ICP did not change until the 3mg/kg dosing level was reached. At 3 and 5 mg/kg, ICP fell by 15 mmHg +/- after the first dose, and +/- 6 mmHg after the second dose, thus improving cerebral perfusion pressure. (Figure 1)

Effect on CBF and Global Cerebral Oxygen Uptake:

CGS19755 exerted no discernible effect upon middle cerebral artery Doppler velocity, $JVSatO_2$, or $AVDO_2$, at any of the dose levels administered.

Neurological Effects and Outcome:

Ventilator "weaning" was not influenced by therapy with the drug. Only one patient died, and 85 percent of the patients were in the top two outcome categories of the Glasgow Outcome Scale, by six months. Three patients recalled formed visual hallucinations when they were interviewed as outpatients. In all three, these were brief, transient and not unpleasant.

DISCUSSION:

Over one hundred stroke patients, and about sixty severely head injured patients have received CGS19755. In conscious stroke patients, the maximum tolerated dose was 1.5 mg/kg. In severely head injured patients, the dose at which physiologic effects were seen was 5 mg/kg.[6] This study has therefore shown that CGS19755 is well tolerated at putatively neuroprotective doses in human head injury patients. Hematological, biochemical, and hemodynamic monitoring failed to indicate any adverse events which were clearly drug related.

The most interesting indication of possible beneficial effect in this study however, comes from the ICP and CPP data. This compound appears to demonstrate an ICP lowering effect, which is achieved without jeopardizing mean arterial pressure, so that cerebral perfusion pressure was improved. We speculate that this beneficial effect may be achieved by stabilizing the ionic flux which occurs as a consequence of the effect of glutamate upon the effect of the NMDA-gated ion channel. This may result in reduced potassium uptake by astrocytes, and reduced calcium and sodium influx into neurons.

Further safety and efficacy studies are in progress to determine whether this ICP lowering effect is related to outcome. Definitive efficacy studies with this compound, are due to commence in Europe and the United States in the last quarter of 1994.

This preliminary evidence of favorable effect upon ICP in humans with TBI, taken together with the broad spectrum of laboratory "neuroprotection" achieved by this compound, and others in this category, lead us to conclude that NMDA antagonists may be ideal neuroprotective drugs for use in severe human head injury.

REFERENCES

1. McCulloch J, Bullock R, Teasdale GM (1991) Excitatory amino acid antagonists: opportunities for the treatment of ischemic brain damage, in Excitatory Amino Acid Antagonists. B Meldrum (Ed), Blackwell Scientific: Oxford, p 287-326.

2. Ozyust E, Graham DI, Woodruff GN, McCulloch J (1988): Protective effect of the glutamate antagonist MK801 in focal cerebral ischemia in the cat. J Cereb Blood Flow Metab 8:138-143.

3. Hayes RL, Jenkins LW, Lyeth BG (1992): Neurotransmitter mediated mechanisms of traumatic brain injury: acetylcholine and excitatory amino acids. J Neurotrauma 9:173-187.

4. Chen MH, Bullock R, Graham DI, Miller JD., McCulloch J (1991): Ischemic neuronal damage after acute subdural hematoma in the rat: effects of pretreatment with a glutamate antagonist. J Neurosurg 74:944-950.

5. Bullock R, Stout A., Woodward JJ, Tsuji O, Marmarou A, Young HF (1994): Excitatory amino acid release in severe human head trauma: the role of intracranial pressure and cerebral perfusion pressure changes, in Proceedings of the Ninth International Symposium on ICP and It's Related Problems. H Nagai, et al (Eds) (this volume)

6. Grotta J and the CGS19755 Stroke Trial Group (1994): Safety and tolerability of the glutamate antagonist CGS19755 in acute stroke patients. Stroke 25(1):12.

Role of Hypotensive Agents in the Treatment of Post Traumatic Brain Oedema

BOGI ASGEIRSSON[1,2], PER-OLOF GRÄNDE[1,2], and CARL-HENRIK NORDSTRÖM[3]

Departments of [1] Anaesthesiology, [2] Physiology and Biophysics, and [3] Neurosurgery, University and University Hospital of Lund, Sweden

INTRODUCTION

During the traditional treatment of post traumatic brain oedema, cerebral perfusion pressure (CPP) is normally kept at a relatively high level (>70-80mmHg) and, if necessary, with the aid of inotropic support [1,2]. The alternative, that high levels of CPP should be avoided as they may increase the vasogenic oedema due to transcapillary filtration has been discussed in the literature [3,4]. This however is rejected in the traditional clinical practise as ischaemia is supposed to be the main triggering mechanism behind the post traumatic brain oedema and the severity of the outcome. Still, there may be an optimal CPP for each patient; too low CPP may be deleterious by inducing ischaemia, and too high CPP by increasing intracranial pressure (ICP) through transcapillary filtration. Transcapillary filtration, caused by increase in hydrostatic capillary pressure, presupposes that the normally semi-permeable blood-brain barrier is open for solutes, as also shown to be the case after head injury [5].

Based on the assumption that the optimal CPP level in fact may be lower than normally recommended, hypotensive therapy could be a useful tool to drain the interstitial space through lowering of hydrostatic capillary pressure, thereby reducing the ICP. This approach in fact has been part of our therapy of post traumatic brain oedema during the last few years in the most severely head injured patients (GCS<8) with a persistent raised ICP above 20-25 mmHg [6]. The hypotensive drugs used for this purpose are the β_1-antagonist metoprolol at an initial max dose of 0.3mg/kg/24h i.v. and the α_2-agonist clonidine at an initial max dose of 1µg/kgx8 i.v., both normal therapeutical doses for these drugs. These types of drugs are used as they should have less direct influence on cerebral vasculature than other hypotensive agents, most of which causing dilation of the cerebral vessels. Though still not proven in a specific study, according to our experience, this therapy alone causes a slow reduction of an increased ICP. In combination with dihydroergotamine, a drug introduced into brain oedema therapy by us in 1989 [7], hypotensive treatment decreased arterial pressure and ICP simultaneously, causing no significant change in CPP as shown in a previous study [6]. The hypotensive drugs also may be beneficial by protecting against the massive sympathetic and catecholamine outflow known to occur after a head injury [8,9].

In a first study, an attempt was made to verify that a decrease in arterial pressure reduces and an increase in arterial pressure increases the volume of a tissue that is characterised by an increased tissue pressure, impaired autoregulation and capillaries permeable for solutes, features compatible with the traumatised brain. In a second study on severely head injured patients, an attempt is made to analyse whether there are any direct local cerebral vascular effects of clonidine and metoprolol which might influence ICP, besides the postulated hypotensive effect.

MATERIAL AND METHODS

Experimental study

Six cats, anaesthetised with α-chloralose and urethane and mechanically ventilated, were used. The observations were made on the sympathectomised lower leg muscles of the right hind limb. The preparation, with intact vascular supply, was hermetically enclosed in a temperature controlled plethysmograph filled with isotonic Ringer-Acetate solution. The muscle preparation was perfused from the animal via a pressure controlled roller pump and venous blood was returned to the animal via a tubing open to atmosphere, and with the opening placed above a funnel connected to one of the external jugular veins. Arterial inflow pressure could be varied with the roller pump. The plethysmographic (tissue) pressure could be increased by vertical elevation of a water filled reservoir in fluid communication with the plethysmograph. Changes in tissue volume (ΔVol) were recorded as variations in the weight of the reservoir. Pressure from venous micro vessels was recorded by cannulation of the sural vein in retrograde flow direction, a pressure previously shown to represent the venous hydrostatic capillary pressure (P_c) [10]. Blood flow to the muscle (Q) was continuously measured with a flow meter in the arterial shunt.

Clinical study

Fifteen patients with severe traumatic brain injuries were studied. They were all deeply comatose (GCS score <8) and on ventilatory support. Prior to the study 10 of the patients were operated for space occupying lesions. ICP was measured via an intraventricular catheter and arterial pressure via an indwelling catheter in the radial artery. Zero pressure baseline for both ICP and arterial pressure measurements was set at the forehead level. Oxygen saturation in the jugular venous bulb was measured for calculation of the arterio-venous difference in oxygen content ($AVDO_2$) in 13 of the patients. Mean hemispheric cerebral blood flow (CBF) was measured after injection of 0.5GBq ^{133}Xenon into a cubital vein, followed by a rapid injection of 20 ml sterile saline. The ^{133}Xenon clearance was recorded by the Novo Cerebrograph 10a, using 2 extra cranial scintillation detectors, one over each hemisphere and one air detector reading from the patients expired air. The CBF was calculated as the initial slope index (ISI). Steady state CBF was measured before and 10 minutes after an intravenous bolus dose of clonidine of 1μg/kg (6 patients) and of metoprolol of 0.1 mg/kg (9 patients) respectively.

Statistics

Values in the figure and in the table are presented as mean ± standard error of the mean (SE). In the experimental study (figure), values at mean arterial pressure of 75 and 115 mmHg were compared to values at the control state of 95 mmHg and the differences tested with t-test for Dependent Samples. In the clinical study (table), values after administration of the drugs were compared to values before drug administration and the differences were tested with Wilcoxon Matched Pairs Test. Differences were considered statistically significant when $p<0.05$.

RESULTS

Experimental study

The figure shows hydrostatic capillary pressure (P_c), tissue volume variations (ΔVol), and blood flow (Q) during a raised tissue pressure of 20mmHg and a venous outflow pressure of 5mmHg, at an arterial inflow pressure of 95mmHg, and after an increase of arterial pressure to 115mmHg and a decrease to 75mmHg. At the arterial pressure of 95mmHg the volume curve showed an almost isovolumetric state. An increase in arterial pressure led to an increase in P_c, ΔVol and Q, whereas a decrease in arterial pressure led to a decrease in P_c, ΔVol, and Q.

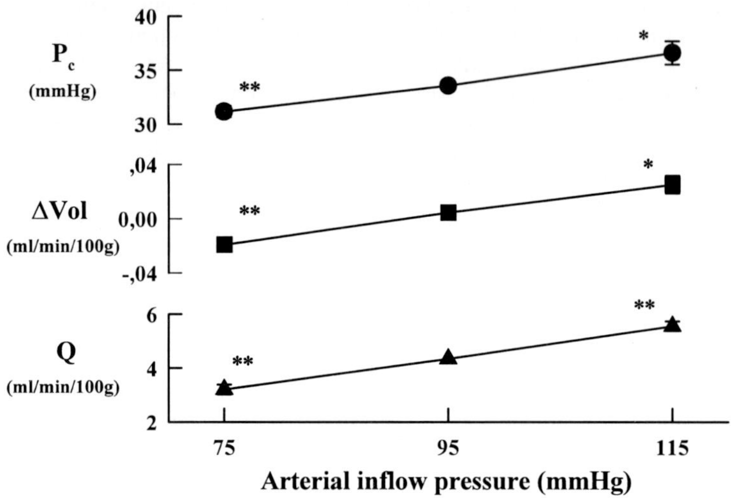

Clinical study

The clinical results are summarised in the table. A bolus dose of clonidine caused a significant decrease in mean arterial pressure (MAP) and a decrease in cerebrovascular resistance (CVR). No significant changes of heart rate, ICP, CBF or $AVDO_2$ were observed. A bolus dose of metoprolol caused a significant decrease in heart rate and MAP, while ICP, CBF, CVR and $AVDO_2$ were unchanged.

Table: Effects of bolus doses of clonidine and metoprolol on systemic and cerebral haemodynamics. Values are mean±SE.

	Clonidine group				Metoprolol group			
	n	Control	Drug	p value	n	Control	Drug	p value
HR	6	74±5	74±4	ns	9	95±7	85±6	<0.01
MAP	6	96±7	87±6	<0.05	9	100±4	94±4	<0.05
ICP	6	24±5	22±5	ns	8	16±2	16±2	ns
CPP	6	72±5	64±2	<0.05	8	85±6	79±6	<0.05
CBF	6	36±6	37±5	ns	9	35±3	35±3	ns
CVR	6	2.2±0.4	2.0±0.3	<0.05	8	2.3±0.2	2.2±0.2	ns
$AVDO_2$	6	3.8±0.9	3.8±0.8	ns	7	4.0±0.9	4.3±1.0	ns

DISCUSSION

As the importance of maintaining a high CPP in order to avoid secondary ischaemic damages to he injured brain is stressed quite extensively in the traditional therapy of a post traumatic brain oedema [1,2], hypotensive therapy is not commonly used in these patients and must be considered controversial. Still hypotensive therapy has been tentatively discussed in the literature for the purpose of decreasing vasogenic oedema [4]. β-blockade is discussed also to protect the heart from adverse effects of the massive catecholamine outflow related to a head injury [8]. Clonidine may also be beneficial in this respect by decreasing the sympathetic outflow from the brain [9].

Increased permeability of the normally semi permeable blood-brain barrier means that not only water, but also solutes more or less freely pass across the capillary membrane. This upsets the normal volume regulating mechanisms of the brain, and instead of depending on the crystalloid osmotic pressure gradient across the capillary membrane [11], fluid transport now becomes dependent on the normally much smaller colloid osmotic and hydrostatic pressure gradients. With impaired autoregulation of cerebral blood flow and hydrostatic pressure [12], increase in arterial blood pressure increases not only the CBF but also the capillary hydrostatic pressure, resulting in increased fluid transport across the capillary membrane into the interstitial space, thereby increasing the interstitial oedema formation. Impaired autoregulation of hydrostatic pressure also implies, that even at normal arterial blood pressure, higher pressures are transmitted into the apillaries, because of the impaired activity of the myogenic control system in the precapillary esistance vessels.

Our experimental study clearly shows, that in a tissue with raised tissue pressure, with impaired utoregulation, and with capillaries permeable for solutes, a decrease in arterial pressure ecreases hydrostatic capillary pressure causing fluid absorption and an increase in arterial ressure increases hydrostatic capillary pressure causing fluid filtration in relation to an isovolumetric state in the control. Simultaneously, there will be a decrease and increase espectively in blood flow. Providing these results can be transferred to the injured brain with npaired autoregulation and capillaries permeable for solutes [5,12] it is apparent that, apart from beneficial tissue volume decreasing effect, hypotensive therapy includes a potential risk of nducing ischaemia in areas with marginal blood supply. Thus, it seems that there may be an optimal arterial pressure level (optimal CPP) as mentioned in Introduction, above which the adverse effects of increasing ICP will influence outcome negatively while below this level the schaemic adverse effects will be predominating for outcome. In our therapeutical regimen to educe an increased ICP due to a post traumatic brain oedema, we have assumed that in most atients arterial pressure, which often is raised, can be decreased without CPP passing below the optimal level. The normal $AVDO_2$ values obtained in this clinical study after the hypotensive eatment and our clinical outcome from a previous study [6] seem to support this assumption. This hypotensive therapy in combination with the vasoconstrictor substance dihydroergotamine, however, by no means needs to imply a decrease in CPP due to the simultaneous decrease in ICP s also shown previously [6]. The vasoconstrictor effect of dihydroergotamine in this respect eems to have other beneficial features than hyperventilation as discussed previously [13].

ased on these considerations, this study also analyses whether β_1-blockade and α_2-stimulation xert any direct local cerebral circulatory effects which may explain a possible ICP reduction by these drugs. This was done by analysing the effects of bolus doses of the drug 10 minutes after its dministration, a time long enough for stabilisation of the circulatory parameters on a steady state vel. Our results show that no cerebral hemodynamic effects were observed either for metoprolol r for clonidine, except a tendency of decrease in CVR for clonidine. Most likely this CVR decrease is simply due to vasodilatation secondary to the lowered blood pressure as autoregulation is not completely abolished. Also, a metabolic influence of these drugs must be small as no significant change in $AVDO_2$ was observed.

Therefore we conclude that if these hypotensive drugs do contribute to reduce a raised ICP after a head trauma as tentatively observed, these experimental and clinical results support the view that the ICP reduction is due to the blood pressure decrease per se rather than to any direct local interference with cerebral circulation.

REFERENCES

1. Rosner MJ, Daughton S (1990) Cerebral perfusion pressure management in head injury. J Trauma 30: 933-941
2. Chan KH, Miller JD, Dearden NM, Andrews PJD, Midgley S (1992) The effects of changes in cerebral perfusion pressure upon middle cerebral artery blood flow velocity and jugular bulb venous oxygen saturation after severe brain injury. J Neurosurg 77:55-61
3. Durward QJ, Del Maestro RF, Amacher AL, Farrar JK (1983) The influence of systemic arterial pressure and intracranial pressure on the development of cerebral vasogenic edema. J Neurosurg 59:803-809
4. Simard JM, Bellefleur M (1989) Systemic arterial hypertension in head trauma. Am J Cardiol 63:32C-35C
5. Todd NV, Graham DI (1990) Blood-brain barrier damage in traumatic brain contusions. Acta Neurochir Suppl 51:296-299.
6. Asgeirsson B, Grände PO, Nordström CH (1994) A new therapy of post-trauma brain oedema based on heamodynamic principles for brain volume regulation. Intensive Care Med 20:260-267
7. Grände PO (1989) The effect of dihydroergotamine in patients with head injury and raised intracranial pressure. Intensive Care Med 15:523-527
8. Cruickshank JM; Neil-Dwyer G, Degaute JP, Hayes Y, Kuurne T, Kytta J, Vincent JL, Carruthers ME, Patel S (1987) Reduction of stress/catecholamine-induced cardiac necrosis by beta1-selective blockade. Lancet ii:585-589
9. Payen D, Quintin L, Plaisence P, Chiron B, Lhoste F (1990) Head injury: clonidine decreases plasma catecholamines. Crit Care Med 18:392-395
10. Björnberg J, Grände PO, Maspers M, Mellander S (1988) Site of autoregulatory reactions in the vascular bed of cat skeletal muscle as determined with a new technique for segmental vascular resistance recordings. Acta Physiol Scand 102:224-230
11. Fenstermacher JD (1984) Volume regulation of the central nervous system. In: Staub NC, Taylor AE (eds) Edema. Raven Press, New York, pp 383-404
12. Muizelaar JP, Ward JD, Marmarou A, Newlon PG, Wachi A (1989) Cerebral blood flow and metabolism in severely head-injured children. Part 2: Autoregulation. J Neurosurg 71:72-76
13. Asgeirsson B, Berntman L, Grände PO, Messeter K, Nordström CH, Ryding E, Sjöholm H (1991) Role of dihydroergotamine in the treatment of raised intracranial pressure after severe head injury Eighth International Symposium on Intracranial Pressure, Rotterdam, the Netherlands, Abstract 173

ACKNOWLEDGEMENTS

This study was supported by grants from the Swedish Medical Research Council (2210) and from the Faculty of Medicine, University of Lund, Sweden.

Cerebrovascular Effects of Dihydroergotamine

SHANKAR P. GOPINATH, CLAUDIA S. ROBERTSON, RAJ K. NARAYAN, and ROBERT G. GROSSMAN

Department of Neurosurgery, Baylor College of Medicine, One Baylor Plaza, Houston, TX 77030, USA

INTRODUCTION

Increased intracranial pressure (ICP) is detrimental to the outcome of the patients with severe head injuries. Significant improvements in both mortality rate and in neurological recovery in survivors, have been achieved with monitoring ICP and treatment of intracranial hypertension.[1,2] Drugs that have been used clinically either regularly or on an experimental basis to control ICP include mannitol, furosemide, tris-hydroxy-methyl-aminomethane (THAM), or barbiturates. All of these measures have been tried and tested; all have advantages and disadvantages, and no single measure is ideal, giving an opportunity to add new drugs.

Cerebral venous capacitance vessels hold greater blood volume than the resistance vessels,[3] and hence constriction of these venous capacitance vessels should reduce an increased ICP. Based on this assumption, a recent study has suggested that dihydroergotamine (DHE) may be effective in lowering ICP,[4] but did not address the effect on cerebral blood flow. The knowledge of cerebral hemodynamics after DHE is sparse especially in the injured brain with areas of altered blood-brain barrier, and ineffective autoregulation.

The purpose of this study was to evaluate the cerebrovascular effects of DHE in head injured patients with intracranial hypertension.

MATERIAL AND METHODS

Eight adult head injured patients admitted to the neurosurgical ICU with a Glasgow Coma Scale (GCS) score of ≤ 8, and an ICP greater than 20 mm Hg for more than 15 minutes despite sedation with morphine and controlled ventilation ($pO_2 > 100$ mmHg, pCO_2 30-35 mmHg) were studied after obtaining consent from the relatives. Patients with a systolic blood pressure greater than 180 mmHg, an ICP greater than 40 mm Hg, or a surgical condition as the cause of the elevated ICP were excluded. No dose of mannitol was given 2 hours prior to the administration of DHE.

ICP (measured through an intraventricular catheter), mean arterial pressure (MAP), cerebral perfusion pressure (CPP), heart rate (HR), cerebral blood flow (CBF - Kety-Schmidt technique), cerebrovascular resistance (CVR), and continuous jugular venous oxygen saturation ($SjvO_2$) using a fiberoptic catheter were measured immediately before and 30 minutes after an intravenous bolus administration of 0.25mg-0.50mg DHE. Three patients received two doses of 0.25 mg DHE , the second dose was given about 10 minutes after the first one. The changes in the physiological variables with DHE administration were compared by paired t-test.

RESULTS

Typical changes in cerebrovascular variables are shown in fig. 1 and 2.

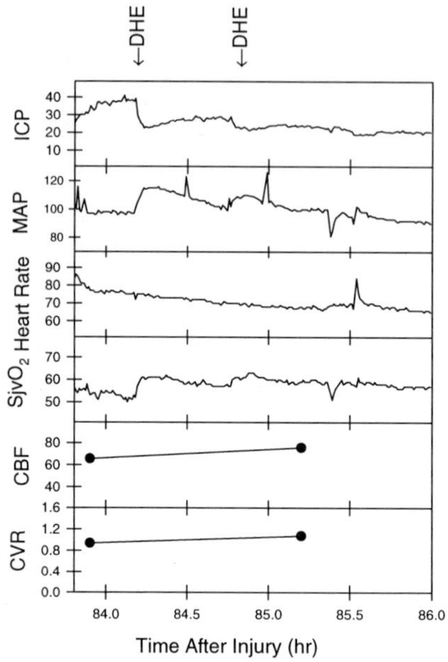

Fig. 1. This patient had a decrease in ICP that was accompanied by an increase in MAP, CBF, CVR, and $SjvO_2$. The reduction in ICP lasted 3 hours.

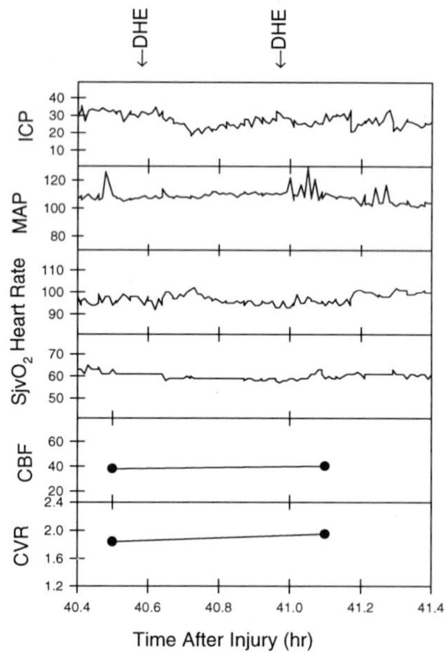

Fig. 2. This patient had a transient decrease in ICP and increase in CVR with no change in MAP, CBF, or $SjvO_2$. The reduction in ICP lasted ~30 minutes.

The mean values of the physiological variables pre- and post-treatment are shown in fig. 3. The changes in ICP after a dose of 0.25 mg DHE was observed within 30-60 seconds. The ICP consistently decreased in all patients after administration of DHE. The mean ICP decreased by an average of 12 mm Hg. This effect lasted for 30-45 minutes in 5 patients, 90 minutes in 2 , and 180 minutes in one. In the three patients who required second dose of DHE, the ICP initially came down to 20mm Hg after the initial dose, but started to rise within next 10 minutes, although it did not reach the baseline high value. Mean arterial pressure increased simultaneously in all patients by an average of 7 mm Hg , while the cerebral perfusion pressure increased by an average of 19 mm Hg. (Table 1). Heart rate and pCO_2 remained unchanged.

There was no significant changes observed in cerebral blood flow, jugular venous oxygen saturation, and arteriovenous oxygen difference after DHE administration. However, there was a significant increase in cerebrovascular resistance by an average of 0.35 ± 0.19 mm Hg/ml/100gm/min, after the administration of DHE.

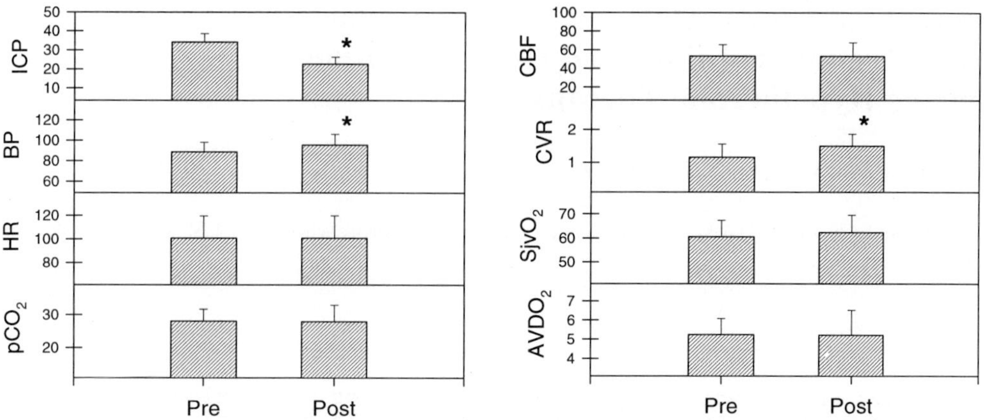

Fig. 3. ICP was significantly decreased, and mean BP and CVR were significantly increased by DHE.

DISCUSSION

Dihydroergotamine is a venoconstrictor but also induces vasoconstriction in resistance vessels,[5] and has been shown to have little effect on cerebral blood flow in healthy people.[6] In the present study none of the patients had either low or high cerebral blood flow, and the blood flow did not change after the last dose of DHE. Similarly, CBF/$CMRO_2$ ratio was not modified as the arteriovenous oxygen difference remain unchanged.

The effects of dihydroergotamine, at least in the doses given in this study, were transient in most of the patients, although a fairly long lasting effect was observed in three patients. Unlike hyperventilation or barbiturates, which also reduce ICP by decreasing cerebral blood volume, dihydroergotamine reduces ICP without decreasing CBF. The decrease in ICP is probably due to the constriction of venous capacitance vessels which hold a greater blood volume than the arterial resistance vessels. The absence of effect on cerebral metabolism and cerebral blood flow, coupled with an increase in cerebrovascular resistance following the administration of DHE, probably signifies its direct constrictive effect on the vessels as the mechanism of reduction of intracranial pressure.

References:

1. Miller JD, Sweet RC, Narayan R, Becker DP (1978) Early insults to the injured brain. JAMA 240:439-442
2. Narayan RK, Kishore PRS, Becker DP (1982) Intracranial pressure: to monitor or not to monitor? A review of our experience with severe head injury. J Neurosurg 56:650-659
3. Mellander S, Johansson B (1968) Control of resistance, exchange and capacitance functions in the peripheral circulation. Pharmacol Rev 20:117-196
4. Grande PO (1989) The effects of dihydroergotamine in patients with head injury and raised intracranial pressure. Int Care Med 15:523-527
5. Mellander S, Nordenfelt I (1970) Comparative effects of dihydroergotamine and noradrenaline on resistance, exchange and capacitance functions in the peripheral circulation. Clin Sci 39:183-201
6. Anderson AR, Refelt-Hansen P, Lassen NA (1987) The effect of ergotamine and dihydroergotamine on cerebral blood flow in man. Stroke 18:120-123

Increase of Cu,Zn-SOD mRNA Expression After Traumatic Injury and Its Preservation During Hypothermic Therapy

T. Fukuhara, Y. Ono, S. Nishio, M. Kawauchi, S. Asari, and T. Ohmoto

Department of Neurological Surgery, Okayama University Medical School, 2-5-1 Shikata-cho, Okayama, 700 Japan

SUMMARY

To analyze the effect of hypothermic therapy on superoxide accumulation after traumatic injury, the expression of Cu,Zn-superoxide dismutase (SOD) mRNA was examined after contusion in rats using Northern blotting. As determined by specific gravity, hypothermic therapy decreased brain edema. The expression of Cu,Zn-SOD mRNA increased at the periphery of the contusion, which may indicate the severity of superoxide injury. This increase was also observed after contusion under hypothermic therapy, which may show that superoxide injury is still severe and the cell's ability to react against the superoxide injury is preserved.

INTRODUCTION

An increase in expression of Cu,Zn-SOD mRNA after reperfusion injury to the brain has been reported [1], and this increase may indicate a protective mechanism against free radical injury. We investigated this expression after traumatic injury, in which the effects of free radicals have also been proved [2]. We also examined the effect of hypothermic therapy on this mRNA expression.

MATERIALS AND METHODS

Thirty SD rats (male, weighing 250-320 g) were divided into 4 groups. In the first group, a traumatic insult was created by dropping a 20 g weight from the height of 30 cm onto a piston resting on the dura of the right parietal portion [3] (Trauma group, n=8). The same insult was carried out under moderate hypothermia in the second group (Hypothermia-Trauma group, n=8). The third group underwent a sham operation in which a burr hole was made in the right parietal portion (Control group, n=8), and the fourth group underwent a sham operation under hypothermia (Hypothermia group, n=6). Six hours after each operation, each rat was decapitated and the cortex was dissected from the core (injured portion, bregma+2~-2), the periphery (posterior to the injury in the same hemisphere, bregma-2~-6) and the distal portion (contralateral hemisphere, bregma-2~-6). The water content of each portion of the cortex was measured using specific gravity method [4]. The expression of Cu,Zn-SOD mRNA of the cortex was analyzed using Northern blotting, according to the single-step method of Chomczynski [5]. The integrity of RNA preparations and the consistency of sample loading were verified with the loading of 5 μg total RNA by staining with ethidium bromide. The probe used for hybridization was 48-mer synthetic oligonucleotide of rat Cu,Zn-SOD cDNA (base 465-512) [6]. After the membranes were hybridized, they were subjected to autoradiography, and the signals of Cu,Zn-SOD mRNA were quantified with densitometric analysis and compared with that of the standard sample loaded on every membrane. Values were expressed as the mean ± standard deviation. All comparisons were performed using analysis of variance (ANOVA) with Scheffe's F test. The results were considered statistically significant if the probability value (p) was < 0.05.

RESULTS

The results of the specific gravity measurements are shown in Table 1. Between the three portions, the specific gravity was small in the core of the Trauma group (core versus periphery; $F=27.3$, $p<0.0001$, core versus distal; $F=107.0$, $p<0.0001$) and in the periphery compared with the distal portion ($F=26.2$, $p<0.0001$). This tendency was also observed in the Hypothermia-Trauma group (core versus periphery; $F=11.9$, $p<0.001$, core versus distal; $F=33.4$, $p<0.0001$ and periphery versus distal; $F=5.4$, $p<0.05$), but the Trauma group had a smaller specific gravity than the Hypothermia-Trauma group in the core ($F=6.4$, $p<0.01$) and in the periphery ($F=3.5$, $p<0.05$). These results indicate that hypothermia decreased the degree of brain edema. Compared with the groups undergoing sham operations, a significant difference was found in the Trauma group in the core ($F=35.1$, $p<0.0001$) and in the periphery ($F=7.9$, $p<0.001$), but a difference was found only in the core of the Hypothermia-Trauma group ($F=10.9$, $p<0.0001$).

Table 1. Specific gravity of rat cortex from each group

Section	Control Group	Trauma Group	Hypothermia Group	Hypothermia-Trauma Group
Core	1.045 ± 0.01	1.035 ± 0.01	1.046 ± 0.02	1.039 ± 0.03
Periphery	1.045 ± 0.01	1.041 ± 0.02	1.045 ± 0.02	1.043 ± 0.02
Distal	1.044 ± 0.01	1.046 ± 0.02	1.045 ± 0.02	1.046 ± 0.01

*; $p<0.05$, **; $p<0.01$, #; $p<0.001$, ##; $p<0.0001$.

The Cu,Zn-SOD mRNA expression is summarized in Table 2. In the peripheral sections of the Trauma and Hypothermia-Trauma groups, the expression increased significantly compared with the core (Trauma; $F=4.1$, $p<0.05$, Hypothermia-Trauma; $F=5.0$, $p<0.05$). When compared with each group undergoing sham operations, the expression in the periphery also increased (Control versus Trauma; $F=4.3$, $p<0.05$, Hypothermia versus Hypothermia-Trauma; $F=3.5$, $p<0.05$). Between the Trauma and Hypothermia-Trauma groups, no significant difference was found.

DISCUSSION

Our results are consistent with earlier reports that hypothermia reduces brain edema [7,8]. But hypothermia is known to depress the metabolism of cells [9] and to decrease some gene expressions [10]. These aspects of hypothermia could have a negative effect on the treatment of injury if the protective mechanism is reduced. Our results indicate that the protective gene expression against free radical injury is preserved during hypothermia, which may support the beneficial aspect of hypothermic therapy. But whether the increase of Cu,Zn-SOD mRNA leads to an actual increase of superoxide scavenging

Table 2. The expression of Cu,Zn-SOD mRNA in each group

Section	Control Group	Trauma Group	Hypothermia Group	Hypothermia-Trauma Group
Core	1.092 ± 0.183	1.045 ± 0.180	0.968 ± 0.144	0.989 ± 0.190
Peripheral	0.97 ± 0.165	1.347 ± 0.299	1.063 ± 0.085	1.431 ± 0.208
Distal	1.004 ± 0.231	1.068 ± 0.225	1.175 ± 0.187	1.071 ± 0.200

*; $p<0.05$.

activity is still uncertain. In ischemic injury, this increase did not lead to the synthesis of SOD [1]. In an earlier report using a modified microdialysis technique [11], we also failed to find an actual increase of superoxide scavenging activity in ischemic injury [12]. This increase in expression can be seen as an indicator of the severity of superoxide injury because superoxide is believed to stimulate the expression of SOD mRNA [13]. Indeed, hypothermia may reduce brain edema, but the decrease of free radical injury may not be the major mechanism. These two speculations -- that the synthesis of SOD is not so dominant even if the mRNA expression increases, and that free radical injury may be still severe under hypothermia -- perhaps justify using hypothermia to increase the scavenging of superoxide.

REFERENCES

1. Matsuyama T, Michishita H, Nakamura H, Tsuchiyama M, Shimizu S, Watanabe K, Sugita M (1993) Induction of copper-zinc superoxide dismutase in gerbil hippocampus after ischemia. J Cereb Blood Flow Metab 13: 135-144
2. Chan PH, Longar S, Fishman RA (1987) Protective effects of liposome-entrapped superoxide dismutase on posttraumatic brain edema. Ann Neurol 21: 540-547
3. Feeney DM, Boyeson MG, Linn RT, Murray HM, Dail WG (1981) Responses to cortical injury: I. Methodology and local effects of contusions in the rat. Brain Res 211: 67-77
4. Marmarou A, Poll W, Shulman K, Bhagavan H (1978) A simple gravimetric technique for measurement of cerebral edema. J Neurosurg 49: 530-537
5. Chomczynski P, Sacchi N (1987) Single-step method of RNA isolation by acid guanidinium thiocyanate-phenol-chloroform extraction. Anal Biochem 162: 156-159
6. Delabar J-M, Nicole A, D'Auriol L, Jacob Y, Meunier-Rotival M, Galibert F, Sinet P-M, Jerome H (1987) Cloning and sequencing of a rat CuZn superoxide dismutase cDNA. Correlation between CuZn superoxide dismutase mRNA level and enzyme activity in rat and mouse tissue. Eur J Biochem 166: 181-187
7. Clifton GL, Jiang JY, Lyeth BG, Jenkins LW, Hamm RJ, Hayes RL (1991) Marked protection by moderate hypothermia after experimental traumatic brain injury. J Cereb Blood Flow Metab 11: 114-121
8. Jiang JY, Lyeth BG, Kapasi MZ, Jenkins LW, Povlishock JT (1992) Moderate hypothermia reduces blood-brain barrier disruption following traumatic brain injury in the rat. Acta Neuropathol Berl 84: 495-500

9. Frizzell RT, Fichtel FM, Jordan MB, Weprin BE, Borchers DJ, Allen EC, Pogue WR, Batjer HH (1993) Effects of etomidate and hypothermia on cerebral metabolism and blood flow in a canine model of hypoperfusion. J Neurosurg Anesthesiol 5: 104-110
10. Chopp M, Li Y, Dereski MO, Levine SR, Yoshida Y, Garcia JH (1992) Hypothermia reduces 72-kDa heat-shock protein induction in rat brain after transient forebrain ischemia. Stroke 23: 104-107
11. Fukuhara T, Gotoh M, Kawauchi M, Asari S, Ohmoto T (1994) Superoxide scavenging activity in vitro and in the cerebral extracellular space measured by microdialysis. J Neurosci Methods, in press
12. Fukuhara T, Gotoh M, Kawauchi M, Asari S, Ohmoto T (1994) Endogenous superoxide dismutase activity in reperfusion injuries. Acta Neurochir (Wien) (Suppl.)60: 250-252
13. Uyama O, Matsuyama T, Michishita H, Nakamura H, Sugita M (1992) Protective effects of human recombinant superoxide dismutase on transient ischemic injury of CA1 neurons in gerbils. Stroke 23: 75-81

Importance and Treatment of Post Ischemic Hypoperfusion Following Removal of Acute Traumatic Intracranial Hematoma

AKIHIKO YABUKI[1], YASUYUKI UEKI[1], TOKIWA SAKAKIBARA[1], and KIYOSHI SATO[2]

[1] Department of Neurosurgery, Tokyo Metropolitan Hiroo Hospital, Tokyo, Japan
[2] Department of Neurosurgery, Juntendo University School of Medicine, Tokyo, Japan

(INTRODUCTION)

Ischemia due to brain compression by the intracranial hematoma is very closely related to the outcome. While the brain compression prior to the surgery being the most influencing factor, we have been focusing on the importance of secondary ischemia due to delayed hypoperfusion immediately following the craniotomy. The type of ischemia which we consider to be occurring by same mechanism as in arterial occlusion and reperfusion.

In this study, we attempt to seek the presence and frequency of delayed hypoperfusion in 30 clinical cases, following the removal of the intracranial hematoma. In addition, the effect of the treatment especially aimed to treat the delayed hypoperfusion, will be accessed in comparison with the conventional treatment aimed merely to reduce the intracranial pressure.

(MATERIAL AND METHOD)

Cases been studied: The study was performed on the patients whose Glasgow Coma Scale was less than 8 points, defined as severe head injury. Only cases below 70 years old were included. All of these patients showed sizable intracranial hematoma on the preoperative CT scan with considerable brain compression. Main cause of their consciousness disturbance were brain compression by the clot. No case of diffuse injuries were included.

Craniotomy and removal of the intracranial hematoma was performed in all cases. Considerable decompression was achieved at the end of surgery, and ICP remained under 20 mmHg for at least 24 hours. Cases with unsuccessful decompression resulting in acute brain swelling were excluded because we considered that delayed hypoperfusion cannot be accessed under the influence of markedly reduced cerebral perfusion pressure.

Monitoring: Continuous monitoring of all parameters were started in the intensive care unit within 2hours of surgery. Intracranial pressure (ICP) was measured as the tissue pressure in all cases by Camino transducer. Systemic blood pressure (ABP) was recorded from the arterial line. Cerebral perfusion pressure (CPP) was calculated as the difference of mean arterial pressure and mean ICP. PaO_2 and $PaCO_2$ were either directly measured by blood sampling, or indirectly by pulsoxymetry and endotidal capnometry.

Treatment: The patients were divided into two groups with 15 cases in each. Group 1, was managed by the conventional treatment. They were ventilated with muscle paralysis with $PaCO_2$ between 35 to 40 mmHg. If ICP exceeded 20 mmHg for more than 5 min. hyperosmotic agents were given. If this failed to reduce ICP, then barbiturates were given to maintain burst and suppression pattern on the EEG. On the other hand, patients in Group were treated as follows. Under controlled ventilation as in group1, continuous ventricular drainage was performed at pressure of 10 mmHg. If SjO_2 was lower than 60 mmHg barbiturates was started to maintain burst and suppression pattern on the EEG. Also hyperosmotic agents were given in large doses, such as 900ml of glycerol and 900ml of mannitol per day. If hypotension co-existed with low SjO_2, blood pressure was corrected a quick as possible, and if the SjO_2 was still low with stabilized blood pressure, barbiturate as well as the hyperosmotic agents were started in the manner mentioned above.

	Group 1	Group 2
No. of Cases	15	15
Age	51.5±13.9	47.5±13.6
GCS prior to Surgery	6.84±1.6	6.19±1.7
Presence of SDH and/or ICH	12/15(80%)	12/15(80%)
Isolated EDH	3/15(20%)	3/15(20%)
Barbiturate Therapy	7/15(46.7%)	12/15(80%)
Surgical Decompression to Barbiturate Therapy (hrs)	20±15.4	4.71±2.14
Continuous Ventricular Drainage	0(0%)	10/12(73.3%)

Table 1. Comparison of two groups of patients.

(RESULT)

Table 1 shows the intergroup comparison of patient background and treatment. Age and GCS prior to the surgery were identical in both groups. The nature of the intracranial lesions which may influence the outcome, such as incidence of subdural hematoma and/or traumatic intracerebral hematoma and uncomplicated extradural hematoma was also same in both groups.

Barbiturates were administered in 80% of cases in group2 and 46.7% in group 1. Also, timing of starting barbiturates after surgery was much more earlier in Group2.

Continuous ventricular drainage was not performed in Group 1, while performed in majority of patients (73.3 %) in group2.

Fig. 1 shows the number of the patients who showed favorable outcome. Sum of good recovery and moderately disabled cases by Glasgow outcome scale, was 73.3%in Group 2 as compared to 46.7% in Group 1.

Fig. 2 shows the time course of average SjO_2, CPP, and $PaCO_2$ of all 30 cases for first 24 hours following the decompression. Desaturation of the jugular vein, indicating ischemia, continued for 6 hours after the decomperssion. This prolonged ischemia was not accompanied by reduced CPP or hypocapnia.

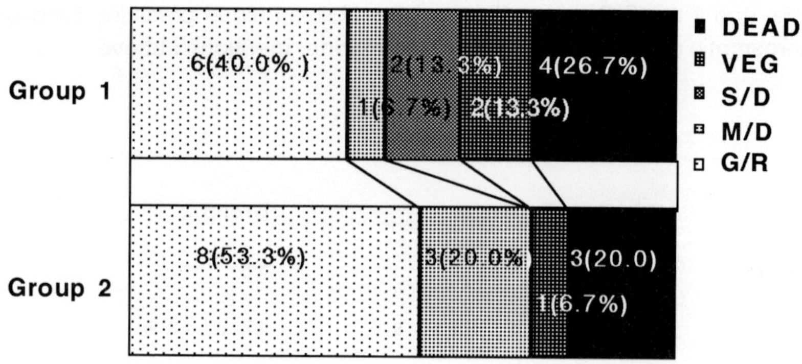

Fig.1 Outcome of two groups

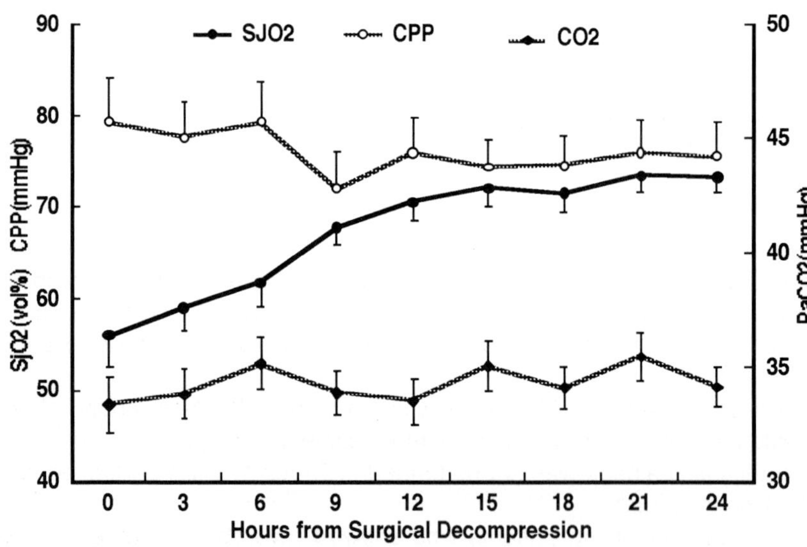

Fig.2 Time course of SjO_2, CPP, and $PaCO_2$ following decompression.

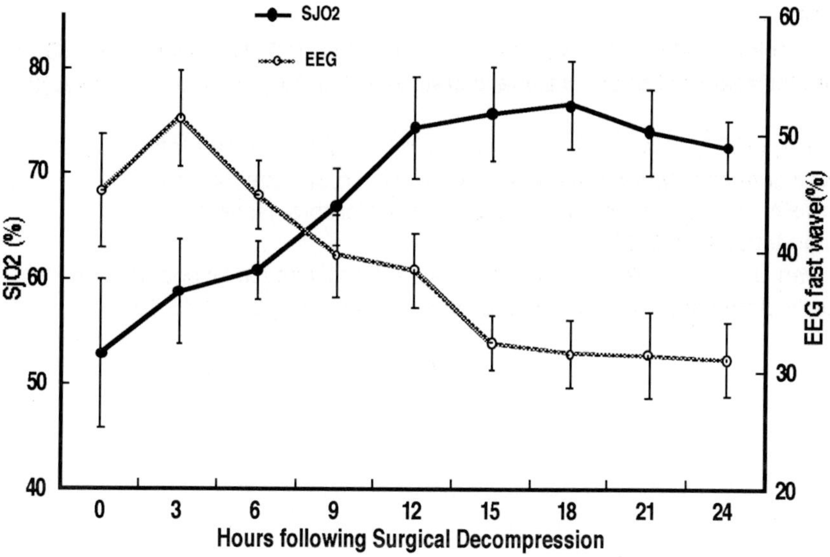

Fig.3 Time course of SjO_2 and fast wave component of EEG (%)

Fig. 3 shows 8 cases from group 2. Fast wave component of EEG recovered up to 40 to 50 % soon after decompression, indicating recovery of brain metabolism, while SjO_2 remained low. Treatment by barbiturate decreased fast wave component, indicating reduction of cerebral metabolism, and simultaneous rise in SjO_2 was seen.

(DISCUSSION)

We have reported in animal experiment, that marked reduction of CBF can occur in the absence of reduced CPP or hypocapnia, after global ischemia by severe brain compression and reperfusion[1]. We regarded this to be equivalent to delayed postischemic hypoperfusion reported by Hossman, Levy, and others[2] [3] [4] , where unproportional recovery of cerebral metabolism is mismatched by poor recovery of CBF. The prolonged ischemia, which we had observed in present study, had shown quite similar attitude. Therefore, we speculate that delayed postischemic hypoperfusion exist in majority of cases undergoing removal of large intracranial hematoma, and it is likely to be give unfavorable influence to ongoing cerebral damage.

Therefore the treatment aimed to reverse the ischemic condition starting within 6 hours of decompression, irrespective of ICP, is likely to improve the outcome as seen in this study. Treatment of choice should include every effort to increase CBF and reduce $CMRO_2$, such as continuous ventricular drainage and maintenance of systemic blood pressure to keep CPP constantly in the autoregulatory range, large dose of hyperosmotic agents to directly increase CBF, and barbiturate therapy to reduce $CMRO_2$.

(REFERENCE)

1. Yabuki A, Mishina H, Miyazaki, Maeda M, Sato K, Ishi S (1991) $AVDO_2$ and EEG as Indicators for treatment of posttraumatic brain swelling. Neurol Med Chir(Tokyo)31:568-574
2. Hosmann KA, (1977) Total ischemia of the brain.In Brain and Heart Infarct. (Zurich KJ,Kaufmann W,Hosmann K-A V,eds), Berlin,Springer,pp 107-227,
3. Hossmann KA, (1982) Treatment of Experimental Cerebral Ischemia. J CBF and Metabolism 2:275-297
4. Levy DE, Van Uitert RL, Pike CL, (1979) Delayed Postischemic Hypoperfusion: A potentially Damaging Consequence of Stroke, Neurology 29:1245-1253

Session XIII: Microdialysis

Chairmen: L.A. Persson and T. Hayakawa

Microdialytic Monitoring of Ischemic Changes During Brain Retraction for Aneurysm Surgery

A. Mendelowitsch[1], H. Langemann[2], H. Landolt[3], and O. Gratzl[1]

[1] University Neurosurgical Clinic, [2] Section of Neurosurgery, Department of Research, Cantonal Hospital, CH-4031 Basel, Switzerland
[3] Neurosurgical Clinic, Cantonal Hospital, CH-5000 Aarau, Switzerland

INTRODUCTION

It is known that self-retaining brain retractors, as required for adequate exposure during many intracranial procedures, can cause local ischemia. The incidence of damage has been estimated as 10% in cranial base procedures and 5% in aneurysm surgery [1]. Monitoring of retractor blade pressure, brain electrical activity and cerebral blood flow can provide information about physiological parameters during retraction. However, intracerebral microdialysis, which has been shown to be feasible intraoperatively [2], is the only method capable of monitoring brain metabolism directly. Changes of levels in the brain extracellular fluid (ECF) of a variety of biochemical parameters, reflecting various aspects of brain metabolism, can be measured at several time points during the operation. Parameters suitable for monitoring retractor damage are those whose ECF levels have been shown to be influenced by ischemic conditions in experimental models. These include pH [3], glucose (Glu), lactate (Lac)[4], and the antioxidants ascorbic acid (Asc), glutathione (GSH), cysteine (Cys) and uric acid (UA)[5]. We now report findings of microdialytic monitoring for ischemia during 6 aneurysm operations, in which the parameters listed above were determined.

METHODS

Measurements were carried out in 6 patients operated on for aneurysm of the carotid circulation (three, asymptomatic; two, 14 days after subarachnoid hemorrhage; one, 24h after subarachnoid hemorrhage). Immediately after the craniotomy, before basal opening of the dura, a 1cm cut was made in the dura and the probe (4mm membrane, 0.5mm diameter), which had been previously sterilised at 60°C with ethylene dioxide, was inserted into the frontal cortex. In one patient, a second probe was placed in the temporal lobe. The probes were perfused with sterile 0.9% saline at 2μl/min until the dura was closed. In 5 of the patients the on-line pH of the dialysate was recorded [3]. Fractions of 40 or 50μl were collected. After the end of the operation the in vitro relative recoveries for all parameters were measured at room temperature using the same probe, flow rate and perfusion medium as in the operation. Relative recovery is defined as the ratio (%) between the concentration of a substance in the perfusion outflow to that of the same substance in the solution surrounding the probe.

Asc, UA, GSH, and Cys were determined in the dialysate (5μl) by reverse phase HPLC and electrochemical detection. Lac and Glu were determined enzymatically, each in 15μl or 20μl. To partially compensate for possible changes in microdialysis conditions during measurement, the ratio of glucose to lactate (Glu / Lac) was calculated for each fraction.

RESULTS AND DISCUSSION

Asc was increased in 4 patients during retraction, as was GSH in 5 patients. In two cases both these parameters showed considerable increases, of up to 7-fold for Asc and 15-fold for GSH (Figs.1A and 2), whereas in the others increases were smaller. Basal levels of Cys were not generally measurable; however this parameter could be detected in 2 patients during retraction (e.g. Fig 1A). Lac was increased in 5 patients, with a concomitant fall in Glu and reduction in Glu / Lac ratio (see Figs 1B and 2). Corresponding changes in all these parameters have been found in microdialysates from the ischemic zone of rats subjected to middle cerebral artery occlusion [4, 5]. In addition, similar results (increased Cys, reduced Glu, increased Lac) were found in microdialysates from a patient with severe head injury, where there was practically no cerebral perfusion [6].

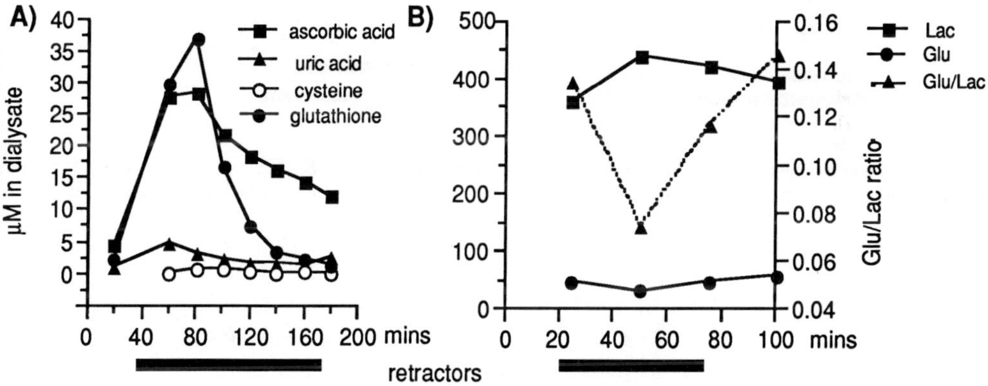

Fig.1 Intraoperative microdialysis in A) patient E.V., measurement of antioxidants; in B) patient B.M.,glucose, lactate and glucose / lactate ratio

In the patient with two probes, frontal effects were much greater than temporal ones for all measured parameters (see Fig. 2). This is an important finding, showing that the changes of levels in the dialysates are not artefacts, but are related to the duration and pressure of retraction, factors which were both less temporally than frontally. The two probes used had very similar recovery characteristics.

The measurement of the pH of the dialysate (see Fig.3) is of special interest because the pH meter is on-line, providing information from the cortex of the patient with a time-lag of only 12-18 min (variable, depending on the length of the tubing from the patient to the pH meter). Values fell up to 0.3 units in the 5 patients with on-line measurement, in accordance with experimental findings (3). After removal of the retractor, pH started to rise.

In one patient, who was not included in the evaluation, there was a typical decrease in pH (to 6.78) during 90 mins of retraction, followed by a sudden rapid unexplained increase of pH to 7.31. Later we found greatly increased UA and Glu/Lac ratio in the fractions collected during and after the pH rise.The patient recovered normally, but a routine postoperative CT showed a tiny hemorrhage near to the probe insertion point. The increase in pH and other changes can thus probably be explained by the presence of blood in the ECF.

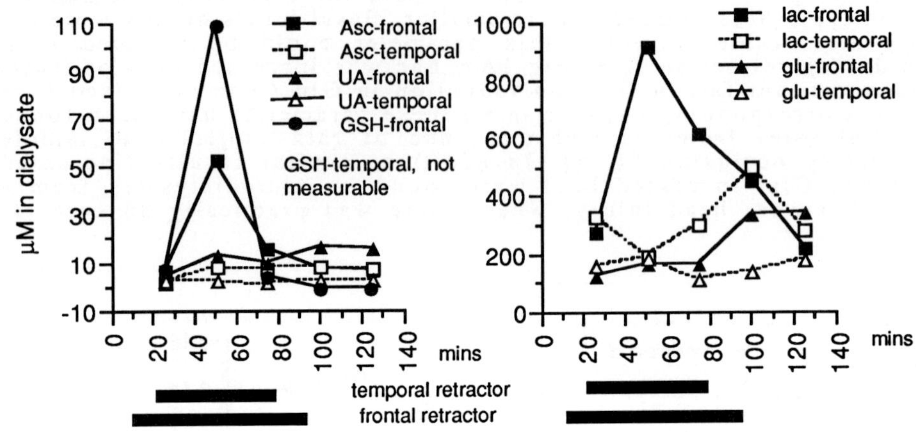

Fig. 2 Intraoperative microdialysis of patient K.K. with two probes (temporal and frontal). Measurement of antioxidants, glucose and lactate.

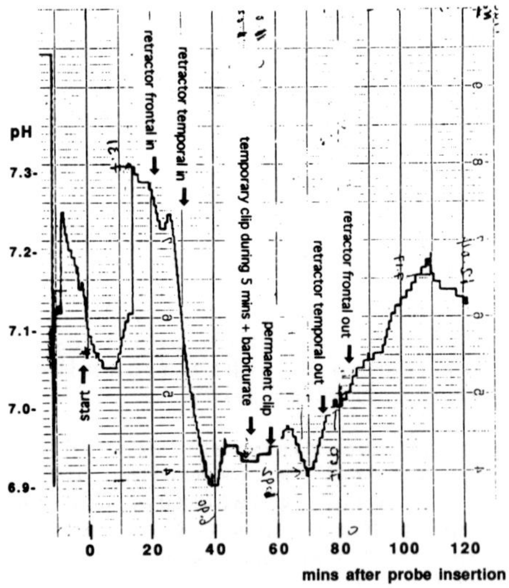

Fig. 3 Original trace showing changes in the pH of the dialysate during the operation on patient K.K. (frontal probe)

Increases or decreases in the parameters were only temporary, and in most cases values began to return before the removal of the retractor (see Figs). This is in accordance with the experimental finding that the brain can adjust itself to retraction pressure (monitored retraction pressure dropped to 50% of its original value after 6-12 mins)[1].

Because of our interest in cerebral monitoring in trauma patients, we wanted to get an idea of basal levels of our parameters in dialysates from minimally disturbed brain. Values before operation were not available, as the interval between probe insertion and application of retractor was often too short for equilibrium to be reached. However, in the patient with 2 probes, levels in the last fraction before probe removal were similar frontally and temporally although the severity of the retractor insult had differed greatly (Fig 2). We can therefore assume that levels in these fractions, which are shown in Table 1 (mean for all six patients), approximate to the above-mentioned basal levels. The values for Asc, GSH and Lac are similar to those found by us [6] and other authors [2].

Table 1: Concentrations (μM) in the last dialysate sample before probe removal, and recovery (%) Mean ± S.E.M.(n = 7) in both cases.

Parameters	Asc	UA	GSH	Glu	Lac	glu/lac	pH
Conc.	6.9 ± 2.9	5.3 ± 2.0	0.72 ± 0.28	247 ± 39	252 ±35	1.08 ± 0.2	7.09 ±0.08
Recovery (%)	11.6 ±3.8	20.5 ± 2.6	3.2 ± 0.9	25.5 ± 1.7	21.6 ± 2.1		

We have thus confirmed that microdialysis is a sensitive tool for detecting metabolic changes intraoperatively. In most of our patients retraction was followed by neurochemical changes similar to those obtained during ischemic events; however, as retraction was routinely intermittent (frequent changes of position) return to normal was relatively rapid. Correspondingly, neurological and postoperative CT findings did not indicate any ischemic changes frontally. The values of our parameters which would indicate permanent damage are not known. Our aim is, with more experience, to be able to monitor ischemic changes with on-line measurements, so that when these critical values are reached, retraction can be modified.

REFERENCES

1. Andrews RJ, Bringas JR (1993) A review of brain retraction and recommendations for minimizing intraoperative brain injury. Neurosurg 33:1052-1064
2. Hillered L, Persson L, Pontén U, Ungerstedt U (1990) Neurometabolic monitoring of the ischemic human brain using microdialysis. Acta Neurochir (Wien) 102: 91-97
3. Landolt H, Langemann H, Gratzl O. (1993) On-line monitoring of cerebral pH using microdialysis. Neurosurg 32: 1000-1004
4. Hillered L, Persson L, Ponten U, Ungerstedt U (1989) Dynamics of extracellular metabolites in the striatum after middle cerebral artery occlusion on the rat monitored by intracerebral microdialysis. J Cereb Blood Flow Metab 9: 607-616
5 Landolt H, Lutz TW, Langemann H, Stäuble D, Mendelowitsch A, Gratzl O. (1992) Extracellular antioxidants and amino acids in the cortex of he rat: monitoring by microdialysis of early ischemic changes. J Cereb Blood Flow Metab 12: 96-102
6. Landolt H, Langemann H, Mendelowitsch A, Gratzl O (1994) Neurochemical monitoring and on-line pH measurements using brain microdialysis in patients in intensive care. Acta Neurochir [Suppl] (Wien) 60:475-478

Excitatory Amino Acid Release After Severe Human Head Trauma: Effect of Intracranial Pressure and Cerebral Perfusion Pressure Changes

R. BULLOCK, A. ZAUNER, O. TSUJI, J.J. WOODWARD, H.F. YOUNG, and A.T. MARMAROU

Division of Neurosurgery, Medical College of Virginia, Richmond, VA, USA

INTRODUCTION:

The role of excitatory amino acids (EAA's) in the pathobiology of acute cerebral damage due to both stroke and head trauma has become the focus of much recent interest [1]. EAA release, associated with both structural damage and behavioral abnormalities, has now been shown in several animal models [2]. These changes may be reversed by administration of EAA antagonists, and this has led to trials of glutamate antagonists in severe human head injury [3]. Release of EAA's has recently been measured in 17 acutely head injured patients at MCV, with the aim of determining the circumstances responsible for glutamate release as a factor causing secondary brain damage after severe head injury. In this report, we have prospectively addressed the hypothesis that an increase in intracranial pressure, or a decrease in cerebral perfusion pressure, is responsible for release of EAA's following severe head trauma.

PATIENTS AND METHODS:

The characteristics of the patients studied are shown in Table 1.

Table 1: Patient Characteristics

Patient Category	No. of Patients	GCS	Outcome
Diffuse Injury	6	4 - 9	2 deaths, 2 SD
Subdural Hematoma	6	3 - 10	2 deaths, 1 VEG, 2 SD
Epidural Hematoma	1	10	GR
Contusion	4	6 - 10	MD = 1 GR = 4
Secondary Insult	6	3 - 8	2 deaths, 1 VEG, 2 SD

Microdialysis:

A 10 mm flexible microdialysis probe with external diameter of 0.75 mm was used. The active portion of the probe was inserted into cortex, either at craniotomy, or via a ventriculostomy twist drill site, and probes were profused at 2 microliters per minute using sterile 0.9% saline. 60 μl dialysates were collected every 30 minutes, into sealed glass tubes using a CMA 170 refrigerated collector system [4^0 c]. Clinical events which took place during microdialysis were logged into a mainframe computer. EAA's and threonine, serine were measured, using HPLC.

ICP and CPP Measurement:

Ventriculostomy ICP data, and mean arterial blood pressure, were continuously acquired by a VAX mainframe computer system, and smoothed to yield graphs for each physiologic parameter for 12 hour epochs. The EAA data was superimposed on these graphs, for analysis.

RESULTS:

Patterns of EAA Release and Intracranial Pathology:

In general, glutamate and aspartate release fluctuated together. In patients with focal cerebral contusions [n = 3] EAA release was 6-20 times above the normal level. [±2mM]. In these patients, EAA levels in extracellular fluid remained elevated, and constant though slowly declining over the entire period of microdialysis - up to four days [Figure 1, a and b]. In diffuse cerebral injury, without secondary insults, such as ischemic events, low CBF, or reduced CPP [n = 4] the pattern of EAA release was remarkably constant. EAA levels were initially 3-4 times above normal (2μmol) but declined over ±6 hrs. to within the normal range. The highest levels of EAA's were seen in patients with severe diffuse injuries, and a prior ischemic event, [n = 6]. In these, EAA's ranged from 20 to 50 times normal.

Relationship Between ICP, CPP and EAA Release:

During 1,648 hours of microdialysis in the 17 patients, only 2 patients demonstrated sustained elevations of ICP for greater than 30 minutes. Both these patients died, and in these two patients EAA's trended steadily upward to extremely high levels - greater than 50 times normal. In 6 patients, 18 brief episodes [less than 5 minutes] of ICP above 40 mm Hg were seen. However, none of these episodes were associated with increases in EAA's. Conversely, 4 episodes of increased EAA release were seen [increase of greater than 100 percent over "basal"] yet none of these episodes were associated with changes in CPP or ICP.

DISCUSSION:

In 1990, Persson et al demonstrated that long term monitoring of the extracellular micro environment was feasible using microdialysis in the intensive care unit [4]. We have modified these techniques for continuous use over up to four days. These early descriptive studies allow us to draw the following general conclusions:

The pattern of EAA release is determined more by the magnitude and nature of the initial injury, together with early secondary events which occur in the few hours prior to stabilization in the intensive care unit. In patients with uncomplicated diffuse injuries, subdural hematomas and epidural hematomas, where microdialysis was performed in brain which appeared normal on CT scan, EAA release trended downward within the first six hours to lie within the normal range. The highest levels of EAA's were seen in the six patients with significant secondary insults in the form of documented global cerebral hypoperfusion, or sustained increases in ICP which failed to respond to therapy. Within this group, patients were of two types: those with initially high EAA release which trended downward as the patients recovered [6-20 times normal] and those in who EAA release began at very high levels [20 -30 times above basal, and rose as the patient progressed from uncontrollable ICP to brain death. In these patients, death occurred as CPP fell below ±20 mm of mercury, and EAA levels 50 - 60 times above normal levels were then recorded [Figure 1]. In six

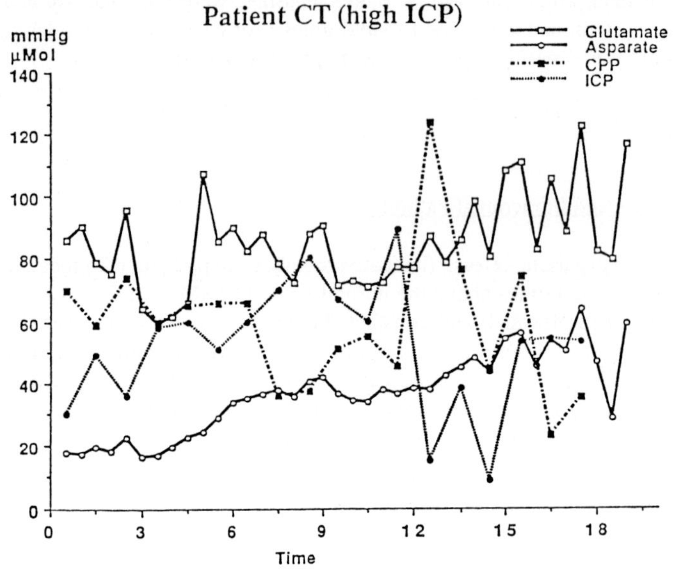

Figure 1: CPP, ICP and EAA's in a patient with severe brain swelling, after a global ischemic insult. Glutamate increased to 50 times normal [2μ mol].

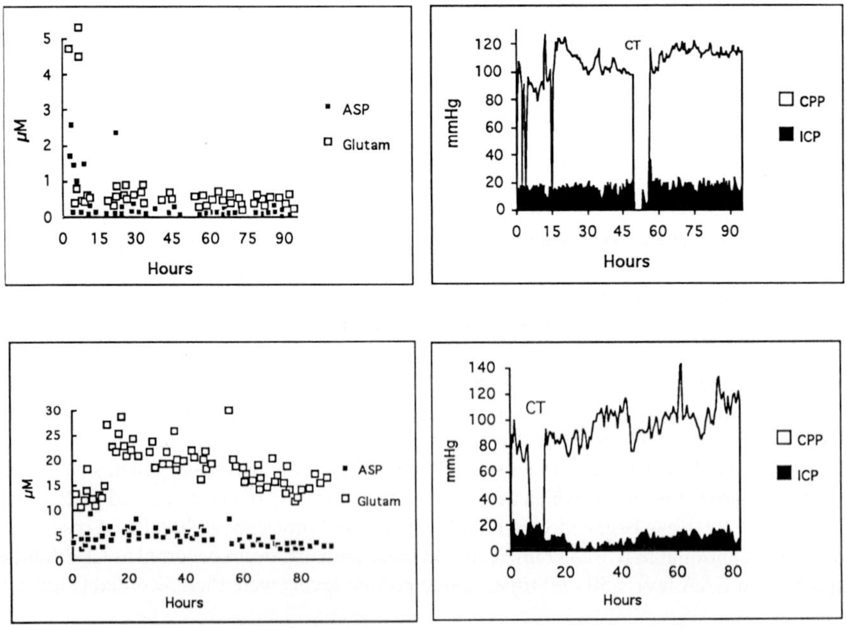

FIGURE 2: RELATIONSHIP BETWEEN ICP AND EAA RELEASE, IN 2 PATIENTS.
TOP:-- PATIENT WITH BRIEF EPISODES OF REDUCED CPP, DUE TO HYPOTENSION, WITHOUT CONCOMMITANT MARKED INCREASE IN EAA'S.(5 MICROMOL.)
BOTTOM:-- PATIENT WITH MARKEDLY INCREASED EAA'S, AND STABLE CPP.

patients, 18 episodes of briefly increased ICP and decreased CPP [less than 40 mm Hg] were seen, but these were unassociated with EAA changes. We thus conclude that in general, patients stabilized in the intensive care unit do not manifest increases in EAA release following brief ICP increases after head injury, and we speculate that in those patients that progress through uncontrollable ICP to brain death, prior severe insult and secondary events act in concert to derange ionic flux, and metabolic substrate delivery, such that ionic homeostasis is not restored, cell swelling is exacerbated, and brain swelling, neuronal necrosis, and high ICP develops, as part of a "cycle of destruction."

REFERENCES:

1. Bullock R, Fujisawa H. (1992) The role of glutamate antagonists for treatment of CNS injury. J Neurotrauma 9: Suppl 2: 5443-5462.

2. Katayama Y, Becker DP, Tamura T, Hovda DA (1990) Massive increases in extracellular potassium and the indiscriminate release of glutamate following concussive brain injury. J Neurosurg 73: 889-900

3. Bullock R, Teasdale GM, Stewart L, Wagstaff A, Kotake A (1994) Experience with the glutamate antagonist CGS 19755 in severe human head injury: Evidence for ICP lowering effect. (This volume, in press)

4. Persson L, Hillered L (1992) Chemical monitoring of neurosurgical intensive care patients using intracerebral microdialysis. J Neurosurg 76: 72-80

Microdialysis Detection of Electrolytes and Amino Acids Changes Following Head Impact Acceleration Injury Coupled with Secondary Insult

OSAMU TSUJI, ANTHONY MARMAROU, and ROSS M. BULLOCK

Division of Neurosurgery, Medical College of Virginia, Richmond, VA, USA

INTRODUCTION

In the severely head injured patient, it has been clearly established that secondary insult including hypoxia an hypotension worsens outcome.[1] In a previous study, we showed that the combination of hypoxia an hypotension remarkably aggravates brain edema formation in traumatized rats which could be a contributin factor to developing brain swelling and ischemia.[2, 3] This edema, it was hypothesized, may be a result of neurotoxic process. In this study, our objective was to determine the effect of secondary insult on ioni homeostasis and release of EAA which may contribute to the neurotoxic component of brain swelling.

MATERIAL and METHODS

All surgical procedures were approved by our internal review board and were in compliance with NII guidelines. Thirty five adult male Sprague-Dawley rats, weighing 350~400 gr (373 ±7.1 gr), wer anesthetized and ventilated through endotracheal tube by mixture of 30% oxygen, 50% nitrous oxide, 1~1.5% Halothane and balanced nitrogen. Both femoral arteries and unilateral femoral vein were cannulated fo continuous measurement of blood pressure and blood gas and exsanguination of blood. After positioning on stereotaxic apparatus, three burr holes were made for insertion of two microdialysis probes (CMA/12, BAS Inc.) into bilateral striatum and an ICP sensor into parietal subcortical white matter. During the experiment, th rectal temperature of animals was maintained at 37°C via a heating lamp.
Animals were divided into 5 groups ; 1) sham operation (n=5), 2) hypotension only (Group I, n=7) , 3 hypotension and hypoxia (Group II, n=9), 4) trauma plus hypotension (Group III, n=5), and 5) trauma plu both of hypoxia and hypotension (Group IV, n=9). Hypotension was induced by exsanguination of arteri blood and mean blood pressure was kept at 35 mmHg for 30 min. The average amount of bloo exsanguinated to maintain mean arterial blood pressure at 35 mmHg was 8.0 ml in Group I and III and 6.5 m in Group II and IV. Hypoxia was induced by manipulating oxygen concentration of the gas mixture, lowerin to 10% and balanced with nitrogen increase. PaO2 during hypoxia was 45±6.2 and 44±4.7 mmHg in Grou II and IV. Hypotension and hypoxia were induced 60 min post trauma and maintained for 30 min. Traum was produced by dropping of a weight (450 gr) from a height of 2 m. Two microdialysis probes wer perfused, using a microinfusion pump (CMA/100, BAS Inc.), with physiological saline at the rate o 2.0µl/min . Dialysate was collected every 7.5 min respectively and analyzed for ions (sodium and potassium by flamephotometry and excitatory amino acids (Glu, Asp) by HPLC. At 3 hours after resuscitation, animal were sacrificed by clamping of the ascending aorta. Animals were excluded from analysis if intracerebra hemorrhage or acute hydrocephalus was noticed in brain slices.

RESULTS

ICP

In the control group, ICP was 6.7±0.8 mmHg initially and 6.4±2.3 mmHg at the end of experiment. Th initial ICP in Group I and II was 6.9±1.5 mmHg and 5.4±2.1 mmHg respectively, showing no significan difference from the control group. In Group III and IV, initial ICP was elevated to 44.1±17.9 mmH ($p<0.01$) and spontaneously decreased to 19.9±4.8 mmHg prior to the secondary insult. In some cases thi ICP elevation was associated with massive subarachnoid hemorrhage. The ICP at the end of experiment wa 6.9±2.6 mmHg, 7.2±2.8 mmHg and 15.2±7.2 mmHg in groups 1, 2 and 3 respectively. In 4 of 9 rats (44% of Group IV, very rapid increase of ICP was observed after resuscitation and reached an average level o 42.2±10.2 mmHg. Subsequently, a rapid drop of blood pressure occurred synchronous with brai herniation.The final ICP of the remaining animals in this group averaged 14.8±3.7 mmHg.

Electrolytes

Extracellular potassium concentration 30 min prior to secondary insult (30 min post trauma in Group III and IV) showed no significant difference among the groups (average : 1.92±0.14 mM). Although, in all groups, extracellular potassium increase was noticed during hypoxia and/or hypotension, the magnitude of potassium increase varied remarkably among each group. In Group I and II, potassium increase reached 117% and 121% of baseline respectively. In Group III, potassium increase reached 166% of baseline ($p<0.05$, to Group I). In these groups however, the potassium increase was transient and returned to base line immediately after resuscitation. In Group IV, potassium increase was sustained at 247% of baseline ($p<0.01$, to Group II). (Fig.1) In animals with remarkable brain swelling, potassium increase reached 288% of baseline. In contrast, in this model, no remarkable change was noticed in extracellular sodium concentration prior to and after secondary insult.

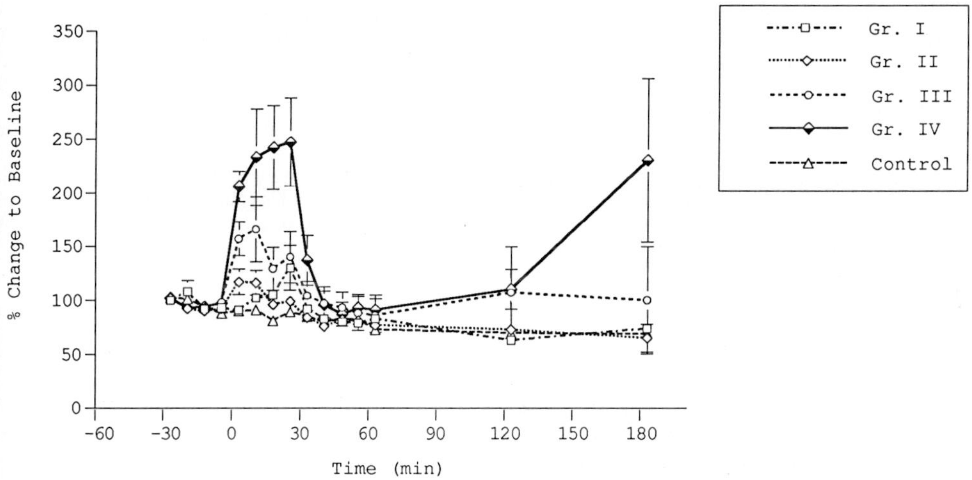

Fig. 1 Extracellular pottasium changes during secondary insult measured by microdialysis. During insult, traumatized group III and IV showed prominent potassium efflux compared to non-traumatized group I and II respectively. ($p<0.05$), mean±SE

Excitatory Amino Acids

The basal levels of Glu and Asp in SHAM operated animals were 3.01 and 1.08 μM respectively. The results obtained from groups I and II exhibited no significant difference. In Group III and IV, the average values of Glu and Asp 30 min after impact acceleration injury were 6.62 and 1.91 μM (III), and 5.65 and 1.56 μM (IV) respectively. These values showed a 50~100% increase in comparison to the control group. During ischemia, Glu and Asp concentrations were elevated in all groups. The magnitude of the EAA's released closely reflected the trends observed in potassium efflux. (Fig. 2)

Fig. 2

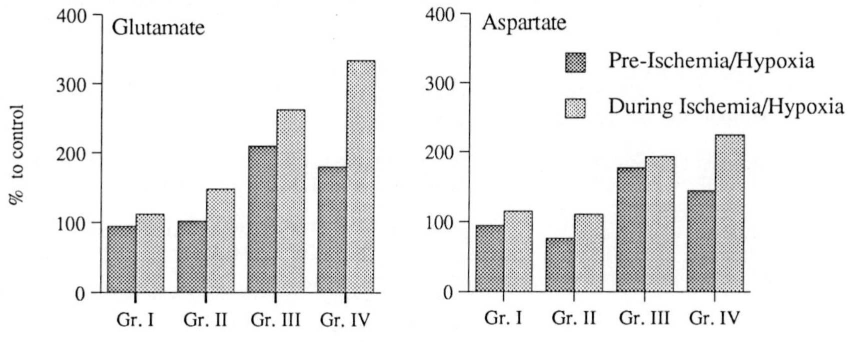

DISCUSSION

It is well known that potassium efflux and excitatory amino acid release occurs during brain ischemia and that traumatized brain is more vulnerable to the ischemic insult. [4, 5] The result of the present study demonstrated that the combination of hypotension and hypoxia exacerbates efflux of potassium and release of excitatory amino acids in the impact acceleration injury model thereby setting the stage for rapid development of acute brain edema. The increase of brain water content and subsequent reduction of cerebral blood volume in this model, following secondary insult has been confirmed in a previous report. [2] In this impact acceleration injury model, by virtue of the accelerating skull, it is not possible to study the ionic alteration and excitatory amino acids dynamics at the time of impact. Thirty minutes after impact, we observed a 150% elevation of Glu and Asp levels lasting 30 min. This is similar to the magnitude of EAA levels associated with microdialysis studies of the fluid percussion model. [6] We suspect that beyond the initial impact, restoration of ionic homeostasis is in occurring but additional ischemic/hypoxic insults can easily disrupt ionic balance. Although the magnitude of the secondary insult applied in this experiment is not of sufficient severity to develop a large potassium efflux in non-traumatized brain, it is of sufficient magnitude to disable the energy dependent ion channel in traumatized brain. Brain metabolic stores may be exhausted by the initially increased demand which takes an hour or more to recover after experimental head injury.[7] This experiment demonstrates that energy metabolism of the traumatized brain is in critical balance for hours.

After resuscitation, in all groups, rapid normalization of extracellular potassium levels was observed. However, almost half of Group IV animals showed a continuous elevation of ICP and extracellular potassium after initial recovery suggesting that derangement of ionic and water balance may be produced by mechanisms other than energy failure. [8] Recent studies have emphasized the role of excitatory amino acids in the development of brain edema.[9] Our results show that excitatory amino acid release is also exacerbated by the combination of ischemia and hypoxia adding to the continued instability.

REFERENCE

1. Chesnut RM, Marshall LF, Klauber MR, Blunt BA, Baldwin N, Eisenberg HM, Jane JA, Marmarou A, Foulkes MA (1990) The role of secondary brain injury in determining outcome from severe head injury. J Trauma 34(2): 216-22.

2. Kita H, Marmarou A (1994) The cause of acute brain swelling after the closed head injury in rats. Acta Neurochir 60 : 452-455

3. Marmarou A, Foda M, Brink W, Campbell J, Kita H, Demetriadou K (1994) A new model of diffuse brain injury in rats. Part I J Neurosurg. 80 : 291-300

4. Harris RJ, Symon L (1984) Extracellular pH, potassium and calcium activities in progressive ischemia of rat cortex. J Cerebral Blood Flow Metabol 1: 203-209

5. Katayama Y. Tamura T. Becker D P. Tsubokawa T. (1991) Calcium-dependent component of massive increase in extracellular potassium during cerebral ischemia as demonstrated by microdialysis in vivo. Brain Res 13; 567(1): 57-63

6. Faden AI, Demediuk P, Panter SS, Vink R (1989) The role of excitatory amino acids and NMDA receptors in traumatic brain injury. Science 244 : 798-800

7. Ishige N, Pitts LH, Pogliani L, Hashimoto T, Nishimura BS, Bartkowski HM, James TL (1987) Effect of hypoxia on traumatic brain injury in rats : Part 2. Changes in high energy phosphate metabolism. Neurosurgery 20 : 854-858

8. Kempski OS, Staub F, Rosen F, Zimmer M, Neu A, Baethmann A (1988) Molecular mechanisms of glial swelling in vitro. Neurochem Pathol 9: 109-125

9. Schneider GH, Baethmann A, Kempski O (1992) Mechanisms of glial swelling induced by glutamate. Can J Physiol Pharmacol 1992; 70 Suppl: S334-43

Session XIV: Imaging

Chairmen: M.J. Caron and D.A. Hovda

Effect of Xenon Gas Inhalation on Intracranial Pressure During Xenon CT CBF Measurement

M. Matsuda, H. Lee, K. Kuribayashi, A. Shiino, and J. Handa

Department of Neurosurgery, Shiga University of Medical Science, Seta, Ohtsu, Shiga, 520-21 Japan

INTRODUCTION

Cerebral blood flow (CBF) measurement using computed tomography (CT) with stable xenon (Xe) inhalation is now one of the routine examinations in patients with neurological and neurosurgical diseases. There are reports that the inhalation of stable Xe gas caused a significant increase in the intracranial pressure (ICP) [1,2], while others reported no such increase in ICP [3,4]. We evaluated the ICP changes during Xe gas inhalation in the Xe CT CBF study.

MATERIALS AND METHODS

There were 12 patients; eight with ruptured cerebral aneurysm, one with ruptured arteriovenous malformation and three with meningioma. They were all postoperative patients aged 43 to 64 years. ICP was measured by a transducer-tipped fiberoptic pressure monitoring catheter (Camino Laboratories, San Diego, California, U.S.A.) placed in the subdural space. During the Xe CT CBF study a mixture of gas containing 30% stable Xe, 30-50% oxygen and balance air was delivered for 5 minutes under spontaneous respiration. The ICP, systemic arterial blood pressure and end-tidal carbon dioxide ($ETCO_2$) were continuously monitored.

RESULTS

In seven patients with baseline ICP of 4-14 mmHg (mean 9.9), ICP slightly increased to 7-16 mmHg (mean 12.3) with maximum increase of 4 mmHg during Xe inhalation. Mean arterial blood pressure (MABP) and $ETCO_2$ were not significantly changed (Table 1). In four patients with baseline ICP of 20-27 mmHg (mean 23.3), ICP increased remarkably to 40-54 mmHg (mean 46.8), and MABP rose from 84 to 102 mmHg, while $ETCO_2$ showed no significant changes (Table 2). Actual records of one of these patients (patient 11) are shown in Figure 1. In one patient whose ICP was controlled at 15 mmHg by ventricular drainage, Xe inhalation caused a remarkable ICP elevation to 40 mmHg. MABP changed from 93 to 113 mmHg and $ETCO_2$ from 5 to 5.8% (Table 3). After the ICP was lowered to 5 mmHg by removing cerebrospinal fluid (CSF) via the ventricular drain, Xe inhalation for 3 minutes raised ICP to 12 mmHg, MABP changed from 92 to 108 mmHg and $ETCO_2$ from 5.5 to 5.8%. No patient deteriorated in neurological condition after the study.

Table 1 Intracranial pressure, mean arterial blood pressure, and end-tidal carbon dioxide before (B) and during (Xe) stable Xe inhalation in patients with ICP within normal range.

Patient	ICP(mmHg)		MABP(mmHg)		ETCO2(%)	
Age/Sex	B	Xe	B	Xe	B	Xe
1) 45/M	14	14	100	106	-	-
2) 54/M	13	13	115	115	4.0	4.1
3) 49/F	12	16	119	125	4.4	4.2
4) 46/M	13	17	88	103	4.1	3.9
5) 60/M	4	7	93	98	4.2	3.9
6) 49/F	5	7	60	87	5.0	4.8
7) 64/F	8	12	105	98	4.6	4.4
mean	9.9	12.3	97.1	104.6	4.4	4.2

Table 2 Intracranial pressure, mean arterial blood pressure, and end-tidal carbon dioxide before (B) and during (Xe) stable Xe inhalation in patients with increased ICP.

Patient	ICP(mmHg)		MABP(mmHg)		ETCO2(%)	
Age/Sex	B	Xe	B	Xe	B	Xe
8) 61/F	27	54	102	143	5.2	4.8
9) 46/M	20	40	63	90	4.6	4.3
10) 43/F	20	50	110	110	3.8	3.9
11) 63/M	26	43	62	68	3.9	4.0
mean	23.3	46.8	84.3	102.8	4.4	4.3

Table 3 Intracranial pressure, mean arterial blood pressure, and end-tidal carbon dioxide before (B) and during (Xe) stable Xe inhalation in a patient with ICP controlled.

Patient		ICP(mmHg)		MABP(mmHg)		ETCO2(%)	
Age/Sex		B	Xe	B	Xe	B	Xe
12) 44/M	1:	15	40	93	113	5.0	5.8
	2:	5	12	92	108	5.5	5.8

1: ventricular drain closed, 5-min inhalation
2: after CSF drained, 3-min inhalation

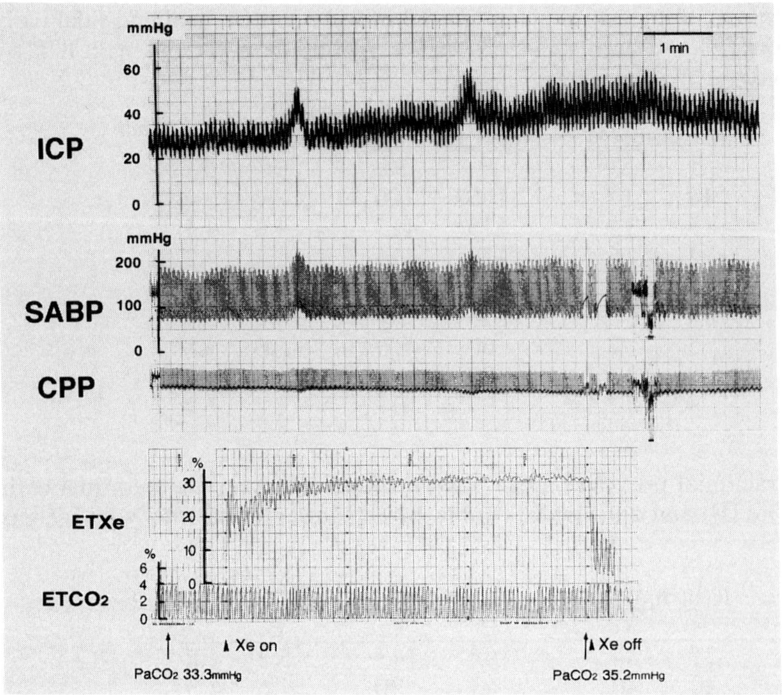

Fig. 1 Record of Patient 11.

DISCUSSION

It is not yet clear whether stable Xe inhalation causes a significant increase in ICP or not. It is observed that Xe inhalation increases CBF [5,6] and accelerates the flow velocity in the middle cerebral artery [7,8]. The latter phenomenon implies an increase in CBF if the vascular diameter is not changed. An increase in CBF results in a rise in ICP. However, it is not always the case, because ICP is more directly related to cerebral blood volume (CBV) than CBF [9]. The effect of Xe on CBV is not known yet. The patients who showed no significant changes in ICP during Xe inhalation were mostly intubated and placed in hypocapnea by mechanically controlled respiration, while our patients were not intubated or mechanically ventilated. There is a possibility that the magnitude of ICP increase may be greater under normocapnea. Xe is known to depress the respiratory center in the pons [10]. Respiratory suppression was observed in some of our patients who showed a remarkable rise in ICP. Possible accumulation of CO_2 and a disturbed venous return due to increased intrathoracic pressure could eventually result in an ICP elevation.

In the present study no clinically relevant increase in ICP was observed during Xe inhalation as long as the baseline ICP was within normal range. In the patients with baseline ICP of 20 mmHg or higher Xe inhalation caused a significant increase in ICP.

These results imply that it is the intracranial comliance that matters. This is well exemplified in Patient 12, whose ICP increase was significant even after it was lowered to the normal level by CSF drainage. Although the ICP was lowered, the amplitude of ICP wave remained high, indicating a decreased intracranial compliance [11].

In conclusion, there is no clinically relevant increase in ICP during the Xe CT CBF study as long as the ICP is within normal range. However, Xe inhalation should be cautiously undertaken in patients with decreased intracranial compliance, even if the ICP was lowered to the normal level. Further investigation of the effect of stable Xe gas and gas delivering system is needed.

REFERENCES

1. Harrington TR, Manwaring K, Hodak J (1986) Local basal ganglia and brain stem blood flow in the head injured patient using stable xenon enhanced CT scanning. In: Miller JD, Teasdale GM, Rowan JO, Galbraith SL, Mendelow AD (eds) Intracranial Pressure VI. Springer, Berlin Heidelberg, pp 680-686
2. Nemati M-N, Dietz H, Holl K, Gaab M, Rzesacz E, Witt JP, Haubitz B, Becker H (1992) Concomitant efffect of acetazolamide and xenon on cerebral blood flow, intracranial pressure, flow velocity, and electroencephalogram: Possible risk for the patient? In: Yonas H (ed) Cerebral Blood Flow Measurement with Stable Xenon-Enhanced Computed Tomography. Raven Press, New York, pp 296-304
3. Darby JM, Yonas H, Pentheny S, Marion D (1989) Intracranial pressure response to stable xenon inhalation in patients with head injury. Surg Neurol 32:343-345
4. Marion D, Crosby K (1991) The effect of stable xenon on ICP. J Cereb Blood Flow Metab 11:347-350
5. Gur D, Yonas H, Jackson DL, Wolfson SK Jr, Rockette H, Good WF, Maitz GS, Cook EE, Arena VC (1985) Measurement of cerebral blood flow during xenon inhalation as measured by the microspheres method. Stroke 16:871-874
6. Hartmann A, Dettmers C, Schuier FJ, Wassmann HD, Schumacher HW (1991) Effect of stable xenon on regional cerebral blood flow and the electroencephalogram in normal volunteers. Stroke 22:182-189
7. Giller CA, Purdy P, Lindstrom WW (1990) Effects of inhaled stable xenon on cerebral blood flow velocity. AJNR 11:177-182
8. Witt J-P, Holl K, Heissler HE, Dietz H (1991) Stable xenon CT CBF: Effects of blood flow alterations on CBF calculations during inhalation of 33% stable xenon. AJNR 12:973-975
9. Muizelaar JP, Marmarou A, DeSalles AAF, Ward JD, Zimmerman RS, Li Z, Choi SC, Young HF (1989) Cerebral blood flow and metabolism in severely head-injured children. J Neurosurg 71:63-71
10. Winkler S, Turski P, Holden J, Koeppe R, Rusy B, Garber E (1985) Xenon effects on CNS control of respiratory rate and tidal volume - The danger of apnea. In: Hartmann A, Hoyer S (eds) Cerebral Blood Flow and Metabolism Measurement. Springer, Berlin Heidelberg New York Tokyo, pp 356-360
11. Van Eijndhoven JHM, Avezaat CJJ (1980) The analogy between CSF pulse pressure and volume-pressure response. In: Shulman K,Marmarou A, Hochwald GM, Brock M (eds) Intracranial Pressure IV.Springer, Berlin Heidelberg New York, pp 173-176

Pericontusional Brain Edema; Evidence for Microvascular Hypoperfusion in Humans

R. Bullock, M.L. Schröder, J.P. Muizelaar, J.B. Salvant, and J.T. Povlishock

Division of Neurosurgery, Medical College of Virginia, Richmond, VA, USA

SUMMARY

Traumatic cerebral contusion causes a zone of peri-focal neuronal necrosis, the cause of which is not known; furthermore, the surgical management of these lesions remains controversial. In order to determine the pathophysiological mechanisms, responsible for brain damage after contusions, we have performed cerebral blood flow (CBF) mapping studies, and related these to changes in local cerebral blood volume (CBV), and ultrastructure. All patients demonstrated pericontusional edema by CT, and significantly reduced CBF. In 11 severely head injured patients with contusions, CBF and CBV were measured in pericontusional areas, using Stable Xenon-CT-CBF. These studies demonstrated a profound reduction in peri-lesional CBF (17.5 ± 4 ml/100g/min), which was always accompanied by a zone of edema, as defined by CT density measurements. CBV in these regions was 2.3 ± 0.4 ml/100g, a reduction to half the value of 4.8 ml/100g in the non-edematous regions, and to thirty five percent of the value of 6.0 ml/100g in normal volunteers.

Ultrastructural analysis of this pericontusional tissue, taken at surgery, in four patients with high ICP showed glial swelling with narrowing of the microvascular lumina due to massive podocytic process swelling. Additionally, some suggestion of vascular occlusion, due to erythrocyte and leucocyte stasis was also seen. These data support the conclusion that microvascular compromise, by compression and/or plugging, is a major event associated with this profound peri-lesional hypoperfusion, which is a uniform finding within edematous peri-contusional tissue, in this series of patients.

INTRODUCTION

Contusions and traumatic intracerebral hematomas are of special importance to neurosurgeons, because the criteria for operative management are still widely debated [11]. Contusions may swell and enlarge over time and lead to increased intracranial pressure and even herniation [2,8]. Although several studies have focused on the mechanisms, pathogenesis, histopathology, quantification, and outcome of patients with cerebral contusions, many aspects remain poorly understood. In particular, the cause of the neuronal pyknosis and astrocyte swelling which extends for several millimeters, or more, into the cortical ribbon adjacent to the hemorrhagic focus, has not been determined [3]. The pattern of neuronal changes is very similar to that which is seen in infarction, yet large vessel occlusion is usually absent [10]. We have therefore studied regional CBF using Stable Xenon-CT-CBF. Our aim was to test the hypothesis that regional CBF is reduced adjacent to focal intraparenchymal traumatic lesions to an extent sufficient to cause ischemic neuronal necrosis. We also report regional cerebral blood volume (CBV) and ultrastructural data which suggests that microvascular compression, and occlusion, explain these CBF findings.

MATERIALS AND METHODS

Eleven patients with a severe closed head injury (GCS $\leq$ 8 or a motor score $\leq$ 5) harboring a cerebral contusion of more than 2 cm. in size were analyzed for this study. On admission to the Emergency Room, patients were immediately intubated, hemodynamically stabilized and rescusitated when necessary. The initial diagnostic head CT scan was immediately followed by a Stable Xenon-CT CBF assessment. In four cases a CBF/CBV study was repeated between the second and fourth days.

To compute CBF in pericontusional zones, a region of interest was drawn freehand around all contiguous low density zones adjacent to the contusion, depicted on the diagnostic CT -scan (Figure 2). The mean CT density, in Hounsfield Units, was calculated for the low density area, as well as for an adjacent brain region of normal density, on the contralateral site. This template was then superimposed on the computerized blood flow map and CBF could then be calculated in the respective 'edematous' and normal brain areas.

In seven patients we also measured regional CBV in the pericontusional low-density areas. CBV was determined according to the central volume principle [7], and computed according to the equation CBV = CBF $\times$ MTT. In order to define CBV in the pericontusional regions we superimposed the identical template as described above on the contrast enhanced dynamic CT scan taken from the same plane. Our normal CBV is 6.0 $\pm$ 0.4 ml/100g [7].

Brain tissue was obtained for the purpose of electron microscopic assessment in four patients who underwent craniotomy for evacuation of focal contusions. All tissue was harvested from those brain regions surrounding the evacuated contusion. Tissue was also taken from "normal" temporal lobes of seizure patients, undergoing resectional surgery for epilepsy. The tissue was immediately immersion fixed in karnoffsky's fixative, and processed for electron microscopy.

RESULTS

Stable Xenon-CT CBF changes

The mean CT density numbers in the pericontusional and normal areas taken from the diagnostic CT-scan are listed in Table 1, together with the corresponding mean CBF and CBV values. The difference in HU between the pericontusional and normal areas was highly significant ($p < 0.001$, Spearman's rank test). Flow values in the pericontusional areas were less than half the values seen in the normal areas ($p < 0.01$). Most of the areas adjacent to contusions had CBF values below the threshold for ischemic damage (CBF ≤ 18 ml/100g/min) [1,9] (Fig. 1). The mean value was 17.5 ml/100g/min (range: 9.5 - 28.5). A significant difference was also found when a comparison was made between CBV in the pericontusional area and the adjacent normal brain (2.3 ml/100g compared to 4.6 ml/100g) ($p < 0.001$, Wilcoxon matched paired rank test). CBV was decreased to 50% in the pericontusional zones.

Table 1. Mean CT number, CBF and CBV values in edematous pericontusional and non-edematous contralateral areas, respectively as determined by CT-scan and Stable Xenon-CT, in 11 patients.

	CT number *(HU)*	CBF *(ml/100g/min)*	CBV *(ml/100g)*
Edema	45.6 ± 4.8	17.5 ± 4.0	2.3 ± 0.4
No edema	54.0 ± 4.3	39.9 ± 11.2	4.6 ± 0.8
Normal*	-	53 ± 13	6.1 ± 0.9

* = global values in normal volunteers.

Figure 1:

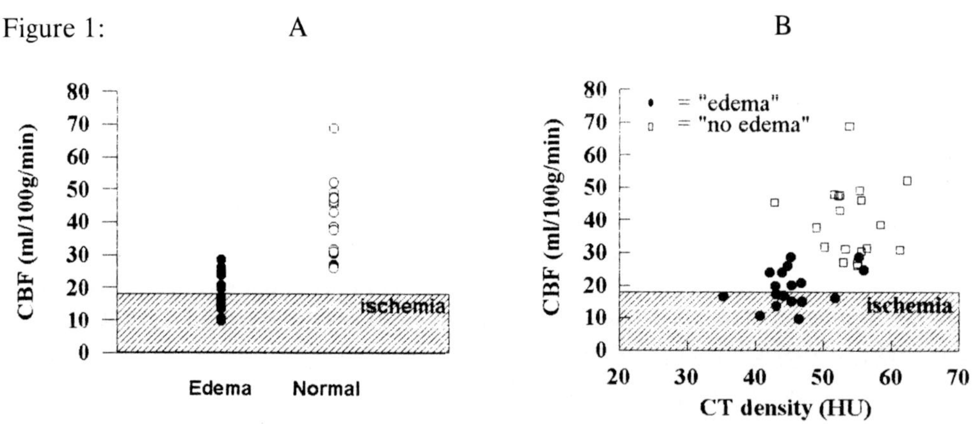

A. The difference in HU between the pericontusional and normal areas was highly significant ($p < 0.01$). B. Flow values in the pericontusional areas were less than half the values seen in the normal areas. Most of the areas adjacent to contusions had CBF values below the threshold for ischemic damage (CBF ≤ 18 ml/100g/min)

Figure 2: Xenon-CT CBF mapping of peri-contusional blood flow.

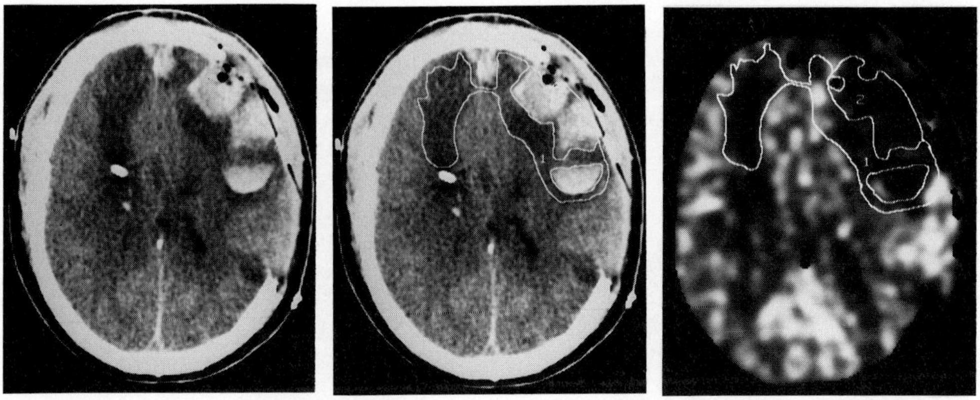

Left panel: Structural CT demonstrating large right frontal contusion and contralateral edema.
Center panel: CT image processing technique used to outline low density areas.
Right panel: Template transferred from structural CT (center) to Xenon-CT CBF map. Mean CBF in the edematous area (labeled 1 on the CBF map) = 16.4ml/100gm/min for this patient.

Ultrastructural vascular changes

All tissue samples showed preservation of neural, glial, and vascular elements. The majority of samples showed evidence of pronounced glial swelling. This was typically found in perivascular loci which revealed distended glial foot processes. Frequently, the adjacent vascular lumina were narrowed. While not all microvessels were affected equally, similar changes were observed throughout the tissue. Erythrocytes and leucocytes were frequently observed within the vascular lumina; however, neither platelet activation nor thrombosis were observed in the specimens studied. Despite the occurrence of this dramatic perivascular swelling and the apparent narrowing of the vascular lumina, the endothelium appeared intact and the endothelial cells were closely adherent to the underlying basal lamina (Figure 3).

Figure 3: A B

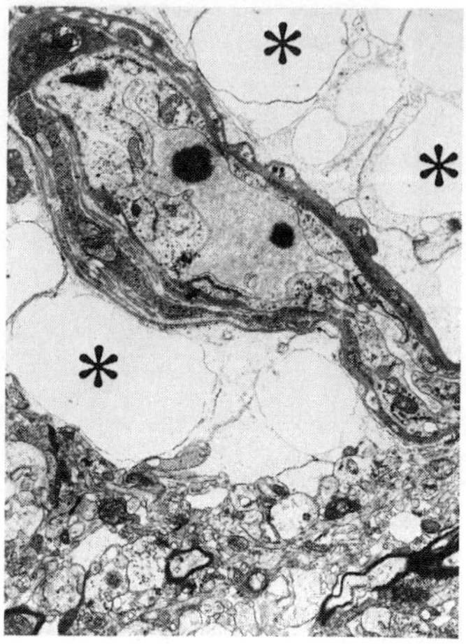

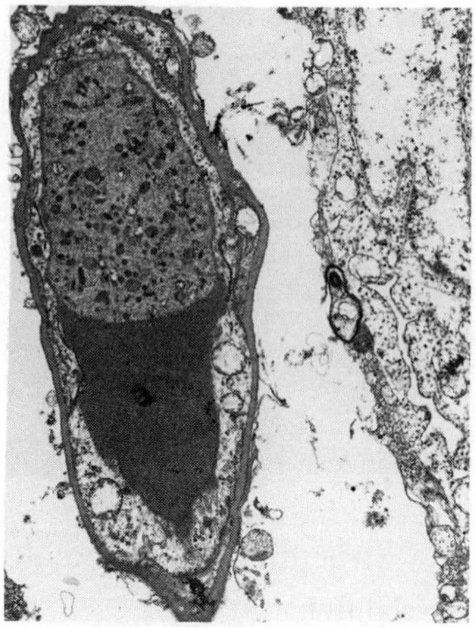

A: In this micrograph prominent perivascular glial swelling is seen. Note the presence of numerous expanded and disrupted astrocytic foot processes (*) which surround this compressed vessel displaying luminal narrowing (×6000). B: This electron micrograph again demonstrates dramatic perivascular glial swelling, which, in this case, is associated with a vessel whose lumen is packed by a circulating leukocyte and red blood cell (×6900).

DISCUSSION

These stable Xenon-CT CBF studies clearly demonstrate profound reductions in blood flow surrounding focal cerebral contusions. Both the CBV data, and the microvessel morphology studies, support the concept that microvascular compromise, via compression and/or leucocytic plugging, is a major factor causing this peri-lesional hypoperfusion. This accords with previous ultrastructural morphology studies, in humans and animal models of focal contusion [36,12]. This study also demonstrates a close relationship between the occurrence of peri-contusional edema and regional CBF. Moreover, CBF did not increase with time, in those patients in whom CBF was measured serially. We postulate that the demonstration of low density areas on CT, after trauma therefore indicates ongoing severe ischemia, and that resection of this tissue, if clinically necessary to control ICP, is indicated. Further studies in these focally injured patients as well as in animal models should be directed at identification of the factors which lead to astrocytic swelling, and polymorphonuclear leukocyte activation.

REFERENCES

1. Ribas GC, Jane JA (1992) Traumatic contusions and intracerebral hematomas. J Neurotrauma 9, supplement 2: s265-s278

2. Bullock R, Maxwell WL, Graham DI, Teasdale GM Adams JH (1991) Glial swelling following human cerebral contusion: an ultrastructural study. J Neurol Neurosurg Psychiatry 54: 427-434

3. MacPherson P, Graham DI (1977) Correlation between angiographic findings and the ischaemia of head injury. J Neurol Neurosurg Psychiatry 41: 122-127

4. Fatouros PP, Schröder ML, Muizelaar JP, Cothran SJ, Shedden A, Kuta AJ (1994) Dynamic CT and cerebral blood volume. In: Tomonaga M, Yonas H, Tanaka A (eds) Xenon/CT CBF in clinical decision making. Mount Hisko, New York, Futura Publishing Company (In Press)

5. Bullock R, Sakas D, Patterson J, Wyper D, Hadley D, Maxwell W (1992) Early post-traumatic cerebral blood flow mapping: correlation with structural damage after focal injury. Acta Neurochir Suppl 55: 14-17

6. Sutton R, Lescaudron L Stein D: Unilateral cortical contusion in the rat (1993) Vascular disruption and temporal development of cortical necrosis. J Neurotrauma 10: 135-149

7. Jones TH, Morawetz RB, Crowell RM, Marcoux FW, Fitzgibbon SJ, DeGirolami U (1981) Thresholds of focal cerebral ischemia in awake monkeys. J Neurosurg 54: 773-782

8. Astrup J, Siesjö BK, Symon L (1981) Thresholds in cerebral ischemia - the ischemic penumbra. Stroke 12: 723-725

Influences of Bone Defect to Cerebral Blood Flow and Metabolism

K. YOSHIDA[1], M. FURUSE[2], H. KUCHIWAKI[1], S. INAO[1], and K. SUGITA[1]

[1] Department of Neurosurgery, School of Medicine, Nagoya University, Japan
[2] Nakatsugawa MGH, Nagoya, Japan

INTRODUCTION

Prolonged improvement in neurological and mental disorders have been seen after only cranioplasty in patients initially treated with external decompression for high intracranial pressure. The objective of this study was, using Xenon CT and 31P Magnetic Resonance Spectroscopy (MRS), to evaluate Cerebral Blood Flow (CBF) and cerebral metabolism before and after cranioplasty.

MATERIALS AND METHODS

Cerebral blood flow and metabolism were evaluated in seven patients (55 - 65 years old) before and after cranioplasty, who had undergone external decompression for uncontrollable intracranial hypertension after acute subarachnoid hemorrhage. They had no neurological deficits and abnormal intensity areas in magnetic resonance imagings before cranioplasty.

Xenon CT system was conducted with a TCT 900s CT scanner (Toshiba Co.Ltd.) and the AZ-723, closed rebreathing xenon inhaler (Anzai Sogyo Co.Ltd.). CBF mapping was created by the end tidal chamber method while the patient inhaled 30% xenon gas over 6 minutes. Region of Interests (ROIs) were placed on the hemisphere, cortex, thalamus, and putamen.

31P MR spectroscopy was performed on a 1.5 tesla whole body system (Shimadzu Co.Ltd.) and the method used to obtain 31P MR spectra was 1D/ISIS ((One Dimensional Image - Selected In - vivo Spectroscopy:Time of repetition (TR) = 2 sec, Average = 400 - 600, Thickness of Volume of interest (VOI) = 30 - 50 mm)) [1,2]. The VOI was placed in the almost whole hemisphere sagittally including grey and white matter, usually at the level of the basal ganglia. Quantification of the spectra was performed by means of area measurements using automated area analysis. The convolution difference method [3] was used to remove the broad signals derived from bone and from tissues in the inhomogeneous profiled magnetic field. In this study, we calculated the ratio of phosphocreatine to inorganic phosphate (PCr/Pi), which is a sensitive ratio that indicates cerebral energy depletion [4], and β-ATP. Tissue pH was calculated from the chemical shift of inorganic phosphate [5, 6].

RESULTS

The CBF values were normalized from 45.4+/-10.2 to 57.4+/-10.2 ml/100g/min. ($p<0.05$) in the thalamus and increased from 27.2+/-3.5 to 29.7+/-3.8 ml/100g/min. in the hemisphere after cranioplasty, on the side with bone defect. Furthermore, PCr/Pi ratio extremely improved from 2.54+/-0.46 to 3.0+/-0.25 ($p<0.05$) after cranioplasty.

Also, on the normal side, the value of CBF and PCr/Pi increased significantly ($p<0.05$) after cranioplasty, and it was speculated this was due to transneural suppression.

Brain tissue pH and β-ATP were unchanged after cranioplasty on the both side.

DISCUSSION

Some patients who underwent external decompression due to acute high intracranial pressure can improve prolonged neurological and mental disorders after only cranioplasty [7]. It was interpreted that EEG changes had well coincided with clinical course. Tabaddor [8] presented that a patient developed contralateral weakness 4 months after surgery which was recovered following cranioplasty. He explained the presumptive mechanism was a gradient between atmospheric and intracranial pressure. Stula [9] suggested the cicatricial changes occurring between the cortex, dura, and the skin, which exerts pressure on the skull contents. Some authors have reported the indication for cranioplasty in addition to cosmetic problem was the post - traumatic syndrome such as headache, dizziness, fatigability, mental depression, and so on [10,11,12]. In animal experiment, craniectomy in the normal brain decreased ICP and increased brain compliance, but facilitated brain edema formation [13,14,15]. In our observations, patients with bone defect had low CBF and metabolism, although they had no neurological deficits and abnormal intensity areas in magnetic resonance imagings before cranioplasty. Possibly brain deformity and unusual condition such as low ICP due to bone defect lead to brain metabolism suppression and subsequently CBF reduction. Furthermore, it is noteworthy that PCr/Pi ratios were suppressed in the contralateral side of hematoma. We speculated this was transneural suppression, because patients had no midline shift on the MR imagings.These results suggest that cranioplasty should be done as soon as the edema has disappeared, since the bone defect itself can decrease CBF and suppress cerebral metabolism.

REFERENCES

1. Ordidge RJ, Connelly A, Lohman LAB (1986) Image-selected in vivo spectroscopy (ISIS). A new technique for spatially selective NMR spectroscopy. J Magn Reson 66:283-294
2. Ordidge RJ, Bowley RM, Mchale G (1988) A general approach to selection of multiple cubic volume elements using the ISIS technique. Magn Reson Med 8:323-331
3. Gonzalez-Mendez R, Litt L, Koretsky AP, Colditz J, Weiner MW, James TL (1984) Comparison of 31 P NMR spectra of in vivo rat brain using convolution difference and saturation with a surface coil. Source of the broad component in the brain spectrum. J Mag reson 57:526-533
4. Yoshida K, Marmarou A (1991) Effects of tromethamine and hyperventilation on brain injury in the cat. J Neurosurg 74:87-965.
5. Petroff OAC, Prichard JW, Behar KL, Alger JR, Hollander JA, Shulman RG (1985) Cerebral intracellular pH by 31 P nuclear magnetic resonance spectroscopy. Neurology 35:781-788
6. Thulborn KR, Boulay GH, Duchen LW, Radda G (1982) A 31 P nuclear magnetic resonance in vivo study of cerebral ischemia in the gerbil. J Cereb Blood Flow Metab 2:299-306
7. Yamaura A, Makino H (1977) Neurological deficits in the presence of th sinking skin flap following decompressive craniectomy. Neurol Med Chir 17 : 43 - 53
8. Tabaddor K, LaMorgese J (1976) Complication of a large cranial defect. Case report. J Neurosurg 44 : 506 - 508
9. Stula D (1985) Intrakranielle druckmessung bei grobn schadelkalottendefekten. Neurochirurgia 28 : 164 - 169
10. Gardner WJ (1945) Closure of defects of the skull with tantalum. Surg Gynecol Obstet 80 : 303 - 312
11. Grant FC, Norcross NC (1939) Repair of cranial defects by cranioplasty. Ann Surg 110: 488 - 512
12. Woodhall MB (1945) Tantalum cranioplasty for war wounds of the skull. Ann Surg 121 : 649 - 668
13. Shapiro K, Fried A, Takei F, Kohn I (1985) Effect of the skull and dura on neural axis pressure - volume relationships and CSF hydrodynamics. J Neurosurg 63 : 76 - 81
14. Hatashita S, Koike J, Sonokawa T, Ishii S (1985) Cerebral edema associated with craniectomy and arterial hypertension. Stroke 16 : 661 - 668
15. Hatashita S, Hoff JT (1987) The effect of craniectomy on the biomechanics of normal brain. J Neurosurg 67 : 573 - 578

Diffuse Axonal Injury (DAI): Utility of MRI, ICP, $SvJO_2$

L. Beretta[1], G. Citerio[1], A. Dell'Acqua[1], L. Sacchi[1], M. Cenzato[2], and N. Anzalone[3]

[1] NeuroIntensive Care Unit, [2] Department of Neurosurgery, [3] Department of Neuroradiology, IRCCS Hospital S. Raffaele, via Olgettina 60, 20122 Milano, Italy

INTRODUCTION

The term "Diffuse Axonal Injury (DAI) is used to describe a situation of post traumatic coma with absence of mass lesions or ischemic insults. Admission CT scan can be normal or show typical findings like small contusion or hemorrhages of the corpus callosum, basal ganglia, periventricular and subcortical regions.
In our region, Lombardia, (population 9 million) there are available only 48 intensive care beds dedicated to neurosurgical patients. For these reasons, a great number of patients suffering from head injury are admitted to general hospitals or to general ICU if they did not present, at the first CT scan, lesions that need surgical evacuation. The number of patients that are not admitted in dedicate Neuro Intensive Care [F. Procaccio, unpublished data] is about 20% of the total number of severe head injury, every year. This group of patients are considered to be at low risk of developing an intracranial hematoma or intracranial hypertension.
The aim of this study was to determine if specific monitoring can differentiate evaluation or medical therapy.
We studied:

- MRI images that can be useful to detect deep lesions and non hemorragic contusion,
- ICP to know the exact risk to develop high ICP (HICP),
- Cerebral extraction of oxygen via continuous monitoring of the jugular bulb saturation ($SvjO_2$) to identify alterations in the ratio between metabolic demand and supply ($CMRO_2$/CBF).

MATERIAL AND METHODS

We selected severe head injury patients admitted to our department from January 1991 to August 1993 (20 males, 3 females; medium age 24 yrs; range 17-44 yrs) which fulfilled these inclusion criteria:

- GCS of 8 or less (no eye opening, no obeying orders for at least 6 hours),
- CT scan normal or without mass lesions, midline shift, obliterated or compressed perimesencephalic cisterns. The diagnostic categories of all the patients were: Diffuse injury I and Diffuse Injury II [1],
- No hypotension (defined as systolic blood pressure $\leq$ 90 mmHg),
- No hypoxia (defined as $PaO_2 < 60$ mmHg),
- Admission to hospital 4 hours post-trauma.

All the patients underwent first CT scan within 4 hours post-trauma and an MRI study within 48 hours post-trauma. Patients with a GCS of 7 or less (12/23 patients) ICP and $SvjO_2$ were continuously recorded. ICP monitor, arterial pressure monitor and fiberoptic jugular catheters were connected to a A/D converter (Mac Lab 4, World Precision Instruments, Saratoga FL) and to an Apple Macintosh personal computer to allow storage and trend analysis in digital form.

The patients were managed in a 5 bed Neuro Intensive Care Unit. Ventilation was selected to maintain a $PaO_2 > 100$ mmHg and $PaCO_2$ more than 30 and less than 40 mmHg. Blood pressure was maintained to permit a CPP > 70. Early physiotherapy and enteral nutrition was started.
All MR examinations were performed on a 1.5 T unit (Magnetom, Siemens), using spin-echo (SE) sequences with 550/14 (TR/TE) and 2500/15-90 and a matrix size of 256x256; axial and sagittal sections, both T1 and T2 weighted, with slice thickness of 5 and 6 mm were obtained in all cases.
CT studies were performed on a Somatom HiQ (Siemens) obtaining axial sections of 8 mm thickness.
Essential monitoring included EKG, BP, $EtCO_2$, SpO_2; all were ventilated and sedated.
Intracranial Pressure was measured in patients with a GCS < 8 (12/23 patients).
We utilized 5 intraparenchimal devices (Camino fiber optic transducers, Camino Laboratories, San Diego, California), 4 ventricular (Camino fiber optic transducers and fluid filled catheters) and 3 subdural catheters (fluid filled catheters). Arterial pressure was measured with a 4F intra-arterial cannula. CPP was calculated (MAP-ICP). Continuos monitoring of $SvjO_2$ was provided with a 4 F fiber optic device (Oximetrics Abbott, Abbott Laboratories, North Chicago, Illinois). The right internal jugular vein was retrograde cannulated percutaneously and the position of the catheter tip was confirmed by 2 projection x-ray film. Twelve hourly the catheter was calibrated in vivo. We recorded the $SvjO_2$ value only if adequate light intensity was present (indicator of the correct position of the catheter tip).

RESULTS

CT scan was performed within 4 hours of injury in all the patients.
CT (assessed by a neuroradiologist) was normal in 3 patients (Diffuse Injury I) and was not normal in 2 (Diffuse Injury II).

TABLE 1. Number of patients in relation to the lesions detected with CT and MRI

	CT	MRI
CORTICAL - SUBCORTICAL	17	20
PERIVENTRICULAR AND BASAL GANGLIA	3	10
CORPUS CALLOSUM	8	20
BRAINSTEM	3	11
SUBARACNOID BLOOD	9	9
CEREBELLAR	0	1

MR studies demonstrated lesion in all the patients (table 1) and the difference in the ability to detect hemorragic and non hemorragic contusion is reassumed in Fig. 1.

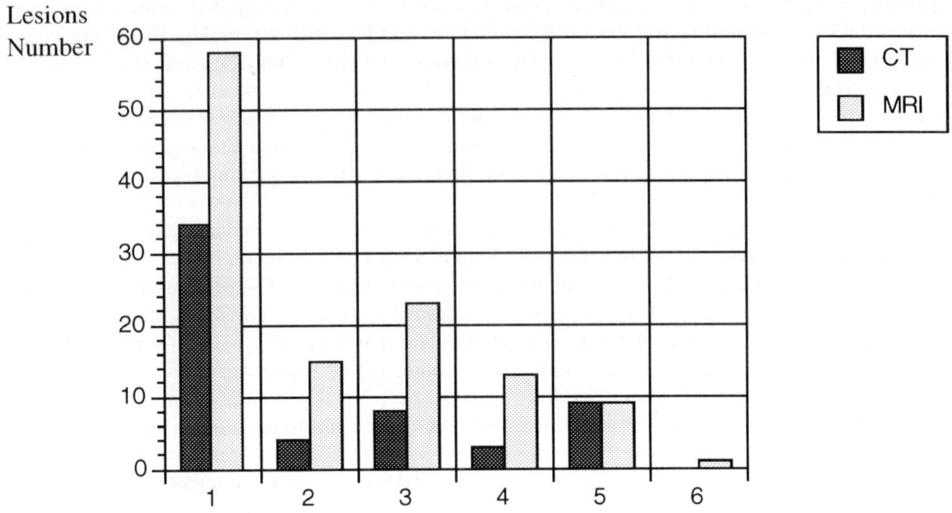

Fig. 1. Difference in number of lesions in different sites.
1= Cortical+Subcortical; 2= Periventricular and basal ganglia;
3= Corpus Callosum; 4= Brainstem; 5= Subaracnoid blood; 6= Cerebellar

Mean monitoring time of intracranial pressure was 4±2 days. Total monitoring time was 1255 hours. 11/12 patients did not demonstrate ICP value higher than 20 mmHg for more than 15 minutes. All the episodes of abnormal ICP, the evidentiate causes (pain, nursing, agitation, posture) were identified and treated with success.
One patients developed episodes of HICP (3 episodes with values higher than 20 for more than 15 minutes requiring specific therapy, mannitol infusion).
Mean monitoring time of SjO_2 was 6±1 days. Only 55% of the total monitoring time had a correct intensity signal and was evaluated. Severe desaturations (< 0.5) were not recorded.
Outcome was determined at 6 months according to the Glasgow Outcome Scale (GOS): 16 patients had good recovery , 7 had moderate disability.

DISCUSSION

Magnetic Resonance appears to be sensitive in detecting areas of brain injury. This study involved MR abnormalities during the acute phase of trauma in patients in coma, with incongruous radiological findings (CT). Great differences in lesions are detected in deep sites as: basal ganglia, corpus callosum and brainstem.
Intracranial Pressure was studied in patients with normal CT or without sign of HICP (mass lesion, shift, absent or compressed basal cisterns and if many authors conclude that the risk of developing intracranial hypertension is low [2, 3], not all data are in agreement [4]. In our group the incidence of HICP is low, but our patients have specific characteristics: not present hypotension, hypoxia, delay in hospital admission [5].

$SvjO_2$, appears to be useful to predict the ratio between $CMRO_2$ and CBF [6]. In this group we did not observe important desaturation phenomena (< 0.5) that had to be treated aggressively. $SvJO_2$ in these patients can lead to optimize ventilation and can be useful in detection of incorrect general management.

REFERENCES

1. Marshall LF, Marshall BS, Klauber MR, Clark MVB, Eisenberg HM, Jane JA, Luerssen TG, Marmarou A, Foulkes MA (1991) A new classification of head injury based on computerized tomography. J Neurosurg 75, S 14 - 20.
2. Narayan RK, Kishore PRS, Becker DP (1982) Intracranial Pressure: to monitor or not to monitor? A review of our experience with severe head injury. J Neurosurg 56: 650-659.
3. Kobayashi S, Yokota H, and Nakazawa S (1993) ICP monitoring of severe diffuse axonal injury. In Avezaat CJJ, van Eijndhoven JHM, Maas AIR, and Tans JTJ (eds) Intracranial Pressure VIII. Springer, Berlin Heidelberg New York Tokyo, pp 564-5673.
4. O' Sullivan MG, Statham PF, Jones PA, Miller JD, Dearden NM, Piper IR, Anderson SI, Housley A, Andrews PJ, Midgley S, Corrie J, Toker JI, Sellar R (1994) Role of intracranial pressure monitoring in severely head-injured patients without signs of intracranial hypertension on initial computerized tomography. J Neurosurg 80: 46-50.
5. Marmaru A, Anderson R, Ward JD, Choi SC, Jung HF, Eisenberg HM, Foulkes MA, Marshall LF, Jane A (1991) Impact of ICP instability and hypotension on outcome in patients with severe head trauma. J Neurosurg 75, S 59- 66.
6. Robertson CS, Narayan RK, Gokaslan ZL (1989) Cerebral arteriovenous oxygen difference as an estimate of cerebral blood flow in comatose patients. J Neurosurgery 70: 222-230.

CSF Dynamics in Increased ICP on Cardiac-Gated Cine MR: MR Signal Analysis of Intracranial CSF Flow in Hydrocephalus

C. KADOWAKI[1,2], M. HARA[2], K. TAKEUCHI[2], and I. SAITO[2]

[1] Division of Neurosurgery, Kugayama Hospital, Kita-Karasuyama, Setagaya, Tokyo, 157 Japan
[2] Department of Neurosurgery, Kyorin University School of Medicine, Shinkawa, Mitaka, Tokyo, 181 Japan

SUMMARY

To evaluate the changes in intracranial CSF dynamics in increased ICP, we studied the changes in CSF flows within ventricles on cine MR imaging utilizing MR signal analysis in acute progressive hydrocephalus, either non-communicating or communicating, comparing them with normal subjects. In aqueductal stenosis, the MR signal ratios [SRs] of CSF within the lateral ventricles and the third ventricle decreased during a cardiac systole, and fluctuated greater than in cases of normal CSF circulation, resulting from the pulsatile and forceful turbulant CSF flow. In the fourth ventricle, however, the MR SRs of CSF fluctuated randomly with no correlation between them in the third ventricle indicating obstructed aqueduct. In communicating hydrocephalus, the MR SRs fluctuated in the same patterns as in normal CSF circulation only with greater amplitude. Chronological changes during an R-R interval in relative MR signal ratios of CSF within ventricles on cine MR images can act as an indicator of abnormal intracranial CSF dynamics in increased ICP.

INTRODUCTION

In spite of the great deal of research to clarify the intracranial and intraspinal cerebrospinal fluid [CSF] flow dynamics, it has not yet been satisfactorily evaluated. Magnetic resonance [MR] imaging non-invasively provides visual images of normal and abnormal intracranial and intraspinal CSF flow [1, 2]. Of particular importance, regardless of some limitations presented later, cardiac-gated cine MR imaging can demonstrate the actual pulsatile CSF flow stimulated by cardiac pulsation [3, 4].

We, therefore, have utilized the MR signal intensities [SIs] and the relative MR signal intensity ratios [SRs] of CSF within ventricles to fat tissue on cine MR imaging to analyse the intracranial pulsatile CSF flow [5, 6].

To evaluate the changes in intracranial CSF dynamics in increased intracranial pressure [ICP], we studied the changes in MR SIs and relative MR SRs of CSF in cases of acute progressive hydrocephalus, either non-communicating or communicating, comparing them with normal CSF circulation in normal ICP.

METHODS AND MATERIALS

Cine MR study and MR signal analysis

Cine MR images were performed on a 0.5-T MR system (MRT-50A, Toshiba Medical Co., Tokyo), utilizing a cardiac gated, field echo study in the mid-sagittal plane including the aqueduct of Sylvius. The pulse sequence was TR 45-48 msec (determined by the R-to-R interval) and TE 14 msec. Multiple images, or "cine frames", in the same plane were obtained during an R-R interval, beginning immediately after the R-wave on electrocardiogram [ECG], and serial successive images were acquired at 50-msec intervals up until about 200 msec before the next R-wave. MR signal analysis was carried out to measure the MR SIs of the CSF within ventricles in the regions of interest [ROI] on each cine image. We have adopted the analysis technique of utilizing the relative SRs of MR signal intensities of the CSF to the fat tissue within the skull bone marrow as well as the MR SIs in each image. Chronological changes in MR SIs and SRs during a cardiac cycle are compared to the actual CSF flow visualized on real cine images [5]. When analysing, combining and comparing the changes in MR SIs and SRs of CSF during a cardiac cycle, the real delay time scales from the R-wave have been normalized to the same percentile within an R-R interval among patients with different heart beats [6, 7].

Subjects

We examined a total of nine cases: five healthy adults with normal CSF circulation with a mean age of 52.6 years; two patients, a 12-year-old girl and a 8-year-old boy, with obstructive hydrocephalus caused by non-neoplastic aqueductal stenosis; and other two patients, a 23-year-old female and a 38-year-old male, with acute progressive communicating hydrocephalus. Upon the investigation, the ICP values in cases of hydrocephalus had increased to more than 15-20 Torr.

RESULTS

1) Aqueductal stenosis: The changes in MR SRs fluctuated in quite different patterns as compared to those with normal CSF flow. MR SRs in the lateral ventricles decreased immediately after the trigger of an R-wave to a point at 45-50% of an R-R interval due to forceful CSF flow to the foramina of Monro and consequent CSF turbulence within the lateral ventricle caused by ventricular constriction [Fig. 1].

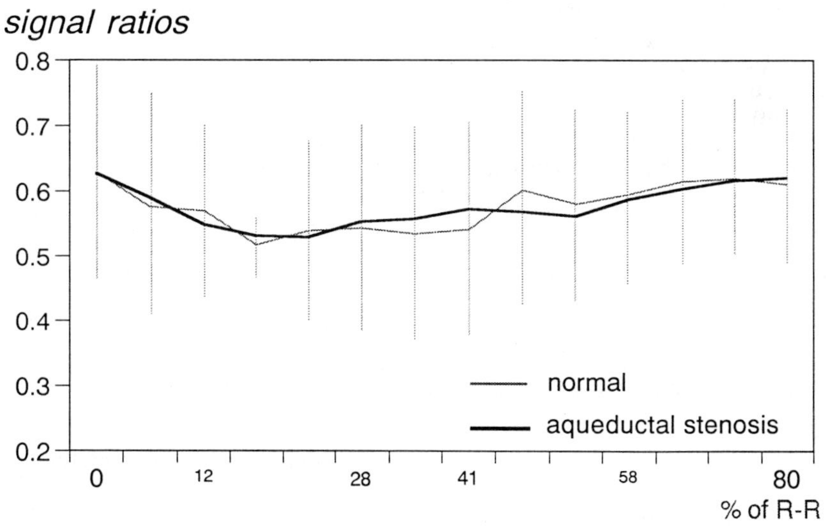

Fig. 1. Changes in MR signal ratios of CSF within lateral ventricles in aqueductal stenosis.

MR SRs in the third ventricle decreased at 10-40% of the R-R interval due to downward CSF flow during cardiac systole, and decreased again from late cardiac systole to diastole due to caudal CSF flow and CSF turbulence/stagnancy within the third ventricle. In the fourth ventricle, MR SRs fluctuated independently of the changes in MR SRs in the third ventricle, and reduced during cardiac systole correlating to upward flow of CSF through the foramina of Luschka and the foramen of Magendie [Fig. 2].

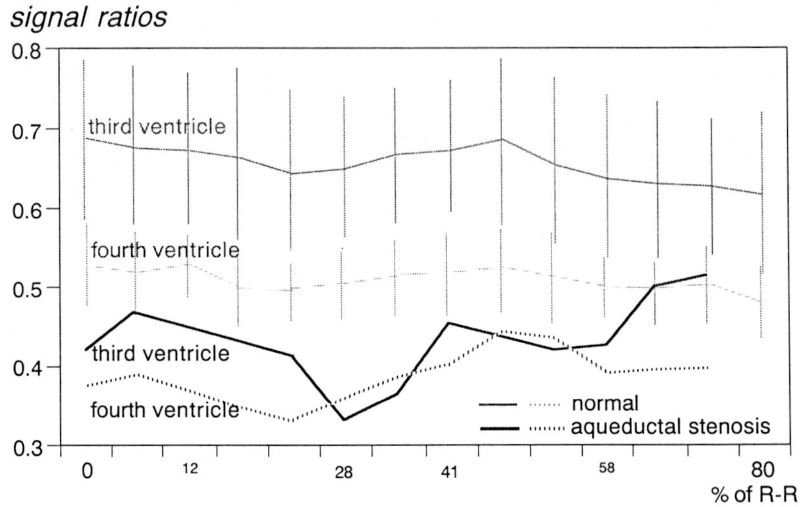

Fig. 2. Changes in MR signal ratios of CSF within third ventricle and fourth ventricle in aqueductal stenosis.

Finally MR SRs in the ventricles also fluctuated much greater than those in cases of normal CSF circulation.
2) Communicating hydrocephalus: The changes in MR SRs in the ventricles were similar to those in normal CSF circulation, but MR SRs fluctuate greater than those in normal CSF circulation [Fig. 3 & 4].

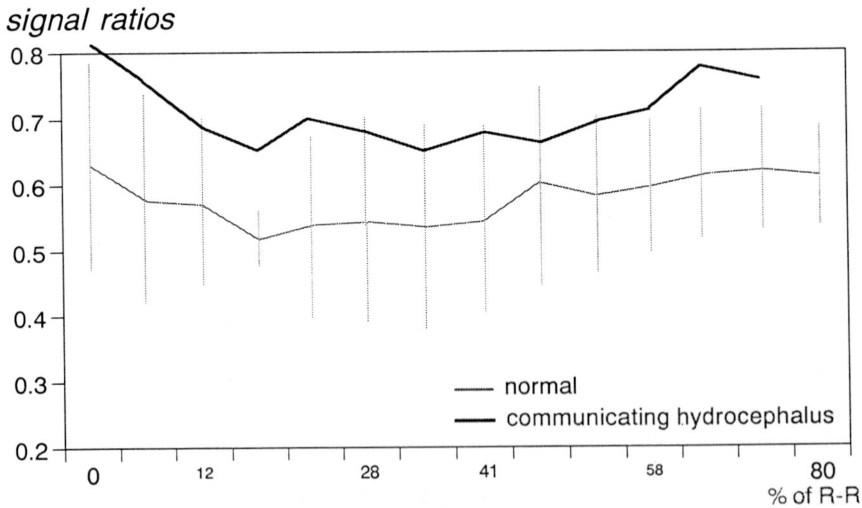

Fig. 3. Changes in MR signal ratios of CSF within lateral ventricles in communicating hydrocephalus.

Especially in the fourth ventricle, the changes in MR SRs are related to the strong CSF streams which flow upward during early cardiac systole and downward during cardiac diastole.

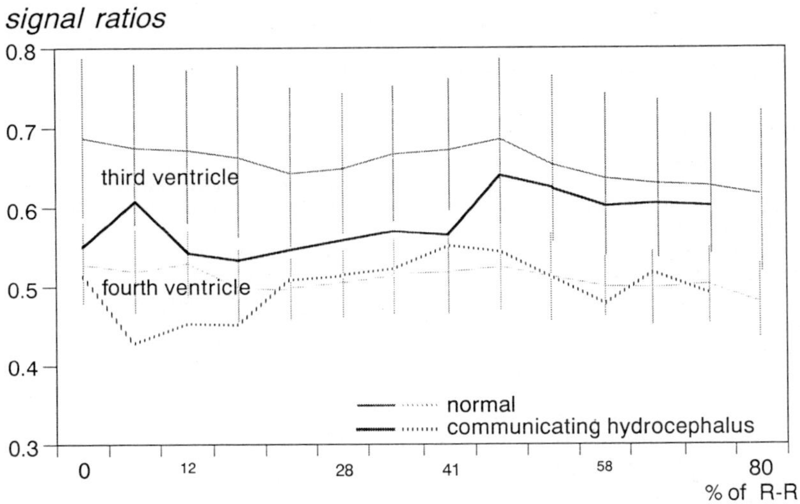

Fig. 4. Changes in MR signal ratios of CSF within third ventricle and fourth ventricle in communicating hydrocephalus.

DISCUSSION

Since the 1980s, which marked the start of the MR era, MR imaging, which permits reassessment of human physiology, can have been used to evaluate the intracranial and intraspinal CSF flow non-invasively [8]. Up to now, cardiac-gated cine MR imaging has been one of the standard techniques to evaluate intracranial pulsatile CSF flow during a cardiac cycle in normal and abnormal conditions. Because, although CSF flow within ventricles is complex and multidirectional, cine-MR imagings can noninvasively provide visual images of the pulsatile CSF flow within ventricles [7, 9, 10] resulting from cardiac pulsations causing brain expansions/retractions and ventricular constrictions [4, 11, 12].
To clarify the intracranial CSF flow objectively on cine MR images, we have utilized a qualitative analysis, analysing changes in MR SRs of CSF within ventricles to fat during a cardiac cycle [5, 6], and we have normalized the delay time with regard to the gating trigger of each frame [6]. In this study, we compared normal CSF flow and altered CSF flow in hydrocephalus by a qualitative analysis on cine MR images. Our results showed that the derangement of CSF flow within ventricles in cases of obstructive hydrocephalus with increased ICP led to greater fluctuations in MR SRs related to strong turbulent and stagnant CSF flows showing different chronological patterns in an R-R interval compared to those in normal conditions. In particular, the changes in MR SRs within the fourth ventricle in cases of aqueductal stenosis had no correlation to those within the third ventricle. These findings clearly indicated no CSF flow through the aqueduct of sylvius from the third ventricle to the fourth ventricle. And, in progressive communicating hydrocephalus with increased ICP, the MR SRs also fluctuated greater than those for normal circulation, which indicated the strong CSF streams within ventricles resulting from greater brain pulsations and ventricular constrictions.

CONCLUSION

The relative MR signal intensity ratios of CSF within ventricles fluctuate in correlation to the intracranial pulsatile CSF flows during a cardiac cycle.

In conclusion, the chronological changes in MR signal ratios of CSF within ventricles to fat on cine MR images act as an indicator of the pathophysiology of intracranial CSF dynamics.

REFERENCES

1. Quencer RM, Donovan Post MJ, Hinks RS (1990) Cine MR in the evaluation of normal and abnormal CSF flow: intracranial and intraspinal studies. Neuroradiol 32: 371-391.
2. Quencer RM (1992) Intracranial CSF flow in pediatric hydrocephalus: Evaluation with cine-MR imaging. AJNR 13: 601-608.
3. Schroth G, Klose U (1989) MRI of CSF flow in normal pressure hydrocephalus. Psychiatry Research 29: 289-290.
4. Kadowaki C, Hara M, Numoto M, Takeuchi K, Saito I (1993) CSF dynamics on cine MR. Video J Jpn Neurosurg 1.
5. Kadowaki C, Hara M, Numoto M, Takeuchi K, Saito I (1993) Qualitative analysis of intracranial CSF flow on cine-MR imaging, with special reference to signal ratio of CSF to fat tissue. Nerv Syst in Child (Shoni no Noshinkei, Jpn) 18: 45-52.
6. Kadowaki C, Hara M, Takeuchi K, Saito I (1994) Intracranial CSF flow on cine-MR: 2. Qualitative analysis in CSF dynamics using MR signal ratio of CSF to fat tissue. Studies in normal conditions and aqueductal stenosis. Nerv Syst in Child (Shoni no Noshinkei, Jpn) 19 (in press).
7. Enzmann DR, Pelc NJ (1991) Normal flow patterns of intracranial and spinal cerebrospinal fluid defined with phase-contrast cine MR imaging. Radiology 178: 467-474.
8. Bradley WG, Kortman KE, Burgoyne B (1986) Flowing cerebrospinal fluid in normal and hydrocephalic stste: appearance on MR images. Radiology 159: 611-616.
9. Ciraola L, Mascalchi M, Bucciolini M, Dal Pazzo G (1990) Fast multiphase MR imaging of aqueductal CSF flow: 1. Study of healthy subjects. AJNR 11: 589-596.
10. Mascalchi M, Ciraolo L, Bucciolini M, Inzitari D, Arnetoli G, Dal Pazzo G (1990) Fast multiphase MR imaging of aqueductal CSF flow: 2. Study in patients with hydrocephalus. AJNR 11: 597-603.
11. Greitz D, Wirestam R, Franck A, Thomsen C, Ståhlberg F (1992) Pulsatile brain movement and associated hydrodynamics studied by magnetic resonance phase imaging. Neuroradiology 34: 370-380.
12. Naidich TP, Altman NR, Gonzalez-Arias SM (1993) Phase contrast cine magnetic resonance imaging: Normal cerebrospinal fluid oscillation and applications to hydrocephalus. Neurosurg Clin N Am 4: 677-705.

Effects of Acetazolamide on Human Brain Tissue pH and CBF

SUGURU INAO[1], HIROJI KUCHIWAKI[1], KAZUO YOSHIDA[1], KENICHIRO SUGITA[1], AKIRA IZAWA[2], and MASAHIRO FURUSE[2]

[1] Department of Neurosurgery, Nagoya University School of Medicine, Japan
[2] Department of Clinical Imaging Laboratory, Nakatsugawa Municipal General Hospital, Japan

INTRODUCTION

Although acetazolamide increases cerebral blood flow, the mechanism for this effect has remained unknown. Acetazolamide blocks carbonic anhydrase in red blood cells, thereby decreasing the removal of CO_2 from blood and tissue. The increased CO_2 in blood and tissue, by inducing extracellular fluid acidosis, may cause cerebral vasodilation [1]. However, other mechanisms have been suggested; acetazolamide may act on carbonic anhydrase within the media of arteries to induce vasodilation [2], or there may be a direct action on vascular smooth muscle, independent of inhibition of carbonic anhydrase [3]. In this experiment, we measured human brain intracellular pH and CBF continuously after intravenous administration of acetazolamide to clarify its vasodilating mechanism.

MATERIALS AND METHODS

Four healthy volunteers (mean age 43 years) were examined for this study. Acetazolamide, 1000 mg in 10 ml distilled water was injected intravenously over 1-2 minutes. CBF and brain intracellular pH were measured in separate experiments by MR imaging and spectroscopy (Shimazdu SMT 150, 1.5 tesla) before and after injection of acetazolamide at 10-minute intervals for 30 minutes. Brain intracellular pH was measured by ^{31}P-MR spectroscopy. The phosphorus spectra were obtained from whole brain, and brain pH was calculated from the chemical shift of inorganic phosphate and Petroff's equation. Within 3 days of the pH measurements, CBF was detected by superior sagittal sinus (SSS) flow velocity using MR-Direct Bolus Imaging (DBI) technique. SSS flow velocity was found to be correlated to hemispheric blood flow obtained by Xe-enhanced CT in our previous report [4]. Arterial blood gas analysis was performed in each experiment.

RESULTS

SSS flow velocity increased immediately after administration of acetazolamide with a peak at 10 minutes (43.7±6.8 cm/sec from 30.9±6.5 cm/sec, mean±SD, $p<0.05$), then gradually decreased, but remained higher than the baseline level for 30 minutes after acetazolamide administration (Table). Brain intracellular pH was 7.11±0.04 before acetazolamide infusion, and slightly increased 10-15 minutes after administration (7.18±0.07), returning to the baseline within 30 minutes. This brain pH increase was not a significant change. Arterial blood gas including pH and PCO_2 did not change significantly during the entire experimental period.

Table: SSS flow velocity (cm/sec), brain pH, and arterial pH after administration of acetazolamide

Time (min)	Velocity	Brain pH	Arterial pH
pre	30.9±6.5	7.11±0.04	7.41±0.01
0	37.6±5.3	7.14±0.05	7.42±0.02
10	43.7±6.8	7.18±0.07	7.42±0.02
20	40.6±7.3	7.14±0.08	7.42±0.02
30	36.5±7.6	7.11±0.04	7.41±0.02

DISCUSSION

In all cases, acetazolamide caused an increase in CBF, but in no case was a fall in brain intracellular pH found; in fact, slight alkalosis was seen in all the spontaneously respiring normal subjects. Our results indicate that there is a some mechanism to maintain nearly stable intracellular pH in the brain after administration of acetazolamide, whether the extracellular pH decreased or not. These results also suggest that the mechanism for the cerebral vasodilating effect of acetazolamide is unrelated to its specific effects as a carbonic anhydrase inhibitor in human brain tissue.

REFERENCES

1. Gotoh F, Meyer JS, Tomita M (1966) Carbonic anhydrase inhibition and cerebral venous blood gases and ions in man. Arch Intern Med 117: 39-46

2. Ehrenreich DL, Burns RA, Alman RW, Fazekas JF (1961) Influence of acetazolamide on cerebral blood flow. Arch Neurol 5: 227-232

3. Hauge A, Nicolaysen G, Thorensen M (1983) Acute effects of acetazolamide on cerebral blood flow in man. Acta Physiol Scand 117: 233-239

4. Inao S, Kuchiwaki H, Sugita K, Izawa A, Yoshida K, Furuse M (1993) Measurements of cerebral venous sinus flow velocity by magnetic resonance imaging. in Brain Edema Symposium 1993, Tokyo, Abstract Book: pp 82

CSF Pulsatile Flow and Intracranial Compliance in Experimental Hydrocephalus—MRI Study

MITSUHITO MASE[1], HAJIME NAGAI[1], TAKASHI MATSUMOTO[1], TSUNEYUKI FUKUSHIMA[1], SHIGEKI OHARA[1], and TATSUO BANNO[2]

[1]Department of Neurosurgery, [2]Department of Radiology, Nagoya City University Medical School, Mizuho-ku, Nagoya, Aichi, 467 Japan

INTRODUCTION

Pulsatile movement of the cerebrospinal fluid (CSF) is well-known and demonstrated easily on magnetic resonance imaging (MRI) as the signal-void phenomenon [1]. However, the meaning of the CSF flow pattern in various intracranial pathologies has not yet been established. CSF pulsatile movement may be a passive motion caused by brain pulsation, and CSF could be an important mediator for transmission of intracranial pressure (ICP) pulse wave to the whole craniospinal cavity. Therefore, it may also be affected by intracranial compliance. To clarify these questions, we analyzed CSF pulsatile flow and the movement of ventricular walls using cine MRI, measuring pulse pressure (PP) of ICP and Pressure-Volume Response (PVR) in Hochward's hydrocephalic model (right-left difference in ventricle size is clearly due to hemicraniectomy) [2].

MATERIALS AND METHODS

Animal preparations

6 adult mongrel dogs of both sexes were anesthetized with intravenous thiopental sodium (10 mg/kg) for endotracheal intubation and intermittent intramuscular ketamine hydrochloride (10 mg/kg) for maintenance. Hydrocephalus was induced by an intracisternal injection of a Kaolin powder solution to the animals which were divided into 4 groups; 1) group A(n=1, control): kaolin induced hydrocephalus without craniectomy, 2) group B(n=1): kaolin induced hydrocephalus with right craniectomy, 3) group C(n=2): kaolin induced hydrocephalus with right craniectomy and dural resection, 4) group D(n=2): kaolin induced hydrocephalus with right craniectomy, dural resection and temporal muscle resection. After these procedures, the animals recovered from the anesthesia.

MRI study

Three weeks after Kaolin injection, electrocardiogram (ECG)-triggered cine MRI using gradient echo (TR 50 msec, TE 11 msec, flip angle 25°) was performed (Shimazu, SMT150, Japan, 1.5 Tesla) under similar anesthesia. Changes in signal intensities every 50 msec after R-wave of ECG were measured by setting the region of interest (ROI) at the bilateral foramen of Monro and the third ventricle in each animal. As a short excitation time (50 msec) makes signal intensities decrease gradually, the ROI was set for the reference in the temporal lobe and the ratio between the signal intensities of the CSF spaces and the reference were calculated to estimate the CSF flow pattern. In group B and D, the pulsatile movement of the lateral ventricular walls were also analyzed using the Dv/Dc ratio (Dv: the distance between the inner and outer wall of the lateral ventricle, Dc: the distance from the midline to the outer edge of the cortex) [Fig.1].

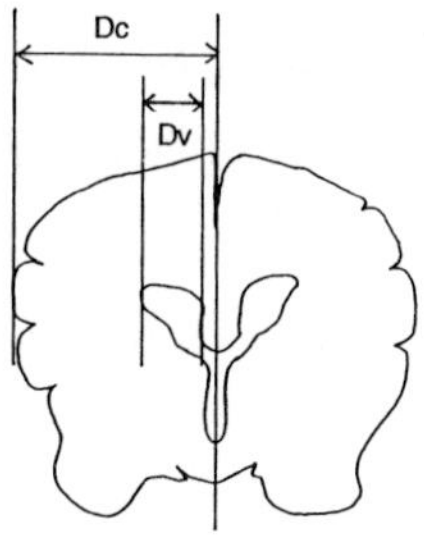

Fig.1. Ventricle / Brain ratio = Dv / Dc X 100. Dv: the distance between the inner and outer wall of the lateral ventricle, Dc: the distance from the midline to the outer edge of the cortex.

ICP measurement

One day after the MRI study, the animals were anesthetized by a similar method, supplemented by the intravenous infusion of alcuronium chloride (0.3 mg/kg/hr) for mechanical ventilation. The ICP pulse wave and PVR [ICP changes after a bolus injection of saline (0.5 ml/sec) into the both lateral ventricles] were measured with two fiber optic ICP sensors (Camino, USA) which were placed in the bilateral lateral ventricles. Arterial blood pressure was continuously monitored. Arterial blood gases were controlled within normal limits by ventilator adjustment.

RESULTS

Ventricular size

The same degree of symmetrical dilatation of the lateral ventricles was identified on MRI in all groups except for group D. Group D alone demonstrated a difference in ventricular size (larger on the side of the craniectomy than on the other).

CSF flow pattern

In group A, CSF flow peaks (about 50 and 200 msec) were not significantly different in each measuring area [Fig.2.left]. Group B showed a similar pattern to group A. However, in group C, CSF flow peaks at the foramen of Monro on the craniectomy side (100 and 250 msec) were delayed in comparison with those on the non-craniectomy side (50 and 150 msec) [Fig.2.right]. The peaks at the third ventricle was also delayed. Group D showed a similar flow pattern to group C.

Pulsatile movement of ventricular walls

The movement of both lateral ventricular walls in group B was symmetrical [Fig.3.left]. However, group D showed that the movements of both ventricles were paradoxical, or that only the ventricle on the craniectomy side had pulsatile movement [Fig.3.right].

ICP and intracranial compliance

There was no significant difference in mean ICP in all groups. The amplitude of PP and PVR decreased stepwise from group A to group D. There was no difference in each area between the right and left lateral ventricles in the amplitude of PP and PVR [Table 1].

Table 1. ICP data of each animal. The right craniectomy was done in group B, C and D. Intracranail pressure (ICP), pulse pressure (PP), pressure-volume response (PVR).

Group	(Animal number)	ICP(mmHg) right	ICP(mmHg) left	PP(mmHg) right	PP(mmHg) left	PVR(mmHg) right	PVR(mmHg) left
A	(No.1)	12.5	11.1	1.7	1.6	47.2	44.8
B	(No.2)	16.5	20.2	1.4	1.3	31	29
C	(No.3)	11.4	13.3	0.6	0.7	9.2	9.2
	(No.4)	13.8	9.3	0.8	0.8	12	12.6
D	(No.5)	1.6	4.1	0.6	0.4		
	(No.6)	11.7	7.9	0.4	0.5	2.8	3.2

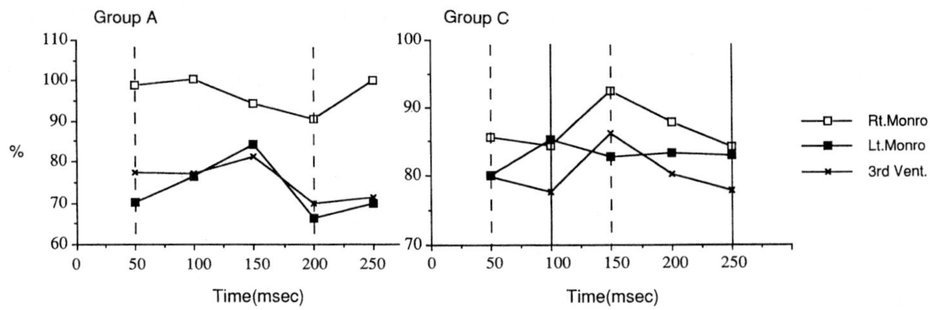

Fig.2. CSF flow pattern at the bilateral foramen of Monro and third ventricle. The changes of the ratio between signal intensity of the CSF spaces and the reference (the temporal lobe) are shown. ***left***: Group A, ***right***: Group C.

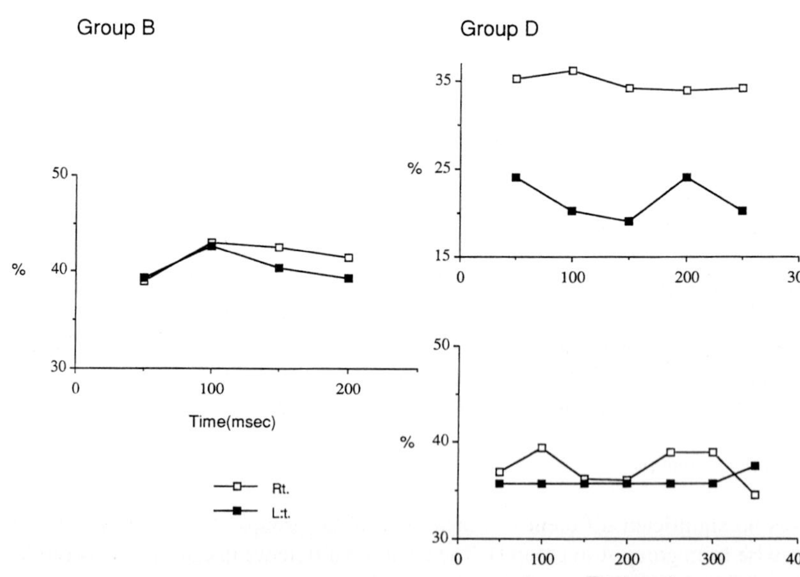

Fig.3. Changes of Dv / Dc ratio. ***left***: Group B, ***right upper***: Group D (animal No.5), ***right lower***: Group D (animal No.6)

DISCUSSION

Though PP is affected by many factors in intracranial pathologies [3], it is thought to be one of the indexes which reflects the intracranial compliance [4]. PVR also reflects the intracranial compliance [5]. In this experiment, the removal of the container of the brain (skull, dura and temporal muscle) made PP and PVR decrease, which meant that the intracranial compliance increased stepwise from group A to D. But the CSF flow pattern did not change step by step. Group C and D similarly had shifts of CSF flow peaks in each measuring area. In this model, the value of the compliance between group B and C could be a break point where the CSF flow pattern might have changed. Considering the paradoxical movement of ventricular walls in group D, CSF may flow to the craniectomy side. This is due to the herniation of the intracranial contents because the elastic coefficient of the craniectomy side is relatively smaller than the other part.

This study could also answer for the question whether a pressure difference existed in CSF spaces in chronic hydrocephalus. As shown in results, there was no difference in ICP, PP and PVR between the right and left ventricles even in the group D which had asymmetric hydrocephalus. This may experimentally prove that there is no pressure difference in CSF spaces in chronic hydrocephalus. If there is no obstruction in CSF spaces and CSF can flow freely, the movement of CSF may be very fast. This compensatory movement of CSF can be detected by MRI as changes of regional CSF flow pattern. There is a possibility that a regional difference of the intracranial compliance can be evaluated by CSF flow study using MRI. However, because of small number of the experimental animals, it cannot be concluded that a general relationship between the compliance and CSF flow pattern in various intracranial pathologies. This will be a subject for the further investigation.

In conclusion, 1) When a container surrounding the brain has a portion where the elastic coefficient is relatively smaller, CSF flow pattern may change, resulting in shifts of regional CSF flow peaks on MRI. 2) If there is a regional difference of intracranial compliance, CSF tends to flow to the region where the compliance is relatively larger in order to compensate for the regional difference of the compliance and keep it constant.

REFERENCES

1. Ohara S, Nagai H, Matsumoto T, Banno T (1988) MR imaging of CSF pulsatory flow and its relation to intracranial pressure. J Neurosurg 69:675-682

2. Hochwald GM, Epstein F, Malhan C, Ransohoff J (1972) The role of the skull and dura in experimental feline hydrocephalus. Dev Med Child Neurol 14(Suppl 27):65-69

3. Mase M, Nagai H, Ueda Y, Matsumoto T, Kamiya K (1993) Influence of intracranial components on epidural pulse pressure. In: Avezaat CJJ, van Eijndhoven JHM, Maas AIR, Tans JThJ (eds) Intracranial Pressure VIII. Springer-Verlag, Berlin, pp 398-401

4. Szewczykowski J, Sliwka S, Kunicki A, Dytko P, Korsak-Sliwka (1977) A fast methods of estimating the elastance of the intracranial system. J Neurosurg 47:19-26

5. Marmarou A, Shulman K, LaMorgese J (1975) Compartmental analysis of compliance and outflow resistance of the cerebrospinal fluid system. J Neurosurg 43:523-534

Session XV:
Causes of Increased or Decreased ICP (4)

Chairmen: G. Salar and T. Asano

The Contribution of Raised ICP and Hypotension to Reduced Cerebral Perfusion Pressure in Severe Brain Injury

ANTHONY MARMAROU[1], ROSS BULLOCK[1], HAROLD F. YOUNG[1], HOWARD M. EISENBERG[2], LAWRENCE MARSHALL[3], JOHN JANE[4], and MARY A. FOULKES[5]

[1] Division of Neurosurgery, Medical College of Virginia, Richmond, VA, USA
[2] University of Maryland Hospital, Baltimore, MD, USA
[3] UCSD Medical Center, San Diego, CA, USA
[4] University of Virginia, Charlottesville, VA, USA
[5] Department of Health & Human Services, National Institutes of Health, Bethesda, MD, USA

INTRODUCTION

Previous studies from the Traumatic Coma Data Bank (TCDB) have demonstrated that the outcome from severe head injury is proportional to the time above 20 mmHg and mean arterial pressure less than 80 mmHg.[1] These studies were among the first to provide substantive data identifying the treatment threshold for ICP of 20 mmHg. However, the observation that head injured patients experienced periods of hypotension during the management period (Fig. 1) was not anticipated, and as a result of these findings, vigilance for hypotensive episodes in the intensive care setting has been heightened during the acute management period. Moreover, the importance of maintaining adequate cerebral perfusion pressure (CPP) in the head injured patient is further emphasized from the studies of Rosner.[2, 3] On the basis of our TCDB studies, the mathematical difference between critical thresholds of 80 mmHg blood pressure and 20 mmHg ICP, which was found to be prognostic, yields a critical perfusion pressure threshold of 60 mmHg.

In the present studies, the objective was to determine which factor, raised ICP or hypotension, was most responsible for the reductions in CPP when these periods occurred during the course of management.

METHODS

The population under study consisted of 386 severely injured patients (GCS < 8) obtained from the combined data banks of TCDB and Medical College of Virginia Neurocore. The demographics of this cohort is described in Table 1. End hour values of ICP and Mean arterial pressure (MAP) were recorded on standardized forms and analyzed by computer. From these respective data bases, we determined the percentage time CPP was less than 60 mmHg during the first 72 hours of monitoring as a function of admission GCS and GOS. Having established these periods of reduced CPP we determined the percentage time average blood pressure (MAP) was below or above 80 mmHg and the percentage time ICP was above or below 20 mmHg.

Table 1 Patient Cohort: TCDB combined with MCV Neurocore (n=386)

Gender :	295 males, 91 females
GCS :	3 (17.4 %), 4-6 (53.9 %), 7-8 (28.2 %)
ETOH :	Positive or suspected (43.3 %),
Age (yrs) :	Mean 30.1, range 0.5-87, S.D. 16.5 yrs
Time from Injury to Hospital :	Mean 3.0 hrs S.D. 4.6
Mass Lesions :	31.3%
Diffuse Injury :	58.8%

RESULTS

The distribution of time CPP was less than 60 mmHg is shown in table 2 for the first three days post injury as a function of the GCS.

Table 2. Percent Time CPP Less than 60 mmHg

GCS	Day 1	Day 2	Day 3
3	18.6	14.6	11.0
4-6	13.8	13.1	13.5
7-8	9.9	7.0	6.4

As can be seen from Table 2, the time below CPP 60 mmHg is related to the severity of injury. Of these periods of low CPP described in Table 2, the percentage time that blood pressure was less than 80 mmHg is shown in Fig. 1.

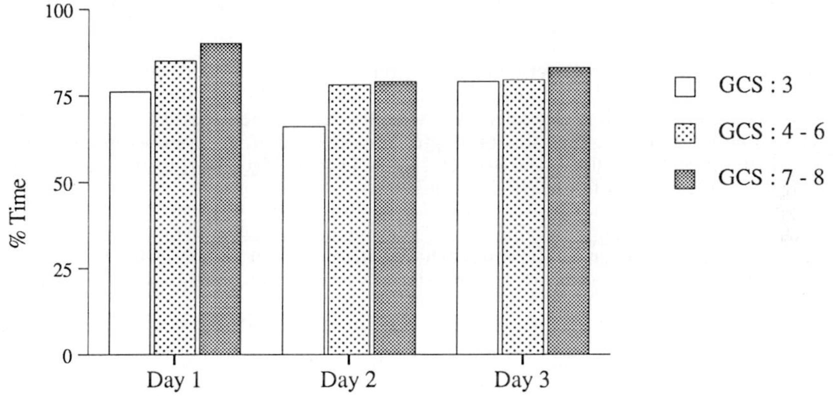

Fig. 1 Percent time that hypotension was associated with CPP< 60 mmHg of periods described in Table 2.

We then processed the percentage of time that ICP was elevated above and below 20 mmHg for patients with CPP less than 60 mmHg and in whom mean blood pressure was less than 80 mmHg. (Fig. 2)

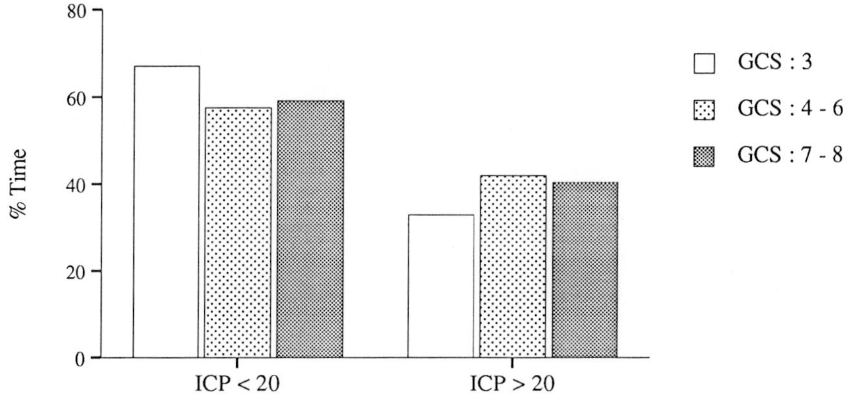

Fig. 2 Percent time that ICP was above and below 20 mmHg for patients in whom CPP < 60 mmHg and BP < 80 mmHg on Day 1.

According to figure 2.0, for those periods of CPP less than 60 mmHg , ICP was elevated above 20 mmHg in approximately 38.6% of the time during the first 24 hours post injury and that ICP remained below 20 mmHg the remaining 61.4 % of the time.

DISCUSSION

This retrospective study shows that the percentage of time that cerebral perfusion pressure is compromised during the acute management period is proportional to the severity of injury as defined by the GCS. For the entire cohort, the percentage of time that CPP was compromised below the critical threshold of 60 mmHg equaled 14.2 percent. Secondly, the incidence of hypotension during these intervals on day 1 ranged from 76.6 % to 89.5 % dependent upon the GCS. Thirdly, from figure 2.0, the incidence of raised ICP during periods of compromised CPP ranged from 33 to 40.7 percent. On the basis of these results, it appears that reduced blood pressure is the predominant cause of reduced CPP and that the hypotension is accompanied by raised ICP approximately 1/3 of the time.

If indeed a CPP of 60 mmHg was critical , these data infer that the critical systolic blood pressure for the head injured patient should be elevated beyond the generally accepted treat threshold of 90 mmHg systolic. The basis for this is as follows. It is generally recognized that the difference in systolic to diastolic arterial pressure is approximately 50 mmHg. With this pulse pressure differential, the systolic pressure corresponding to the critical mean arterial pressure of 80 mmHg equals 114 mmHg. Thus, to maintain a level of 80 mmHg, systolic pressure should not fall below 114 mmHg.

In conclusion, this study suggests that for a CPP threshold of 60 mmHg, arterial pressure should not be allowed to fall below a mean of 80 mmHg which corresponds to a systolic level of 114 mmHg. It suggests that the now accepted definition of hypotension (systolic < 90 mmHg) which is widely used should be altered.

REFERENCES

1. Marmarou A, Anderson RL, Ward JD, Choi SC, Young HF, Eisenberg H, Foulkes MA, Marshall LF, and Jane JA (1991) Impact of ICP instability and hypotension on outcome in patients with severe head trauma, The Traumatic Coma Data Bank, Supplement to J Neurosurg:S59-S66

2. Rosner MN, Daughton S (1990) Cerebral perfusion pressure management in head injury. J Trauma 30:933-941

3. Chesnut RM, Marshall LF, Klauber M, Blunt B, Baldwin N, Eisenberg H, Jane JA, Marmarou A, and Foulkes MA (1993) The role of secondary brain injury in determining outcome from severe head injury. J Trauma 34:216-222

Posttraumatic Hydrocephalus Following Impact Acceleration in the Rat

MONTASSER A. FODA and ANTHONY MARMAROU

Division of Neurosurgery, Medical College of Virginia, Richmond, VA, USA

INTRODUCTION

In the clinical setting, the separation between hydrocephalus and brain atrophy as the two possible causes of posttraumatic hydrocephalus (PTH) has been difficult [1] and has been complicated by the contradictory postmortem pathologic reports.[2] In a companion report, the application of CSF dynamic studies is useful as a diagnostic tool and helps in understanding the various trends in CSF dynamics in patients. Unfortunately, an animal model of PTH has been lacking and as a result, experimental studies of this problem have been limited.

Thus, the first objective of this study was to develop an experimental model of traumatic induced ventriculomegaly. The second objective was to document the CSF dynamics and morphologic changes to help distinguish between brain atrophy and absorptive deficits leading to posttraumatic ventriculomegaly.

METHODS

Adult rats (n=43) were anesthetized with a mixture of Isofluorane (1-2 %), Nitrous Oxide (66 %) and oxygen (33 %) and subjected to either moderate or severe impact acceleration injury using a recently developed weight drop model.[3] As subarachnoid hemorrhage is a complicating factor in head injury, a third uninjured group was injected with autologous blood into the cisterna magna. A fourth group served as sham operated control. Six weeks after the primary insult, all rats were anesthetized and fixed in the stereotaxic frame. The cisterna magna was exposed and CSF dynamics were studied using the bolus injection technique for measurement of PVI and Ro. Following study, the rats were deeply anesthetized and sacrificed for perfusion fixation . Ventricular size was assessed visually in a coronal section at the foramen of Monro and the ventricular brain ratio was calculated. Morphologic studies were also performed utilizing conventional H&E staining and immunocytochemical methods.

RESULTS

Baseline ICP equaled 4.5 mmHg ± 1.3 mmHg in the sham group and 4.9 ± 1.7, 5.1 ± 1.95 and 5.0 ±1.4 mmHg in mild brain injured, severe brain injured and SAH groups, respectively. The differences between these groups were not statistically significant. In addition, PVI measured 0.12 ± 0.02 in sham and in injured groups. On the other hand, the PVI of the SAH group was significantly enhanced. (p=0.03)(Fig. 1)

Fig. 1

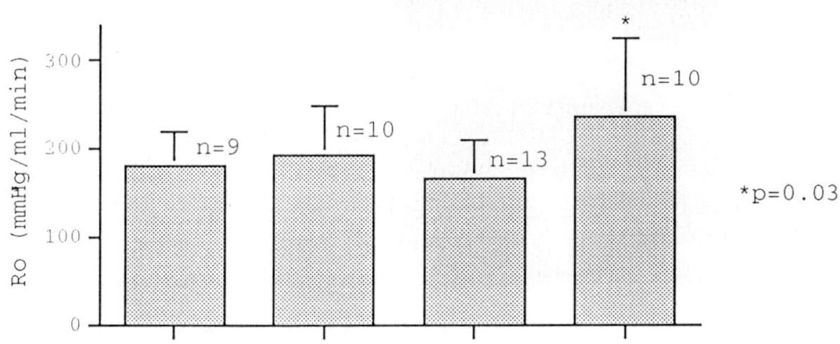

Morphologic Findings

The supraventricular cortical thickness was significantly reduced in mild and severely injured groups (p=0.02 0.01 respectively) compared with that of control. On the other hand, the cortical thickness in the SAH grour was similar to that of control. In addition, the neuronal density of the supraventricular cortex was significantly reduced in mild (81 % of control) and severely injured groups.(78 % of control) (p=0.01 for both), while that in the SAH group was very close to control values. Using GFAP immunoreactivity, a graded reactive astrocytosis was observed in the supraventricular cortical areas of brain but not in the SAH groups. The degree of astrocytosis was directly related to the severity of injury.

Ventricular Size

The average a/b ratio was 0.26 ± 0.02 in the sham group, 0.30 ± 0.05 in the moderate injury and 0.36 ± 0.08 in the severely injured group, and 0.32 ± 0.03 in the SAH group. (Fig. 2) When compared to control, the increase in a/b ratio was significant at p=0.01. However, not all animals in these groups showed ventricula dilation. Approximately 50 % of animals in mild and SAH developed PTV whereas where an a/b ratio large than 0.3 was observed, only in 4 of 10 animals in the mild injured group, 9 of 14 in the severely injure group and 5 of 10 rats in the SAH groups.

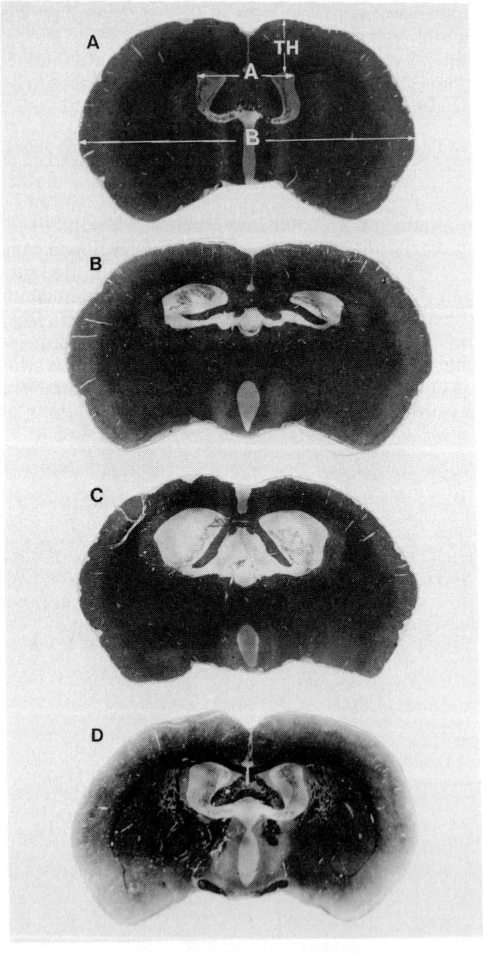

Fig. 2 Photographs of coronal sections at the leve of foramen of Monro in brains representing (A) sham operated, (B) one meter injury (C) two meter injury, and (D) subarachnoi hemorrhage (SAH) groups to demonstrat the changes in ventricular size, as estimate by the A/B ratio, and in the thickness (TH of the supraventricular cerebral cortex i these groups 6 weeks after insult.

DISCUSSION

Within the vast amount of literature on anatomo-pathological changes of the brain after severe head injury in human and animal, posttraumatic ventriculomegaly has not deserved a single complete study. In the postmortem studies of such patients, it has been difficult to distinguish between primary traumatic lesions and secondary alternations caused by hydrocephalus, if any. Recently, we have developed a model of closed head injury in rats that produces diffuse brain injury without any focal lesions in the cerebral hemispheres. When these rats were allowed to survive for six weeks, ventricular dilatation was noticed in 40% of mild injured rats and 64% of the severely injured ones. This incidence of PTV in our model figures are similar to those observed in human.[4] Also, in our study, 50% of rats in the SAH group developed ventricular dilatation, a figure similar to that reported by others.[5] The association of post-SAH ventriculomegaly with a normal baseline ICP in our material is not surprising since it has been shown in longstanding post-SAH hydrocephalus, both in human and experimental animals, the baseline ICP would return to normal levels in the vast majority of cases. Morphologically, the impact of such a mild degree of ventricular dilatation after SAH on the periventricular white matter and hence on the PVI was minimal.

An elevated CSF outflow resistance has been the key finding to make the diagnosis of an active hydrocephalic process and in our study, an elevated CSF outflow resistance was observed in 80% of animals with longstanding post-SAH ventriculomegaly. On the other hand, ventricular dilatation developed as a result of head trauma was associated with a normal baseline ICP, a normal neural axis-buffering capacity and a normal CSF outflow resistance. The observation of normal CSF dynamics in association with PTV would preclude the presence of an active hydrocephalic process in these animals. Ventriculomegaly in the brain-injured rats was associated with significant decrease in the neuronal density and in the thickness of cerebral cortex together with an increase in the astrocytic density (reactive astrocytosis) that were limited to the supraventricular cortical area. These findings are not surprising as the morphological studies performed in these rats in the first few days after trauma showed that the supraventricular cortex suffered the maximum neuronal injury. On the other hand, in the SAH group, neuronal count and cortical thickness in the supraventricular area were similar to those in the control rats. These observations would relate the neuronal loss and thinning of the cerebral cortex in brain-injured rats developed as a result of the initial trauma and not as a result of an active hydrocephalic process. In summary, a model of posttraumatic ventriculomegaly has been developed in rats. Morphological characterization of this model supports the notion that PTV develops to compensate for the reduction in the bulk of the brain caused by the degeneration in the white and gray matter after head injury and not as a result of an active hydrocephalic process.

REFERENCES

1. Beyerl B, Black P (1984) Posttraumatic hydrocephalus. Neurosurgery 15:257-261

2. Adams JH, Doyle D, Ford I, Gennarelli TA, Graham DI, McLellan DR (1989) Diffuse axonal injury in head injury: definition, diagnosis and grading. Histopath 15: 49-59

3. Marmarou A, Abd-elfattah Foda M, van den Brink W, Campbell J, Kita H, Demetriadou K (1994) A new model of diffuse brain injury in rats Part I: Pathophysiology and Biomechanics. J Neurosurg 80:291-300

4. Cope D, Date E, Mar E (1988) Serial computerized tomographic evaluations in traumatic head injury. Arch Phys Med Rehabil 69: 483-486

5. Kaufman H, Dujovny M, Huchton J, Kossovsky N, Miller M, Carmel P (1980) "Natural" canine model of infantile hydrocephalus. Neurosurgery 6: 142-148

Relationships Between Jugular Oxygen Saturation, Cerebral Lactate Production and Intracranial Pressure in Patients with Severe Traumatic Brain Injury

T. Kano, Y. Katayama, K. Kinoshita, T. Hirayama, T. Kawamata, and T. Tsubokawa

Department of Neurological Surgery, Nihon University School of Medicine, Tokyo, 173 Japan

SUMMARY

Monitoring of the jugular bulb venous oxygen saturation (SjO2) is widely used to detect circulatory disturbance to the level at which cerebral blood flow (CBF) fails to meet cerebral metabolic demand. In order to determine whether a critical level of SjO2 which accelerates anaerobic metabolism can be defined or not in patients suffering from traumatic brain injury, we measured SjO2 and the arteriovenous difference of lactate content (AVDlac). The results obtained indicated that an increased lactate production was often seen without a reduced SjO2, especially in the early period after trauma. This finding suggests that the critical level of SjO2 was raised to various degrees in patients with traumatic brain injury.

INTRODUCTION

Reduced CBF is one of the major causes of the secondary injury process in patients suffering from traumatic brain injury. Previous studies have indicated that a decreased SjO2 is a sensitive indicator of inadequately reduced CBF for given cerebral metabolic demand [1, 2]. Thus, a decrease in SjO2 below 50 - 60% has been suggested to represent a critical level for ischemic brain injury. Consistent with this concept, an increase in cerebral lactate production is observed when this level of SjO2 is reached during ischemia. In order to determine whether or not such a relationship between SjO2 and cerebral lactate production exists in traumatic brain injury, we measured SjO2 and AVDlac values in patients with severe traumatic brain injury.

MATERIALS AND METHODS

Patient population and clinical management

The best Glasgow Coma Scores of 16 patients ranged from 3 to 8 upon admission to hospital. The mechanism of trauma was traffic accident in all cases. We excluded data from 6 patients with traumatic injuries of multiple organs who demonstrated elevated arterial lactate levels far above the normal range, since the AVDlac value doesnot necessarily reflect the cerebral lactate production in such patients [3]. 10 patients were thus included in the study, of which 5 patients had diffuse brain injury (DBI), 4 patients had acute subdural hematoma (ASDH) and 1 patient had cerebral contusion. Surgical interventions were carried out in 4 cases for either ASDH or intracerebral hematoma. Except in 1 patient, the intracranial pressure (ICP) was well controllable below 20 mmHg, hyperventilation was avoided and normoventilation (PaCO2: 30 - 40 mmHg) was carried out. Arterial oxygen saturation was maintained at over 99 % in all cases, and blood transfusion was given when Hb fell below 10 g / dl.

Measurement of AVDlac and SjO2

SjO2 was monitored continuously by a 5 Fr opticath placed in the dominant jugular bulb employing Oximetrix 3 (Abott). AVDlac was determined from the blood of arteries and the jugular bulb. SjO2 and AVDlac data were obtained 5 times during the initial 48 hours posttrauma with intervals of approximately 12 hours. The average time of starting observations was 4.6 hours after admission. SjO2 values were averaged for a 1 - hour period, and AVDlac values were expressed as the average of 4 blood samples taken during the same 1 - hour period. All patients also underwent continuous monitoring of ICP.

RESULTS

As shown in Fig. 1 and Table 1, out of the total of 48 AVDlac values obtained, 13 were abnormally elevated (> 3 mg / dl) [2].

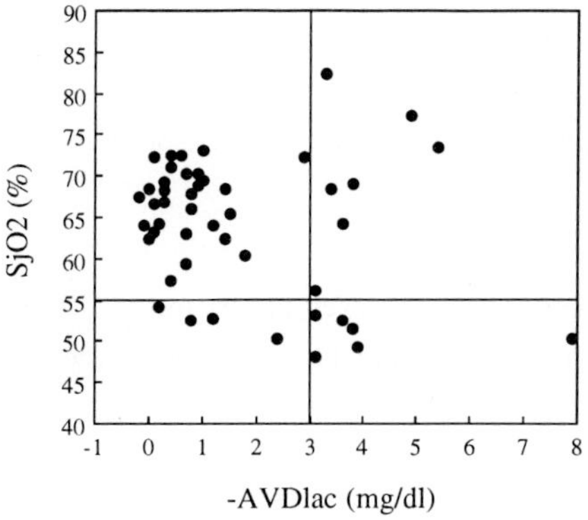

Fig. 1 Relationship between AVDlac and SjO2 at 48 points

Table 1 Classification of 48 points according to AVDlac and SjO2

AVDlac > 3 mg / dl 13 / 48 (28%)

SjO2 ≧ 55% : Traumatic Pattern 7 / 48 (15%)

SjO2 < 55% : Ischemic Pattern 6 / 48 (13%)

AVDlac ≦ 3 mg / dl 35 / 48 (72%)

SjO2 < 55% : Compensated Hypoperfusion 4 / 48 (8%)

55% ≦ SjO2 ≦ 80% : Normal 31 / 48 (64%)

SjO2 > 80% : Hyperemia 0 / 48 (0%)

Among them, 6 were associated with SjO2 values reduced to below 55%: this pattern is thought to be observed in ischemic brain injury (ischemic pattern). The remaining 7 were not associated with a reduced SjO2: this pattern might be characteristic of traumatic brain injury (traumatic pattern). The other 35 AVDlac values were within the normal range. Among them, 4 were associated with SjO2 values reduced to below 55%. This pattern might represent compensated hypoperfusion [1]. Fig. 2 shows the ratio of the 4 patterns at each observation point.

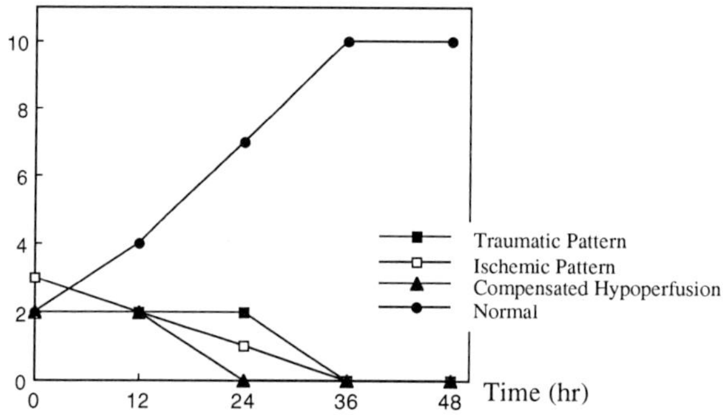

Fig. 2 Ratio of 4 patterns at each observation point

At the starting point, each pattern existed almost equally. We observed the traumatic pattern and ischemic pattern only within the first 24 hours. The increase in AVDlac values displayed no clear relationship to either the decrease in SjO2 values (r = 0.03) or ICP (r = 0.08).

DISCUSSION

The present findings suggest that a critical level of SjO2 for cerebral lactate production cannot be defined in traumatic brain injury. This indicates that cerebral lactate production is also induced by mechanisms other than ischemia. Accelerated anaerobic metabolism due to an increased energy demand may be one of such mechanisms [4, 5, 6]. Although SjO2 reflects the changes occurring in the brain as a whole, conditions are not necessarily uniform in each region of the brain. In such a case with focal brain injury, CBF is reduced in the regions around contusional necrosis [7], and anaerobic metabolism is presumed to be accelerated. Furthermore, in DBI, mechanically injured regions and viable regions are mixed. In such instances, reduction of the CBF is more critical for the viable regions. Especially in the early period after trauma, conditions frequently exist in which the balance between CBF and energy demand readily collapses. Clinical interventions which reduce the CBF, for example hyperventilation, should be avoided when ICP is controllable.

REFERENCES

1. Robertson CS, Narayan RK, Gokaslan ZL, Pahwa R, Grossman RG, Caram P and Allen E (1989) Cerebral arteriovenous oxygen differences as an estimate of blood flow in comatose patients. J Neurosurg 70: 222 - 230
2. Unterberg A, Helden A, Schneider GH and Lanksch W (1991) Combined monitoring of ICP and cerebrovenous oxygen saturation to estimate cerebral blood flow. Intracranial Pressure VIII: 288 - 290
3. Nemoto NA, Hoff JT and Severinghaus JW (1974) Lactate uptake and metabolism by brain during hyperlactatemia and hypoglycemia. Stroke 5: 48 -53
4. Andersen BJ, Marmarou A (1989) Isolated stimulation of glycolysis following traumatic brain injury. In: Intracranial Pressure VII (Hoff JT, Betz AL, eds), Berlin, Springer - Verlag 575 - 580
5. Kawamata T, Katayama Y, Hovda DA, et al (1992) Administration of excitatory amino acid antagonist via microdialysis prevents the increase in glucose utilization seen immediately following concussive brain injury. J Cereb Blood Flow Metab 12: 12 - 24
6. Yoshino A, Hovda DA, Kawamata T, et al (1991) Dynamic changes in local cerebral glucose utilization following fluid-percussion injury: evidence of a hyper- and subsequent hypometabolic state. Brain Res 561: 106 - 119
7. Bouma GJ, Muizelaar JP, Choi SC, et al (1991) Cerebral circulation and metabolism after severe traumatic brain injury: the elusive role of ischemia. J Neurosurg 75: 685 - 693

Blood Volume Change Corresponding to pCO_2 Alterations in Severely Head Injured Patients

M. YOSHIHARA, K. BANDOH, and A. MARMAROU

Division of Neurosurgery, Medical College of Virginia, Richmond, VA, USA

[INTRODUCTION]

Cerebral vasodilatation and vasoconstriction in response to arterial hypercapnia or hypocapnia leads to cerebral blood volume change and this response defines the CO_2 reactivity of cerebral vessels. The ability of the vessels to respond to hyperventilation in cases of marked ICP rise is key to ICP management, however the amount of blood volume change necessary to provoke a rise in ICP or reduction in response to hypocapnia remains unknown.

Recently, a new method was introduced as a simple measurement of CO_2 reactivity termed Blood Volume Responsivity (BVR)[1,2]. It was based on the principle that the change in pCO_2 will alter the ICP according to the slope of the pressure volume curve. Knowledge of the Pressure Volume Index (PVI) would then allow calculation of the blood volume change corresponding to the ICP change. As the ability to reduce ICP by hyperventilation in head injured patients is essential, the first objective was to characterize this response quantitatively and determine the amount of blood volume change corresponding to changes in pCO_2. A second objective was to examine the relationship between the blood volume responsivity and outcome.

[MATERIALS and METHODS]

(Study Population)

Forty nine severely head injured patients (GCS $\leq$ 8) admitted to Medical College of Virginia Neuroscience Intensive Care Unit were involved in this study. All patients remained intubated, paralyzed and mechanically ventilated during the study according to standard head injury protocol in our unit. ICP was measured using a fluid filled ventricular catheter connected to a bedside monitor and end-tidal pCO_2 was measured with a capnometer (Hewlett Packard 47210A) which was installed through the endothoracheal tube. The radial artery was cannulated for blood pressure measurements which were followed continuously by a bedside monitor.

(Calculation of Blood Volume Change)

Capnic stimuli were induced in patients by altering ventilation and resulted in small changes (3 or 4mmHg) of end-tidal pCO_2. At first, baseline ICP, PVI and end-tidal pCO_2 were obtained. Following this procedure, an increase of end-tidal pCO_2 by three or four mmHg was performed by lowering the respiratory rate. After reaching the new steady state, ICP, PVI and end-tidal pCO_2 were determined. The respiratory rate was returned to baseline level and new baseline values for mild hypocapnia were obtained by hyperventilating the patient.

The estimated blood volume (EBV) corresponding to these maneuvers was computed from the equation EBV = PVI x Log (Pp / Po)where Pp is the pressure equilibrium reached following the capnic stimuli and Po the baseline pressure. The blood volume responsivity (BVR) was defined as the change in blood volume per torr change in pCO_2 or BVR = EBV/Δ pCO_2. Substituting for EBV, the BVR is given by BVR = [PVI x ΔLog ICP] / ΔpCO_2 where Δlog(ICP) and ΔpCO_2 were values obtained during the capnic changes produced by mild hyper and hypo ventilation. Using these equations, two indices were defined: (BVRr) the blood volume response to hypercapnia and (BVRo) the blood volume response to hypocapnia expressed in ml/mmHg. These studies were performed and BVR's were determined within 24 hours post injury.

(Assessment of outcome)

Outcome at three months was assessed by independent observers according to the five level Glasgow Outcome Scale (GOS) categories: good recovery, moderate disabled, severely disabled, vegetative and dead. These data were examined to determine their correlation with BVR at day 1 calculated by the data from the capnic studies.

[RESULTS]

(Stability of PVI during pCO_2 manipulation)

It is essential for accuracy of blood volume estimates that PVI remain constant during $pC0_2$ manipulation. The average data for ICP, PVI and end-tidal pCO_2 obtained before and during mild hypo and hyper capnia is summarized in Table 1. Although ICP changed remarkably in response to alteration of pCO_2, the PVI remained stable during these maneuvers.

Thus the assumption that PVI remains constant for estimation of blood volume change is reasonable with changes of 3 or 4 mmHg end-tidal pCO_2. This indicated that the data from mild hypo and hyper capnic study could be applied to EBV and BVR equation. The BVR for each patient was calculated using the mild hypo and hyper capnic data, which resulted in an average BVR for hypercapnia of 0.806ml/mmHg and for hypocapnia of 0.404ml/mmHg and this difference was significant, ($P<0.01$: unpaired Student T test).

Table 1. Average values for ICP, PVI and end-tidal pCO2 before and during mild hypo and hyper capnia

	Hypercapnia		Hypocapnia	
	Before	During	Before	During
Patient (n)	48		49	
ICP	14.9 ± 5.18	18.9 ± 6.65	16.8 ± 5.27	14.8 ± 5.41
PVI	21.1 ± 6.05	21.1 ± 6.17	20.9 ± 6.28	20.4 ± 5.77
end-tidal pCO_2	28.3 ± 4.77	31.4 ± 5.28	30.6 ± 5.12	26.9 ± 4.33

(ICP change produced by alteration of blood volume)

The average ICP changes produced by alteration of blood volume by these measures for mild hypercapnia and hypocapnia were 3.92 ± 0.55mmHg and -1.97 ± 0.28mmHg, respectively. The average EBV for mild hypercapnia and hypocapnia were 1.97 ± 0.28ml and -1.11 ± 0.15ml as shown in Fig.1. Dividing EBV by ΔICP, the blood volume necessary to alter 1mmHg of ICP was calculated. It was found that, with hypercapnia, only 0.5ml of blood volume change was necessary to produce an ICP change of 1mmHg while a slightly greater amount (0.56ml) was required with hypocapnia. The average PVI for these data equaled 21.1ml for hypercapnia and 20.9ml for hypocapnia. This would imply that from the baseline ICP values of 15mmHg, only 2.5ml change in blood volume is necessary to reach critical ICP levels of 20 mmHg. Moreover, the amount of blood volume required to increase 1mmHg of ICP in the patients with PVI less than 15ml was much less than that of greater than 15ml as illustrated in Fig.2.

Fig. 1 ICP change produced by alteration of blood volume

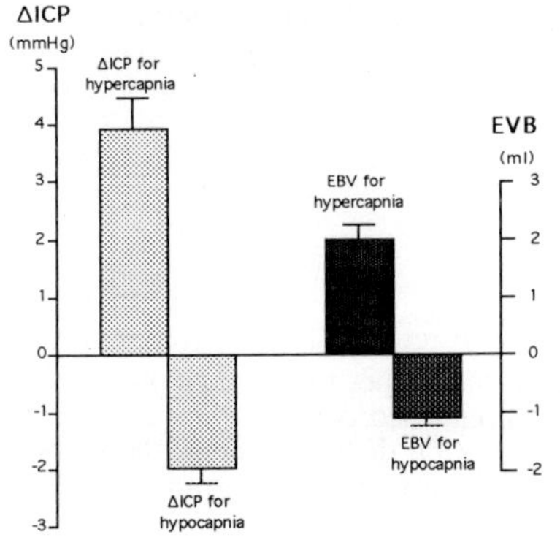

Fig.1 This figure demonstrated that the average alteration of ICP caused blood volume change produced by mild hypo and hyper capnia. It suggested that a small amount of blood volume change affected ICP response.

Fig.2 Blood volume required to increase ICP

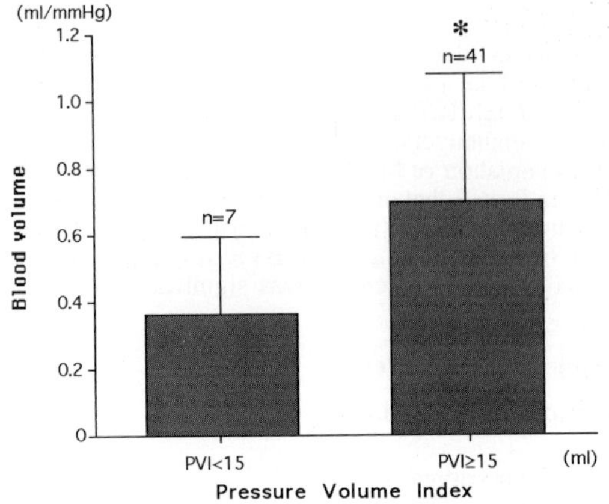

Fig.2 This figure describes the amount of blood volume required to increase 1mmHg of ICP in different PVI groups. The smaller the PVI, the less blood volume necessary to increase ICP. *This relation was statistically significant at $p<0.05$ (unpaired Student-t test).

(Relationship of BVR and Outcome)

Patients were divided into two groups based on their outcomes (GOS) after 3 months post injury. The average BVR values for hypercapnia in the favorable outcome group (GOS: good recovery and moderate disabled) was higher than that in poor outcome group (GOS: severe disabled, vegetative and dead) as indicated in Fig.3. This difference was statistically significant at $p < 0.01$. On the other hand, the difference in BVR values for hypocapnia between these groups was not significant.

Patients were also divided into three groups based on their BVR values for hypercapnia (BVRr): a less reactive BVRr group (BVRr<0.6), a moderately reactive BVRr group (0.6≤ BVRr<0.8) and a higher reactive BVRr group (0.8≤BVRr). As illustrated in Fig.4, in the group of 17 patients with higher reactive BVRr, 59% of patients had favorable outcomes while 41% were associated with poor outcome. Less favorable outcome was associated with reduced BVRr. In the group of 17 patients with less reactive BVRr, outcome in 12% was favorable while 88% remained in the poor outcome category. The relationship between BVRr and the dichotomized GOS was analyzed by a chi square test of trend and the correlation was significant at $p<0.03$.

Fig.3 Average BVR at day 1 vs Outcome

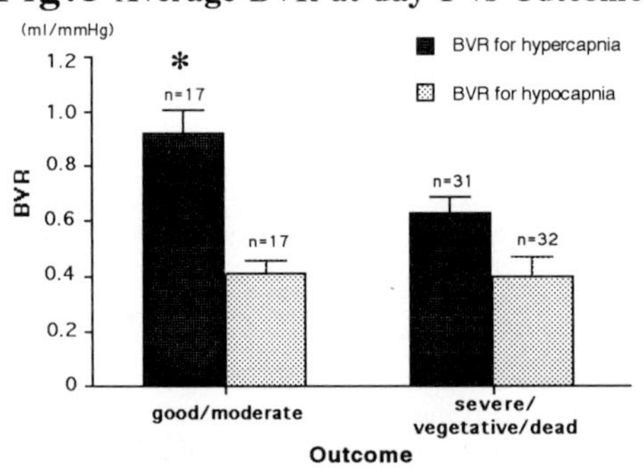

Fig.3 BVR for hypercapnia in favorable outcome group was much higher than that of poor outcome group, while BVR for hypocapnia was no different between two groups. *This relation was statistically significant at $p<0.01$ (unpaired Student-t test).

[DISCUSSION]

(Establishment of the methodology to calculate BVR)

The equation of BVR were derived from the equation of PVI. Under the assumption that PVI remains constant during the alteration of pCO_2, blood volume change per torr change of pCO_2 can be calculated by BVR equation. In our studies, the average PVI remained constant during 3 or 4mmHg changes of end-tidal pCO_2. This indicates that mild alteration of pCO_2 does not change the shape of the pressure volume curve itself, but ICP shifts along the same curve in response to changes in blood volume.

Fig.4 Percentage of favorable outcome in different BVR values for hypercapnia

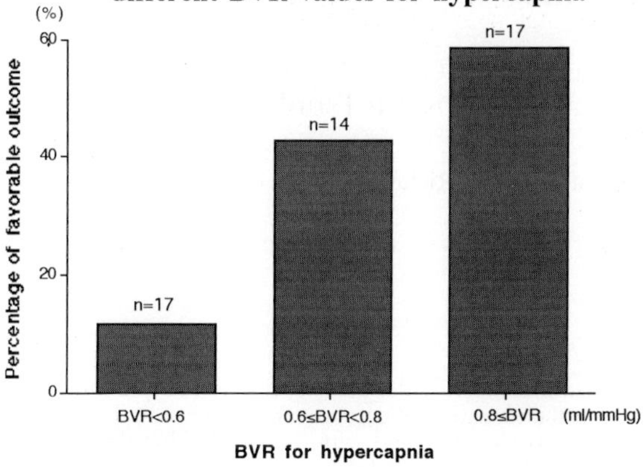

Fig.4 The higher the BVR values, the better the percentage of outcome. This trend was statistically significant at $p<0.03$ (Chi square test of trend).

(ICP change produced by alteration of blood volume)

The ICP response caused by alteration of blood volume depends upon both of brain compliance (PVI) and baseline ICP. In general, the higher the baseline ICP and reduced compliance, the less blood volume is necessary to produce a significant ICP rise. This was illustrated in our study where patients with PVI less than 15 ml only required approximately 4 ml of blood to raise ICP by 10 mmHg while nearly double that volume was required to raise ICP the same amount in patients in whom PVI was greater than 15 ml. According to these concepts, the blood volume change necessary to raise ICP is reduced in direct proportion to reduction of PVI as the brain swells. This clearly emphasizes the importance of maintaining adequate volume reserve and not allowing ICP to exceed 20 mmHg[3].

(Relationship of BVR and Outcome)

According to our results, the BVR values for hypocapnia was markedly reduced and we believe this was partially due to a sustained vasoconstriction by hyperventilation and/or trauma. Based on the observation by many investigators that CO_2 reactivity correlates well with outcome[4,5,6] we analyzed our data and determined the threshold separating poor and favorable outcome. Poor outcome was associated with BVRo values less than 0.6 ml/mmHg while favorable outcome was associated with BVRr's above 0.8 ml/mmHg. We think that CO_2 reactivity assessed by BVR correlates with outcome and an estimated value of 0.7ml/mmHg may be considered the critical level in our study. Thus, we conclude that BVR values for hypercapnia determined within 24 hours of injury may be useful as prognostic index in severely head injured patients.

[REFERENCES]

1. Marmarou A, Wachi A: Blood Volume Responsivity to ICP Change in Head Injured Patients. Intracranial Pressure VII, Springer-Verlag:688-690, 1988

2. Marmarou A: Increased Intracranial Pressure in Head Injury and Influence of Blood Volume. J Neurotrauma 8 (Supplement 2):301-306, 1991

3. Marmarou A, Anderson RL, Ward JD, et al: Impact of ICP instability and hypotension on outcome in patients with severe head trauma. J Neurosurg 75 (Supplement):59-66, 1991

4. Enevoldsen EM, Jensen FT: Autoregulation and CO_2 responses of cerebral blood flow in patients with acute severe head injury. J Neurosurg 48:689-703, 1978

5. Overgaard J, Tweed WA: Cerebral circulation after head injury. Part 1: Cerebral blood flow and its regulation after closed head injury with emphasis on clinical correlations. J Neurosurg 41:531-541, 1974

6. Schalén W, Messeter K, Nordström CH: Cerebral vasoreactivity and the prediction of outcome in severe traumatic brain lesions. Acta Anaesthesiol Scand 35:113-122, 1991

Direct Measurement of Sagittal Sinus Pressure in Head Injured Patients

ANTHONY MARMAROU[1], ANTON VALAVANNIS[2], HANS-GEORG IMHOF[2], MICHELE H. JOHNSON[1], MASAAKI YOSHIHARA[1], and OSAMU TSUJI[1]

[1] Neurosurgery and Radiology, Medical College of Virginia, Richmond, VA, USA
[2] University Hospital Zürich, Switzerland

Introduction

Previous studies in head injured patients have shown that the vascular contribution to ICP predominates ove the CSF contribution and these investigations suggested elevation of cerebrovenous pressure. [1] Subsequen studies confirmed that pressure in the jugular bulb was elevated, and with the assumption that jugular bul pressure was close to that of the sagittal sinus, these results contradicted the generally held concept that Sagitta sinus pressure remains constant and independent of the ICP. [2] In this study, we report for the first time th direct measurement of sagittal sinus pressure in head injured patients.

Methods

After obtaining informed consent and internal review board approval, mechanically ventilated and sedated hea injured patients (n=2) were transferred to the angiographic suite and radiologic procedures were used t position micro-catheters via the femoral vein into the superior sagittal sinus. The angiographic micro-catheter were immersed in saline columns and connected to conventional disposable strain gauge transducers. Afte confirming position of the catheter by radiographic technique ,pressures in the sagittal sinus, torcular Herophil straight sinus and jugular bulb were monitored by repositioning the catheter and recording pressur continuously on computerized strip chart along with ventricular fluid pressure monitored by convention methods.

Results

The studies were completed with no complication. The SSSP was pulsatile with respiratory and cardia components. The respiratory peak to trough level equaled 3 mmHg and equaled the respiratory pulse level c the ICP. The SSSP of patient A averaged 13 mmHg and was slightly below the VFP of 15 mmHg. At constant VFP level of 15 mmHg, torcula Herophili and jugular bulb pressures measured 12 and 10 mmH respectively. In patient B, mean ICP during the study equaled 40 mmHg with adequate CPP of 70 mmHg. Th SSSP under these conditions equaled 20 mmHg. Pressure in the torcular Herophili and transverse sinus we very close to the SSSP and pressure in the Jugular bulb equaled 19.5 mmHg.

Discussion:

In previous investigations, we determined the contribution of CSF and Vascular components of ICP as give by the equation ICP = (If x Ro + Pv) where If equaled rate of formation, Ro the outflow resistance to CSF an Pv the vascular component of pressure.[1] In these studies, conducted in head injured patients, we found th the CSF component accounted for approximately 1/3 of the ICP rise while the vascular component was th predominant factor contributing 2/3 of the ICP elevation. The measurement of Pv was determined indirectly, b withdrawing fluid at the rate of CSF formation, thereby canceling the contribution of the CSF component (If R). In theory, the Pv should be the pressure of the sagittal sinus. Thus, these studies inferred that Pv must b elevated. Heretofore, our attempts to measure Pv were accomplished by measurement of jugular bulb pressure and we confirmed that indeed they were elevated. In fact, if one averages the ICP and Jugular hourly average in head injured patients, the levels are approximately equal (Table 1), further confirming the elevation of veno outflow close to the ICP level.

Table 1. Percent Time avove 20 mmHg : Jugular Bulb

Day	n (Pts)	Jugular Bulb Press. (mmHg) Mean	S.D.	% Time > 20mmHg
1	53	16.0	8.8	16.0
2	57	16.5	8.2	18.8
3	57	16.5	7.2	18.4
4	53	17.0	8.3	22.1
5	45	16.4	7.4	18.6

n these studies, we measured for the first time the pressure of the sagittal sinus and observed that sagittal inus pressure was elevated confirming that venous outflow pressure is increased with increasing ICP. urther the small gradient between sinus and jugular bulb indicates that jugular bulb pressures may be onsidered close to the SSSP. The observation that cerebrovenous exit pressure is elevated in the head injured atient has important implications to our current understanding of the pathophysiology of raised ICP. Under ormal conditions, venous valves located at the thoracic inlet impede the transmission of intrathoracic pressure o the jugular vein. It is possible that these valves are less functional in the head injured patient thereby ncreasing the coupling of airway pressure through the venous pathways to the jugular bulb pressure. Moreover, it further suggests a dysregulation or maximal dilation of the bridging veins. In summary, the bservation that cerebrovenous pressure is elevated in the head injured patient has important implications to ur current understanding of the pathophysiology of raised ICP.

Reference

1. Marmarou A, Maset A, Ward J, et al. (1987) Contribution of CSF and Vascular factors to elevation of ICP in severely head injured patients. J. Neurosurg. 66:883-890

2. Marmarou, A., Abdelfattah Foda, Bandoh K., Stocchetti N., Yoshihara MI, Young H.F.(1993) Elevated Venous Outflow Pressure in Head Injured Patients. In. ICP VIII eds. C.J.J. Avezaat, J.H.M. van Eijndhoven A.I.R. Maas, and J.T.J. Tans Springer Verlag NY.

Post-Traumatic Hydrocephalus—
A Multi-Center Retrospective Survey

MASATSUNE ISHIKAWA and HARUHIKO KIKUCHI

Department of Neurosurgery, Kyoto University, 54 Kawaharacho, Shogoin, Sakyoku, Kyoto, 606 Japan

SUMMARY

A multi-center retrospective survey of post-traumatic hydrocephalus was done to study clinical factors in intractable hydrocephalus after head trauma. The present study revealed that subarachnoid hemorrhage was the commonest disorder in post-traumatic hydrocephalus and that a high incidence of brain edema preceded the hydrocephalus. The outcome of post-traumatic hydrocephalus was closely correlated with symptoms of normal pressure hydrocephalus, pre-shunt activity, shunt effect within 3 months and extent of brain damage. Results can be predicted with three parameters; shunt effect within 3 months, pre-shunt activity and age.

INTRODUCTION

Head trauma is one of the major causes of hydrocephalus. Although primary brain damage is an important factor in the outcome, post-traumatic hydrocephalus developing in the chronic stage can also affect the outcome. In contrast to subarachnoid hemorrhage after ruptured aneurysm, little is known about the outcome of post-traumatic hydrocephalus. As a part of the research on intractable hydrocephalus from various causes, a multi-center retrospective survey of post-traumatic hydrocephalus investigated critical factors in the outcome.

MATERIALS AND METHODS

A questionnaire on hydrocephalus developing in the chronic stage of head trauma was sent to 43 affiliated hospitals of Kyoto University. The subjects of this study were patients hospitalized with head trauma between January 1988 and December1992. The questionnaire consisted of multiple questions about 1) head trauma, 2) clinical state at admission and clinical courses, 3) hydrocephalus, 4) laboratory examinations, 5) shun surgery, and 6) post-shunt clinical course. One hundred and nine cases were collecte from 23 hospitals. Among these, 58 cases fulfilled the following criteria: 1) hydrocephalus developed more than 3 weeks after head trauma, 2) clinical course was evident , 3) CSF shunt was performed, 4) postoperative shunt effect was assessed within 3 months, and 5) there was no subdural fluid collection.

The outcome was classified into four grades; good, fair, poor, death. Glasgow Outcome Scale was partly modified; "severely disabled " and "vegetative survival" wer grouped into the "poor" category. All items were classified into these four grades. Statistical analysis was performed on thirty-three items, which included age, sex, Glasgow Coma Scale, cause of head trauma, duration of unconsciousness, clinical symptoms on admission, degree of ventricular enlargement, brain edema, subarachnoic hemorrhage, laboratory examinations including cerebral blood flow and intracranial pressure measurement, pre-shunt activity, modality and number of shunt procedures, complications, effect of shunt operation within 3 months, and contribution of brain damage assessed by the physician.

Wilcoxon U-test or Kruskal-Wallis H test was applied for each item. Multiple regression analysis was also done for evaluating prognostic factors. For this purpose, fourteen items were selected, which are of full data, objective and independent. They were age, sex, mechanism of head trauma, Glasgow Coma Scale, treatment modality for head trauma, subarachnoid hemorrhage, intraventricular hemorrhage, widening of cerebral sulci, parenchymal abnormality on CT, pre-shunt activity, interval from trauma to shunt surgery, number of shunt operations, complication and effect of shunt operation within three months. Statistical significance was set at $p<0.05$.

RESULTS

One hundred nine cases were collected in 8368 hospitalized patients. Among these, the above criteria were fulfilled in 58 cases. The incidence of post-traumatic hydrocephalus was 1.1 $\pm$1.5% of 8317 patients. There were 38 males and were 20. females. Mean age was 58.8 years old. Commonest type of head trauma was subarachnoid hemorrhage (32 cases), followed by acute subdural hematoma(30 cases) and brain contusion(29 cases) (Fig. 1) .

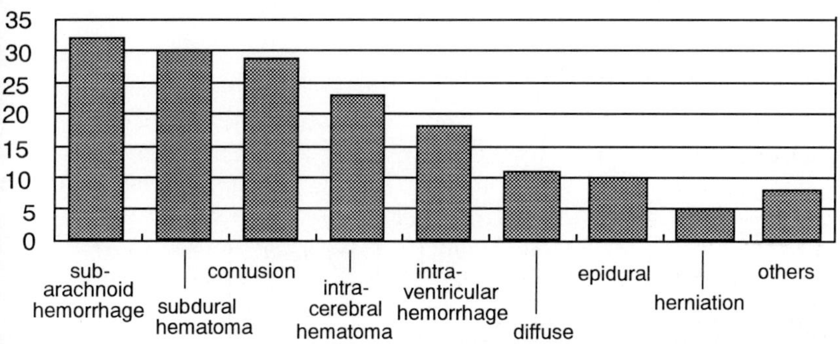

Fig. 1 Type of head trauma (multiple selection)

The number of patients with a Glasgow Coma Scale under 8 was 33(57%), 9 to 11 was 11(19%) and 14 (24%). Brain edema was noted in 49/54 (91%); none 5, mild 27, moderate 10, severe 12. Symptoms of normal pressure hydrocephalus (more than two of the triad) were none in 3, mild in 11 and severe in 25. Improvement of symptoms after shunt surgery was noted in 27 (47%). The outcome within 3 months was good in 7 patients (12%), mildly disabled in 21 (36%), markedly disabled in 16 (28%) and dead in 14 (24%).

Statistical analysis revealed that a significant difference was noted in only 4 items; symptoms of normal pressure hydrocephalus, pre-shunt activity (Fig. 3), shunt effect within 3 months(Fig. 4) , and extent of brain damage. There were no statistical differences in signs, symptoms and causative factors at the acute stage of head trauma. In contrast to the physician's general estimation of brain damage, individual CT findings including subarachnoid hemorrhage, brain contusion, brain edema and degree of ventricular enlargement did not correlate with the outcome.

Multiple regression analysis was performed with fourteen items. It revealed the following formula;

Y = 0.665X1 + 0.699X2 + 0.331X3 - 1.655 (proportion = 0.597, p<0.001; regression coefficiency: 0.773, p<0. 01), where Y = outcome, X1 = effect of shunt surgery, X2 = pre-shunt activity, X3 = age.

CT or MRI images were obtained in all cases, and lumbar tap was done in 62.9%. However, other studies including cisternography, CSF pressure measurement and cerebral blood flow, were rarely performed. Therefore, such data were unavailable for statistical assessment.

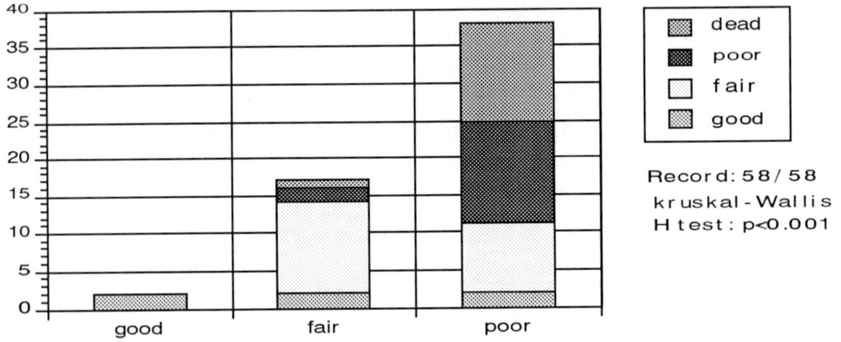

Fig.2. Pre-shunt activity

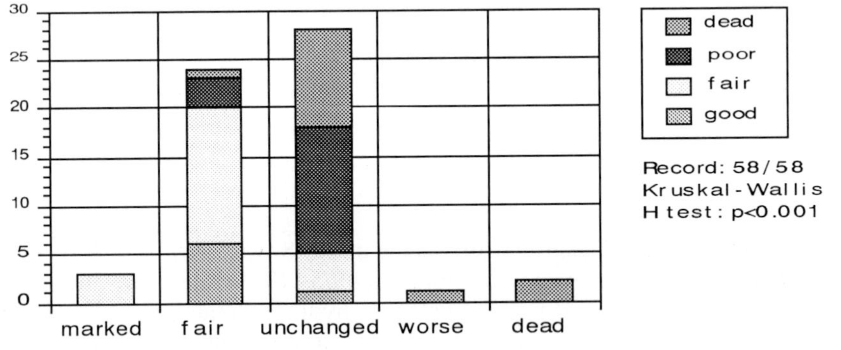

Fig. 3. Shunt effect within 3 months

DISCUSSION

Although this survey has some drawbacks in the homogeneity of population because of different policies for treatment and handling of "unknown" data, etc., it provided useful information on post-traumatic hydrocephalus.

The incidence of post-traumatic hydrocephalus in severe head trauma was about 5% [1,2]. Present study showed lower incidence, which was probably due to inclusion of milder cases. Thus, post-traumatic hydrocephalus is a rare sequelae of head trauma.

Subarachnoid hemorrhage is the commonest cause of normal pressure hydrocephalus. The present study revealed it was also an important cause of post-traumatic hydrocephalus. It suggests that development of post-traumatic hydrocephalus would share the same pathophysiology as that after ruptured aneurysm.

Brain edema might cause delayed brain atrophy, which would be related to the development of post-traumatic hydrocephalus [3]. The present study also showed a high incidence of brain edema. However, no data was obtained to support this view.

The present study revealed that the outcome was well correlated with symptoms of normal pressure hydrocephalus, pre-shunt activity and effect of shunt surgery within 3 months. Extent of brain damage as estimate d by the physician was also highly correlated, although individual CT findings such as subarachnoid hemorrhage, brain contusion and brain edema did not show a high correlation with it. These findings suggest that a good outcome can be expected only if the initial brain damage is not great enough to cause irreversible damage of higher brain function and normal pressure hydrocephalus is a major factor for clinical symptoms in the chronic stage. The present study revealed that age was also important in predicting outcome.

REFERENCES

1. Kishore PRS, Lipper MH, Miller JD, Girevendulis AK, Becker DP, Vines FS (1978) Post-traumatic hydrocephalus in patients with severe head injury. Neuroradiology 16:261-265
2. Kawakami K, Kawamura Y, Kawamoto K, Ikeda Y, Oka N, Matsumura H, Matsumoto A (1983) Post-traumatic normal pressure hydrocephalus following severe head injury. Neurol Med Chir (Tokyo) 23:945-951
3. Tjuvajev J, Eelmae J, Tomberg T, Tikk A (1991) Traumatic Brain Edema in the pathogenesis of post-traumatic hydrocephalus. In: Matsumoto S and Tamaki N (eds) Hydrocephalus-pathogenesis and Treatment. Springer-Verlag Tokyo, pp. 311-323

ACKNOWLEDGMENTS

This survey was perfromed tto investigate "intractable hydrocephalus" . We deeply appreciate the help of The Ministry of Health and Welfare of Japan and the cooperation of the affiliated hospitals of Kyoto University in this post-traumatic hydrocephalus survey.

Session XVI: Causes of Increased or Decreased ICP (5)

Chairmen: C.P. McGraw and H. Chigasaki

Role of Necrosis Area in Development of the Mass Effect of Cerebral Contusion and Elevated Intracranial Pressure

YOICHI KATAYAMA, ATSUO YOSHINO, TSUNEO KANO, HIDEHIKO KUSHI, and TAKASHI TSUBOKAWA

Department of Neurological Surgery, Nihon University School of Medicine, Tokyo, 173 Japan

SUMMARY

The present study investigated changes in the intracranial pressure (ICP) caused by the presence of contused brain tissue within the intracranial space. The frontal lobe of the rat was isolated by transection, taken out from the intracranial space and then contused. The contused brain tissue was returned into the cavity from which it had been obtained. While isolation of the brain tissue naturally causes interruption of blood supply, we employed this procedure in order to exclude vasogenic edema component. The results were compared with those from rats in which the brain tissue was returned without inducing contusion. It was found that more pronounced ICP elevation was induced when the brain tissue was contused prior to returning into the intracranial space. A greater increase in water content was also observed ($p<0.01$) in contused brain tissue. When the brain tissue was incubated in Ringer solution, an accumulation of water was more rapid ($p<0.01$) in contused brain tissue as compared to non-contused brain tissue. These findings suggest that cytotoxic edema contributes the mass effect of cerebral contusion. In actual cerebral contusion, water can be supplied through the capillaries with increased cerebrovascular permeability. Thus, the mass effect of cerebral contusion may be regarded as the result of synergistic effect of vasogenic and cytotoxic edema components.

INTRODUCTION

Cerebral contusions in head trauma patients cause progressive edema, sometimes leading to uncontrollable elevation of the intracranial pressure (ICP) and clinical deterioration [1]. Experimental studies have demonstrated that cerebral contusions are associated with an increased cerebrovascular permeability and a resultant vasogenic edema [e.g., 2]. Contusion edema in head trauma patients extends along the white matter fibers which is a characteristic of vasogenic edema. In addition, there are several lines of evidence indicating that a large amount of fluid is produced in the extracellular space within cerebral contusions [1,3,4]. Intravenous slow infusion of gadolinium-DTPA and delayed magnetic resonance imaging reveals evidence of an increased cerebrovascular permeability in patients with cerebral contusions [5]. These findings support the widely held view that vasogenic edema is responsible for development of the mass effect of cerebral contusion and elevated ICP.

It is not certain, however, whether or not the increased cerebrovascular permeability is an exclusive cause of the mass effect of cerebral contusion. In ischemic injury, an increase in plasma membrane permeability causes cytotoxic edema. Mechanical injury may also increases plasma membrane permeability of the cells which eventually undergo contusion necrosis. It is, therefore, probable that some component of contusion edema is cytotoxic in nature. The present study tested the hypothesis that cytotoxic edema significantly contributes development of the mass effect of cerebral contusion and elevated ICP.

MATERIALS AND METHODS

In the present study, we first isolated the frontal lobes of the rat bilaterally by transection and took them out from the intracranial space. The isolated brain tissue was then contused. Changes in the ICP were investigated when such a brain tissue was returned into the cavity from which it had been obtained. In addition, edema occurring in the isolated brain tissue was examined. We compared these changes between contused and non-contused brain tissue. While isolation of the brain tissue naturally causes interruption of blood supply, we employed this procedure in order to exclude vasogenic edema component.

In vivo experiment

Young Wistar rats weighing 250-300 g were anesthetized with a mixture of 33% oxygen, 66% nitrous oxide and 1% halothane. With the rectal temperature kept at 37.0-38.0 °C with a heating pad, the animals were placed in a stereotaxic frame, the calvarium was exposed and a craniotomy was performed. The frontal lobe was isolated bilaterally by transection at the level 2.5 mm rostral to the bregma and taken out from the intracranial space. Hemorrhage from the transection surface was controllable with gentle compression with cottonoid. Coagulation was not necessary. The olfactory bulb was left intact to avoid causing uncontrollable hemorrhage and leakage of cerebrospinal fluid. The removed brain tissue was contused with weight-drop method and was returned to the cavity from which the brain tissue had been obtained. The craniotomy site was water-tightly sealed by silicon plate. In a separate group of animals, the cavity was filled with isolated but non-contused brain tissue. ICP was continuously monitored from the cisterna magna for 12 hours. The animals were decapitated at 12 hours and water content of the brain tissue was evaluated by specific gravity technique.

In vitro experiment

Animals were prepared similarly as those for the above-mentioned experiment. The frontal lobe was isolated bilaterally by transection and taken out from the intracranial space. The isolated brain tissue was contused with weight-drop method. The contused brain tissue was then incubated in Ringer solution maintained at 37.0 °C. Water content of the brain tissue was evaluated by specific gravity technique after various periods of incubation. The same experiment was performed with isolated but non-contused brain tissue.

RESULTS

Changes in Intracranial Pressure

A slight increase in ICP was observed when non-contused brain tissue was returned into the intracranial space. The ICP was gradually elevated and reached an equilibrium level at 2-3 hours (Fig. 1). More pronounced increase in ICP was observed when the brain tissue was contused prior to returning into the intracranial space. The ICP was elevated more rapidly, and reached a level significantly greater ($p<0.01$) than the level observed in the experiment with non-contused brain tissue at 6-12 hours (Fig. 1).

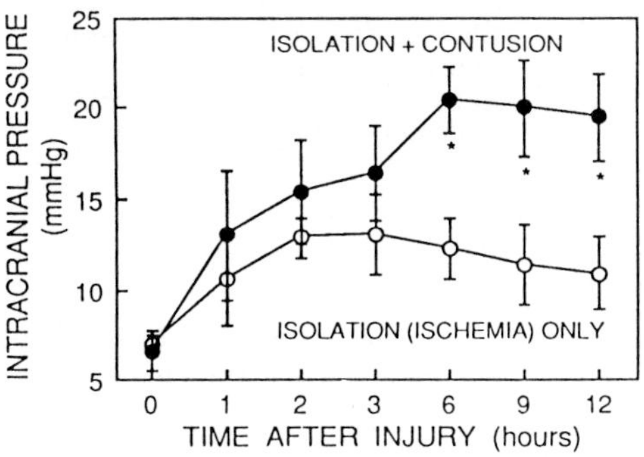

Fig. 1 Changes in ICP in rats in which either contused (solid dots, n=5) or non-contused (open circles, n=5) brain tissue was returned into the intracranial space. * $p<0.01$

Changes in Water Content

An increase in water content was observed in the isolated brain tissue which had been placed in the intracranial space for 12 hours. The increase in water content of contused brain tissue was significantly more pronounced ($p<0.01$) as compared to that of non-contused brain tissue (Fig. 2). In contrast, there was a trend that the water content of remaining brain areas was lower when contused brain tissue was returned. Similar results were obtained in the in vitro experiment. A progressive increase in water content of the isolated brain tissue was observed during incubation in Ringer solution. The increase in water content was significantly more rapid ($p<0.01$) in contused brain tissue as compared to non-contused brain tissue (Fig. 3).

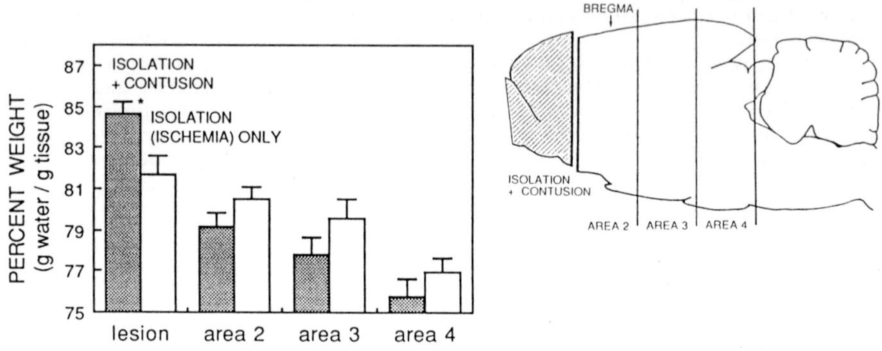

Fig. 2 Changes in water content of respective brain areas (indicated in the left) of the rats in which either contused (hatched column, n=5) or non-contused (open column, n=5) brain tissue was returned to the cavity from which the brain tissue had been obtained. The brain tissue was placed in the intracranial space for 12 hours. * $p<0.01$

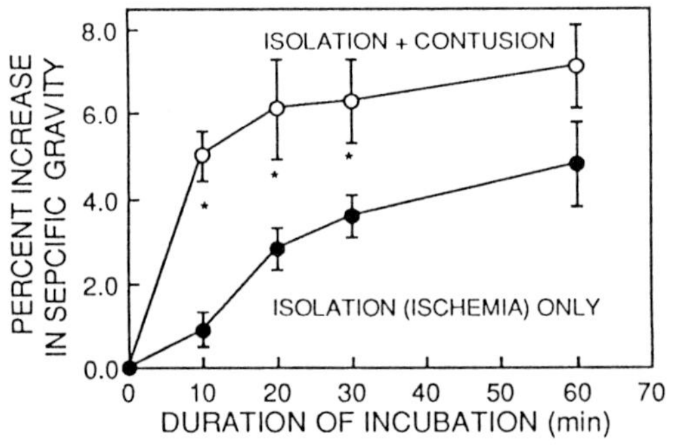

Fig. 3 Time courses of changes in water content of contused (open column, n=5 for each) or non-contused (hatched column, n=5 for each) brain tissues during incubation in Ringer solution.
* $p<0.01$

DISCUSSION

The present study demonstrated that isolated brain tissue accumulates water when returned into the cavity from which the brain tissue had been obtained. Isolation of the brain tissue can be regarded as equivalent to complete ischemia. Such a brain tissue has a potential to swell as far as water is supplied. As expected, water content of isolated brain tissue increased rapidly during incubation in Ringer solution. While the major source of water within the brain is normally the blood, water may also be supplied from adjacent brain tissue and cerebrospinal fluid space. The water accumulation within the isolated brain tissue may be responsible for the observed ICP elevation.

The present study further demonstrated that the magnitude of water accumulation within the isolated brain tissue and the ICP elevation was significantly augmented when it was contused prior to returning into the intracranial space. This augmentation may be caused by either an increased water supply or a greater increase in plasma membrane permeability, or both. If the extracellular space is enlarged by cerebral contusion, the tissue compliance is increased and more water may be supplied. The enlarged extracellular space may also provides a larger effective surface area for water movement through the plasma membrane. In addition, it appears possible that mechanical injury causes greater changes in plasma membrane permeability as compared to ischemic injury.

The present finding suggests that cytotoxic edema contributes the mass effect of cerebral contusion. Water can be supplied by the blood in actual cerebral contusion. This may be enhanced by increased cerebrovascular permeability. Thus, the mass effect of cerebral contusion may be regarded as the result of synergistic effect of vasogenic and cytotoxic edema components.

There is no established medical treatment for the mass effect of cerebral contusion. The most effective therapy for ameliorating the potentially fatal mass effect is surgical excision of contused brain tissue. The effect of such surgical excision of contused brain tissue may be partially accounted for by an increased space compensation for the mass lesions. The excision of the contused brain tissue does also mean the removal of the source of edema fluid. In addition, the present finding suggests that the excision of contused brain tissue represents the removal of the reservoir of edema fluid.

REFERENCES

1. Katayama Y, Tsubokawa T, Miyazaki S, Kawamata T and Yoshino A (1990) Oedema fluid formation within contused brain tissue as a cause of medically uncontrollable elevation of intracranial pressure in head trauma patients. *Acta Neurochir* suppl 51: 308-310
2. Sutton RL, Hovda DA, Adelson PD, Benzel EC and Becker DP (1994) Metabolic changes following cortical contusion: Relationships to edema and morphological changes. *Acta Neurochir* suppl 60: 446-448
3. Marmarou A, Maset AL, Ward JD, Choi S, Brooks D, Lutz H, Moulton RJ, Muizelaar JP, DeSalles A and Young HF (1987) Contribution of CSF and vascular factors to elevation of ICP in severe head-injured patients. *J Neurosurg* 66: 883-890
4. Katayama Y, Tsubokawa T, Kinoshita K and Himi K (1992) Intra-parenchymal fluid-blood levels in traumatic intracerebral hematomas. *Neuroradiology* 34: 381-383
5. Kushi H, Katayama Y, Shibuya T, Tsubokawa T and Kuroha T (1994) Gadolinium DTPA-enhancement magnetic resonance imaging of cerebral contusions. *Acta Neurochir* suppl 60: 472-474
6. Marmarou A, Takagi H and Shulman K (1980) Biomechanics of brain edema and effects on local cerebral blood flow. In: *Advances in Neurology*, Vol 28, Raven Press, New York, pp 345-358

Intracranial Pressure and Cerebral Plasma Volume Immediately After Closed Head Injury in the Rat

H. Nawashiro, K. Shima, and H. Chigasaki

Department of Neurosurgery, National Defense Medical College, Namiki, Tokorozawa, Saitama, 359 Japan

SUMMARY

In the present study, we investigated intracranial pressure (ICP) and cerebral plasma volume (CPV) using a newly developed impact acceleration injury model to elucidate the acute pathophysiology of closed head injury. In this experimental model that is quite different from the fluid-percussion injury model, increased CPV did not result in a prolonged increase in ICP. Decreasing compliance could occur due to existing traumatic SAH, however, an increment of CPV, about 50% of control values, caused no significant prolonged rise in ICP. Intact BBB soon after trauma may play an important role to protect from a vicious circle that might lead to acute brain swelling.

INTRODUCTION

Transient rises in ICP and mean arterial blood pressure (MABP) concomitant with a traumatic impact has been demonstrated in the fluid-percussion injury model. In the fluid-percussion injury, a prolonged increase in ICP coupled with immediate breakdown of blood-brain barrier (BBB) was noted even at the moderate injury level. In the present study, we investigated ICP and cerebral plasma volume (CPV) using a newly developed impact acceleration injury model [1] to elucidate the pathophysiology of closed head injury.

MATERIALS AND METHODS

Male Sprague-Dawley rats weighing 400 to 450 g (about 12 weeks of age), maintained on a normal diet, were used in the present study. Each animal was anesthetized with a mixture of 1% halothane, air, and oxygen delivered by a closely fitting face mask. The femoral arteries and veins were catheterized for arterial blood sampling and continuous monitoring of arterial blood pressure, and for intravenous injection of drugs.

Trauma Model

In the present study, a new experimental model for closed head injury introduced by Marmarou et al. [1] was used. Soon after discontinuing halothane inspiration, each animal was mounted in a prone position on a foam bed and was placed under hollow plexiglass tubing. A blunt head injury was delivered by dropping a brass weight (450 g) through the tubing from a height of 1 meter, which was adjusted to represent a moderate injury level. Three separate experiments were done as follows.

Experiment 1

ICP and MABP monitoring before and after trauma were performed continuously (n=5). ICP was measured by a Camino fiber optic device placed in the subdural space and anchored by dental cement onto the frontal bone.

Experiment 2

Experiments were carried out on 9 rats. RCPV was determined as the ^{14}C-sucrose space, (dpm/g brain)/(dpm/ml plasma), soon after intravenous ^{14}C-sucrose injection. In the trauma group (n=5), 3.7 Mbq of ^{14}C-sucrose was administered simultaneously with the traumatic impact. Samples of arterial blood were withdrawn to determine the average tracer concentration and hematocrit. Each rat was decapitated at 30 sec. The brain was removed quickly and then frozen and cut into 20-μm-thick sections. Each of the sections were mounted on glass coverslips, dried on a hot plate and placed in an X-ray cassette with calibrated ^{14}C-methylmethacrylate standards (Amersham Corp., Arlington Heights, IL) against X-ray film (SB-5, Kodak) for 14 days. The optical densities of cerebral structures were determined using a microdensitometer (PDS-15, Sakura). In the sham operated control animals (n=4), rCPV was measured in the same manner as described above.

Experiment 3

BBB permeability (n=5) was measured autoradiographically using ^{14}C-alpha-aminoisobutyric acid (^{14}C-AIB, New England Nuclear Corp., Boston; specific activity 1.48-2.22 Gbq/mmol) [2]. ^{14}C-AIB (3.7 Mbq/one rat), dissolved in 1 ml of saline and adjusted to pH 7.4, was administered simultaneously with the traumatic impact. Timed arterial blood samples were rapidly taken and plasma radioactivity was measured by a liquid scintillation counter. At 10 min, each rat was decapitated. The brain was rapidly removed, frozen and cut into 20- μm-thick sections. Serial histology slices were picked up and processed for light microscopic analysis to match autoradiograms with the histology. Each of the sections were mounted on glass coverslips, dried on a hot plate and placed in an X-ray cassette with calibrated ^{14}C-methylmethacrylate standards (Amersham Corp., Arlington Heights, IL) against X-ray film (SB-5, Kodak) for 14 days. The optical densities of cerebral structures were determined using a microdensitometer (PDS-15, Sakura).

RESULTS

Gross Pathology

In the trauma groups, apart from a mild subarachnoid hemorrhage (SAH) in the basal cisterns, brains looked normal without any contusions or focal lesions. Macroscopic intraparenchymal hemorrhage was not found in any of the animals.

ICP and MABP

Before injury, baseline ICP values ranged from 6 to 12 mmHg in all animals . Immediately after trauma, ICP increased synchronously with blood pressure to levels in excess of 100 mmHg and quickly returned to baseline values. MABP rapidly increased by 20% in the trauma groups, and returned to baseline values within 30 sec.

CPV

All brain regions showed varied increase in rCPV at 30 sec after trauma , and the increase was particularly significant in the frontal cortex, parietal cortex, thalamus, and hypothalamus ($P<0.05$). Mean increment of CPV was 46% of control values.

BBB permeability

The transfer constant for AIB was less than 0.1 ml/kg/min for all brain regions except those with a relatively leaky BBB.

DISCUSSION

It is well known that cerebral blood volume (CBV) is one of the determinants of ICP, and increased CBV may contribute to intracranial hypertension. In our experimental model that is quite different from the fluid-percussion injury model [3,4], increased CPV did not result in a prolonged increase in ICP. Values of rCPV in sham operated control animals were nearly similar to those reported previously for conscious rats [5]. Decreasing compliance could occur due to existing traumatic SAH, however, an increment of CPV, about 50% of control values, caused no significant prolonged rise in ICP. Intact BBB soon after trauma may play an important role to protect from a vicious circle that might lead to acute brain swelling.

REFERENCES

1. Marmarou A, Foda MAA, van den Brink W, Campbell J, Kita H, Demetriadou K (1994) A new model of diffuse brain injury in rats. J Neurosurg 80: 291-300

2. Blasberg RG, Fenstermacher JD, Patlak CS (1983) Transport of α–aminoisobutyric acid across brain capillary and cellular membranes. J. Cereb. Blood Flow Metab. 3: 8-32

3. Dewitt DS, Jenkins LW, Wei EP, Lutz H, Becker DP, Kontos HA (1986) Effects of fluid-percussion brain injury on regional cerebral blood flow and pial arterial diameter. J. Neurosurg. 64: 787-794

4. Wei EP, Dietrich WD, Povlishock JT, Navari RM, Kontos HA (1980) Functional, morphological, and metabolic abnormalities of the cerebral microcirculation after concussive brain injury in cats. Circulation Research 46: 37-47

5. Ohno K, Pettigrew KD,,Rapoport SI (1978) Lower limits of cerebrovascular permeability to nonelectrolytes in the conscious rat. Am. J. Physiol. 235: 299-307

Attenuation of Elevated Intracranial Pressure in a Rat Cerebral Contusion Model by Excitatory Amino Acid Antagonist

TATSURO KAWAMATA, YOICHI KATAYAMA, ATSUO YOSHINO, and TAKASHI TSUBOKAWA

Department of Neurological Surgery, Nihon University School of Medicine, Itabashi-ku, Tokyo, 173 Japan

SUMMARY

In order to clarify whether or not excitatory amino acids are involved in the elevation of ICP following contusional brain injury, the effects of kynurenic acid (KYN), a broad spectrum glutamate antagonist, on ICP were investigated in a rat contusion model. The contusion injury was inflicted in the frontoparietal cortex using a controlled cortical impact device (diameter of injury tip = 5 mm, velocity = 6 m/sec, penetration depth = 3 mm). At 30 min before the injury induction, KYN (800 mg/kg) was administered intraperitoneally. In another group of animals, saline vehicle was injected as a control. In the control animals, the ICP rose rapidly immediately after the injury induction. Within 5 min after the induction, it returned to a near-normal level and then progressively increased up to 10-15 mmHg after 3 hours. Systemic pretreatment with KYN did not affect the initial rapid rise in ICP. However , the secondary ICP elevation was significantly attenuated by the KYN treatment. Similarly, the edema formation in brain areas adjacent to the contusion was attenuated by the KYN treatment. These findings suggest that EAAs may induce edema formation surrounding the contusion, resulting in a second ICP elevation following contusional brain injury.

INTRODUCTION

Cerebral contusions are associated with progressive edema formation in the surrounding brain areas, resulting in an elevation of the intracranial pressure (ICP). The edema formation associated with brain contusion has been considered to be due to an increase in vasopermeability. We demonstrated previously that excitatory amino acids (EAAs) are released from contused brain tissue to adjacent brain areas[1]. It has also been reported that EAAs induce cellular swelling in experimental models of cerebral concussion[2][3] and/or ischemia[4][5]. EAAs may thus play a role in eliciting edema formation and ICP elevation following contusion[6]. Little is currently known, however, concerning the role of EAAs in ICP elevation[7]. In the present study, in order to clarify the relationship between EAAs and an elevated ICP in contusional brain injury, the effects of EAA antagonist on ICP were investigated in a rat contusion model.

MATERIALS AND METHODS

Preparation of animals

Young adults rats weighing 250-300 g were anesthetized with a mixture of nitrous oxide, oxygen and halothane. The rectal temperature was maintained at 37-38°C. The systemic arterial pressure (SAP) was monitored from the femoral artery. Each rat was placed in a stereotaxic frame and craniectomy was performed on the frontoparietal bone. Contusion injury was inflicted using a controlled cortical impact device. The tip of the device was 5 mm in diameter, and its velocity and penetration depth into the cortex were predetermined (velocity = 6 m/sec, penetration depth = 3 mm). Details of this controlled cortical impact model have been described previously elsewhere[8]. At 30 min prior to the injury induction, kynurenic acid (KYN; 800 mg/kg), a broad spectrum glutamate antagonist, was administered intraperitoneally. In another group of animals, saline vehicle was injected as a control. The bone window was closed water-tightly with plastic film immediately after the injury induction.

Measurement of ICP and edema formation

The ICP was monitored continuously via a cannula placed in the cisterna magna or a Camino catheter placed in the occipital lobe. At 3 hours after injury induction, the animals were sacrificed with overdose pentobarbital. The edema formation was estimated by the dry weight method (% brain water) in the injured and contralateral hemispheres, and by the specific gravity method in the contused and surrounding brain areas (2 and 4 mm distant from the edge of the contusion) in separate groups of animals.

RESULTS

In the control animals, ICP rose rapidly from 5.1±1.2 mmHg (mean±SD) to 12.2±4.7 mmHg immediately after the injury induction, and returned to a near-normal level (5.3±2.1 mmHg) within 5 min. It then increased gradually and reached a plateau level (Fig. 1). The ICP level at 3 hours after injury induction was 14.1±1.9 mmHg in the control animals. The SAP rapidly increased from 82.6±3.2 to 118.3±8.9 mmHg and returned to a neat-normal level (79.1±5.7 mmHg) within 5 min. Following the initial elevation, the SAP showed no significant changes during the 3-hour investigation period.

In the KYN-treated animals, immediately after the injury induction, ICP rose rapidly from 4.9±1.4 to 11.8±3.8 mmHg, i.e. to almost the same level as in the control animals, and returned to a near-normal level within 5 min. It then increased gradually and reached a plateau level. However, the ICP level at 3 hours after injury induction was 9.8±1.5 mmHg, which was significantly lower than that in the control animals ($p<0.01$) (Fig. 1). The baseline level of SAP was 81.7±4.7 mmHg and immediately after injury induction, the SAP increased to 116.1±9.8 mmHg in the KYN-treated animals. The changes in SAP exhibited no significant difference as compared to those in the control animals.

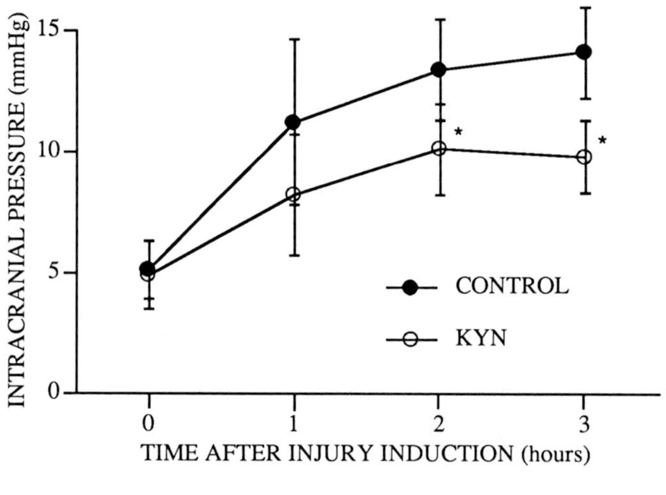

Fig. 1 ICP changes following injury induction. The ICP in the control animals was elevated and reached a plateau level (closed circles). This elevation was attenuated in the KYN-treated animals (open circles). *$p<0.01$.

The % brain water of the injured hemisphere was significantly higher than that of the contralateral hemisphere (80.2±0.61% vs. 78.4±0.25%) in the control animals, and this increase in % brain water was attenuated in the KYN-treated animals (79.4±0.42%). The specific gravity of the contused brain tissue showed no significant difference between the KYN-treated and control animals. However, the specific gravity of the brain tissue at 2 mm from the edge of the contusion was significantly higher in the KYN-treated animals than that in the control animals (1.051±0.003 vs. 1.046±0.006). (Fig. 2).

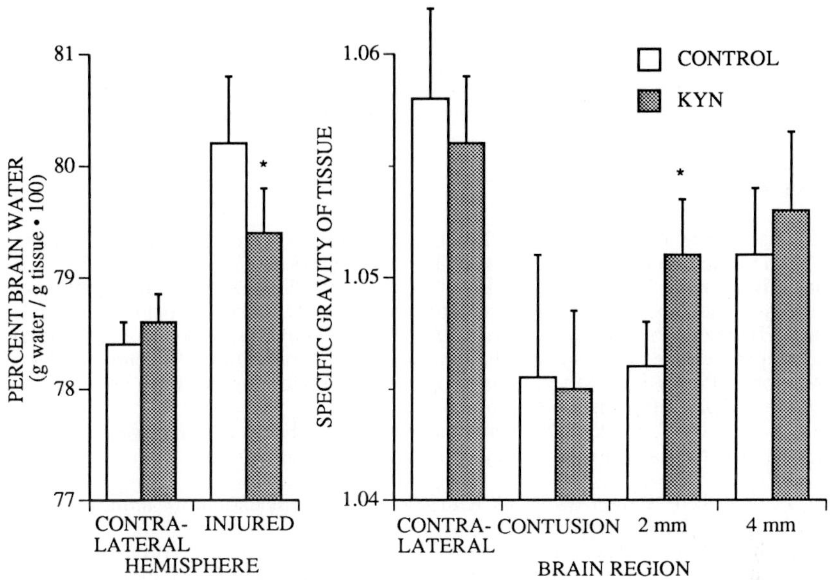

Fig. 2 The % brain water in the injured hemisphere was significantly increased as compared to that in the contralateral hemisphere. This increase in % brain water was significantly attenuated by KYN treatment (left panel). The specific gravity of the contused brain tissue and of the brain tissue adjacent to the contusion was decreased as compared to that of the contralateral cortex. This decrease in specific gravity was attenuated by KYN treatment in the brain tissue at 2 mm distant from the contusion (right panel). *p<0.01.

DISCUSSION

The results of the present study demonstrate that controlled cortical contusion can induced a biphasic elevation of ICP. The initial ICP elevation had a small magnitude and short duration. This rapid elevation was probably due to the accompanying increase in SAP, since ICP and SAP changed almost in parallel. The second elevation of ICP was of large magnitude and long duration, and formed a plateau. This elevated ICP was not associated with any SAP changes. The water content of the injured hemisphere was increased, indicating that the second ICP elevation was due to edema formation following the contusional brain injury. The attenuation of the ICP elevation and edema formation by KYN treatment suggests that EAAs may be involved in the secondary ICP elevation.

We have demonstrated that EAAs are released from contused brain tissue and induce metabolic derangement in the surrounding brain tissue[1]. It has also been reported that EAA antagonist can attenuate the cellular swelling that occurs after cerebral concussion and/or ischemia by blocking ionic shifts via EAA-coupled ion channels[2][3][4][5]. EAAs release from contused brain tissue to surrounding brain areas may thus induce cellular swelling due to ionic fluxes via EAA-coupled ion channels. Such a mechanism appears to contribute to the secondary ICP elevation following contusional brain injury.

The present data show that KYN attenuated edema formation in the tissue surrounding the contusion, but not significantly in the contused brain tissue itself. These findings imply that EAAs are, at least in part, involved in the edema formation occurring within the brain tissue surrounding the contusion. Different mechanisms could exist for the edema formation within the contused brain tissue itself. One possibility is indicated by the results of a recent study showing that contused brain tissue accumulates water because of its high osmotic potential [9].

In conclusion, following experimental contusional brain injury induced with a controlled cortical impact device, the ICP increased biphasically. Administration of KYN, a broad spectrum glutamate antagonist, attenuated the second ICP elevation as well as the edema formation in the brain tissue adjacent to the contusion. These observations suggest that EAAs are involved in the ICP elevation following contusional brain injury, and imply a possible therapeutic effect for EAA antagonist in clinical cases of brain contusion.

REFERENCES

1. Tanaka H, Katayama Y, Kawamata T, Tsubokawa T (1994) Excitatory amino acid release from contused brain tissue into surrounding brain areas. Acta Neurochir [Suppl] 60: 524-527
2. Katayama Y, Becker DP, Tamura T, Ikezaki K (1990) Early cellular swelling in experimental traumatic brain injury: A phenomenon mediated by excitatory amino acids. Acta Neurochir [Suppl] 51: 271-273
3. Katayama Y, Becker DP, Tamura T, Hovda DA (1990) Massive increases in extracellular potassium and indiscriminate release of glutamate following concussive brain injury. J Neurosurg 54: 773-782
4. Choi DW, Koh J, Peters S (1988) Pharmacology of glutamate neurotoxicity in cortical cell culture: attenuation by NMDA antagonists. J Neurosci 8: 185-196
5. Katayama Y, Tamura T, Becker DP, Tsubokawa T (1992) Early cellular swelling during cerebral ischemia in vivo is mediated by excitatory amino acids release from nerve terminal. Brain Res 577: 121-126
6. Faden AI, Demediuk P, Panter SS, Vink R (1989) The role of excitatory amino acids and NMDA receptors in traumatic brain injury. Science 244: 798-800
7. Kinoshita K, Katayama T, Kano T, Hirayama T, Tsubokawa T (1994) Attenuation of hemispheric swelling associated with acute subdural hematomas by excitatory amino acid antagonist in rats. Acta Neurochir [Suppl] 60: 505-507
8. Dixon CE, Clifton GL, Lighthall JW, Yaghmai AA (1991) A controlled cortical impact model of traumatic brain injury in the rat. J Neurosci Methods 39: 253-262
9. Katayama Y, Yoshino A, Kano T, Kushi H, Tsubokawa T (1994) Role of contusion necrosis in development of the mass effect and elevated intracranial pressure. presented in 9th International Symposium on ICP (Nagoya, Japan)

Analysis of 37 Patients with Evolving Intracranial Lesions in the First 12 Hours After Trauma: Value of ICP Monitoring

F. SERVADEI[1], A. NANNI[2], M.T. NASI[1], D. ZAPPI[2], G. VERGONI[3], C. STURIALE[1], and A. ARISTA[1]

[1] Division of Neurosurgery, [2] Intensive Care Unit, [3] Neuroradiological Service, Ospedale M. Bufalini, Cesena, Italy

INTRODUCTION

Since the introduction of CT scanning in management of head injuries it became clear that serial examinations (1) are required to show either an evolution of an already present lesion or the appearence of new lesions.Even if progressive worsening is more frequent, recent papers described also a rapid disappearence of extracerebral postraumatic collections without a surgical treatment and with clinical improvement(2).The biochemical basis of a delayed cerebral damage are related to the presence of oxygen free radicals , to exitatory aminoacids such as aspartate and glutamate(3) and to coagulopathy (4).Also concerning surgery and future medical therapies (3),the crucial point is patients' monitoring and timinig of investigations.In this paper we study a group of comatouse patients with "early"evolving intracranial postraumatic lesions in order to find the best method to detect lesions' evolution before clinical deterioration.

MATHERIAL AND METHODS

Our Neurosurgical Intensive Care Unit is the referring Centre for an area populated by aproximately 1200000 inhabitants.There are in the same area 7 other regional hospitals without Neurosurgery but with a 24 hrs available CT scanning and a General Intensive Care Unit. An Emergency medical service is available both with elicopters and with ambulances carrying Casualty doctors.From 1/1/90 to 30/4/93 412 patients were admitted in coma following an head injury to our Intensive Care Unit.Thirty seven (9%) patients were retrospectively identified as harbouring lesions evolving within 12 hrs from admission.We define early lesions' evolution as increasing or decreasing of an already present haematoma or as appearence of a totally new lesion which occurred within 12 hrs from injury.Because of the presence of CT scans in many peripheral hospitals and of a well organized transport system,all these cases were submitted to the first examination within 3 hrs from injury (and 32 ouf of 37 within 2 hrs).The second CT examination was obtained from 2 to 12 hrs after trauma because of clinical deterioration,of a scheduled CT control or of an increasing ICP (defined as ICP >25 mmHg or CPP <70 mm Hg). Clinical criteria for inclusion in this study are GCS from 4 to 8 and at least one reacting pupil on admission.On the contrary,all patients presenting evolving lesions and a clinical deterioration are included independently from the depth of coma at treatment.Immediate laboratory tests obtained on admission included a complete blood count,platlets, prothombin time and partial thromboplastine time.

RESULTS

Our study group is therefore constituted by 37 patients either comatouse on admission or following clinical deterioration.In these patients a second CT examination showed evolving intracranial postraumatic lesions within 12 hrs from injury.There are 25 males and 12 females,mean age is 34.9 yrs(from 5 to 72 yrs) and the trauma was caused by road traffic accidents in 32 cases (86.5%).Ten patients (27%) presented significant associated injuries,9 (24.3%)patients were reported as having had at least one episode of shock (defined as sist.BP persistently below 80) and only 6 cases (16.2%) had a verified coagulopathy on admission.Mean GCS on admission was 6.8 (from 4 to 14),12 (32.4%)cases presented with abnormal pupils,13(35.1%) patients showed clinical deterioration .
The first CT examination, obtained from 30' to 3 hrs from trauma showed a subdural haematoma (SH) in 31 cases (with a thickness ranging from 4 to 23 mm),an Extradural Haematoma (EH) in 7 cases (thickness from 8 to 35 mm) and an hemorragic contusion/Intracerebral Haematoma (ICH) in 14 cases (Volume >25 cc only in 1 case).It is to be noted that many patients harboured more than one lesion.
Our casework material is then divided into 3 different cathegories according to the CT classification of the Trumaumatic Coma Data Bank(5):1) Fifteen patients with an initial diagnosis of Diffuse Injury (DI,grading from 1 to 4) with evolving lesion but within the same cathegory (DI>DI) 2)Fifteen patients with an initial diagnosis of Diffuse Injury evolving into an Evacuated Mass Lesion (EML) (DI>EML)3) Seven patients already operated because of an acute postraumatic lesion showing a second surgical lesion within 12 hrs from injury.(EML>EML)

Tab 1:Demographics and clinical parameters in 3 different cathegories

	age	RTA	shock	ass.inj.	abn.coag	GCS	abn.pup.	clin.det
Cat 1 (DI>DI)	27.2	83%	13.3%	26.6%	13.3%	6.4	40%	/*
Cat 2 (DI>EML)	39.1	83%	40%	13.3%	13.3%	7.8	20%	73.3%*
Cat 3 (EML>EML)	42.4	86%	28.5%	14.2%	28.5%	5.7	43%	28.5%*

Note that all the paramethers,apart from mean age and GCS, are expressed as percentage of patients showing road traffic accident,shock on admission,abnormal coagulation,abnormal pupils and clinical deterioration;*p<0.01

Median timing of the second CT examination was 9 hrs in Cat 1 (DI>DI),6 hrs in Cat 2 (DI>EML) and 10 hrs in Cat 3 (EML>EML).This difference is statistically significant (p<0.05).
Among the first group (DI>DI) there are 15 cases of disappearence or of significant reduction of an acute SH,3 cases of unchanged lesion (one SH and 2 ICHs).In 7 cases a totally new lesion appeared:3 ICHs,3 patients showing landmarks of Diffuse Axonal Injury (DAI) and one patient with a small (15cc) EDH.
Among the second group of patients (DI>EML) there are 4 cases of desappearence of a SH,10 cases of increased lesions (6 ICH,2 SH,2 EDH) and 8 cases of new lesions (4 ICH and 4 EDH).Out of 4 new EDH,2 were delayed Haematoma with a normal CT scanning and a state of shock on admission.
In the last group (EML>EML) the first surgical intervention was the evacuation of a SH in 5 patients and of an EDH in 2 cases.The second surgical approach was always (exept for a cerebellar ICH) related to a controlateral lesion (6 ICH,3 EDH and 1 SH).Four of these haematomas were already present in the first CT scanning but with a smaller volume.
There is a statistically significant difference in lesions' evolution (p<0.01,chi square test) being SH more prone to reabsorption and ICH to increase or to appear as a new lesion.

If we consider how we monitored our patients, in 16 cases we recorded ICP.In 11 of these either an increase of ICP or a decrease of CPP led us to repeat a CT scanning.There were no deaths in these group.In 16 other patients the diagnosis was due to a scheduled CT control (5 deaths) and in the remaining 10 cases a clinical deterioration led to a new examinations (4 deaths).
The outcome was evaluated at 6 months according to the GOS.Twenty-four patients had a good recovery (64.8%),4 were left severly disabled (11.9%) and 9 died (24.3%).

DISCUSSION

The danger of an early CT examination in evaluating severe head injuries has been stressed by several authors (6).Common risk factors leading to delayed haematomas are the presence of shock on admission (7) as in 2 of our cases,an already present small lesion and surgical decompression in case of haematoma in the postoperative period (8),a coagulopathy on admission (4),but this observation is not confirmed in our material.Whereas delayed EDH are not uncommon (6),usually acute SH tend to reach its maximum size within a few hours from trauma(9).The timing of the evolution of ICH is more controversial:at 12 hrs from trauma from 84% to 26%
of haematomas were already present in 2 different series (10,11).Also in our material ICH are the lesion more prone to enlarge or to appear as a new haematoma .On the contrary there is a statistically significant tendency toward reabsorption or decrease in size of subdural collections together with resolution of an immediate midline shift (patients in the cathegory DI>DI).Furthermore ,also in the group of patients evolving toward a mass lesion (DI>EML)there are 4 cases of SH's disappearence.Even if we had 2 cases of increase of the SH requiring surgery,careful conservative management of small (thickness <10mm always) subdural collections with ICP monitoring seems appropriate.Aggressive surgical treatment in such cases can be unjstified (9) and can lead to miss (as in 4 of our patients)the real "surgical evolving lesion" or (as in other 3 cases) the presence of signs of DAI which explain part of the bad outcomes intially related to small SH.Patients moving form the DI group to the surgical group (EML) tend to present clinical deterioration earlier (median 6 hrs from trauma,$p<0.05$).Concerning then the best method to monitor patients' evolution,there are no bad outcomes among the group of patients followed by an ICP monitoring even if not to a statistically significant degree.Immediate ICP monitoring was unusual in our Center since we preferred in cases with normal basal cysterns and normal third ventricle (5) to follow the patient with serial CT and eventually to insert later an ICP monitoring.The high rate of clinical deterioration with bad results in the very first hours postrauma (group DI>EML) conviced us that in presence of comatouse patients with intracranial lesions or with normal CT scanning but with a state of shock ,ICP monitoring should be initiated immediatly after the first assessment.

REFERENCES

1)Roberson FC,Kishore PR,Miller JD,Lipper MH,Becker DP:The value of serial Computerized Tomography in the management of severe head injury Surg Neurol 12,161-167,1979
2)Polman CH,Gijsbers CJ,Heimans JJ,Ponssen H,Valk J:Rapid spontaneous resolution of an acute subdural hematoma
Neurosurgery 19,446-448,1986
3)McIntosh:Novel Pharmacological therapies in the treatment of experimental traumatic brain injury J Neurotrauma 10,215-259,1993
4)Stein SC,Young GS,Talucci RC,Greenbaum BH,Ross SE:Delayed brain injury following head trauma: significance of coagulopathy Neurosurgery 30,160-165,1992
5)Marshall LF,Bowers Marshall S,Klauber MR,Van Bernum Clarke M:
A new classification of head injury based on computed tomography
J Neurosurg. 75,S14-S20,1991
6)Poon WS,Poon CYS, Li AKC:Traumatic extradural hematoma of delayed onset is not a rarity

Neurosurgery 30,681-686,1992
7)Bucci MN,Phillips TW,McGillicuddy JE:Delayed epidural hemorrhage in hypotensive multiple trauma patients Neurosurgery 19,65-68,1986
8)Reale F,Biancotti R:Acute bilateral epidural hematoma
Surg Neurol 24,260-262,1985
9)Mathew P,Oluoch-Olunya L,Condon BR,Bullock R:Acute subdural haematoma in the conscious patient:outcome with initial non-operative management Acta Neurochir. 121,100-108,1993
10)Soloniuk D,Pitts LH,Lovely M,Bartkowski H:Traumatic intracerebral hematomas:timing of apperence and indications to operative removal J Trauma 26,787-793,1986
11)Yamaki T,Hirakawa K,Ueguchi T,Tenjin H,Kuboyama T,Nagakawa Y:
Chronological evaluation of acute traumatic intracerebral haematoma Acta Neurochir. 103, 112-115,1990

Secondary Growth of a Primary Brain Tissue Necrosis from Focal Trauma

J. Eriskat[1], O. Kempski[2], L. Schürer[3], S. Berger[4], F. Staub[1], and A. Baethmann[1]

[1]Institute for Surgical Research, [3]Department of Neurosurgery, Klinikum Großhadern, Ludwigs-Maximilians-University, 81336 Munich, Germany
[2]Institute for Neurosurg. Pathophysiology, [4]Department of Pediatric Surgery, Johannes-Gutenberg-University, 55131 Mainz, Germany

SUMMARY

Secondary brain damage developing from a primary lesion in head injury or cerebral ischemia is of major significance for the outcome of afflicted patients. Understanding of underlying processes is required in order to devise specific, i.e. more effective methods of treatment. Novel information has been obtained by this laboratory that a primary brain tissue necrosis resulting from a focal lesion is liable to increase secondarily. Presently, its growth kinetics has been investigated more closely during a posttraumatic period of 24 hours. For that purpose a highly standardised focal cold injury of the brain was induced in rats. Area as well as volume of the resulting parenchyma necrosis were quantitatively determined by histomorphometry after increasing periods of survival, reaching from 5 minutes to 24 hours after trauma. The maximal plane of the necrosis in histological sections was increasing by 45 % ($p < 0.001$) within the total posttraumatic observation period. Growth of necrosis was not limited to the early period, but continued between 12 and 24 hours, amounting then to 29 % ($p < 0.05$). As based on integration of the histologically determined areas of necrosis, it was found that its volume was also increasing by 45% within 24 hours. The present findings confirm that a primary focal brain lesion, corresponding to a contusion focus in severe head injury, is significantly growing within 24 hours after trauma, longer periods of survival were not investigated yet. Nevertheless, quantitative assessment of the phenomenon makes possible not only to study mechanisms which are involved, but also to develop therapeutical methods to inhibit growth of the lesion.

INTRODUCTION

Development of secondary brain damage in acute cerebral lesions from trauma or ischemia is highly significant for the outcome of afflicted patients (1). Pertinent examples to elucidate this point are formation of brain edema and impairment of the cerebral blood flow in head injury, resulting among others in intracranial hypertension and ischemic brain damage. The increase of a primary brain tissue necrosis from a focal lesion, for example a contusion focus in head injury, may be considered as manifestation of secondary brain damage having the potential of therapeutical inhibition. Understanding of underlying mechanisms, however, is required for that purpose, making necessary availability of suitable experimental models. The report presents recent findings of this laboratory analyzing growth of a brain tissue necrosis at high temporal and spatial resolution (cf. 3, 8, 9). Attempts of inhibiting this process by interfering with glutamate excitotoxicity were included.

MATERIALS AND METHODS

Male Sprague-Dawley rats (280 ± 40 g b.w.; n = 59) were anesthetized by ether following premedication by subcutaneous atropin. Anesthesia was continued by i.p. chloralhydrate (360 mg/kg b.w.). The spontaneously room-air breathing animals were supplied with additional oxygen. The skull was fixed in a stereotactic frame for exposure of the left parietal brain by craniotomy of 3 mm Ø. A dental drill was utilized for that purpose under continuous cooling of the skull surface and employment of an operating microscope. The dura mater which was frequently moistened with isotonic saline remained undamaged. The insult was made by a metal probe (1 mm Ø) attached to a stainless steel cylinder and cooled to -68° C by dry ice/acetone mixture. The metal probe was fixed to a stereotactic device powered by a computer-controlled stepper motor for its precise placement and control of the duration of freezing. Cold injury was induced according to KLATZO (4) through the craniotomy during a freezing period of 10 sec. Histological studies of the resulting lesion were demonstrating a clearly demarcated necrosis of cerebral cortex. The body temperature was maintained at 37.5° C - 38.5°C during anesthesia by a feed-back controlled heating pad. Animals were distributed in six different experimental groups with increasing survival after trauma, i.e. from 5 min to 3, 6, 12, 18 or 24 hrs, respectively allowing characterization of the dynamics of lesion growth during the posttraumatic course. Following sacrifice animals were rapidly thoracotomized for perfusion fixation of the brain through the left cardiac ventricle, commencing with isotonic saline followed by 2 % buffered paraformaldehyde (pH 7.4) for 20 min. In two additional groups of animals (n: 9 - 10) surviving trauma for 24 hrs, the AMPA-receptor blocking agent NBQX was administered as bolus followed by continuous infusion at two different dose levels (total dose: 7, or 70 mg/kg b.w.).

Animals surviving longer periods after trauma were allowed to recover from anesthesia after suturing the skin flap over the skull. Anesthesia was introduced again after respective survival for perfusion fixation of the brain. This was followed by decapitation with placement of the head in 10 % formalin at 4° C overnight. The brain was carefully removed then from the skull and again stored in 10 % formalin prior to histological preparation after dehydration and embedding in paraffin. Coronal serial brain sections of 3 - 5 µm were made at 100 µm intervals throughout the brain containing lesion. The histological sections were stained with cresyl violet (Nissl). The plane of necrosis was quantitatively assessed in sections demonstrating presence of the traumatic lesion. The maximal lesion area was determined by this approach, and the integral of all areas of necrosis of a brain was used for calculation of the necrosis volume according to the "Basic volume estimator" (7). The results are given as mean ± standard error of the mean. Differences between groups were tested by the Kruskal-Wallis test with Conover´s multiple comparisons according to Theordorsson-Norheim (6). Part of the results were reported by Eriskat et al. (1994).

RESULTS

The primary size of the maximal area of necrosis and its subsequent growth are shown in table 1 together with the volume calculated from the integer of all areas of necrosis. As seen, the plane of necrosis was increasing within 3 hrs after the insult by 20 %, i.e. from 0.75 ± 0.06 mm^2 to 0.90 ± 0.05 mm^2. No active growth of necrosis occurred between 3 and 12 hrs thereafter. Subsequently, however, the area of necrosis was growing again between 12 and 24 hours, from 0.85 ± 0.05 mm^2 to 1.09 ± 0.08 mm^2 ($p < 0.05$). Hence, the maximal area of necrosis was growing in total by 45 % within 24 hrs after trauma ($p < 0.001$). The corresponding volume of necrosis obtained by utilizing the lesion areas of serial brain sections was increasing from 0.78 ± 0.09 mm^3 at 5 min after lesion to 1.13 ± 0.09 mm^3 at 24 hrs later. The increase in necrosis volume of 45 % is in perfect agreement with that of the maximal necrosis plane within this observation period. Due to deviation of individual data, however, differences in the necrosis volume between 5 min and 24 hrs were stastistically not significant. Administration of NBQX was not found to inhibit the secondary increase of the focal tissue necrosis within 24 hrs after lesion, neither as low- nor high dose regimen.

Table 1. Maximal plane and volume of necrosis of the brain in rats with a focal cold lesion *

Survival Time	n	Maximal area (mm^2)	Necrosis volume (mm^3)
5 min	9	0.75 ± 0.06^{c}	0.78 ± 0.09
3 h	8	0.90 ± 0.05	1.02 ± 0.09
6 h	10	0.85 ± 0.05^{b}	0.97 ± 0.11
12 h	7	0.85 ± 0.05^{b}	1.04 ± 0.10
18 h	10	0.94 ± 0.06^{a}	1.07 ± 0.07
24 h	15	1.09 ± 0.08	1.13 ± 0.09

^{a} $p < 0.05$ vs. 5 min; ^{b} $p < 0.01$ vs. 24 h; ^{c} $p < 0.001$ vs. 24 h.; * from (3).

DISCUSSION

The current results provide a clear answer to the question, whether an acute irreversible brain lesion is liable to increase during the posttraumatic course. Respective observations made in other forms of brain damage, such as laser injury are in agreement with the present findings (2, 5). The dynamic analysis of lesion growth indicates that spread of the brain tissue necrosis occurred during two distinguishable periods, an early phase up to 3 hrs after trauma and a delayed from 12 to 24 hrs. Quantitative histological morphometry provided the basis to assess the progressive destruction of brain parenchyma following the freezing insult. The primary lesion was limited by purpose to the grey matter of cerebral cortex to facilitate distinction between irreversibly damaged tissue and viable perifocal parenchyma in histological sections. Spread of the lesion in the histological preparations was additionally studied by assessment of the density of viable nerve cells in perifocal brain tissue areas (data not shown). These findings confirm that growth of the necrotic lesion is attributable to a progressive demise of cells and not to mere expansion of necrotic tissue by swelling (9).

Various factors may be considered to contribute to the increase of irreversibly damaged brain parenchyma. Among others, deterioration of the cerebral blood flow might be involved from progressive damage of the arterial blood supply to the lesion proper and perifocal tissue. Further, activation of cytotoxic processes might be implicated secondary to formation and/or release of neurotoxic mediator compounds, such as glutamate, arachidonic acid and its many metabolites, and the development of tissue acidosis. The present failure of the AMPA-receptor blocking agent to inhibit lesion growth within 24 hrs after trauma does not rule out, however, that processes relating to glutamate excitotoxicity were involved. More conclusive data are expected by testing other types of glutamate receptor antagonists.

The technical approach utilized for this analysis and the emerging data demonstrating increase of a primary tissue necrosis after trauma at a quantitative level is an important step. It provides a basis not only for elucidation of underlying mechanisms, but also for development and evaluation of specific methods of therapeutical inhibition. Since it can be assumed that, e.g. formation of vasogenic brain edema is a function of the mass of irreversibly destroyed tissue, therapeutical inhibition of lesion growth would have clinical consequences for the improvement of specificity of treatment of secondary brain damage.

ACKNOWLEDGEMENTS

The technical and secretarial assistance of Ann Hedblom, Helga Kleylein and Daniele Gehrke is gratefully acknowledged.

REFERENCES

1. Baethmann A, Maier-Hauff K, Kempski O, Unterberg A, Wahl M, Schürer L (1988) Mediators of brain edema and secondary brain damage. Crit Care Med 16: 972-978

2. Eggert HR, Kiessling M, Kleihues P (1985) Time course and spatial distribution of neodymium: yttrium-aluminium-garnet (Nd: YAG) laser-induced lesions in the rat brain. Neurosurgery 16: 443-448

3. Eriskat J, Schürer L, Kempski O, Baethmann A (1994) Growth kinetics of a primary brain tissue necrosis from a focal lesion. Acta Neurochir (Suppl) 60: 425-427

4. Klatzo I, Piraux A, Laskowski EJ (1958) The relationship between edema, blood-brain barrier and tissue elements in a local brain injury. J Neuropathol Exp Neurol 17: 548-564

5. Lindsberg PJ, Frerichs KU, Burris JA, Hallenbeck JM, Feuerstein G (1991) Cortical microcirculation in a new model of focal Laser-induced secondary brain damage. J Cereb Blood Flow Metab 11: 88-98

6. Theodorsson-Norheim E (1986) Kruskal-Wallis test: BASIC computer program to perform nonparametric one-way analysis of variance and multiple comparisons on ranks of several independent samples. Comp Meth Prog Biomed 23: 57-62

7. Uylings HBM, van Eden CG, Hofman MA (1986) Morphometry of size/volume variables and comparison of their bivariate relations in the nervous system under different conditions. J Neurosci Meth 18: 19-37

8. Vonhof S (in preparation) Autoradiographische Untersuchungen des Gehirns über das sekundäre Nekrosewachstum nach primärem Trauma. Thesis, Ludwig-Maximilians-Universität München

9. Wyrwich W (1994) Die Entwicklung einer sekundären Hirngewebsnekrose nach primärem Trauma. Thesis, Ludwig-Maximilians-Universität München

Closed Head Injury as a Model of Alzheimer Disease

BRUCE J. ANDERSEN[1], W. SUE T. GRIFFIN[1], and SVETLANA V. PRAVDENKOVA[2]

[1] University of Arkansas for Medical Sciences, Little Rock, AR, USA
[2] Sklifosovsky Institute of First Aid, Moscow, Russia

SUMMARY

Alzheimer Disease is functionally characterized by slow but progressive deterioration of memory and cognition. Histologically it is characterized by increased numbers of neurofibrillary tangles and amyloid deposition in brain. Immunohistochemically, it is characterized by increased amounts of the glia derived cytokine IL-1α, and increased expression of S100ß and ß-APP proteins. The underlying cause of this disease is unknown but recently, reports suggest that closed head injury may be an inciting factor in the later development of Alzheimer Disease (AD).

Although Alzheimer Disease affects a significant portion of the adult population, no animal model of the disease exists, severely hampering examination of both causative and therapeutic factors. Since head trauma in humans produces immunohistochemically identical pathology to that seen in classic Alzheimer Disease, we adapted an easily administered, reproducible, and minimally invasive head injury for use in weanling Fischer 344 rats then examined the brains of these animals at various time post injury for expression of IL-1 and S100ß. These two proteins are expressed in both Alzheimer Disease and in humans suffering from "dementia pugilistica", a premature development of Alzheimer type histopathology brought about by closed head injury. If this model of close injury is able to cause expression of IL-1 and S100ß in surviving animals, prognostic and possible therapeutic measures referable to Alzheimer Disease may be developed using this animal model of the disease.

INTRODUCTION

Head injury has been shown to be the most consistent environmental factor predisposing persons to the early development of Alzheimer Disease, [1-3] and a significant association between head injury and Alzheimer Disease has been shown in up to 20% of Alzheimer Disease cases [4]. Histologically, ß amyloid precursor proteins are thought to be critical in the development of classic human Alzheimer Disease [5]. Roberts [6] has shown that ß-APP is produced in previously normal post-traumatic brain tissue, and has observed that the chronic progressive dementia ("dementia pugilistica") suffered by persons subjected to repeated closed head injuries clinically mimics the symptoms of early onset Alzheimer Disease [7]. Furthermore, the ß-APP seen in head injured persons is immunohistochemically identical to that seen in classic Alzheimer Disease [2].

From these data, researchers have inferred that closed head injury may be an event which predisposes persons to develop Alzheimer Disease at an early age, and that the severity of the head injury may correlate with the amount of ß-APP expressed [8]. Additionally, intervening with the IL-1 cascade (hypothesized to stimulate ß-APP expression) with IL-1 antagonists may be a potential therapeutic strategy to decrease ß-APP expression and to slow the onset of Alzheimer Disease [8,9].

Identification of whether or not isolated closed head injury acts as an inciting event remains to be shown in an experimental situation. Furthermore, whether the severity of the head injury correlates with the degree of protein expression or the speed of onset remains to be quantitated. Finally to be answered is the question of whether or not specific antagonists or other agents, given at appropriate times, can actually decrease protein expression or slow the onset of Alzheimer Disease.

To attempt to provide answers to these questions we used a closed head injury of varying severity as an inciting event to produce the histopathologic changes characteristic of Alzheimer Disease and identify the chronology of their development and elevation following injury.

The type of head injury model selected for use in this project needs to fulfill a number of criteria:

1. It must mimic human head injury as closely as possible in order to allow reasonable extrapolation of the data from experimental to clinical situations.

2. Its morbidity must be easily controlled to allow changes in the degree of injury delivered without altering the entire experimental paradigm.

3. Administration of the head injury must involve minimal surgical manipulation of the animal to maximize post-traumatic survival.

4. Survivors must be able to care for themselves without outside intervention.

5. Immunohistochemical assays for S100ß, IL-1α, and ß-APP must be reliably performed and show positive results following trauma.

The reason this model is ideally suited for this investigation is as follows:

1. This device produces diffuse axonal injury (DAI) & hydrocephalus without hematomata or brain stem damage [10,11]. Most currently used models of head injury (eg. fluid percussion, pneumatic stunners, projectiles) produce intraparenchymal contusions or hemorrhages in the course of the injury, and require or produce an opening in the skull. None of these are desirable if a colony of long term survivors is to be produced, as they introduce secondary insults which confound the analysis of the effects of the initial concussion. Histopathologically, diffuse axonal injury and post-traumatic ventriculomegaly are frequently seen in this model, paralleling the most commonly reported pathologic findings in human head injury, [10,11] further supporting the use of this particular model as one that closely mimics human head injury.

2. The weight drop, closed head injury model proposed for this project has well defined morbidity and mortality that are easily varied by changing the impact force either by weight or height changes, thereby allowing animals to be injured at different severity levels without changing the overall biomechanics of the device (see chapter entitled "A Survivable Closed Head Injury Model in Weanling Rats" by Andersen et al. in this volume).

3. The preparation involves only a small scalp opening and leaves the skull intact, making recovery and incorporation into a long term maintenance colony feasible.(see methods)

4. In our pilot data (see chapter entitled "A Survivable Closed Head Injury Model in Weanling Rats" by Andersen et al. in this volume), we have seen no short term changes in the normal weight gain of our rats surviving LD_{25}, LD_{50}, and LD_{75} injury levels without skull fractures. This suggests that although a significant head injury has been delivered, neurologic functions vital to long term survival are not affected by the injury.

METHODS

The weight drop model of closed head injury in rats recently reported by Marmarou [10,11]was adapted for use in weanling Fischer 344 rats by decreasing the delivered force. This model of consists of a vertical tube though which weights are dropped. The weight drops onto a stainless steel button cemented to the vertex of the animal's skull. This metal button distributes the force evenly, prevents any rotational component, and decreases the incidence of skull fractures. The animal is supported on a contoured foam rest of specific density to allow approximately 2-3 cm of neck flexion upon impact (no additional immobilization is used). This degree of neck flexion has been shown not to produce spinal cord injury or cervical spine fractures, yet allows a small motion component to be a part of the injury model, which more closely approximates the human condition of head injury than a static impact paradigm.

The surgical preparation is minimal, requiring only exposure of the vertex and cementing the steel cap to the exposed skull. This incision is easily closed and well tolerated by the animals, making this an ideal model for survivor experiments to examine the long term sequelae of closed head injury (see chapter entitled "A Survivable Closed Head Injury Model in Weanling Rats" by Andersen et al. in this volume). The expression of S100ß was examined immunohistochemically.

RESULTS

We found an increased immunoreactivity to S100ß protein and increased staining of astrocytic processes as early as three hours following an LD_{50} impact level. Furthermore, we found approximately a 150% increase in the expression of S100ß protein over similar aged control rats within the first week following trauma.

We also found that animals which survive the trauma without skull fractures have no neurologic dysfunction that prevent them from feeding, grooming, moving, or gaining weight. Animals of both sexes that survived the injury without fracture gained weight at the same rate that non-injured control animals did (see chapter entitled "A Survivable Closed Head Injury Model in Weanling Rats" by Andersen et al. in this volume).

DISCUSSION

The significance of these data is two-fold: it shows that this closed head injury model results in abnormal protein expression similar to those seen in clinical head injured and Alzheimer's Disease patients, and when combined with the normal growth pattern in survivors, suggest that this weight drop model of closed head injury in Fischer 344 rats may be used to establish colonies of long term closed head injury survivors to evaluate the effect head injury has upon the premature development of Alzheimer type neuropathology.

REFERENCES

1. Corsellis JAN, Ambler MW, Freeman-Brown D (1973): The aftermath of boxing. **Psychol Med 3**: 270-273.

2. Roberts GW (1988): Immunocytochemistry of neurofibrillary tangles in demential pugilistica and Alzheimer's Disease: evidence for a common genesis. **Lancet 2(8626-8627)**: 1456-1458.

3. Van duijn CM, Hofman A, Kay DWK (1991): Risk factors for Alzheimer's Disease: a collaborative analysis of case-control studies. **Int J Epidemiol 20**: S4.

4. Mortimer JA, Van Duijn CM, Chandra V (1991): Head trauma as a risk factor for Alzheimer's Disease: a collaborative re-analysis of case-control studies. **Int J Epidemiol 20**: S28.

5. Joachim CL, Selkoe DJ (1992): The seminal role of ß-amyloid in the pathogenesis of Alzheimer Disease. In: **Alzheimer Disease and Associated Disorders**, Raven Press New York, pp. 7-34.

6. Roberts GW, Allsop D, Bruton CJ (1990): The occult aftermath of boxing. **J Neurol Neurosurg Psychiatry 53**: 373-378.

7. Roberts GW (1969): **Brain Damage in Boxers**, Pitman, London.

8. Roberts GW, Gentleman SM, Lynch A, Murray L, Landon M, Graham DI (1993): ß-amyloid protein deposition in the brain following severe head injury: Implications for the pathogenesis of Alzheimer's Disease. **J Neurol Neurosurg Psychiatry** in review.

9. Royston MC, Rothwell NJ, Roberts GW (1992): Alzheimer's Disease: pathology to potential treatments? **TIPS 13**:131-133.

10. Marmarou A, Foda MA, van den Brink W, Campbell J, Kita H, Demetriadou K: (1994): A new model of diffuse brain injury in rats. Part I: Pathophysiology and biomechanics. **J Neurosurg 80**: 291-300.

11. Foda MA, Marmarou A (1994): A new model of diffuse brain injury in rats. Part II Morphological characterization. **J Neurosurg 80:** 301-313.

Session XVII: Effects of Increased ICP (3)

Chairmen: P. Reilly and H. Yamada

High Cerebral Perfusion Pressure Is Not a Synonym to Preserved Cerebral Blood Flow

E. SHALMON, M.J. CARON, N.A. MARTIN, D.A. HOVDA, and D.P. BECKER

Division of Neurosurgery, Brain Injury Research Center, UCLA School of Medicine, Los Angeles, CA, USA

INTRODUCTION

The maintenance of adequate cerebral circulation is considered critical in the treatment of any head-injured patient. This circulation is governed by a pressure gradient existing between the inflow and the outflow divided by the total resistance. The concept of cerebral perfusion pressure (CPP) has consequently been defined as the difference between mean arterial blood pressure (MABP) and intracranial pressure (ICP).

In 1970, Zwetnow (13) and Haggendal et al. (2) proposed that ICP was equal to the cerebral venous pressure and therefore adopted ICP as the outflow pressure of the brain. In their studies they found that CBF was stable until CPP fell to 40 mm Hg. Two years later, Miller et al. (4) confirmed these studies and established the relationship between CBF and CPP in intact and defective autoregulatory states. Thereafter, CPP was calculated as the difference between MABP, as an indicator of the arterial pressure, at the site the vessels entering the subarachnoid space, and ICP, as an indicator of the pressure in the venous outflow pressure as the veins enter the dural sinuses. In recent years, studies have emphasized that effective cerebral circulation depends on adequate cerebral perfusion pressure above 70 mm Hg (1, 8). The purpose of this study was to correlate simultaneous measurements of CPP and CBF in severely head-injured patients, and to assess the ability of predicting CBF from CPP. The concern addressed in the present study is that physicians may have a sense of false security of adequate cerebral circulation if they rely solely on CPP maintenance.

METHODS

Subjects: Fifty two consecutive head-injured patients were prospectively evaluated for this study (44 males and 8 females; mean age 35 years, ranging 18 - 74). Initial Glasgow Coma Scale score was 3 to 12, (mean 6.8). One hundred and five studies were conducted when patients had GCS 3-8 and 25 studies were conducted when patients had GCS 9 and above. Patients were treated according to the circumstances with intubation, early evacuation of mass lesion or conservative treatment. Intracranial pressure was monitored with a ventricular catheter in 46 patients and by an intraparenchymal device in the remaining 6 patients. ICP was treated according to the therapy intensity level concept with sedation, paralysis and ventricular CSF drainage, followed by mild hyperventilation and mannitol. Gunshot injured patients and patients who received barbiturates as part of ICP treatment were excluded.

Cerebral perfusion pressure and blood flow measurements: CPP was constantly monitored during the acute period by subtraction of mean ICP from MABP. Routine measurements of CBF were performed within the first 24 hours of admission and every other day thereafter. Cerebral blood flow measurements were performed by the ^{133}Xe intravenous technique. Global CBF-15 was calculated from the clearance curve with 5 detectors over each hemisphere by the Novo-10a Cerebrograph.

RESULTS

A total of 130 measurements of CBF were obtained across all patients. These measurements revealed a wide spectrum of CBF-15 from "reduced flow" to "absolute hyperemia" (23-77 ml/100gm/min). Since ICP and MABP were intensively treated, CPP values were well controlled above 70 mm Hg in 121 of the 130 studies. Figure 1 represents the relationship between simultaneous measurements of CPP and CBF. In 14% of the observations, ICP was above 20 mm Hg and in 22% MABP was below 90 mm Hg. This data discloses a poor correlation (0.016) between CBF and CPP over wide range of CPP (57-128 mm Hg). Consequently, in the lower, as well as in the higher CPP range, high and low CBF values were equally possible. Regression analysis confirms this observation (R^2 - 0.008, n.s.). Figure 2 represents the comparison between simultaneous measurements of CBF and ICP. These data reveal that patients exhibiting low levels of ICP could also exhibit a wide variety of CBF rates. Higher ICP levels tended to have a narrower range of CBF, although there was no evidence of a significant predictive value from one variable to the other (R^2 - 0.011).

Fig.1

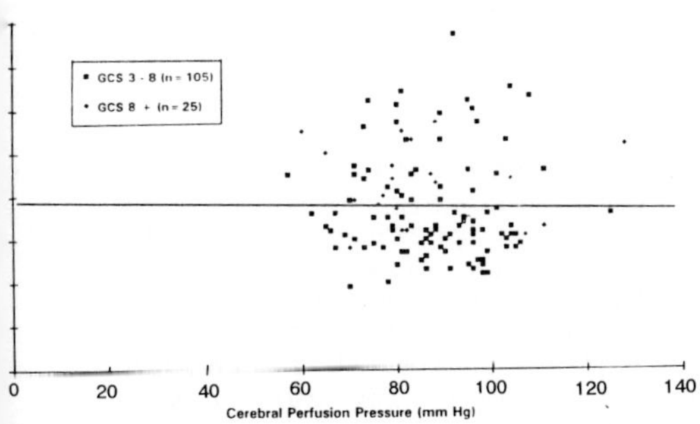

Fig. 2

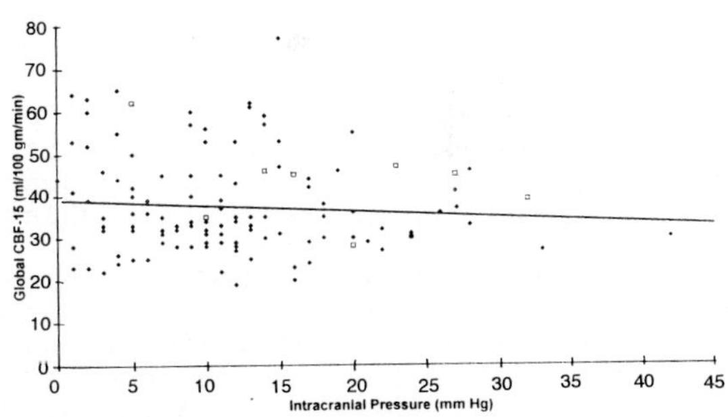

Fig. 1) Correlation between CBF-15 and CPP (n=130). Correlation = 0.016, R^2 = 0.0008, slope = -0.014.
Fig 2) Correlation between CBF-15 and ICP (n=130). Open squares - CPP below 70 mm Hg. Closed diamonds - CPP above 70 mm Hg. Correlation = 0.107, R^2 = 0.011, slope = -0.16.

DISCUSSION

The data presented in this study suggest that CPP and CBF are poorly correlated in head-injured patients. Consequently, in the patient population represented in the current study, relying on CPP to evaluate CBF would have been, at best, an approximation. Perhaps the lack of predictability could be explained in terms of our general lack of understanding of the physiological and anatomical relationship associated with the calculation of CPP. In order to calculate the CPP, the anatomical sites for determination of the inflow and outflow of cerebral vessels need to be defined, and the pressure within these vessels measured. For the measurement of the inflow pressure, the systemic MABP measured in the brachial artery has been used in experimental studies in dogs (4). However, in order to estimate the BP at the arteries as they pierce the dura, the systemic MABP at the foramen of Monro has been used (8). Changes in the caliber of these vessels results in predictable changes in vascular resistance. For example, BP drops by about 50% from the aorta to the small arteries, and therefore, MABP can only provide a relative reflection of the actual BP the brain is exposed to. Shulman found that the pressure in small arteries with an outer diameter of 0.4-0.7 mm is less than half that in the aorta (10). Other studies confirmed these findings demonstrating a linear relationship between the aortic pressure and the intravascular pressure in pial arterioles over the range of 40-200 mm Hg (3, 11). The gradual decline of arterial pressure within the subarachnoid space from large to smaller arterioles, implies that different sites of blood pressure determination most likely would result in different values. Nevertheless, regardless of the exact anatomical site of BP measurement, the different thresholds of the autoregulatory mechanisms and their effect on microcirculatory flow should be considered.

As with inflow pressure, determination of the anatomical site for outflow pressure (as well as the relationship between pressure along the venous tree and ICP), in normal and intracranial hypertension conditions, is important. Shulman considered the subarachnoid veins as a part of a collapsible system of vessels whose thin-walls are highly sensitive to progressive external compression as the extravascular pressure exceeds the intraluminal pressure (9, 10). Furthermore, pressure gradients along the superior sagittal sinus (SSS) in the dog have been reported, with the pressure within the anterior-membranous portion of SSS being approximately 60% of ICP compared to 30% of ICP inside the bone-enclosed torcular Herophili. It is thought that this pressure gradient allows rapid blood flow out of the subarachnoid veins and "venting" blood to the jugular bulb. These findings were later confirmed by other studies describing a linear relationship between cortical venous pressure and ICP, with SSS pressure being low regardless of ICP level (5, 12). Similarly, in another animal study, SSS pressure was found to be lower than ICP, with the difference becoming more pronounced with increasing ICP (7). It is important to note that the lowest SSS pressure values were monitored during hypovolemic and hypotensive episodes. In serial cerebral angiograms Shulman demonstrated direct communication between the subarachnoid veins and SSS (9). Consequently with the lack of valves in the venous system between the right atrium and the cortical subarachnoid veins, the cerebral drainage system is sensitive to hydrostatic effects. In an attempt to incorporate these findings, Permutt and Riley introduced a theoretical hemodynamic model from which they developed the hypothesis that the pressure-flow relationship of waterfall could be applied to the cerebral circulation (6). In more recent modeling, Portnoy and Chopp proposed that the pressure within small arteries and arterioles, is the balance between the vasomotor tone (which tends to collapse) and transmural pressure (which tends to distent) the vessel wall (7). In summary, these models, as well as the previous cited studies, indicate that MABP may not represent the inflow pressure of the brain. Furthermore, the outflow pressure of the brain can be represented by ICP, however, its best estimation of the outflow pressure occurs in normal pressure conditions.

CONCLUSION

1. Cerebral perfusion pressure, as defined by the difference between MABP and ICP, dose not by itself predict CBF.
2. Frequent determinations of CBF are important to assess the cerebral circulation.
3 . Maintaining MABP above 90 mm Hg and preventing intracranial hypertension above 20 mm Hg are among the main principles in neurosurgery but they do not insure adequate CBF in severely head-injured patients.

Acknowledgements supported by NS30308.

REFERENCES

[1]. Chan K-H, Miller JD, Dearden NM, Andrews PJD, Midgely S: The effect of changes in cerebral perfusion pressure upon middle cerebral artery blood flow velocity and jugular bulb venous oxygen saturation after severe brain injury. J Neurosurg 77:55-61, 1992.
[2]. Haggendal E, Lofgren J, Nilsson NJ, Zwetnow NN; Effects of varied cerebrospinal fluid pressure on cerebral blood flow in dogs. Acta physiol scand 79:262-271, 1970.
[3]. Kontos HA, Wei EP, Navari RM, Levasseur JE, Rosenblum WI, Patterson JL: Responses of cerebral arteries and arterioles to acute hypotension and hypertension. Am J Physiol 234:H371-H383, 1978.
[4]. Miller JD, Stanek K, Langfitt TW: Concepts of cerebral perfusion pressure and vascular compression during intracranial hypertension. Prog Brain Res 35:411-432, 1972.
[5]. Nakagawa Y, Tsuru M, Yada K: Site and mechanism for compression of the venous system during experimental intracranial hypertension. J Neurosurg 41:427-434, 1974.
[6]. Permutt S, Riley, RL: Hemodynamics of collapsible vessels with tone: the vascular waterfall. J App Physiol 18:924-932, 1963.
[7]. Portnoy HD, Chopp M, Branch G: Hydraulic model of myogenic autoregulation and the cerebrovascular bed: The effects of altering systemic arterial pressure. Neurosurg 13:482-498, 1983.
[8]. Rosner MJ, Daughton S: Cerebral perfusion pressure management in head injury. J Trauma 30: 1990.

[9]. Shulman K, Yarnell P, Ransohoff J: Dual sinus pressure in normal and hydrocephalic dogs. Arch Neurol 10:575-80, 1964.
[10]. Shulman K: Small artery and vein pressures in the subarachnoid space of the dog. J Surg Res 5:56-61, 1965.
[11]. Stromberg DD, Fox JR: Pressures in the pial arterial microcirculation of the cat during changes in systemic arterial blood pressure. Circul Res 31;229-239, 1972.
[12]. Yada K, Nakagawa Y, Tsuru M: Circulatory disturbance of the venous system during experimental intracranial hypertension. J Neurosurg 39:723-729, 1973.
[13]. Zwetnow, NN: Effects of increased cerebrospinal fluid pressure on the blood flow and on the energy metabolism of the brain. Acta Physiol Scand, Suppl 339:1-31, 1970.

Relationship of Cerebral Blood Flow, Cerebral Metabolism and Fast Component of EEG to Outcome in Acute Experimental Compression Ischemia: CBF-Index as in New Indicator

H. Mishina[1], A. Yabuki[1], M. Maeda[1], B.N. Xu[2], M. Miyazaki[2], and S. Ishii[2]

[1] Department of Neurosurgery, Juntendo University Izunagaoka Hospital, Japan
[2] Juntendo Casualty Center of Izunagaoka Hospital, Japan

INTRODUCTION

The pathophysiolosy of brain swelling (edema) following removal of the acute space-occupying lesion is not clearly understood. Now, conventional methods cannot monitor exact value of CMRO2 and CBF continuously at the bed side. We aimed to estimate the exact value of cerebral blood flow and metabplism, by calculating the fast wave component of EEG in combination with AVDO2, as substitute for CMRO2. We made simultaneous observation of the early postischemic changes in cerebral blood flow and metabolism, following global ischemia and reperfusion. Also,we evaluated the effect of barbiturates on secondary cerebral ischemia.

MATERALS AND METHODS (Figure 1)

Experiments were performed on 30 adult cats. Animals were anesthetized and respired artificially. The ICP was monitored by a fiber optic transducer inserted into the subcortical resion of the right occipital lobe. EEG recordings were made using a screw electrode located epidurally over the bilateral sensorimotor cortex. EEG data were transferred to an EEG trend monitor for fast Fourier transform (FFT) % specrtrum band analysis. Regional CBF was measured by the hydrogen clearance method that needle electrodes were inserted into the bilateral thalami stereotaxically. The clearance curve was analysed by the height over-area method for the CBF values. Arteriovenous oxygen difference(AVDO2) and CMRO2 were measured in all cats. The superior sagittal sinus was cannulated anteroposterioly towards the confluence. The AVDO2 was cadlculated as the difference in O2 content between arterial and superior sagittal sinus samples taken simultaneously using:

$$AVDO2 = \{Sat(a)O2 - Sat(v)O2\} \times 1.34. \times Hb / 100 + 0.0031$$

where Hb = hemoblobin and Sat O2 = oxygen saturation. The CMRO2 was estimated from the AVDO2 and the mean CBF: $CMRO2 = AVDO2 \times CBF / 100$

A small rubber balloon located in the right frontal epidural space was gradually inflated using with saline to increase the ICP by 10mmHg per 10 minutes. The ICP was raised until the EEG become completely isoelectric, and hydrogen clearance ceased. This was defined as "global ischemia" to be maintained for 5 minutes in all cats and the balloon was then deflated and removed. All parameters were recorded intermittently. Continuous venous injection of thiopental as 10-15 mg/hr was started after EEG recovery following balloon deflation in seven cats. This was the minimum dose to maintain the burst and suppression EEG pattern. No thiopental was administered after decompression in 13 cats. Wilcoxon test was used for comparison within groups. A calculated difference of $p<0.01$ was considered to be statistically significant.

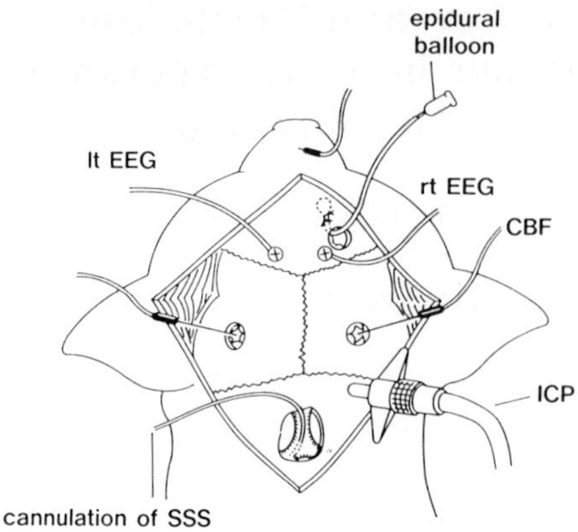

Fig.1

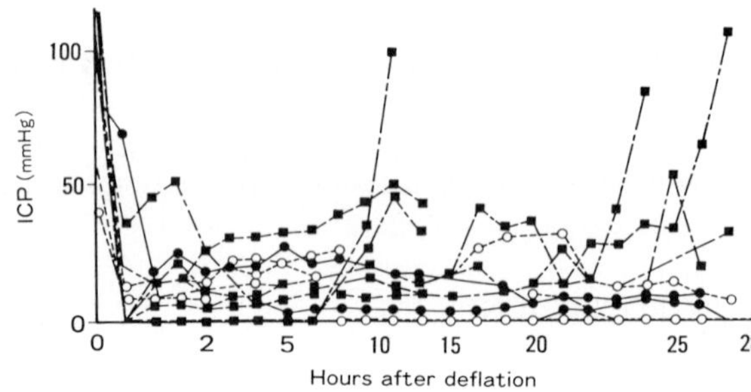

Fig.2

Fig.1 Diagram of experimental arrangement, showing typical recording locations. SSS: superior sagittal sinus

Fig.2 Changes in ICP for each animal in no swelling(●), delayed swelling(■) and barbiturate no swelling group(○).

Results

Figure 2 shows the changes in ICP after balloon deflation. These can be classified into two groups: no or only minimal increase in ICP (no swelling group), and fatal brain swelling after deflation (delayed swelling group). Of 13 cats undergoing 5 minutes global ischemia, six cats were in no swelling group(46%) and seven in delayed swelling group(54%). All seven cats receiving barbiturate after 5 minutes global ischemia, demonstrated no rises in ICP(barbiturate no swelling group). Figure 3A shows the change in thalamic CBF. CBF marked increase just after balloon deflation. One hour after balloon deflation, the CBF fell down significantly in all three groups($p<0.01$). The CBF then gradually recovered in no swelling group. In delayed swelling group, the CBF was remained the low value for 8 hours, and gradually fell. In barbiturate no swelling group, the values obtained during administration of thiopental within 5 hours were slightly low, but then recovered afterwards. Figure 3B shows the time course of the AVDO2 values after deflation of balloon. The AVDO2 decreased and a rapid increase occurred, and remained high for 8 hours in all three groups. No swelling and barbiturate no swelling group showed that the AVDO2 increased after 9 hours. Delayed swelling group showed a rapid decrease of AVDO2 after 8 hours($p<0.01$). Figure 3C shows the time course of the CMRO2. In no swelling group, the CMRO2 values had rapid recovery. In delayed swelling group, the CMRO2 values failed to continuously increase after the initial rapid recovery and decrease significantly after 12 hours($p<0.01$). In barbiturate no swelling group, the CMRO2 had rapid and progressive recovery as in no swelling group, after 5 hours of suppression during thiopental administration, and maintained the same value after 8 hours. Figure 4 shows the time course of the % fast wave component($\alpha + \beta$) from % power spectrum EEG band analysis. The time course is simlar to that of the CMRO2. The % fast wave component recovered quickly in no swelling and delayed swelling group initially, the delayed swelling had a rapid fall after 11 hours. In the barbiturate no swelling, remained low during thiopental administration, and quickly recovered afterwards. Figure 5 shows the time course of the CBF index which is defined as the % fast wave component divided by the AVDO2 values. The CBF index coursed closely the measured CBF values .

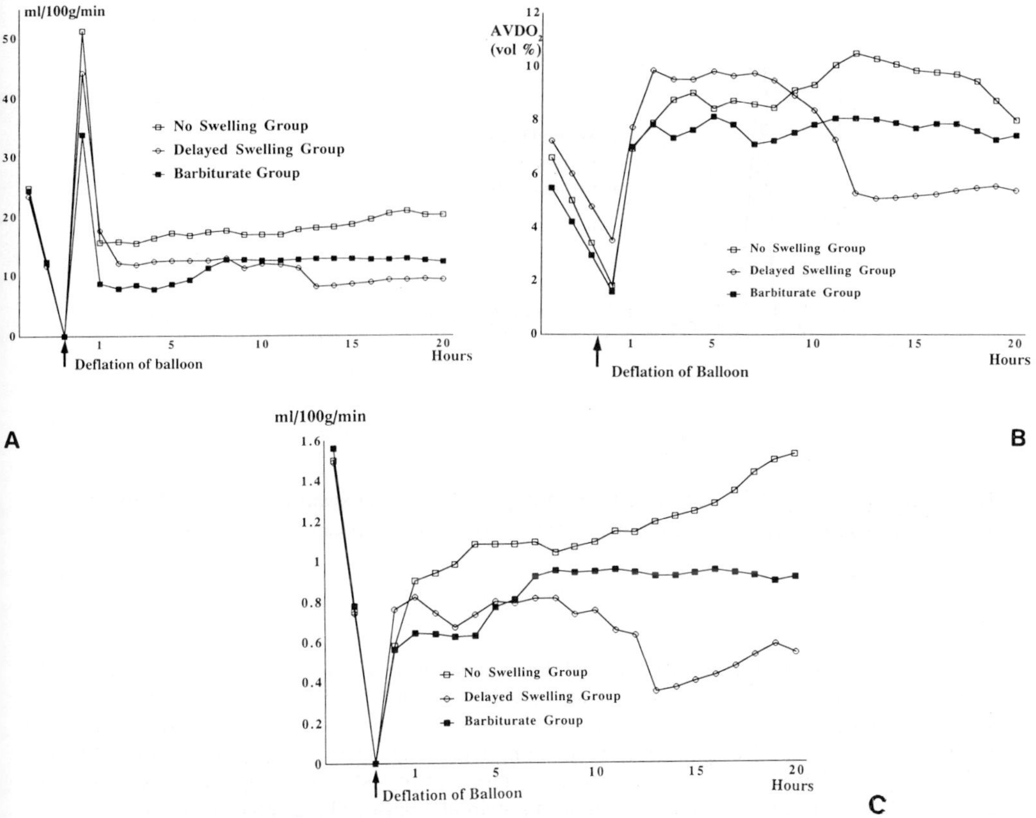

Fig.3 Changes in CBF (A), AVDO2 (B) and CMRO2 (C) during and after balloon inflation and deflation in no swelling (□), delayed swelling(○) and barbiturate no swelling group(■).

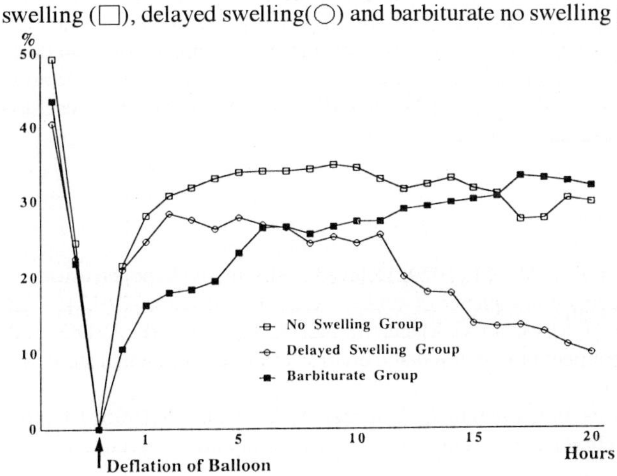

Fig.4 Time course of % fast wave component ($\alpha + \beta$) in no swelling(□), delayed swelling(○) and barbiturate no swelling group(■).

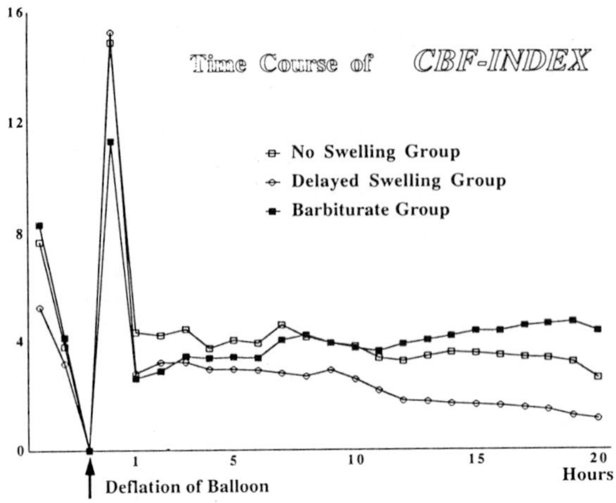

Fig.5 Time course of CBF index in no swelling (□), delayed swelling (○) and barbiturate no swelling group (■).CBF index is defined as the % fast wave component divided by AVDO2.

DISCUSSION

In the arterial occulusion-reperfusion model, hyperemia initially, following delayed hypoperfusion with postischemic hypermetabolism may develop[2]. The compression ischemia model used in this study, may induce many types of insult other than pure ischemia. Our study shows that serial measurement of AVDO2 allows some evaluation of the changes in CBF[3]. We substituted EEG monitoring for CMRO2. The EEG slow-wave component persist longer with increased severity of ischemic damage following global ischemia and recirculation[4]. The greater fast wave component related to higher CMRO2[5]. The % fast wave($\alpha + \beta$) component coursed similar to that of CMRO2. Also, the CBF index closely resembled changes in the CBF. Administration of barbiturate should be effective to reduce of hypermetabolism for improving the relative ischemia following brain compression. We consider that the effect of barbiturates in clinical cases can be expected by earlier administration at the stage of ischemic metabolism is characterized by: 1) rapid recovery of % fast wave component, 2) high AVDO2, and 3) low CBF index. We confirm the usefulness of CBF index with AVDO2 for the estimation of CBF

REFERENCE

1.Levy DE, Van Uitert RL, Pike CL(1979):Delayed postischemic hypoperfusion: A potentially damaging consequence of stroke. Neurology(Minneap)29:1245-1253

2.Yabuki A, Mishina H, Miyazaki M, Maeda M, Sato K, Ishii S(1991):AVDO2 and EEG as indicators for treatment of post-traumatic brain swelling:Experimental study.Neurol Med Chir (Tokyo)31:568-574

3.Hockaday JM, Potts FD, Epstein E, Bonazzi A, Schwab RS(1965):Electroencephalographic changes in acute cerebral anoxia frpm cardiac or respiratory arrest.Electroenceph Clin Neurophysiol 18: 575-586

4.Maekawa T, Takeshita H, Sakabe T, Miyauchi Y, Tateishi A, Matsumoto K(1985):EEG,cerebral circulation and metabolism following cardio pulmonary resuscitation. Rinsho Niha 27:703-709(in Japanese)

The Relationship Between Cerebral Blood Flow and Metabolism in Severely Head-Injured Patients

E. Shalmon, M.J. Caron, N.A. Martin, E.S. Blander, D.A. Hovda, and D.P. Becker

Division of Neurosurgery, Brain Injury Research Center, UCLA School of Medicine, Los Angeles, CA, USA

INTRODUCTION

Cerebral metabolism can be assessed by the Fick principle as the product of cerebral blood flow (CBF) and the arterio-venous differences (AVD) of metabolites consumed and produced by the brain (6, 7). In normal conditions, CBF is closely coupled to cerebral metabolism, and changes in CBF are accompanied by reciprocal alterations in oxygen and glucose extractions, as can be calculated by AVD of oxygen ($AVDO_2$) and glucose (AVD-Glu). However, in ischemic conditions, extraction of oxygen and glucose increase in order to compensate for the low CBF (2, 6). Following severe head injury, cerebral metabolic rates of oxygen ($CMRO_2$) and glucose (CMR-Glu) are reduced by as much as 50%. In these patients, as opposed to ischemic patients, metabolic dysfunction presumably occurs as a result of cellular injury, rather than by ischemia (7, 9). If so, cellular demand for oxygen and glucose by the injured brain is low, and therefore, lower uptake is expected.

The purpose of this study was to assess the association between oxygen and glucose utilization in conjunction with CBF in severely head-injured patients. Furthermore, this study examines the hypothesis that the cerebral supply of these metabolites is sufficient for metabolic demand.

MATERIALS AND METHODS

Subjects: Fifteen severely head injured patients (4 females and 11 males; mean age 39.5 years, ranging 19-80 years) were prospectively studied. Initial Glasgow Coma Scale score was 3-7 (mean 4.7). Gunshot injured patients were excluded. All patients were intubated and resuscitated upon admission. Initial CT scan revealed an operative mass lesion in 9 patients and a non-operative brain contusion, hematoma or edema in 6 patients. Intracranial pressure was treated according to the therapy intensity level concept with sedation, paralysis and ventricular drainage followed by mild hyperventilation and mannitol. Patients receiving barbiturates were excluded.

Cerebral blood flow and AVD measurements: CBF measurements were performed by Novo 10a Cerebrograph, utilizing the ^{133}Xe intravenous technique, within the first 24 hours of admission and every day thereafter. Arterial and jugular blood samples were obtained simultaneously for determination of AVD of oxygen and glucose and lactate (AVD-Lact). CBF-15 was calculated and correlated to these AVD measurements, and to $CMRO_2$ and CMR-Glu.

RESULTS

The data indicate that these patients exhibited a wide range of CBF (23-77 ml/100 gm/min). Figure 1a illustrates that regardless of CBF, patients exhibited stable $AVDO_2$ levels (mean = 1.94, S.D. = 0.49 μ mol/ml) with a horizontal slope (-0.006). Lactate production was not related to low CBF or oxygen consumption. Patients with higher CBF exhibited a lower extraction of oxygen (small $AVDO_2$). In the lower CBF range, oxygen extraction did not increase. Therefore, in spite of the low CBF, hyperemic conditions were encountered by $AVDO_2$ criteria.
Figure 1b illustrates a similar pattern for glucose utilization. Regardless of CBF, homogeneous AVD-Glu levels were calculated (mean = 0.38, S.D. = 0.34 μ mol/ml) and a slope of -0.0008.

Fig 1a.

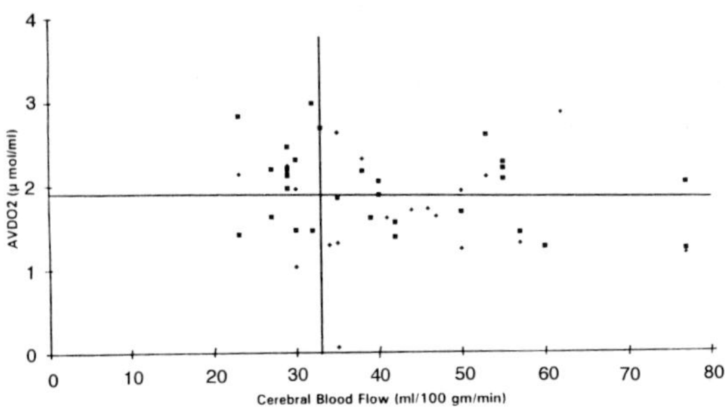

Fig 1b.

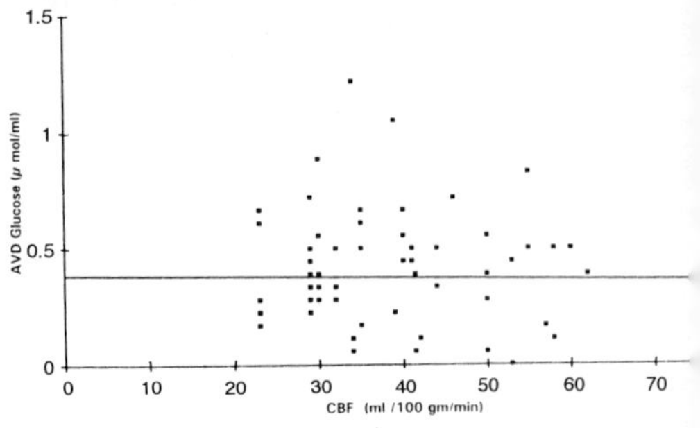

Fig. 1a) Correlation between $AVDO_2$ and CBF-15 (n=93). Vertical line at CBF 32.9 ml/100gm/min. Squares-lactate consumption, diamonds-lactate production. Correlation = 0.097, R^2 = 0.000541, slope = -0.006.
Fig. 1b) Correlation between AVD Glu and CBF (n = 72). Correlation = 0.029, R^2 = 0.013, slope = -0.0008.

Figures 2a and 2b illustrate that low CBF range (below 30 ml/100 gm/ min) was associated with low $CMRO_2$ and CMR-Glu. Generally, as the cerebral metabolic rate of oxygen and glucose improved, CBF improved. This improvement in metabolism was higher for $CMRO_2$ (slope 1.67), reaching levels close to the normal range, while CMR-Glu increased slightly above the injured level (slope 0.43).

Fig 2a.

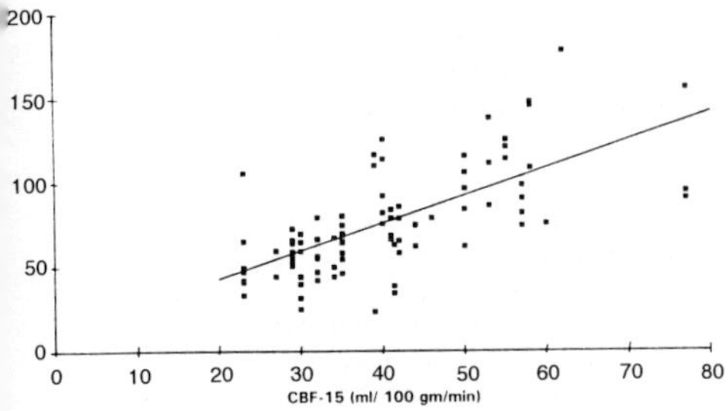

Fig 2b.

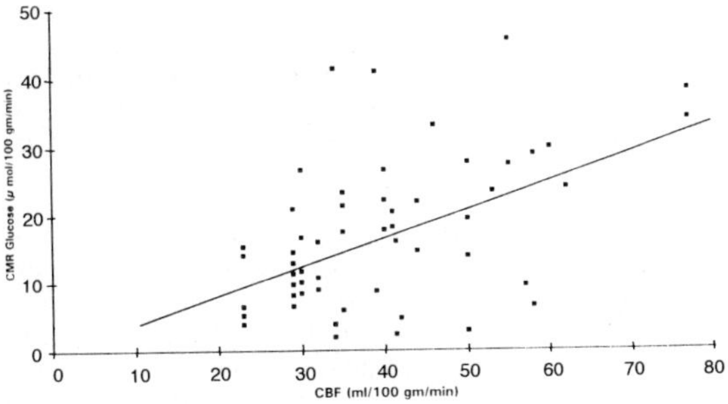

Fig 2a) Correlation between CBF-15 and $CMRO_2$ (n = 93). Correlation = 0.684, $R^2 = 0.462$, slope = 1.666.
Fig. 2b) Correlation between CBF=15 and CMR Glu (n=64). Correlation = 0.523 $R^2 = 0.261$, slope = 0.43.

DISCUSSION.

The results suggest that in severely head-injured patients oxygen and glucose extractions are independent of CBF. Within a wide range of CBF, the patients exhibited a consistent and marked unchanged level of $AVDO_2$ and AVD-Glu, with no correlation to CBF. Even in the low CBF range, where compensatory extraction of oxygen was expected, low-normal $AVDO_2$ values were found. Significant correlations between $CMRO_2$ and CMR-Glu and CBF were found utilizing the Fick equation (5). Gradual increasing $CMRO_2$, from a low rate to a normal rate of 150 μ mol/100 gm/min, and of CMR-Glu, as CBF improved may indicate coupling of CBF to metabolic requirements in these patients.

Several factors can affect oxygen extraction. Among them include the brain's requirements and the oxygen provided by CBF. Cruz et al. used the Fick principle to confirm the inverse relationship between CBF and $AVDO_2$ in severely head-injured patients (2, 3). This ratio led them to suggest that profound hyperventilation could be used to treat uncontrolled ICP, as long as large $AVDO_2$ values were prevented.

In another study by Robertson et al, a diagrammatic model for the relationship between CBF and metabolism in comatose patients was developed (6). This model suggested that, as long as the $CMRO_2$ is constant, a reciprocal correlation exists between CBF and the amount of oxygen extracted by the brain. At low CBF levels, two groups of comatose patients were identified. The first group consisted of patients who were able to compensate for low CBF by extracting more oxygen from the blood, resulting in a higher $AVDO_2$. Therefore, these patients did not suffer ischemia and did not produce lactate. Patients in the second group were unable to compensate for low CBF by increased extraction of blood oxygen and had low-normal $AVDO_2$. These patients suffered ischemia identified by lactate production.

In the current study, patients with low CBF would have belonged to Robertson et. al's second group. Their low $AVDO_2$ indicated that they were unable to compensate for low CBF with improved extraction of oxygen. Nevertheless, many of them did not produce lactate. Consequently, it appears that some patients had low $AVDO_2$, which indicates preserved perfusion in association with low CBF.

The reason for the inability of some "ischemic" patients to compensate for low CBF with an increased extraction of oxygen (and increase $AVDO_2$) is not entirely clear. We hypothesize that in these patients the $AVDO_2$ was low due to injury induced changes in cellular metabolic demand. This results in a metabolic depression at the cellular level which alters the utilization of oxygen and glucose. It is an interesting possibility, that in these specific patients, low CBF may not play a major roll in their pathogenesis (4). Therefore, improved CBF as well as better oxygenation may not improve incorporation of oxygen to the brain, given a reduction in demand. The same situation appears to apply to glucose consumption since it's supply is abundant and rarely falls to hypoglycemic levels.

CONCLUSION

1) Traumatic brain injury alters the metabolic demands of cells and hence adjusts the uptake of oxygen and glucose accordingly.

2) Low uptake of oxygen and glucose results in small $AVDO_2$ and AVD-Glu regardless of their supply.

3) $CMRO_2$ and CMR-Glu are often coupled to CBF in severely head-injured patients.

Acknowledgements supported by NS 30308.

REFERENCES

[1]. Cruz J, Miner ME, Allen SJ, Alves WM, Gennarelli TA: Continuous monitoring of cerebral oxygenation in acute brain injury: injection of mannitol during hyperventilation. J Neurosurg 73:725-730, 1990.

[2]. Cruz J, Miner ME, Allen SJ, Alves WM, Gennarelli TA: Continuous monitoring of cerebral oxygenation in acute brain injury: assessment of cerebral hemodynamic reserve. Neurosurg 29:743-749, 1991.

[3]. Cruz J: On-line monitoring of global cerebral hypoxia in acute brain injury. Relationship to intracranial hypertension. J Neurosurg 79:228-233, 1993.

[4]. Marion DW, Darby J, Yonas H: Acute regional cerebral blood flow changes caused by severe head injuries. J Neurosurg 74:407-414, 1991.

[5]. Robertson CS, Clifton GL, Grossman RG, OU C-H, Goodman JC, Borum P, Bejot S, Barrodale P: Alteration in cerebral availability of metabolic substrates after severe head injury. J Trauma 28:1523-1532, 1988.

[6]. Robertson CS, Narayan RK, Gokaslan ZL, Pahwa R, Grossman RG, Caram P, Allen E: Cerebral arteriovenous oxygen difference as an estimate of cerebral blood flow in comatose patients. J Neurosurg 70:222-230, 1989.
[7]. Siesjo BK: Pathophysiology and treatment of focal cerebral ischemia. Part 1: Pathophysiology. J Neurosurg 77:169-184, 1992
[8]. Sheinberg M, Kanter MJ, Robertson CS, Contant CF, Narayan RK, Grossman RG: Continuous monitoring of jugular venous oxygen saturation in head-injured patients. J Neurosurg 76:212-217, 1992
[9]. Zwetnow NN, Kjallquist A, Siesjo BK: Cerebral blood flow during intracranial hypertension related to tissue hypoxia and to acidosis in cerebral extracellular fluids. Prog Brain Res 30, Cerebral Circulation: 87-92, 1968.

Remote and Local Effects on CBF in Patients with Supratentorial Mass Lesions

S. Inao[1], H. Kuchiwaki[1], K. Yoshida[1], K. Sugita[1], A. Izawa[2], H. Koida[2], and M. Furuse[2]

[1] Department of Neurosurgery, Nagoya University School of Medicine, Japan
[2] Department of Clinical Imaging Laboratory, Nakatsugawa Municipal General Hospital, Japan

INTRODUCTION

When the brain is compressed by a supratentorial mass lesion, local cerebral blood flow (CBF) does not always decrease in an adjacent area, but often decreases in a remote area. We analyzed the relationships between brain displacement and local CBF reduction in the cortex and thalamus, and clarified the local and remote effects on these parameters of supratentorial mass lesions.

SUBJECTS AND METHODS

Forty-five cases (age range 58 - 87 years, mean 71.9 ± 8.4) of unilateral chronic subdural hematoma were studied. Patients were categorized into 3 groups; I: headache without any neurological defecit (n=16); II: paresis of the extremities (n=14); and III: altered mental status with or without paresis (n=15). T1 weighted MR images were obtained in all patients preoperatively. Quantitative values of hematoma thickness and brain rotation angle (the incline of the third ventricle and the axis of brainstem) were obtained on coronal MR images. The midline shift (septum pellucidum and pineal body) was measured on axial MR images. In 21 cases, local CBF was measured by Xe enhanced CT. CBF values were obtained in selected regions of interest: frontal cortex, thalamus, and whole hemisphere on both the hematoma and contralateral side.

RESULTS

The clinical symptoms related to the brain deformity, which showed the patients with headache alone had less thickness of hematoma and septum shift, the patients with paresis had a thicker hematoma and a moderate septum shift, and the patients with altered mental status had the thickest hematoma and greatest septum shift. Local CBF decreased linearly in all the areas corresponding to the degree of brain deformity. The magnitude of the decrease was larger in the thalamus than in the cortex. The cortical flow decrease had the best linear correlation to the hematoma thickness (r=0.57), whereas the decrease in the thalamic flow had the most significant correlation with the pineal shift (r=0.65) and the third ventricle incline (r=0.67). In the paresis patients, cortical and thalamic flow decreased significantly on the hematoma side (p<0.05). The patients with altered mental status showed a significant decrease of blood flow in the thalamus on both sides (p<0.01), but the decrease in cortical flow was only on the side with the hematoma (see Table).

Table: Local CBF in cortex and thalamus.

	cortex		thalamus	
group	hematoma	contralateral	hematoma	contralateral
headache	35.0±1.5	34.5±2.1	50.8±4.6	51.4±3.9
paresis	31.0±1.6*	32.8±1.9	39.3±2.9*	42.9±3.1
mental change	28.8±1.5**	30.5±1.5	34.7±2.4**	31.1±2.6**

*p<0.05, **p<0.01

DISCUSSION

In acute intracranial mass lesions, brain deformity changes anticipated or confirmed clinical signs, but there was less correlation clinically and anatomically in chronic illness [1][2]. However, we previously reported the mechanism of the chronic brain compression and correlation between cerebrum and brainstem displacement when the cerebrum was compressed by the chronic subdural hematoma [3]. In this study, we analyzed the chronic mass effects (brain deformity) on local CBF change in adjacent and remote areas in evaluating the clinical signs. Our data indicated that altered mental status (consciousness disturbance) occurs when thalamic flow is decreased bilaterally by the transtentorial brain herniation or deep brain structural deformity associated with supratentorial lesions. The data also indicated that the paresis of the extremities results from cortical flow reduction by direct compression due to the hematoma. This study might provide data useful in evaluating the clinical symptoms of patients with a supratentorial mass lesion.

REFERENCE

1. Reich JB, Sierra J, Camp W, Zanzonico P, Deck MDF, Plum F (1993) Magnetic resonance imaging measurements and clinical changes accompanying transtentorial and foramen magnum brain herniation. Ann Neurol 33: 159-170

2. Ropper AH (1986) Lateral displacement of the brain and level of consciousness in patients with an acute hemispheral mass. N Engl J Med 314: 953-958
3. Inao S, Kuchiwaki H, Kanaiwa H, Sugita K, Banno M, Furuse M (1993) Magnetic resonance imaging assessment of brainstem distortion associated with a supratentorial mass. J Neurol Neurosurg Psychiatry 56: 280-289

Session XVIII: Effects of Increased ICP (4)

Chairmen: M.J. Rosner and K. Hashi

Hyperventilation Reduces Intracranial Volume Tolerance as Estimated by Pressure Volume Index

W. JOHN GRAY[1] and MICHAEL J. ROSNER[2]

[1] Department of Neurosurgery, Royal Victoria Hospital, Belfast, Northern Ireland, UK
[2] Division of Neurosurgery, University of Alabama at Birmingham, Birmingham, AL, USA

INTRODUCTION

Previous studies have shown that pressure volume index (PVI) is not a constant, but varies with changes in cerebral perfusion pressure (CPP)[1,2]. Hyperventilation has been a well established therapeutic modality for the treatment of intracranial hypertension for many years, and is often used as the primary therapy for reducing intracranial hypertension following cerebral trauma. However, hyperventilation is not without hazards. It may reduce cerebral blood flow (CBF) to threshold levels and some studies have suggested that outcome following trauma may be worse in patients treated by hyperventilation compared to patients who are ventilated without reducing $PaCO_2$ to low levels[3]. We tested the hypothesis that hyperventilation would decrease the pressure volume index of the neuraxis and render the brain less tolerant of volume change.

METHODS

Twelve adult cats were anesthetized with Methohexital (10 mg/kg). The animals were paralyzed with pancuronium bromide (0.2 mg/kg), intubated endotracheally and ventilated with a 70% N_2O, 30% O_2 mixture. Polyethylene catheters were placed in the abdominal aorta and inferior vena cava and connected to strain gauge transducers for pressure monitoring. The animals were held in a stereotactic frame and intracranial pressure (ICP) was measured using 22 gauge needles placed stereotactically in each lateral ventricle. All transducers were zeroed to the level of the ear bars. Cerebral blood flow was measured via the hydrogen clearance method. Using insulated platinum electrodes, diameter 0.007" with the bare tip of 2 mm, electrodes were placed bilaterally in the caudate nucleus and the deep frontal white matter. The electrodes were polarized to +450 mV. 10% hydrogen gas was introduced into the inspired gas mixture until the electrode currents were stable and the ensuing washout curves were recorded. Regional cerebral blood flow for each electrode was calculated from the equation: CBF mls / 100 gm / min = 69.3/T 1/2 where T 1/2 = the time in minutes required for the electrode current to fall to half of its original value. CO_2 reactivity was assumed to be normal if there was a change in CBF of 30% with a change in $PaCO_2$ of 10 mmHg.

The bolus technique for pressure volume index was utilized[4]. 0.1 mls of 0.9% NaCl solution was injected over a period of 1 second into a lateral ventricle and the maximum pressure reading from the contra-lateral ventricle was recorded. The PVI was calculated by the equation:

$$\text{PVI (ml)} = \frac{\Delta V}{\text{Log } P_p / P_o}$$

where V = volume of fluid injected, P_p = peak ICP after injection and P_o = ICP before injection.

Ventilation of the animals was adjusted to allow PVI measurements to be recorded at $PaCO_2$ levels of 40, 30 and 20 mmHg. After measurements had been made at baseline CPP levels, the CPP was reduced in six animals using an infusion of adenosine triphosphate (ATP) (5 mg/ml, infusion rate 0.2 to 2 mg/min) and increased in six animals using an infusion of norepinephrine bitartrate (160 μg/ml, infusion rate 3 to 15 μg/min). The infusion rates were adjusted so that perfusion pressure was maintained towards the upper and lower limits of autoregulation. Further measurements of cerebral blood flow and pressure volume index were taken at these new perfusion pressure levels. The PaO_2, pH and hematocrit were monitored. The core temperature was monitored with an oesophageal probe. An infrared heat lamp was used to keep the temperature between 38.5°C and 39°C. An infusion of 8.4% sodium bicarbonate was used to keep pH constant within the normal range. Hematocrit was maintained at baseline levels by infusion of packed cells or 0.9% saline as required.

RESULTS

At all levels of CPP, PVI varied directly with $_pCO_2$ (Table 1). The reduction in PVI with reduction in $_pCO_2$ was most marked at high levels of CPP where volume tolerance has previously been shown to be maximal (Figure 2).

Table 1.

CPP LEVEL	PVI	N	r
63.4 ± 5.7 mmHg	$PVI = 0.002 + 0.005\ PaCO_2$	55	0.43
104 ± 11.4 mmHg	$PVI = 0.289 + 0.004\ PaCO_2$	93	0.36
149 ± 8.8 mmHg	$PVI = 0.074 + 0.009\ PaCO_2$	41	0.81

Figure 1

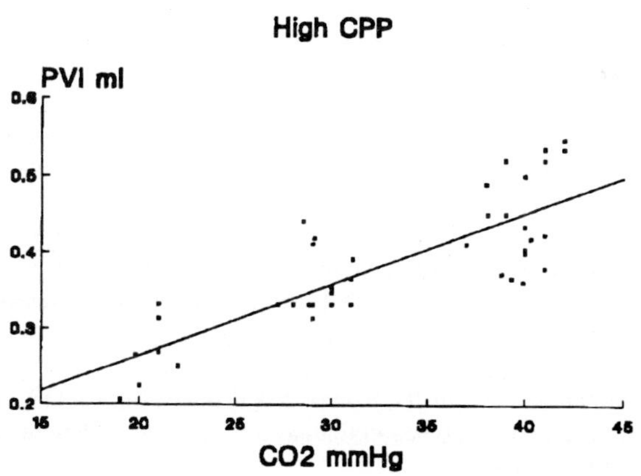

There was a small rise in baseline ICP measurements (not statistically significant) with falling CPP.

Table 2. Baseline ICP Levels (mmHg)

	CPP Low	CPP Normal	CPP High
CO_2 20 mmHg	9.61 ± 3.1	7.96 ± 1.6	7.14 ± 1.1
CO_2 30 mmHg	7.77 ± 2.9	7.13 ± 1.9	6.17 ± 2.5
CO_2 40 mmHg	7.19 ± 2.6	7.04 ± 2.2	7.00 ± 2.1

DISCUSSION

These results indicate that the volume tolerance is lowest in this preparation at low level of $PaCO_2$. There are a number of possible explanations for this apparent discrepancy. It has been shown that cerebrospinal fluid (CSF) volume changes during hypercapnia and hypocapnia[5]. At high levels of CPP and low $PaCO_2$, vaso-constriction is at its maximal and presumably CSF volume is maximized. The resultant response to a volume load under these conditions would maximize the contribution of the CSF space compared to the response of the vascular tree. As CO_2 levels rise, the vessels progressively dilate, leading to a decrease in CSF volume and a reduction in CVR. The increase in PVI under these conditions may reflect the fact that the vascular response to the volume load is buffered better than the CSF response. In addition, although we did not measure CSF lactate levels and kept blood pH within a constant range during measurements, it is possible that a change in CSF pH with falling CO_2 may have had further effects on the intracranial vasculature and caused a change in response to a volume load.

It would appear from these results that hyperventilation, rather than improving volume tolerance, in fact, reduces volume tolerance as measured by the PVI method. These findings have important implications with respect to hyperventilation as a primary treatment modality for raised intracranial pressure.

REFERENCES

1. Gray WJ, Rosner MJ (1987). Pressure-volume index as a function of cerebral perfusion pressure. Part 1: The effects of cerebral perfusion pressure changes and anesthesia. J Neurosurg 67:369-376.

2. Gray WJ, Rosner MJ (1987). Pressure volume index as a function of cerebral perfusion pressure. Part 2: The effects of low cerebral perfusion pressure and autoregulation. J Neurosurg 67:377-380.

3. Muizelaar JP, Marmarou A, Ward JD, Kontos HA, Choi S, Becker DP, Gruemer H, Young HF (1991). Effect of Prophylactic Hyperventilation on Outcome in Patients with Severe Head Injury. J Neurosurg 75:731-739.

4. Marmarou A, Schulman K, Rosende RM (1978). A non-linear analysis of the cerebrospinal system and intracranial pressure dynamics. J Neurosurg 48:332-344

5. Grant R, Condon B, Patterson J, Rowan J, Teasdale GM, (1989). Changes in Intracranial CSF Volume during Hypercapnia and Hypocapnia. In: Hoff, JT, Betz AL (eds) Intracranial Pressure VII. Springer, Berlin Heidelberg, pp 339.340.

The Effect of Positive End Expiratory Pressure (PEEP) on Intracranial Compliance

ZEEV FELDMAN[1], SHANKAR P. GOPINATH[1,2], MONICA CLAYPOOL[1], CLAUDIA S. ROBERTSON[1], JEFF CROUCH[1], CHARLES F. CONTANT[1], and ROBERT G. GROSSMAN[1]

[1] Department of Neurosurgery, Baylor College of Medicine, One Baylor Plaza, Houston 77030, TX, USA
[2] Current address: Soroka Medical Center, Ben-Gurion University, P.O. Box 151, Beer-Sheva 84101, Israel

INTRODUCTION

Acute respiratory distress syndrome (ARDS), is commonly encountered in head-injured patients. The syndrome is characterized by increased physiologic shunting, low functional residual capacity (FRC) and surfactant activity, decreased pulmonary compliance and increased cardiac output.[1] Positive end expiratory pressure (PEEP) is a useful in improving oxygenation. PEEP increases the number of ventilated alveoli, increases the PaO_2 and decreases the alveolar-arterial oxygen tension gradient without increasing the inspired oxygen concentration (FiO_2).[2] PEEP, by increasing intrathoracic pressure, decreases the venous return, the mean arterial pressure (MAP), the cardiac output, and increases jugular vein pressure. There is conflicting evidence in the literature as to the potential effect of PEEP on intracranial pressure (ICP). Cooper et al.[3] and Frost [2], studied the effect of PEEP on ICP in head-injured patients, and could not find a clinically significant rise in ICP after application of PEEP of up to 40 cm H_2O. On the other hand, several authors found that PEEP increased ICP in dogs [4,5,6], and others observed an increase of more than 10 mm Hg after administration of PEEP of 4-8 cm H_2O in 6 of 12 head injured patients.[7]

The effect of PEEP on ICP in the presence of diminished intracranial compliance was studied by Apuzzo et al.[1] and Bruchiel et al.[8] They found a significant increase in ICP with the application of PEEP only in patients who manifested increased cerebral elastance. However, Cooper et al. [3] could not find any increase in ICP after PEEP administration, even in patients with increased baseline ICP, and Huseby et al. [5] studying the effect of PEEP on dogs, found that the presence of intracranial hypertension diminished the increase in ICP seen at a given level of PEEP.

METHODS

Twelve male rabbits weighing 3.5-4.5 kg were used. Each rabbit underwent a tracheotomy, catheterization of the iliac artery, bilateral burr holes over the frontal region, and a right parietal craniectomy. The following parameters were monitored: arterial blood pressure, ICP (intraparenchymal Camino device), pCO_2, and pO_2. A double lumen pediatric Swan-Ganz catheter was placed over the right parietal region, and the craniectomy site, as well as the burr holes were sealed with acrylic. The balloon was filled with water at a rate of 30 μl per minute using an infusion pump. After the point of exponential increase of ICP was reached, the balloon was emptied, and 30 minutes were given for relaxation and equilibration of baseline parameters. A PEEP of 10 cm of water was then applied, and the balloon was inflated again. Each animal served as its own control. For the first 6 rabbits the initial PEEP was 0, and for the rest the initial PEEP was 10 cm.

RESULTS

The mean values of the physiological parameters monitored are given in the following table:

PEEP(cm H_20)	MAP (mm Hg)	pCO_2 (mm Hg)	pO_2 (mm Hg)
0	73±12	32±9	375±106
10	69±12	33±8	366±84
P value	0.001	0.38	0.44

An example of the ICP curves at 0 PEEP and at PEEP 10 cm H_2O are shown in fig. 1. The difference between the volume required to reach the point of exponential rise in ICP at PEEP 0 and at PEEP 10 cm H_2O for the individual animals are shown in fig. 2.

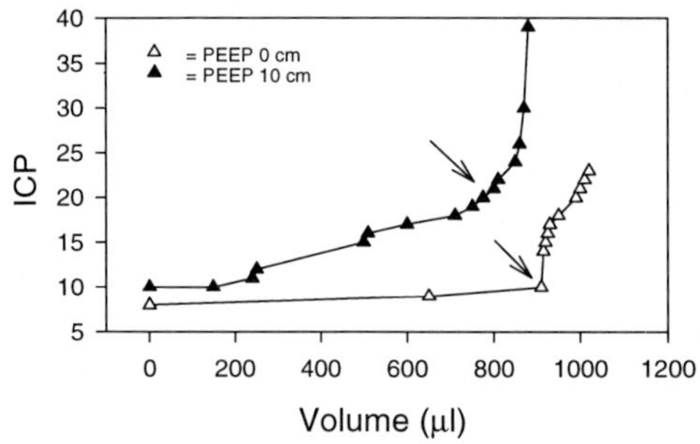

Figure 1. ICP curves at PEEP 0 and at PEEP 10 cm H_2O of animal 4. The arrows mark the exponential rise of ICP, which occurred at lower volume when PEEP is applied.

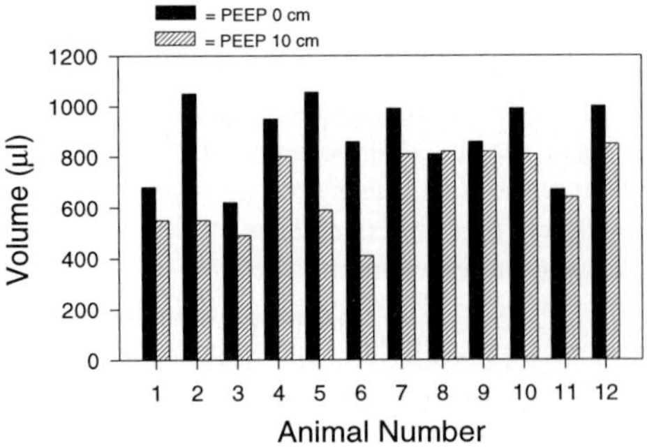

Figure 2. Volume required for ICP exponential rise at PEEP 0 and at PEEP 10 cm H_2O by animals.

The mean volume needed to reach the deflection point of the ICP curve was 883±159 µl when PEEP was 0 cm H_20, and 685±165 µl when PEEP was 10 cm H_20 (p = 0.0023).(Fig. 3).

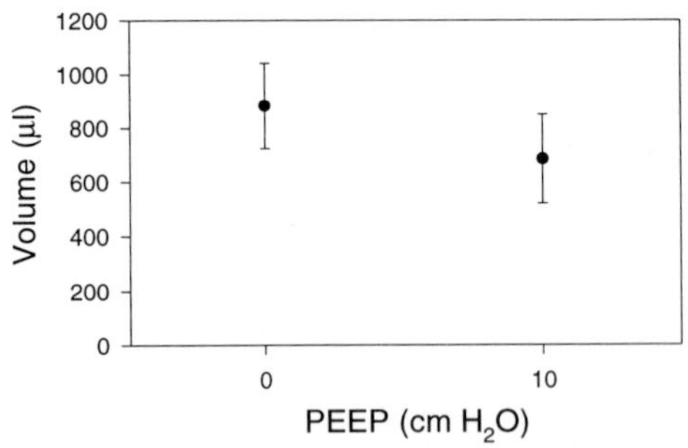

Figure 3: The mean volume needed to reach the deflection point of ICP was significantly less when PEEP was applied (p = 0.0023)

DISCUSSION

The results of the present study demonstrate that PEEP decreases the intracranial compliance, shifts the volume-ICP curve to the left, and results in an increase of ICP at lower volumes of space occupying lesion. PEEP, by increasing the intrathoracic pressure, increases the CVP and reduces the venous return to the heart, and by that, interferes with the compensatory mechanism that helps maintain the ICP, i.e. shifting of blood and CSF from the intracranial compartment. This effect may be manipulated by head elevation which will reduce the pressure in the jugular vein. However, by reducing cardiac output and MAP, PEEP may cause a decrease in cerebral perfusion pressure, and as shown by Shapiro and Marshall, may increase the cerebral blood volume (CBV) and intracranial pressure.[7] Another possible mechanism is the increase pCO_2, observed when PEEP is applied, which by itself will increase the CBV.[3]

We conclude that although PEEP improves arterial oxygenation, it must be applied with utmost care, and patients should be observed for signs of increased intracranial pressure.

ACKNOWLEDGMENTS

This work was supported by NIH grant #PO1-NS27616.

REFERENCES

1. Apuzzo ML, Weiss MH, Petersons V, Small RB, Kurze T, Heide JS (1977) Effect of positive end expiratory pressure ventilation on intracranial pressure in man. J Neurosurg 46: 227-232
2. Frost EAM (1977) Effect of positive end-expiratory pressure on intracranial pressure and compliance in brain-injured patients. J Neurosurg 47: 195-200
3. Cooper KR, Boswell PA, Choi SC (1985) Safe use of PEEP in patients with severe head injury. J Neurosurg 63: 552-555
4. Cotev S, Paul WL, Ruiz BC, Kuck EF, Modell JH (1981) Positive end-expiratory pressure(PEEP) and cerebrospinal fluid pressure during normal and elevated intracranial pressure in dogs. Intensive Care Med 7: 187-191
5. Huseby JS, Luce JM, Cary JM, Pavlin EG, Butler J (1981) Effect of positive end-expiratory pressure on intracranial pressure in dogs with intracranial hypertension. J Neurosurg 55: 704-707
6. Luce JM, Huseby JS, Kirk W, Butler J (1982) Mechanism by which positive end-expiratory pressure increases cerebrospinal fluid pressure in dogs. J Applied Physiol 52: 231-235
7. Shapiro HM, Marshall LF (1978) Intracranial pressure response to PEEP in head-injured patients. J Trauma 18: 254-256
8. Bruchiel KJ, Steege TD, Wyler AR (1981) Intracranial pressure changes in brain injured patients requiring positive end-expiratory pressure ventilation. Neurosurgery 8: 443-449

Multimodal Evaluation of Cerebral Oxygen Metabolism Disturbances Related to Hyperventilation in Patients with Severe Head Injury

T. Shiogai, A. Noguchi, E. Sato, and I. Saito

Department of Neurosurgery, Kyorin University School of Medicine, 6-20-2 Shinkawa, Mitaka, Tokyo, 181 Japan

SUMMARY

Cerebral oxygen metabolism disturbances related to hyperventilation (HV) in 16 comatose patients with severe head injuries were evaluated with a continuous multimodal neuromonitoring system, consisting of jugular bulb venous oxygen saturation (SjO_2) and arterial oxygen saturation (SpO_2), transcranial Doppler (TCD), end-tidal CO_2 partial pressure ($PetCO_2$), intracranial pressure (ICP) and cerebral perfusion pressure (CPP), and Fourier-transformed quantitative EEG (qEEG). The results of CO_2 reactivity tests within two weeks after injury were classified on the basis of minimal SjO_2 during HV into ischemic ($SjO_2 < 55\%$), normal (SjO_2 55-70%), and hyperemic ($SjO_2 \geq 70\%$) groups. Differences among the three groups and correlations with SjO_2 were evaluated in terms of 1) TCD mean velocity in the middle cerebral artery (Vm) and CO_2 reactivity ($\Delta Vm/\Delta CO_2$, $\Delta SjO_2/\Delta CO_2$), 2) ICP and CPP, 3) TCD pulsatility index (PI) and cerebrovascular resistance (CVR = CPP/Vm), and 4) qEEG recorded on the ipsilateral scalp.
a) CO_2 reactivity: No significant differences in response to Vm were observed among the three groups. Response of SjO_2 was significantly high in the order of frequency (ischemic > normal > hyperemic).
b) Correlation with SjO_2: 1) Significant correlations with Vm ($p < 0.05$), CVR ($p < 0.01$), and PI ($p < 0.05$) frequently were observed in the ischemic, followed by the normal groups, but rarely in the hyperemic group. 2) Correlation with ICP also was apparent in the ischemic group. 3) Correlation with CPP noticeably was rare in all three groups. 4) Correlation with qEEG changes (increased TP and decreased α power) was frequent in the ischemic group. To conclude, cerebral ischemia during HV is closely related to decreased cerebral circulation and increased CVR, and less frequently related to ICP and EEG changes. Contributions to cerebral hyperemia, however, are not obvious in patients with severe head injuries.

INTRODUCTION

In the management of severe head injury patients, HV routinely has been used for reduction of ICP or improvement of cerebral acidosis which recently emphasizes the risk of ischemic brain damage [1,2]. This study was aimed to evaluate cerebral oxygen metabolism disturbances related to HV in comatose patients with severe head injuries. To this end, we have introduced and analyzed a computerized multimodal system continuously monitoring SjO_2 and SpO_2, TCD, $PetCO_2$, ICP and CPP, and qEEG [3].

PATIENTS AND METHODS

The subjects were 16 patients with acute head injury: ages, 15-72, mean 41; focal injury, 11 cases, diffuse injury, 5 cases; Glasgow coma scores of 8 or less. Cerebral CO_2 reactivity tests were assessed by cerebral circulation (TCD) and oxygen metabolism (SjO_2), and correlations of SjO_2 with TCD, ICP and CPP, qEEG during HV were analyzed. Data acquisition was carried out every 2 minutes for 30-40 minutes, and this was performed one to five times (total 38 times) within two weeks after injury. SpO_2

was maintained over 97% during the tests. The test results were classified, on the basis of minimal SjO_2 during HV, into an ischemic group ($SjO_2 < 55\%$, n = 13), a normal group (SjO_2 55-70%, n = 13), and a hyperemic group ($SjO_2 \geq 70\%$, n = 12). EEG was recorded in the parietal scalp (P3 - A1 or P4 - A2 montage) ipsilateral to TCD monitoring. qEEG was calculated by power spectral analysis. Differences among the three groups and correlations with SjO_2 were evaluated in terms of 1)Vm and CO_2 reactivity ($\Delta Vm/\Delta CO_2$, $\Delta SjO_2/\Delta CO_2$), 2) ICP and CPP, 3) PI and estimated CVR (= CPP/Vm), and 4) Total power (TP) and α power of qEEG.

RESULTS

a) CO_2 reactivity and other basic data (Table 1):
No significant differences were observed among the three groups with regard to age, Glasgow coma scale score (GCS), barbiturate therapy, mean ICP and CPP, $PetCO_2$ and ΔCO_2. Focal injury was relatively frequent in the ischemic group, but difference in type of injury was not significant among the three groups. Δ ICP and Δ CPP were tended to be high in the normal group, but not high in the ischemic and hyperemic groups. No significant differences in response to Vm also were observed among the three groups. The SjO_2 response, however, was significantly high in the order of frequency (ischemic > normal > hyperemic).

Table 1 Comparison of CO_2 reactivity and basic data in the three groups based on minimal SjO_2 during hyperventilation*.

	group			
	ischemia	normal	hyperemia	p values**
n	13	13	12	
SjO_2 (%)	< 55	55-70	70 ≥	
Age	41 ± 23	38 ± 20	37 ± 15	ns
GCS	5 ± 1.5	4 ± 1.5	4 ± 1.6	ns
type of injury				
focal	10	6	6	ns
diffuse	3	7	6	
barbiturate therapy	6	8	7	ns
mean ICP (mmHg)	16 ± 5.5	14 ± 5.5	17 ± 13	ns
mean CPP (mmHg)	65 ± 16	77 ± 16	63 ± 16	ns
Δ ICP (mmHg)	7 ± 2.7	14 ± 13	8 ± 5.9	ns
Δ CPP (mmHg)	12 ± 6.3	19 ± 13	12 ± 5.1	ns
$PetCO_2$ (mmHg)				
minimal	23 ± 2.5	22 ± 2.0	24 ± 2.8	ns
maximal	33 ± 2.5	32 ± 4.1	34 ± 2.8	ns
ΔCO_2 (mmHg)	10 ± 2.6	9.9 ± 3.0	11 ± 3.2	ns
$\Delta Vm/\Delta CO_2$	4.0 ± 1.9	3.8 ± 2.8	3.4 ± 2.0	ns
$\Delta SjO_2/\Delta CO_2$	1.9 ± 1.0	1.3 ± 0.8	0.8 ± 0.8	< 0.05

* mean ± SD.
** ANOVA, Kruskal-Wallis test, nc = not significant (p > 0.05).

b) Correlation with SjO_2 (Table 2):
1) Significant correlations with Vm ($p < 0.05$), CVR ($p < 0.01$), and PI ($p < 0.05$) were frequently observed in the ischemic group, followed by the normal group, and rarely in the hyperemic group.
2) Correlation with ICP also was frequently identified in the ischemic group. Correlation with CPP noticeably was rare in all three group.

Table 2 Correlation coefficients of TCD parameters, ICP and CPP with SjO_2*

	group			
	ischemia	normal	hyperemia	p values**
Vm (cm/s)	0.62 ± 0.37	0.27 ± 0.35	0.18 ± 0.40	< 0.05
CVR	-0.59 ± 0.28	-0.28 ± 0.29	-0.14 ± 0.40	< 0.01
PI	-0.47 ± 0.27	-0.18 ± 0.30	-0.18 ± 0.37	< 0.05
ICP (mmHg)	0.49 ± 0.49	0.34 ± 0.37	0.02 ± 0.49	ns
CPP (mmHg)	0.11 ± 0.50	-0.01 ± 0.46	-0.07 ± 0.42	ns

* mean ± SD.
** ANOVA, nc = not significant (p > 0.05).

3) Correlation with qEEG changes (increased TP and decreased α power) was observed frequently in the ischemic group. qEEG changes to some degree were identified in all three groups (Fig. 1).

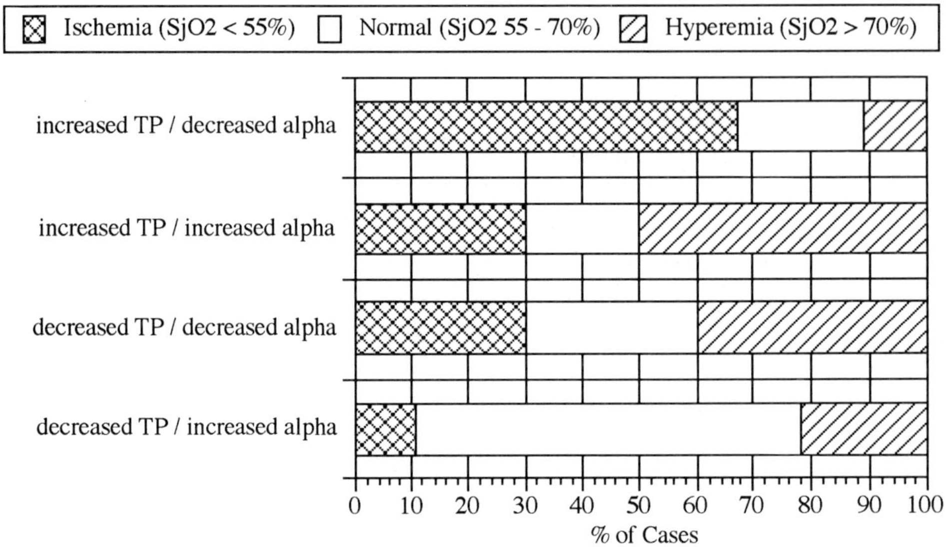

Fig. 1 Correlation between quantitative EEG and SjO_2.
TP: total power of qEEG

DISCUSSION

HV used to control ICP and to ameliorate cerebral acidosis in the management of acute severe head injury can result in a reduction in the cerebral blood flow (CBF), which may produce brain ischemia [2]. The usefulness of SjO_2 monitoring, which can be evaluated by coupling CBF with the cerebral metabolic rate of oxygen ($CMRO_2$), has been emphasized in the early detection of global ischemia during HV[1] . Our results confirmed a strong correlation of cerebral ischemia during HV detected by SjO_2 with decreased CBF and increased CVR [4,5] which is demonstrated by decreased Vm and increased PI. In the experimental development of ischemic brain damage after head injury, the importance of decreased CBF and increased CVR has been pointed out [6]. Increased pulsatility of the Doppler velocity waveform reflects increased downstream vascular resistance during HV [7] or decreased intracranial compliance in relation to CPP [8]. The combined use of TCD and SjO_2 monitoring appears to be extremely useful in detecting early ischemic brain damage and in clarifying the underlying pathophysiology in severe head injury.

In our study, qEEG changes were observed during HV, especially increased TP and decreased α power in the ischemic group, that indicated $CMRO_2$ may change and affect SjO_2 values. This same qEEG pattern has been pointed out in focal ischemia due to chronic cerebrovascular accidents [9]. Generally, it is considered that $CMRO_2$ does not change during HV. These qEEG changes do suggest, however, that the possibility of increased $CMRO_2$ [4,10] or a relation with anaerobic metabolism [11] should be taken into consideration, especially in cases of severe head injury.

Cerebrovascular CO_2 reactivity has a direct relationship with reduction of CBF and ICP [12] and a close relationship with the prognosis [10]. In our study, CO_2 reactivity ($\Delta Vm/\Delta CO_2$) did not demonstrate significant differences among three groups. Preserved CO_2 reactivity in the ischemic group may indicate an inverse steal phenomenon [2], because there was a relatively large number of patients with focal injury. Increased CO_2 reactivity in hyperemic patients has been known and associated with increased ICP [13]. In our study, however, preserved CO_2 reactivity and decreased ICP during HV was observed in the hyperemic group, but not always associated with intracranial hypertension. Our results supported the preserved effectiveness of HV in hyperemic patients.

This work was supported by the Tokyo Institute of Medical Science.

REFERENCES

1. Cruz J, Miner ME (1986) Modulating cerebral oxygen delivery and extraction in acute traumatic coma. In: Miner ME, Wagner KA (eds) Neurotrauma. Treatment, Rehabilitation, and related Issues. Butterworths, Boston.1, pp 55-72
2. Patel PM (1993) Hyperventilation as a therapeutic intervention: do the potential benefits outweigh the known risks? J Neurosurg Anesthesiol 5:62-65
3. Shiogai T, Sato E, Fujii Y, Takeuchi K, Saito I (1993) Continuous monitoring of transcranial Doppler, jugular venous oxygen saturation, and quantitative EEG in severe head injury. In: Nakamura N, Hashimoto T, Yasue M (eds) Recent Advances in Neurotraumatology. Splinger-Verlag, Tokyo, pp297-300
4. Kety SS, Schmidt CF (1946) The effects of active and passive hyperventilation on cerebral blood flow, cerebral oxygen consumption, cardiac output, and blood pressure of normal young men. J Clin Invest 25:107-119
5. Pierce EC, Lambertsen CJ, Deutsch S, Chase PE, Linde HW, Dripps RD, Price HL (1962) Cerebral circulation and metabolism during thiopental anesthesia and hyperventilation in man. J Clin Invest 41: 1664-1671
6. Pfenninger EG, Reith A, Breitig D, Grünert A, Ahnefeld FW (1989) Early changes of intracranial pressure, perfusion pressure, and blood flow after acute head injury: Part 1: An experimental study of the underlying pathophysiology. J Neurosurg 70:774-779
7. Beasley MG, Blau JN, Gosling RG (1979) Changes in internal carotid artery flow velocities with cerebral vasodilation and constriction. Stroke 10:331-335
8. Nelson RJ, Czosnyka M, Pickard JD, Maksymowics W, Perry S, Martin JL, Lovick AHJ (1992) Experimental aspects of cerebrospinal hemodynamics: the relationship between blood flow velocity waveform and cerebral autoregulation. Neurosurgery 31:705-710
9. Slug I (1984) Quantitative EEG as a measure of brain dysfunction. In: Pfurtscheller G, Jonkman EJ, Lopes da Silva FH (eds) Brain Ischemia: Quantitative EEG and Imaging Techniques, Progress in Brain Research, Elsevier, Amsterdam 62: pp65-84
10. Nordström CH, Messeter K, Sundbärg G, Schalén W, Werner M, Ryding E (1988) Cerebral blood flow, vasoreactivity, and oxygen consumption during barbiturate therapy in severe traumatic brain lesions. J Neurosurg 68:424-431
11. Michenfelder JD, Sundt TM (1973) The effect of $PaCO_2$ on the metabolism of ischemic brain in squirrel monkeys. Anesthesiology 38:445-453
12. Marmarou A, Bandoh K, Yoshihara M, Tsuji O (1993) Measurement of vascular reactivity in head injured patients. Acta Neurochir 59 (Suppl):18-21
13. Obrist WD, Lagfitt TW, Jaggi JL, Cruz J, Gennarelli TA (1984) Cerebral blood flow and metabolism in comatose patients with acute head injury. J Neurosurg 61:241-253

Evaluation of Morphologic Recovery of the Brain in Chronic Subdural Hematoma After Decompression

K. YAMANE[1], T. SHIMA[1], Y. OKADA[1], M. NISHIDA[1], S. OKITA[1], T. HATAYAMA[1], and A. YOSHIDA[2]

Departments of [1] Neurosurgery and [2] Critical Care Medicine, Chugoku Rousai Hospital, Kure, Japan

Introduction

Chronic subdural hematoma (Chr SDH) is an intracranial space-occupying lesion that can cause cerebral dysfunction by compressing and displacing the brain. Hematoma compresses the brain not only on the ipsilateral side but also at times on the contralateral side. This compression can produce serious adverse effects on the cerebral circulation.

Chr SDH is generally treated with burr hole and irrigation but there are patients who demonstrate poor morphologic recovery from deformation after decompression.

The purpose of this paper is to assess the possibility to predict brain recovery after irrigation therapy in patients with Chr SDH by measuring epidural pressure (EDP) and monitoring cerebral oxygenation and cerebral blood volume (CBV) using near infrared spectrophotometry (NIRS).

Patients and Methods

Fourteen patients with unilateral Chr SDH (12 males and two female, aged from 39 to 83 years) were studied. Under mild sedation (diazepam and pentazosine) and local anesthesia, a burr hole was placed on the hematoma side with twist drill. EDP was measured by inserting a sensor (CardioSearch Instruments) into the space between the dura mater and the skull through the burr hole. After measurement of EDP, dura was opened and irrigation of hematoma cavity was performed. Changes in oxy hemoglobin (oxy-Hb), deoxy hemoglobin (deoxy-Hb), and total hemoglobin (total-Hb) contents were monitored continuously at the contralateral frontal area using near infrared spectrophotometry (Shimazu OM100A) during the operation.

The methodology of NIRS was described previously in detail [1, 2, 3, 4]. In brief, NIR light from three laser diodes (780, 805, 830 nm) illuminated the frontal head through an optic fiber at about 4 cm lateral to the midline on the non-hematoma side. Transmission of light was received at about 2.5 cm lateral to the illuminator. The level of each hemoglobin was expressed as an index. The relationship among the oxy-Hb, deoxy-Hb and total-Hb contents is described by the following formula.

Total-Hb = oxy-Hb + deoxy-Hb

Changes in oxy-Hb, deoxy-Hb and total-Hb were evaluated after irrigation treatment.

Morphologic recovery of the compressed brain was evaluated by the recovery rate (RR) which was calculated by the following formula.

$$RR\ (\%) = \frac{[V]_{pre} - [V]_{post}}{[V]_{pre}} \times 100$$

[V]pre: hematoma volume before operation

[V]post: hematoma cavity seven days after operation

Hematoma volume was estimated on CT scan [5]:

When RR was more than 50 %, morphological recovery was evaluated as good and when RR was less than 50 % recovery was poor.

The relationship between RR and EDP, and changes in each hemoglobin content were investigated.

Results

The intensity of the hematoma on CT scan varied from hypo to hyperdense. Midline structures of the brain were shifted to the contralateral side in all patients, ranging from 2.5 to 15.6 mm (8.6 ± 4.5,

mean ± SD).
CT scans performed seven days after irrigation demonstrated that nine patients had good morphologic recovery and the remaining five patients had poor recovery.
EDP was ranging from 10 to 71 mm Hg (36.2 ± 19.8, mean ± SD).
There was no significant relationship between EDP and brain recovery (Fig.1).
In four of five patients with poor recovery, no changes in oxy-Hb or deoxy-Hb was observed. Six of nine patients with good recovery demonstrated decrease in deoxy-Hb and increase in oxy-Hb after irrigation of hematoma (Fig. 2).
There was no obvious relationship between brain recovery and changes in total Hb after irrigation.

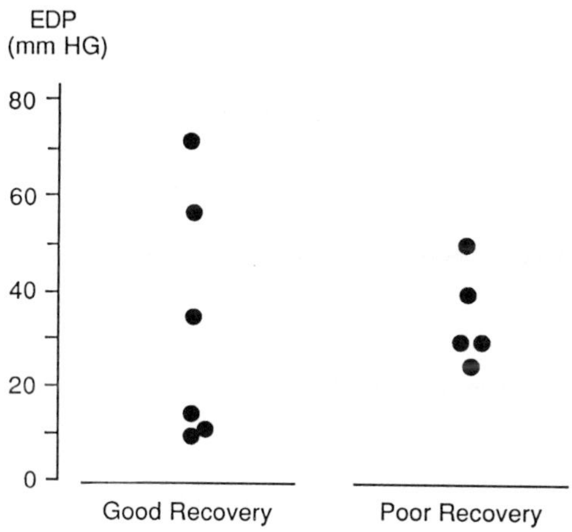

Fig. 1. Relationship between morphological recovery and epidural pressure (EDP). There was not significant relationship between them.

Discussion

Chr SDH, as other intracranial subdural space-occupying lesions, compresses not only the brain but also the cortical arteries and veins. Then compression of these vessels would cause increase in venous blood volume and increase in vascular resistance, resulting in decrease in CBF. These changes may occur in the contralateral hemisphere when midline structures of the brain is displaced to the contralateral side [6, 7]. In the patients who have good recovery from deformation after irrigation treatment, venous blood volume and CBF are expected to decrease and increase, respectively. On the other hand, in the patients who have poor recovery, changes in venous blood volume and CBF are not expected.

NIRS has been introduced as a non-invasive and continuous method of monitoring cerebral oxygenation and CBV by measuring oxy-Hb, deoxy-Hb and total Hb [1, 2, 4, 8, 9, 10].

Content of oxy-Hb indicates oxygenation of the examined cerebral cortex and it increases when oxygen saturation , cerebral blood flow (CBF) , and / or concentration of oxy-Hb increase. Deoxy-Hb responds to changes in oxygen saturation and cerebral hemodynamics. It increases with a fall in oxygen saturation, an obstruction to cerebral venous return, an increase in the inflow of desaturated blood, or an increase in the concentration of deoxy-Hb [4, 8, 11].

In this study, patients with good morphologic recovery after irrigation frequently demonstrated increase in oxy-Hb and decrease in deoxy-Hb. As oxygen saturation and concentration were unlikely to change significantly during irrigation, increase in oxy-Hb can be explained by increase in CBF which may be induced by reduction in vascular resistance and decrease in deoxy-Hb indicated decrease in venous blood volume which may be induced by improvement of venous return.

Total-Hb, which is the sum of oxy-Hb and deoxy-Hb contents, reflects CBV unless hematocrit of the cerebral vessels change. Since hematocrit of the cerebral vessels are unlikely to change, changes in total Hb would indicate change in CBV. In this study, there was no significant relationship between the changes in CBV and morphorogic recovery. The reason of this poor relation may be due to changes in

CBV after irrigation depend on the changes in oxy-Hb and deoxy-Hb which varied from patients to patients.

From this results, patient who demonstrates decrease in deoxy-Hb and increase in oxy-Hb after irrigation is expected to have a good morphologic recovery of the brain.

EDP is determined mainly by hematoma volume, compliance of the brain, and craniocerebral proportion. In the patients with brain atrophy and/ or high compliance, EDP may be low in spite of large hematoma. Though measuring EDP is important for evaluation of intracranial pressure, insignificant relationship between brain recovery and EDP may indicate that EDP is not an indicator for prediction of brain recovery.

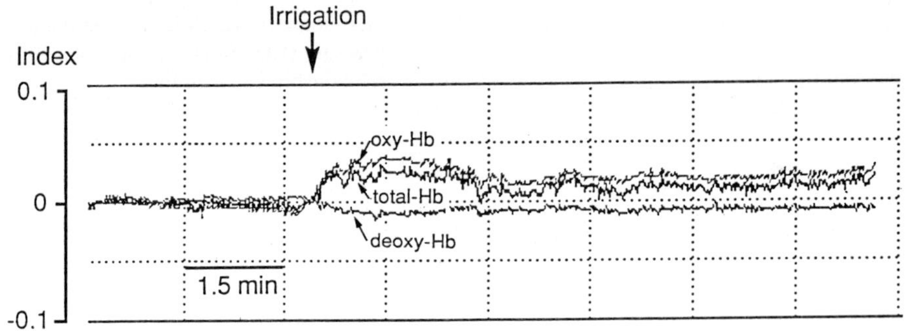

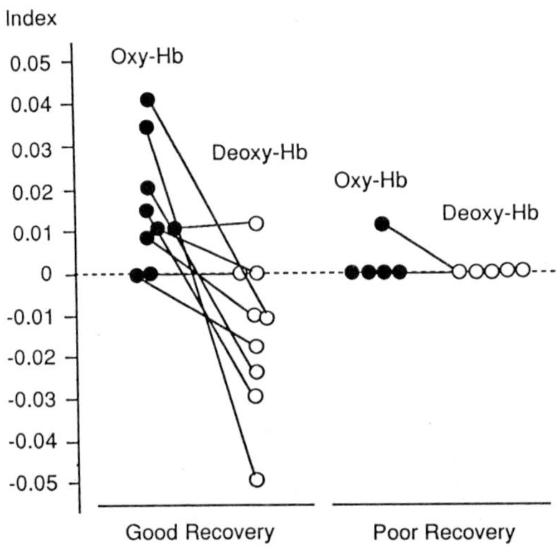

Fig. 2. (upper) Recording of changes in oxy-Hb, deoxy-Hb and total Hb after irrgation therapy in a patient with good recovery. After irrigation, oxy-Hb increased and deoxy-Hb decreased. (left) Relationship between morphological recovery and changes in oxy-Hb and deoxy-Hb after irrigation. Closed and open circles indicate changes in oxy-Hb and in deoxy-Hb, respectively. Patients with good recovery demonstrated that oxy-Hb increased and deoxy-Hb decreased after irrigation. There were not changes in oxy-Hb or changes in deoxy-Hb in patients with poor recovery.

References

1. Giannini I, Ferrari M, Carpi A, Fasella P: Rat brain monitoring by near infrared spectroscopy: and assessment of possible clinical significance. Physiol Chem Phys (1982) 14:295-305.
2. Jobsis FF: , infrared monitoring of cerebral and myocardial oxygen sufficiency and circulatory parameters. Science (1977) 98:1264-1267.
3. McCormick PW, Stewart M, Lewis G, Dujovny M, Ausman: Intracerebral penetration of infrared light. Technical note. J Neurosurg (1992) 76:315-318.
4. Tamura M: Non-invasive monitoring of brain oxygen metabolism during cardiopulmonary bypass by near-infrared spectrophotometry. Jpn Circ J (1991) 55:330-335.
5. Petersen OF, Espersen JO: Extradural hematomas: Measurement of size by volume summation o CT scanning. Neuroradiol (1984) 26:363-367.
6. Ikeda K, Kano A, Hayase H, Yamashita T, Ito H, Yamamoto S: Relationship between symptoms of chronic subdrual hematoma and hematoma volume or regional cerebral blood flow [in Japanese, English abstr]. Neurol Med Chir (Tokyo) (1984) 24: 869-875.
7. Tanaka A, Yoshinaga S, Kimura M: Xenon-enhanced computed tomographic measurement of cerebral blood flow in patients with chronic subdural hematomas. Neurosurg (1990) 27:554-561.
8. Brazy JE: Cerebral oxygen monitoring with near infrared spectroscopy: Clinical application to neonates. Clin Monit (1991) 7:325-334.
9. von Siebenthal K, Bernert G, Casear P: Near-infrared spectroscopy in newborn infants. Brain Dev (1992) 14:135-143.
10. Wyatt JS: Near infrared spectroscopy. Investigation and assessment of perinatal brain injury. Biol Neonate (1992) 62:290-294.
11. Scov L, Pryds O, Greisen G: Estimating cerebral blood flow in newborn infants: Comprison of near infrared spectroscopy and 133Xe clearance. Pediatr Res (1991) 30:570-573.

Kinetics of Atrial Natriuretic Peptide and Cyclic GMP in Cerebrospinal Fluid in Canine Kaolin-Induced Hydrocephalus

TSUNEYUKI FUKUSHIMA[1], TAKUJI TAKAGI[1], and HAJIME NAGAI[2]

[1] Department of Neurosurgery, Nagoya Higashi General Hospital, Wakamizu, Chikusa-ku, Nagoya, Aichi, 464 Japan
[2] Department of Neurosurgery, Nagaoya City University Medical School, Mizuho-ku, Nagoya, Aichi, 467 Japan

INTRODUCTION

Atrial natriuretic peptide (ANP) was first recognized as a peptide produced by atrial myocytes involved in the regulation of body sodium and intravascular volume, and has been identified subsequently in the central nervous system (CNS)[1]. The ANP concentration in CSF has been reported to increase in patients with hydrocephalus[2]. The CSF concentration of 3',5' cyclic guanosine monophosphate (cGMP), which is regarded as a second messenger for ANP, was also reported to increase in patients with intracranial hemorrhage or hydrocephalus[3] prior to the discovery of ANP. However the role of CSF-ANP has not been fully elucidated, and the significance of cGMP in the CSF remains unknown. The present study was designed to evaluate alterations in the CSF and plasma concentrations of ANP and cGMP during the progression of canine kaolin-induced hydrocephalus. The relationship between the CSF-ANP concentration and CSF pressure and that between the CSF-ANP concentration and CSF-cGMP concentration were examined.

MATERIALS AND METHODS

Sixteen adult mongrel dogs(8-10Kg) were used. The animals were anesthetized with ketamine HCl(10mg/Kg) and experimental hydrocephalus was induced by injection of sterile kaolin suspension (50-65mg/Kg) into the cisterna magna. In three control animals, 3cc saline was injected after cisternal puncture. Measurement of cisternal CSF opening pressure above the interaural line (cmH_2O), and CSF and blood sampling were performed before cisternal injection. The presence of ventricular dilatation was evaluated by MRI or postmortem dissection. Animals in which ventricles did not dilate were excluded from the hydrocephalic group.

At 2,7,14,21, and 28 days after cisternal injection, the animals were anesthetized, cisternal CSF opening pressure was measured, and CSF and blood samples were obtained. Plasma ANP, CSF-ANP, plasma cGMP, CSF-cGMP, and plasma ADH(arginine-vasopressin) were measured by radioimmunoassay. Concentration of sodium and osmolarity were measured in CSF and serum samples. Any CSF sample contaminated with blood was excluded. Data were analyzed after being divided into three groups: control, acute (within 2 weeks after intracisternal injection) or chronic (from 3 to 4 weeks after injection) stage of hydrocephalus.

RESULTS AND DISCUSSION

Seven of 13 animals injected with kaolin solution died within 4 weeks. Ventricular dilatation was observed in 11 of 13 kaolin-injected animals. In control animals, ventricular dilatation was not observed at 4 weeks after saline injection.

Table 1 CSF data in canine kaolin-induced hydrocephalus[10]

group	control	kaolin hydrocephalus		sham group	
		acute	chronic	acute	chronic
CSF pressure (cmH2O)	8.9±0.9 (16)	#17.9±0.9 (27)	11.4±1.6 (10)	8.5±0.7 (9)	9.8±0.7 (6)
CSF ANP (pg / ml)	2.9±1.2 (15)	*14.4±2.0 (24)	6.2±1.9 (10)	2.0±0.7 (9)	2.7±1.7 (6)
CSF cGMP (pmol / ml)	11.9±1.2 (15)	*30.1±5.0 (15)	*37.0±9.3 (10)	9.2±0.5 (9)	8.8±0.7 (6)
CSF Na (mEq / l)	151.1±1.4 (14)	153.8±2.6 (12)	150.8±1.1 (5)	152.3±1.0 (9)	152.3±1.6 (6)
Osmolarity (mOsm/KgH2O)	313.9±4.8 (14)	314.0±6.3 (14)	318.0±8.1 (5)	307.0±2.3 (9)	307.0±0.7 (6)

Values are means±SEM. Numbers in parentheses represents the number of specimens.
*Difference: P<0.01, using Wilcoxon rank sum test. #Difference: P<0.01, using t-test.

Table 2 Blood data in canine kaolin-induced hydrocephalus[10]

group	control	kaolin hydrocephalus		sham group	
		acute	chronic	acute	chronic
Plasma ANP (pg / ml)	39.6±5.7 (16)	30.0±2.6 (27)	35.9±4.1 (13)	33.8±9.0 (9)	31.5±7.5 (6)
Plasma cGMP (pmol / ml)	14.5±1.5 (16)	13.0±0.9 (27)	16.1±1.4 (13)	12.4±1.8 (9)	13.8±1.5 (6)
Plasma ADH (pg / ml)	13.5±4.4 (16)	15.4±4.3 (27)	12.2±2.6 (13)	14.4±2.2 (9)	11.8±2.1 (6)
Serum Na (mEq / l)	143.8±1.5 (16)	143.4±1.1 (27)	147.3±2.1 (13)	143.0±1.5 (9)	145.2±0.8 (6)
Osmolarity (mOsm/KgH2O)	299.4±2.5 (16)	295.3±1.6 (27)	298.2±2.9 (13)	298.2±4.4 (9)	297.8±4.6 (6)

Values are means±SEM. Numbers in parentheses represents the number of specimens.

CSF pressure

CSF pressure increased significantly during the acute stage of hydrocephalus (P<0.01,Table1). In the chronic stage, CSF pressure did not differ significantly from that in the control stage. In the sham group, CSF pressure did not change significantly for 4 weeks following cisternal saline injection.

Plasma concentrations of ANP,cGMP, ADH, and Sodium

Plasma concentrations of ANP, cGMP, ADH, sodium and CSF level of sodium were stable and did not vary significantly during the 4 week period following cisternal injection both in the hydrocephalus group and in the sham group (Tables 1,2). Intravascular volume change is a clear stimulus for alteration of the plasma ANP level[4] and, perhaps, CSF-ANP, plasma ADH, and serum sodium levels. It is suggested that since the intravascular volume of the animals was controlled, there was no significant endocrinological effect in the present study.

CSF concentrations of ANP

CSF concentrations of ANP increased significantly during the acute stage of hydrocephalus ($p<0.01$, Table1). In the chronic stage, CSF-ANP levels did not differ significantly from those in the control stage. In the sham group, CSF-ANP levels did not change significantly following cisternal saline injection. A significant positive correlation was seen between the CSF-ANP concentration and CSF pressure ($r=0.664, p=0.0001$, Fig. 1). No significant correlation was seen between plasma ANP and CSF-ANP levels.

Figure 1 Relationship between ANP concentration in CSF and CSF pressure[10]

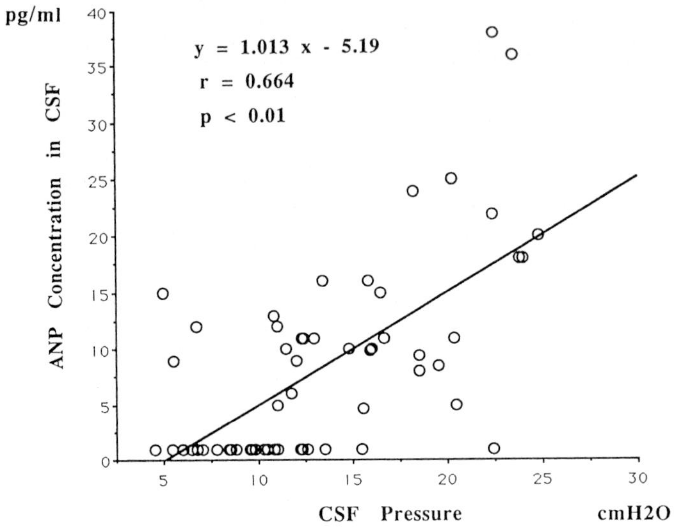

ANP concentrations in CSF have been reported to increase in patients with hydrocephalus[2]. In recent studies, ANP injected into the ventricle has been reported to decrease CSF production in rabbits[5], and to reduce the increased intracranial pressure in experimental hydrocephalus in rats[6]. These data and our results support the hypothesis that the CSF-ANP level increases to compensate for the pathophysiology of hydrocephalus.

The positive correlation between CSF-pressure and CSF-ANP levels suggests that the CSF-ANP level may depend directly or indirectly on CSF pressure in kaolin-induced hydrocephalus. A few mechanisms may explain how CSF-ANP levels are elevated in acute kaolin-induced hydrocephalus. The first hypothesis is that high intracranial pressure or acute stretch of the ventricle walls may trigger ANP release from paraventricular ANP-containing neurons. It is proven that physical stimuli can trigger ANP release. Edwards demonstrated recently that atrial stretch acts as the principle stimulus for cardiac ANP release[7]. Second, ANP may leak into the extracellular space from destroyed paraventricular ANP-containing cells during ventricular dilatation. Our data does not support this mechanism strongly since CSF-ANP levels did not correlate with the degree of ventricular dilatation on MRI in the present study. However, we may conclude that high intracranial pressure without ventricular dilatation can trigger elevation of the CSF-ANP level. Third, some neurotransmission system that results in neural ANP release may be stimulated in acute kaolin-induced hydrocephalus. ANP production in the hypothalamus has been reported to be increased by muscarinic-cholinergic stimulation[8]. However, the intracerebral cholinergic system is thought to be weakened in kaolin-induced hydrocephalus in rats[9]. It is unknown if any other neurotransmitter may be involved in neural ANP release.

CSF concentrations of cGMP

CSF concentrations of cGMP increased significantly during the acute stage of hydrocephalus ($p<0.01$), and remained significantly ($P<0.01$) elevated in the chronic stage (Table1). Compared to control plasma cGMP levels, CSF-cGMP levels were significantly higher during the acute and chronic stages of hydrocephalus ($p<0.01, p<0.01$), although no significant difference was seen between control plasma cGMP levels and control CSF-cGMP levels. In the sham group, CSF-cGMP levels did not change significantly following cisternal saline injection. No significant correlation was seen between CSF-cGMP levels and CSF-ANP levels ($r=0.062$), nor between CSF-cGMP levels and CSF pressure.

Since CSF-cGMP levels did not correlate with CSF-ANP levels in the present study, the CSF-cGMP concentration seems to be independent of the CSF-ANP concentrations. As elevated CSF-cGMP levels were significantly higher than plasma cGMP levels, blood brain barrier destruction should not be related to elevated CSF-cGMP levels. It is obvious that elevated CSF-cGMP concentrations are related to the activation of intracerebral guanylate cyclase. Not only the ANP system, but also the muscarinic cholinergic, alpha adrenergic, H1-histamine, and enkephalin systems are known to cause intracellular cGMP generation. Some of these systems may be activated in kaolin-induced hydrocephalus. Further investigation is necessary to clarify the significance of an elevated CSF-cGMP level in hydrocephalus.

REFERENCES

1. Young VTF, Lai CK, Cockram CS, Teoh R (1991) Atrial natriuretic peptide in the central nervous system. Neuroendocrinol 53(suppl 1): 18-24
2. Tulassay T, Khoor A, Bald M, Ritvay J, Szabo A, Rascher W (1990) Cerebrospinal fluid concentrations of atrial natriuretic peptide in children. Acta Pediatr Hung 30 : 20-207
3. Rudman D, O'Brien MS, McKinney AS, Hoffman JC, Patterson JH (1976) Observations of the cyclic nucleotide concentrations in human cerebrospinal fluid. J Clin Endocrinol Metab 42: 1088-1097
4. Alan L Davis (1989) Atrial natriuretic factor. Adv Pediatr 36: 137-150
5. Steardo L, Nathanson JA: Brain barrier tissues (1987) End organs for atriopeptins. Science 235: 470-473
6. Hashimoto K, Kikuchi H, Isikawa M, Yokoi K, Kimura M (1990) The effect of atrial natriuretic peptide on intracranial pressure in a congenital hydrocephalic model. Brain and Nerve 42: 683-687
7. Edwards BS, Zimmerman RS (1988) Atrial stretch, not pressure, is the principal determinant controlling the acute release of atrial natriuretic factor. Circ Res 62 : 191-195
8. Massi M, Saja A, Polidori C (1991) The release of atrial natriuretic factor induced by central carbacol injection may be mediated by muscarinic M1 receptors. Eur J Pharmacol 195 : 245-250
9. Mori K, Kurisawa M, Kamimura Y, Fujito K (1985) Muscarinic cholinergic receptor in experimental hydrocephalus. Annual report of the Ministry of Health and Welfare "Progressive hydrocephalus" 1984, 13-18
10. Fukushima T (1992) Alteration of Atrial Natriuretic Peptide and Cyclic GMP in CSF in Canine Kaolin-induced Hydrocephalus. Brain and Nerve 44 : 457-462

Session XIX: Drugs and Anesthetic Agents (1)

Chairmen: M. Brock and T. Sakabe

Rebound Phenomenon Following Multiple Doses of Mannitol?

G.-H. Schneider, P. v. Berenberg, A. Unterberg, and W.R. Lanksch

Department of Neurosurgery, Rudolf Virchow Medical Center, Free University of Berlin, Augustenburger Platz 1, D-13353 Berlin, Germany

SUMMARY

Mannitol has successfully been used in the therapy of elevated intracranial pressure (ICP). Recently, it has been suggested that in cases of a damaged blood-brain barrier frequent use of mannitol may aggravate vasogenic cerebral edema. Thus, it was studied whether multiple doses of mannitol infused during the development of vasogenic brain edema affect posttraumatic hemispheric swelling, edema and ICP.

In Sprague-Dawley rats, a cortical freezing lesion was applied to the right parietal region in ketamine-xylazine anaesthesia. In series (A), 9 animals received four doses of mannitol (0.4 g/kg b.w. per infusion) 30 min, 3, 6 and 9 hrs after trauma. 12 hrs post injury the brains were removed for determination of hemispheric swelling and cerebral water content. In a second series (B), 7 rats were treated with eight doses of mannitol 30 min, 3, 6, 9, 12, 15, 18 and 21 hrs following injury. In this series, the hemispheres were removed 24 hrs post trauma. In a third series (C), 8 rats were infused with nine doses of mannitol starting 30 min after injury and then q 3 hrs. In this group, animals were kept for another 12 hrs after the last mannitol administration and were sacrificed 36 hrs after trauma. Additionally, ICP was monitored during the last hour before sacrifice. In all three series (A - C), respective control animals (n = 9, 7, 8) received saline only.

Following four doses of mannitol, hemispheric swelling was slightly lower compared to control animals (7.5 ± 0.4 % vs. 7.9 ± 0.5 %, n.s.). In series (B), hemispheric swelling was reduced by mannitol treatment (eight doses) from 9.8 ± 0.5 % (saline infused animals) to 8.5 ± 0.3 %. Accordingly, the water content of traumatized hemispheres was lower in mannitol treated rats. Water content of control hemispheres was also slightly reduced by mannitol. In series (C), hemispheric swelling was marginally lowered by mannitol. This was mirrored by ICP (mannitol: 7.5 ± 0.7 mmHg vs. saline: 8.0 ± 0.8 mmHg).

These findings indicate that multiple doses of mannitol do not aggravate total hemispheric swelling, nor global hemispheric water content, even when administered during development of vasogenic edema. After discontinuation of mannitol treatment there is no rebound of ICP. On the contrary, there is indication that frequent application of mannitol may even reduce posttraumatic swelling. Taken together, a multiple dose regimen of mannitol in the management of elevated ICP should be favoured, even in the blood-brain barrier is disturbed.

INTRODUCTION

Mannitol is an important instrument in the management of elevated intracranial pressure associated with intracranial masses or cerebral edema. Though, a single dose of mannitol is beneficial for transient reduction of cerebral bulk [1,2,3], it has been speculated for many years that mannitol administration might be responsible for a rebound of ICP after discontinuation of treatment [4]. Moreover, Kaufmann and Cardoso suggested that multiple doses of mannitol might aggravate vasogenic cerebral edema [5]. Treating a cryogenic injury in cats with five doses of mannitol, they reported an accumulation of mannitol in vasogenic edema. This caused a reversal of the osmotic

concentration gradient between edematous brain and plasma and resulted in an increase of cerebral water content in edematous regions. Based on these findings, Kaufmann concluded that the long-term use of mannitol in cases of disturbed blood-brain barrier should be reevaluated [5].
The aim of this study was, therefore, to determine whether multiple doses of mannitol administered during the development of vasogenic brain edema following a cryogenic injury affect posttraumatic hemispheric swelling, edema and intracranial pressure and whether discontinuation of long-term mannitol treatment provokes a rebound of ICP.

MATERIALS AND METHODS

For the experiments 48 male Sprague-Dawley rats weighing 521 ± 17 g were used. In ketamine-xylazine anaesthesia a craniectomy was made over the right parietal region. A standard lesion was applied to the cortex by stereotactically lowering a copper probe (5 mm) cooled to -60 °C by a dry ice/acetone-mixture onto the exposed dura for 30 seconds [6,7]. During the perioperative period mean arterial blood pressure was monitored via a cannula in the tail artery.
The animals were devided into three groups (A - C) which were treated with multiple intravenous doses of mannitol (0.4 g/kg b.w. per infusion). In series A, 9 rats received four doses of mannitol 30 min, 3, 6, and 9 hrs post trauma. Subset B (n = 7) was treated with eight infusions at 30 min, 3, 6, 9, 12, 15, 18, and 21 hrs following cryogenic injury. Group C (n = 8) was infused with a total of nine doses of mannitol starting 30 min after trauma and then q 3 hrs till 24 hrs. In all three series (A - C), control animals (n = 9, 7, 8) were infused with respective volumes of saline, only.
In series A and B, the brains were removed 3 hrs following the last mannitol administration. In order to study whether frequent application of mannitol induces a rebound of intracranial pressure after longer discontinuation of treatment, the animals of group C were kept for a period of 12 hrs after the last dose of mannitol and were sacrificed 36 hrs following the cryogenic injury. In addition, intracranial pressure (ICP) was monitored during the last hour before sacrifice by stereotactic puncture of the left lateral ventricle using a specially prepared 25 gauge needle.
After removal of the brains, hemispheres were carefully separated with the help of an operating microscope and weighed for determination of brain swelling. Thereafter, the hemispheres were dried at 100 °C for 48 hrs and weighed again. Cerebral water content was then calculated as the difference of hemispheric wet- and dryweight.

RESULTS

Treatment with four doses of mannitol (series A) slightly reduced posttraumatic brain swelling compared to control animals (7.5 ± 0.4 % vs. 7.9 ± 0.5 %, n.s., Tab. 1). Accordingly, water content of the traumatized hemisphere was marginally lower in mannitol-infused rats (79.8 ± 0.3 % vs. 80.2 ± 0.3 %, Tab. 1). Non-traumatized left hemispheres of rats treated with mannitol also showed a slight decrease in water content (Tab. 1).
Following eight applications of mannitol in subset B, brain swelling induced by cryogenic injury was significantly reduced by 13 % from 9.8 ± 0.5 % to 8.5 ± 0.3 % ($p < 0.05$; Fig. 1, Tab. 1). In this group, cerebral water content of both hemispheres was found to be lower in animals receiving mannitol (Tab. 1).
In series C where the brains were analyzed 12 hrs after the last of a total of nine doses of mannitol, frequent administration of mannitol, again, marginally reduced posttraumatic hemispheric swelling (Tab. 1). This was mirrored by the slightly lower ICP in mannitol-treated animals during the last hour before sacrifice (Fig. 2). Due to the method of measurement, the initial value is raised a few mmHg by a small volume of saline entering the ventricular system during puncture. The following decrease of ICP depends on the intracranial compliance and ICP then approaches the actual value (mannitol: 7.5 ± 0.7 mmHg vs. NaCl: 8.0 ± 0.8 mmHg). Cerebral water content of both hemispheres was not influenced by mannitol treatment, in this series (Tab. 1).

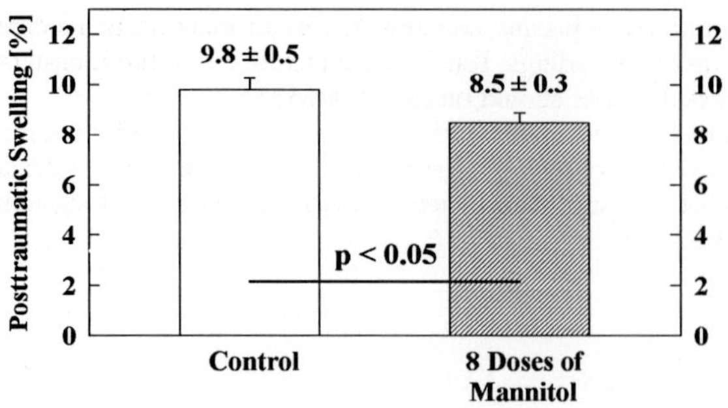

Fig. 1: Posttraumatic hemispheric swelling following eight doses of mannitol - series (B). Siginificant reduction of swelling by treatment.

	Posttraumatic Hemispheric Swelling [%]		Hemispheric Water Content [%]			
			NaCl		Mannitol	
Series	NaCl	Mannitol	traum. Hem.	control	traum. Hem.	control
A	7.9 ± 0.5	7.5 ± 0.4	78.7 ± 0.2	80.2 ± 0.3	78.4 ± 0.2	79.8 ± 0.3
B	9.8 ± 0.5	8.5 ± 0.3 *	78.9 ± 0.2	80.6 ± 0.3	78.7 ± 0.2	80.3 ± 0.2
C	7.3 ± 0.8	7.0 ± 0.8	78.7 ± 0.2	80.2 ± 0.2	78.8 ± 0.1	80.3 ± 0.1

Tab. 1: Posttraumatic hemispheric swelling and cerebral water content in the different treatment groups (A - C); * $p < 0.05$.

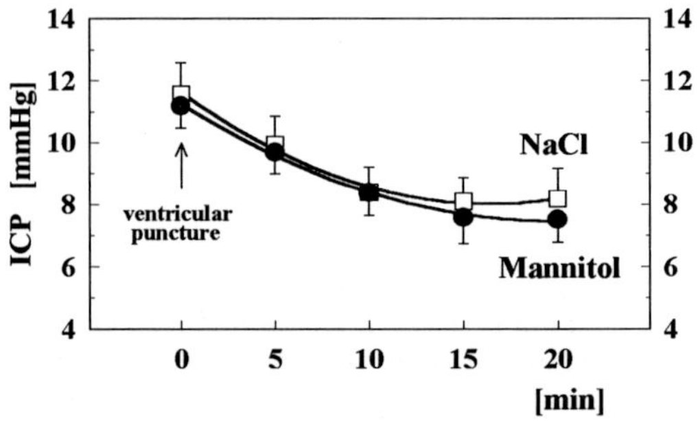

Fig. 2: Intracranial pressure 35.5 hrs post trauma - series (C). Discontinuation of mannitol treatment (nine doses) 24 hrs post cryogenic injury did not lead to a rebound of ICP.

DISCUSSION

Frequent use of mannitol is widely accepted as a basis for treatment of elevated intracranial pressure. Several mechanisms of beneficial effects of mannitol on intracranial compliance have been discussed. Administration of mannitol leads to a transient increase in cerebral blood flow which in turn induces a compensatory vasoconstriction with a consecutive reduction of cerebral blood volume and ICP [1]. Osmotic dehydration of brain tissue is considered as a second mechanism of mannitol [2,5]. Additionally, mannitol may act as a free radical scavenger thus beneficially influencing the development of secondary brain damage [8].

While local accumulation of mannitol with consecutive increase of water content in edematous regions may be true [5], our findings in a model with grossly damaged blood-brain barrier show that repeated application of mannitol does not aggravate total hemispheric swelling, but rather reduces posttraumtic swelling and edema. Additionally, no rebound of ICP was observed after discontination of mannitol infusions. It might be speculated that the possible local increase of tissue water content in edematous regions is more than compensated by other actions of mannitol like osmotic dehydration of non-traumatized brain tissue [2,5] or interference with promoting mediators of secondary brain damage, e.g. free radicals [8].

Taken together, our study favours a multiple dose mannitol regimen in the management of intracranial hypertension, even in cases of a disturbed blood-brain barrier.

REFERENCES

1. Muizelaar JP, Wei EP, Kontos HA, Becker DP (1983) Mannitol causes compensatory cerebral vasoconstriction and vasodilation in response to blood viscosity changes. J Neurosurg 59: 822 - 828

2. Nath F, Galbraith S (1986) The effect of mannitol on cerebral white matter water content. J Neurosurg 65: 41 - 43

3. Hartwell RC, Sutton LN (1993) Mannitol, intracranial pressure, and vasogenic edema. Neurosurgery 32: 444 - 450

4. Kofke WA (1993): Mannitol: Potential for rebound intracranial hypertension? Editorial. J Neurosurg Anesthesiol 5: 1 - 3

5. Kaufmann AM, Cardoso ER (1992) Aggravation of vasogenic cerebral edema by multiple-dose mannitol. J Neurosurg 77: 584 - 589

6. Klatzo I, Piraux A, Laskowski EJ (1958) The relationship between edema, blood-brain barrier and tissue elements in local brain injury. J Neuropath Exp Neurol 17: 548 - 564

7. Schneider G-H, Unterberg A, Lanksch WR (1994) 21-Aminosteroid U-74389F reduces vasogenic brain edema. Acta Neurochir [Suppl] 60: 516 - 518

8. Macgovern GJ, Bolling SF, Casale AS (1984) The mechanism of mannitol in reducing ischemic injury: hyper-osmolarity or hydroxyl scavenger. Circulation 70 [Suppl I]: 191 - 195

Use of Low Dose Mannitol in Vasopastic States

BRUCE J. ANDERSEN[1], SVETLANA V. PRAVDENKOVA[2], and GRANT A. SKIDMORE[1]

[1] University of Arkansas for Medical Sciences, Little Rock, AR, USA
[2] Sklifosovsky Institute of First Aid, Moscow, Russia

PURPOSE

The effects of mannitol on blood viscosity, cerebral blood flow, and intracranial pressure are known, as is the diuretic effect observed at standard clinical doses. In stroke and vasospastic states decreasing blood viscosity to improve microcirculation is desirable but a diuretic effect is not. Dosing mannitol to avoid its diuretic effect but maintain its effect on blood viscosity could be beneficial to patients suffering from vasospasm. To investigate this hypothesis, our study examines the effects of differing doses of mannitol on blood viscosity, cerebral microcirculation, and trans-cranial doppler signals.

METHODS

The dose-response relationship between viscosity and mannitol dosage was determined using whole blood and packed red blood cells from human volunteers. Mannitol corresponding to human doses of 0.125 to 2.0 g/kg were added to aliquoits of blood then viscosity was measured using a rotating plate micro viscometer producing shear rates of 106 sec^{-1}. Hematocrit was also measured. Control aliquoits were diluted to identical hematocrit values using normal saline.

The dose-response relationship between mannitol dosage and cerebral microcirculation was determined *in vivo* using a rodent cranial window model through which a laser doppler flow meter was positioned. Mannitol dosage was varied from 0.125 to 2.0 g/kg in identical volumes. Saline was used for control values. Flow and velocity were monitored for 60 minutes after mannitol or saline bolus.

To determine what effect, if any, varying doses of mannitol has upon trans cranial doppler (TCD) blood flow measurements, a closed circuit containing blood diluted with equal volumes of saline or differing doses of mannitol was pumped at a know velocity and insonated by a standard TCD probe.

RESULTS

The aliquoits of human blood containing mannitol were compared with non-mannitol containing aliquoits diluted to identical hematocrit values using normal saline.A linear dose-response relationship was observed with even the lowest dose of mannitol resulting in a decrease in blood viscosity. The viscosity changes caused by mannitol were significantly greater than those seen by saline dilution alone at similar hematocrit values (p ranged from <0.02 to <0.001).

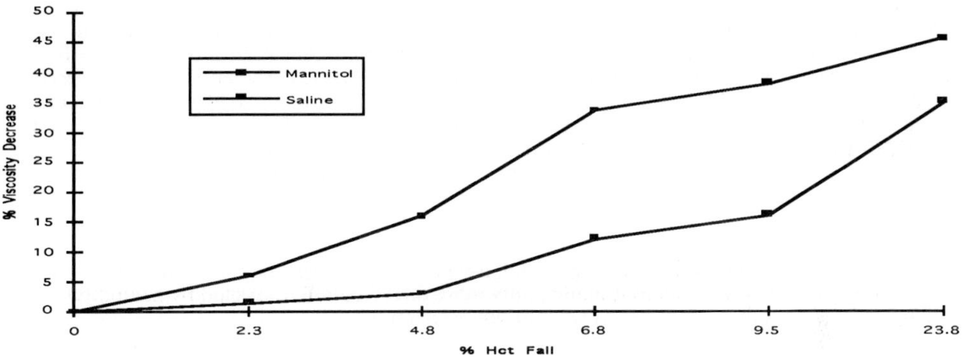

Dose-response effects of mannitol on cerebral microcirculation were then observed *in vivo* in rats using the same mannitol doses as above. All doses of mannitol imparted a statistically significant increase in blood flow and velocity ($p<0.001$). The animal receiving only normal saline showed no increase in blood flow or velocity. The mannitol dose imparting the greatest increase in CBF was 0.25 gm/kg.

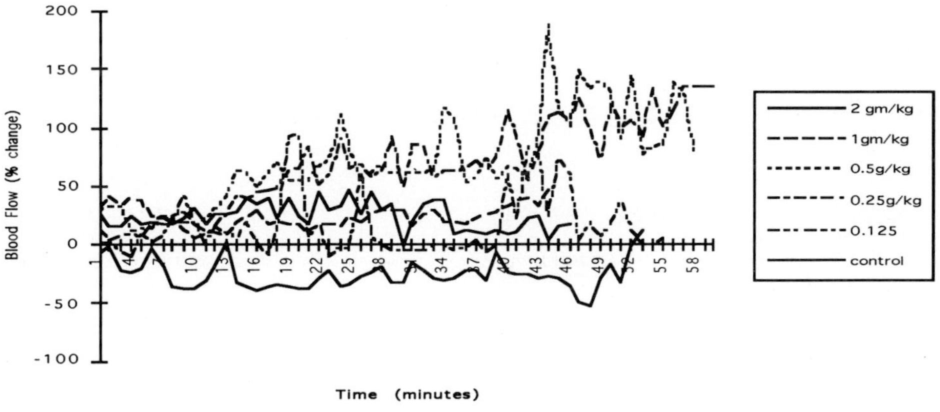

Finally, as transcranial Doppler (TCD) measurements of blood velocity are commonly used to monitor patients in vasospasm, the effects of these doses of mannitol were evaluated as to their effect on TCD signal accuracy. TCD signals were not affected at any mannitol dose.

DISCUSSION

At constant temperature, blood viscosity is influenced by plasma viscosity, red blood cell aggregation, hematocrit, and red blood cell deformity. Mannitol has been shown not to effect plasma viscosity. Heparinization prevented aggregation in this study. The effects of heamtocrit change were controlled for using equal volumes of saline to dilute blood to identical hematocrit values. Thus, the significant effects noted appear to be due to the influence of mannitol on red cell deformability. In this study and others, mannitol clearly decreases the viscosity and increases blood flow. The question is, are these beneficial rheologic factors dose dependent, and if so, what is the lowest effective dose?

We conclude that mannitol, even at very low doses (0.125 gm/kg), improves cerebral blood flow through the microcirculation significantly more than would be expected by hemodilution alone without affecting standard TCD monitoring techniques.

The clinical significance of this finding is that, if dosed low enough to avoid its osmotic diuretic effect, or if urine output is replaced with equivalent intravenous fluids, mannitol could prove useful as a therapy for the treatment of vasospasm and hypoperfusion.

CSF, Sagittal Sinus, and Jugular Venous Pressures During Desflurane or Isoflurane Anesthesia in Dogs

A.A. Artru, K. Powers, and P. Doepfner

Department of Anesthesiology, RN-10, University of Washington School of Medicine, Seattle, WA, USA

INTRODUCTION

Previous studies suggest that desflurane may increase ICP and that the magnitude of the increase is determined in part by the levels of P_aCO_2 and ICP or cerebrospinal fluid (CSF) pressure prior to administration of desflurane [1-3]. However not all P_aCO_2/ICP conditions have been studied and the reported effects of desflurane on ICP are often inconsistent with the effects of desflurane on the factors generally believed to determine ICP such as cerebral blood volume (CBV), CSF volume, brain tissue volume and intracranial compliance.

When ICP and P_aCO_2 initially were normal, administration of 0.5, 1.0 MAC or 1.5 MAC desflurane increased ICP in dogs to values that were higher than those previously reported with < 0.2 MAC halothane, initial exposure to either 1.0 MAC enflurane or 1.0 MAC isoflurane, sufentanil, nitrous oxide and etomidate, but similar to those previously reported with < 0.2 or 2.0 MAC isoflurane. The finding that desflurane causes higher ICP than other inhlational anesthetics under these P_aCO_2/ICP conditions is not consistent with previous reports in dogs that the magnitude of cerebral blood flow (CBF) increase with desflurane was similar to equivalent MAC concentrations with other inhalational anesthetics [1], and that desflurane caused no increase in CSF formation, decrease in CSF reabsorption or increase in brain tissue water content.

There are no reports on the effects of desflurane on ICP under conditions where P_aCO_2 was normal and ICP was increased prior to administration of desflurane. An increase of ICP with desflurane would be consistent with a previous report that desflurane, like other inhalational anesthetics, increases CBF [1].

When ICP initially was normal and hyperventilation was used to decrease P_aCO_2 during administration of 0.5, 1.0 or 1.5 MAC desflurane in dogs, there was no significant change in ICP [2]. The finding that hyperventilation failed to decrease ICP during desflurane anesthesia differs from results with other anesthetics.

When ICP initially was increased and hyperventilation was used to decrease P_aCO_2 during administration of 0.5 MAC desflurane and 50% nitrous oxide in oxygen or 0.8 MAC desflurane in air/oxygen, there was no significant change in ICP of patients with space occupying lesions. Under the same P_aCO_2/ICP conditions and 1.0 MAC desflurane in air/oxygen, ICP increased in patients with space occupying lesions [3].

We hypothesized that some of the inconsistencies between reported effects of desflurane on ICP and reported effects of desflurane on determinants of ICP such as CBV, CSF volume, brain tissue volume and intracranial compliance, may relate to differences in experimental conditions between studies. Accordingly the present study was designed to examine CSF pressure during 4.0 h desflurane anesthesia in dogs using a design that permitted within group comparisons and included a concurrent comparison group (isoflurane) and direct measurement of both intra- and extracranial CSF pressures. Along with CSF pressures, sagittal sinus and jugular venous pressures were examined to determine whether these might affect CSF pressure. CSF, sagittal sinus and jugular venous pressures were measured during 0.5 and 1.0 MAC desflurane and during normo- and hypocapnia to determine whether desflurane concentration or P_aCO_2 state affected the measured pressures or their interrelationships.

METHODS

Twelve unmedicated mongrel dogs (weights 15-21 kg) were anesthetized and surgically prepared for measurement of lateral ventricle and cisternal CSF pressures, sagittal sinus blood pressure, external jugular venous pressure and systemic values. After control measurements were obtained, all dogs were studied during 4.0 h desflurane (n=6) or isoflurane (n=6). With both anesthetics dogs were studied for 1.0 h at each of 4 experimental conditions: 1) 0.5 MAC desflurane or isoflurane and normocapnia, 2) 0.5 MAC desflurane or isoflurane and hypocapnia, 3) 1.0 MAC desflurane or isoflurane and normocapnia, and 4) 1.0 MAC desflurane or isoflurane and hypocapnia. For normocapnia P_aCO_2 was maintained at 35-39 mmHg and for hypocapnia P_aCO_2 was maintained at 20-24 mmHg. The duration of each experimental condition was 60 min.

Systemic values and CSF, sagittal sinus and jugular venous pressures were analyzed using analysis of variance and three-way, repeated measures analysis of variance. Effects of the anesthetic (desflurane vs isoflurane), P_aCO_2 state, time, desflurane or isoflurane dose, and order of presentation of experimental condition were examined for. Change of CSF, sagittal sinus and jugular venous pressures for 4.0 h desflurane or isoflurane anesthesia (independent of P_aCO_2 state or desflurane or isoflurane dose), for 2.0 h at each P_aCO_2 state (independent of desflurane or isoflurane dose) and for 1.0 h at each experimental condition were determined. These post hoc analyses were performed using analysis of variance and Student's t-test for paired samples. Values are tabulated as mean ± SD.

RESULTS

Three-way repeated measures analysis of variance indicated that CSF pressure was significantly affected by the anesthetic, i.e., desflurane vs isoflurane. This analysis also indicated that CSF pressure was significantly affected by P_aCO_2 and by time at each experimental condition, but not by desflurane or isoflurane dose, i.e., 0.5 vs 1.0 MAC. In contrast, sagittal sinus and jugular venous pressures were not significantly affected by the anesthetic (desflurane vs isoflurane), P_aCO_2, time, desflurane or isoflurane dose, or order of presentation of experimental conditions.

CSF Pressure

Baseline ventricular CSF pressure was 10.4 ± 1.8 cmH_2O prior to desflurane and 10.7 ± 1.9 cmH_2O prior to isoflurane. CSF pressure increased significantly during 4.0 h anesthesia with either desflurane or isoflurane. The increase of CSF pressure during 4.0 h desflurane anesthesia (to 40.2±12.7 cmH_2O), was significantly greater than the increase of CSF pressure during 4.0 h isoflurane anesthesia (to 26.2±11.5 cmH_2O).

Because P_aCO_2 was varied during the 4.0 h desflurane or isoflurane anesthesia, the effect of desflurane or isoflurane on CSF pressure during either normocapnia or hypocapnia is indicated by the 2.0 h data at each P_aCO_2 state. CSF pressure increased significantly during 2.0 h of desflurane at normocapnia (by 21.7±15.7 cmH_2O) and during 2.0 h of isoflurane at normocapnia (by 8.6±3.2 cmH_2O). The increase of CSF pressure during 2.0 h of desflurane at normocapnia (from 22.0±12.6 to 43.7±11.1 cmH_2O) was significantly greater than the increase of CSF pressure during 2.0 h of isoflurane at normocapnia (from 17.6±9.9 to 26.2±11.0 cmH_2O). CSF pressure also increased significantly during 2.0 of desflurane at hypocapnia (by 10.9±4.5 cmH_2O) and during 2.0 h of isoflurane at hypocapnia (by 8.8±4.9 cmH_2O). The increase of CSF pressure during 2.0 h of desflurane at hypocapnia (from 17.6±10.6 to 28.5±11.6) was not significantly different from the increase of CSF pressure during 2.0 h of isoflurane at hypocapnia (from 9.7±2.3 to 18.4±7.0 cmH_2O).

The effectiveness of hypocapnia for decreasing CSF pressure during desflurane or isoflurane is indicated by comparison of CSF pressure before and after changing the P_aCO_2 state. At 2.0 h when the transition was made from normocapnia to hypocapnia or vice versa, CSF pressure changed significantly by 15.1±4.1 cmH_2O during desflurane and by 6.8±2.8 cmH_2O during isoflurane. The change of CSF pressure during desflurane was significantly greater than that during isoflurane.

Baseline cisternal CSF pressure was 10.1±1.9 cmH_2O prior to desflurane and 9.7±2.6 cmH_2O prior to isoflurane. During 4.0 h desflurane or isoflurane anesthesia cisternal CSF pressures followed the same pattern as ventricular CSF pressures. The gradient between ventricular and cisternal CSF pressures was not significantly altered by the anesthetic (desflurane vs isoflurane), P_aCO_2, time, desflurane or isoflurane dose, or order of presentation of experimental conditions.

The increase of saggital sinus pressure during 4.0 h desflurane anesthesia (to 27.3±20.3 cmH_2O) was not significantly different from the increase of sagittal sinus pressure during 4.0 h isoflurane anesthesia (to 27.4±14.3 cmH_2O).

Jugular venous pressure was not significantly different between anesthetics and was not significantly changed during 4.0 h desflurane or isoflurane anesthesia.

DISCUSSION

Principal findings of the present study are that ventricular and cisternal CSF pressures and sagittal sinus blood pressure increase when thiopental/halothane anesthesia is replaced by desflurane or isoflurane. The increase of CSF pressure was greater during desflurane than during isoflurane, but the increase in sagittal sinus blood pressure with desflurane was not significantly different from that with isoflurane. Consequently, the ventricular CSF-sagittal sinus pressure gradient and the slope of the relationship between ventricular CSF-sagittal sinus pressure gradient and CSF pressure was greater during desflurane than during isoflurane. The greater increase of CSF pressure during 4.0 h desflurane than during 4.0 h isoflurane was the result of a greater CSF pressure increase during 2.0 h desflurane and normocapnia and a similar CSF pressure increase during 2.0 h desflurane.

The reason for the increase of CSF pressure that occurred during desflurane anesthesia is uncertain. One possible cause for increase of CSF pressure is increase of jugular venous pressure. When jugular venous pressure increases, cerebral venous flow from the sagittal sinus to the jugular vein resumes only when sagittal sinus pressure increases to a level greater than that in the jugular vein. In turn, reabsorption of CSF from the subarachnoid space into the sagittal sinus proceeds only when CSF pressure increases to a level greater than that in the sagittal sinus. However, in the present study desflurane caused no increase in jugular venous pressure. Thus, it is unlikely that this mechanism accounts for the observed increase in CSF pressure with desflurane. Another possible cause for increase of CSF pressure is increase of sagittal sinus pressure. In the present study sagittal sinus pressure increased with both desflurane and isoflurane, consistent with the increase of CBF (and presumably CBV) previously reported to occur with both anesthetics [1]. However, the greater increase of CSF pressure with desflurane than with isoflurane is not explained by cerebral vasodilation because in previous studies the increase of CSF pressure with desflurane was similar to that with isoflurane and in the present study sagittal sinus pressure with desflurane was not different from that with isoflurane. The greater increase of CSF pressure with desflurane also is probably not explained by differences in intracranial compliance because a previous study reported that estimated intracranial compliance with desflurane was not significantly different from that with isoflurane. The greater increase of CSF pressure with desflurane may be explained by a greater increase of CSF volume with desflurane than with isoflurane because a previous study reported V_f values that were 45% greater with desflurane and R_a values that were 2% greater with desflurane than with comparable MAC values with isoflurane.

Another principal finding of the present study is that hypocapnia significantly decreased CSF pressure during both desflurane and isoflurane. The greater decrease of CSF pressure with hypocapnia during desflurane probably occurred because CSF pressure prior to hypocapnia during desflurane was increased compared to that during isoflurane. Thus, the slope of the relationship between intracranial volume and pressure presumably was steeper in the dogs receiving desflurane than in the dogs receiving isoflurane.

REFERENCES

1. Lutz LJ, Milde JH, Milde LN (1990) The cerebral functional, metabolic and hemodynamic effects of desflurane in dogs. Anesthesiology 73:125-131
2. Lutz LJ, Milde JH, Milde LN (1991) The response of the canine circulation to hyperventilation during anesthesia with desflurane. Anesthesiology 74:504-507
3. Muzzi DA, Losasso TJ, Dietz NM, Faust RJ, Cucchiara RF, Milde LN (1992) The effect of desflurane and isoflurane on cerebrospinal fluid pressure in humans with supratentorial mass lesions. Anesthesiology 76:720-724

Intravenous Lidocaine Decreases but Cocaine Does Not Alter the Rate of CSF Formation in Anesthetized Rabbits

A.A. ARTRU, C.M. BERNARDS, and D.S. MAUTZ

Department of Anesthesiology, RN-10, University of Washington School of Medicine, Seattle, WA, USA

INTRODUCTION

During anesthesia and surgery, patients are exposed to numerous drugs and treatments that may alter CNS physiology in general and CSF physiology in particular. One such drug is cocaine. Cocaine may influence CNS physiology as a result of self administration by patients or topical administration by physicians for purposes of analgesia and vasoconstriction. The effects of cocaine on the rate of CSF formation (V_f) and resistance to reabsorption of CSF (R_a) are not known. It is expected that cocaine may alter V_f and/or R_a because cocaine possesses both adrenergic stimulating and local anesthetic properties. While the effects of local anesthetics on V_f and R_a are not known, increased adrenergic activity, either by stimulation of the adrenergic innervation to the CNS or by iv or intraventricular administration of adrenergic agonist drugs, is reported to decrease V_f. There are no previous reports on the effects of increased adrenergic activity on R_a. Accordingly, the present study was designed to examine the effects of cocaine on V_f and R_a.

The effects of lidocaine on V_f and R_a also were studied. Lidocaine was chosen as a comparison drug to cocaine because it posesses local anesthetic properties without causing adrenergic stimulation. A second reason for examining the effects of lidocaine on V_f and R_a is that it is routinely used during the anesthetic management of neuro-surgical patients. Iv lidocaine is recommended to prevent circulatory and ICP responses to laryngoscopy and tracheal intubation. Iv lidocaine also has been proposed as a treatment to minimize ischemic cerebral damage and at our institution is often used as part of a technique of balanced anesthesia for neurological surgery, in particular when the surgery includes cortical stimulation to evoke peripheral motor responses.

Three concentrations of both cocaine and lidocaine were examined in order to determine whether the effects of these treatments (if any) were dose related. The drug doses chosen were those expected to provide comparable local anesthetic potency between cocaine and lidocaine [1]. Because it was not known whether the doses used in this study were close to those needed to cause significant cardiovascular depression, additional doses of cocaine and lidocaine were given at the end of the study to determine the doses needed to produce significant dysrhythmias and hypotension.

METHODS

Thirteen New Zealand white rabbits, weighing 3.5-4.3 kg, were anesthetized and surgically prepared for ventriculocisternal perfusion and determination of the EEG and systemic values. The experimental period began once tracer equilibration was complete. All 13 rabbits were examined at four experimental conditions: 1) control, 2) low dose cocaine or lidocaine, 3) moderate dose cocaine or lidocaine, and 4) high dose cocaine or lidocaine.

In group 1 (cocaine, n=7), control values (condition 1) were obtained during halothane 0.8-1.0% inspired and nitrous oxide 66% inspired in oxygen. For conditions 2-4, cocaine was given iv and halothane/nitrous oxide/oxygen anesthesia was continued. For condition 2, cocaine 0.5 mg/kg was given over 10 min followed by continuous infusion at 1.0 $\mu g \cdot kg^{-1} \cdot min^{-1}$. For condition 3, cocaine 1.5 mg/kg was given over 10 min followed by continuous infusion at 3.0 $\mu g \cdot kg^{-1} \cdot min^{-1}$. For condition 4, cocaine 4.5 mg/kg was given over 10 min followed by continuous infusion at 9.0 $\mu g \cdot kg^{-1} \cdot min^{-1}$. V_f, R_a, EEG, ECG and systemic values were determined at each cocaine dose for comparison with control values for group 1. At the conclusion of each condition arterial blood samples were obtained for determination of plasma cocaine, epinephrine and norepinephrine concentrations.

In group 2 (lidocaine, n=6), control values (condition 1) again were obtained during halothane/nitrous oxide/oxygen anesthesia. For conditions 2-4, lidocaine was given iv and halothane/nitrous oxide/oxygen anesthesia was continued. Initial doses, subsequent infusion rates, and values determined were the same as for group 1.

Plasma samples were stored at -20°C until analysis. Cocaine and lidocaine concentrations were determined separately by gas chromatography with nitrogen-phosphorus detection. Epinephrine and norepinephrine concentrations were determined using high performance liquid chromatography coupled with an electrochemical detector. The limits of detection were 65 and 190 pg/ml for epinephrine and norepinephrine, respectively.

At each condition, three consecutive samples of cisternal outflow were collected (collection time of 5-7 min per sample) for determinations of V_f and the rate of CSF reabsorption (V_a). V_f and V_a were calculated as previously described according to the formulas of Heisey et al. [2]. For these calculations, concentrations of Blue Dextran in samples of the labeled mock CSF being perfused into the ventricle were determined using light absorbance at 620 nm. Values for V_a at two CSF pressure states were used to calculate R_a for each experimental condition. By definition, R_a is a reciprocal measure of the slope relating V_a (expressed as ml/min) to CSF pressure (expressed as cmH_2O).

All data except V_f, V_a and CSF pressure data were analyzed using two factor, repeated measures analysis of variance (ANOVA). For the data analyzed using two factor ANOVA the factors were treatment (cocaine or lidocaine), dose and treatment x dose. Data for V_f, V_a and CSF pressure were analyzed using three factor, repeated measures ANOVA. For these comparison the factors were treatment, dose, CSF pressure state, and the interaction among them. Post hoc comparisons of experimental conditions to the control condition were performed using Dunnett's test with $p < 0.05$ considered significant. Values are tabulated as mean ± SD.

RESULTS

In the cocaine group (group 1), the control V_f values for the two CSF pressure states were 8±2 and 9±2 μl/min. V_f values during the low, medium and high doses of cocaine ranged from 7±1 to 8±2 μl/min and were not significantly different from control values. In the lidocaine group (group 2), the control V_f values for the two CSF pressure states were 8±2 and 9±1 μl/min and were not significantly different from the control values in the cocaine group. V_f values during the low and medium doses of lidocaine ranged from 7±1 to 9±3 μl/min and were not significantly different from control values. In contrast, V_f values at the high dose of lidocaine (4.5 mg/kg) were decreased (by 16% based on mean V_f values) compared to control values.

In the cocaine group, the control R_a value was 852±193 $cmH_2O \cdot ml^{-1} \cdot min$. R_a values during the three cocaine doses ranged from 910±210 to 1118±167 $cmH_2O \cdot ml^{-1} \cdot min$ and were not significantly different from control values. In the lidocaine group, the control R_a value was 525±148 $cmH_2O \cdot ml^{-1} \cdot min$, not significantly different from the control value in the cocaine group. R_a values during the low, medium and high doses of lidocaine ranged from 798±237 to 919±238 $cmH_2O \cdot ml^{-1} \cdot min$ and were not significantly different from control values. At all experimental conditions in both groups, V_a during CSF pressure state 2 (increase of CSF pressure by 6 cmH_2O) was significantly increased as compared to V_a during CSF pressure state 1.

In the cocaine group, plasma cocaine concentration increased as the dose of iv cocaine increased. Plasma cocaine concentrations for doses 1-3 were 2.0±1.5, 2.7±1.8 and 3.0±1.8 μg/ml. In contrast, plasma epinephrine and norepinephrine concentrations decreased as the dose of iv cocaine increased. Plasma epinephrine concentrations for doses 1-3 were 1119±796, 855±442 and 547±359 pg/ml. Plasma norepinephrine concentrations for doses 1-3 were 323±165, 198±168 and 70±85 pg/ml. In the lidocaine group, plasma lidocaine concentration increased as the dose of iv lidocaine increased. Plasma lidocaine concentrations for doses 1-3 were 28±15, 81±35 and 319±152 ng/ml.

Within each group systemic values were not significantly different between experimental conditions with the exception of MAP and heart rate. In the cocaine group MAP increased during the two lower doses of cocaine and heart rate decreased during the two higher doses of cocaine. In the lidocaine group heart rate decreased during the high dose of lidocaine. Systemic values were not different between groups.

When additional doses of cocaine or lidocaine were given at the conclusion of the study, the dose of cocaine causing severe dysrhythmias and hypotension, 7.7±3.3 mg, was significantly lower than the dose of lidocaine that produced severe dysrhythmias and hypotension, 33.5± 11.7 mg.

DISCUSSION

One principal finding of this study was that cocaine did not significantly decrease V_f. Considering that cocaine causes adrenergic stimulation, and previous reports that adrenergic stimulation decreases V_f, we had hypothesized that cocaine may decrease V_f.

There are several possible explanations for the finding in the present study that cocaine did not decrease V_f. It is possible that cocaine did not decrease V_f because the doses of cocaine used were too low to produce adrenergic stimulation. This seems unlikely considering that the low and moderate doses of cocaine caused statistically significant increases in MAP, consistent with increase of adrenergic activity. It is also possible that the dose range of cocaine was too narrow to produce measurable effects. This seems unlikely as the low dose of cocaine increased MAP and, after the high dose of cocaine, rabbits had received 84% of the cocaine dose that caused severe dysrhythmias, profound hypotension and, soon thereafter, death in all rabbits. A third possibility is that the local anesthetic effects of cocaine counteracted its adrenergic stimulating effects so as to reverse the decrease of V_f expected from adrenergic stimulation in the absence of local anesthetic administration. Against this possibility is the finding that with local anesthetic administration without adrenergic stimulation, i.e., the lidocaine group, no increase of V_f occurred. If the local anesthetic effects of cocaine did reverse the adrenergic stimulating effects of cocaine, this action would probably occur at the choroid plexus epithelium and not at choroid plexus blood vessels because local anesthetics, such as lidocaine, cause constriction of cerebral blood vessels just as does adrenergic stimulation. Finally, it is possible that no decrease of V_f occurred with cocaine because rabbits were anesthetized with halothane and nitrous oxide in oxygen. Halothane decreases V_f in rabbits, possibly by stimulating vasopressin receptors which, in turn, reverse halothane-induced increase of choroid plexus blood flow. This state of "relative constriction" of choroid plexus vessels may prevent adrenergic stimulation from causing further vasoconstriction of choroid plexus vessels. Alternatively, general anesthesia may act at the preceding "step" by preventing the CNS sympathoexcitatory response to cocaine.

A second principal finding of the present study was that the high dose of lidocaine decreased V_f, while lower doses of lidocaine caused no significant change of V_f. These effects of lidocaine are similar to those previously reported with sedative-hypnotics and opioids. Pentobarbital, propofol, sufentanil, alfentanil, ketamine, and low doses of thiopental, etomidate, midazolam and fentanyl cause no significant change of V_f. High doses of thiopental, etomidate, midazolam and fentanyl decrease V_f. Lidocaine-induced decrease of V_f may result from decreased choroid plexus blood flow and/or secretory activity at the choroid plexus epithelium. Like the sedative-hypnotic drugs, lidocaine is reported to decrease cerebral blood flow and metabolic rate.

The increase of plasma epinephrine and norepinephrine concentrations with cocaine 0.5 $mg \cdot kg^{-1}$ followed by 1.0 $\mu g \cdot kg^{-1} \cdot min^{-1}$ iv is consistent with that previously reported in rats given cocaine 0.4 mg/kg intraarterially. That plasma epinephrine and norepinephrine concentrations with cocaine 1.5 and 4.5 $mg \cdot kg^{-1}$ decreased from values seen with 0.5 $mg \cdot kg^{-1}$ presumably reflects depletion of releasable catecholamines during repeated "bolus" doses combined with prolonged, continuous iv infusion of cocaine. The decrease of heart rate seen in the present study during cocaine 1.5 and 4.5 $mg \cdot kg^{-1}$ is consistent with depletion of releasable catecholamines. That MAP remained increased during cocaine 1.5 $mg \cdot kg^{-1}$ is consistent with a previous report that increase of MAP in rats given cocaine 0.03-3 mg/kg iv was mainly of CNS origin and that release of norepinephrine from sympathetic nerve terminals and inhibition of sympathetic neuronal uptake of norepinephrine were not critical for the increase of MAP.

REFERENCES

1. Covino BG (1988) Clinical pharmacology of local anesthetic agents. In: Cousins MJ, Bridenbaugh PO (eds) Neural blockade in clinical anesthesia and management of pain. JB Lippincott, Philadelphia, pp 111-144
2. Heisey SR, Held D, Pappenheimer JR (1962) Bulk flow and diffusion in the cerebrospinal fluid system of the goat. Am J Physiol 203:775-781

Effects of Anesthetics on Neurologic Outcome and Blood–Brain Barrier Function Following Acute Subdural Hematoma in Rats

K. Nakakimura[1], R. Uchimoto[1], T. Sano[1], Y. Kuroda[2], and T. Sakabe[1]

[1] Department of Anesthesiology-Resuscitology, Yamaguchi University School of Medicine, 1144 Kogushi, Ube, Yamaguchi, 755 Japan
[2] Department of Anesthesiology, Labour Welfare Cooperation, Yamaguchi Rosai Hospital, 1315-4 Onoda, Onoda, Yamaguchi, 756 Japan

INTRODUCTION

Intracranial hematoma occurs in almost half of severely head injured patients, and the outcome is particularly poor in patients with acute subdural hematoma. Recently, Miller et al. [1] devised a rat model of acute subdural hematoma. Using this model, several studies have been done to explore the cerebral circulatory and metabolic disturbances. However, neurologic outcome after long term recovery of the model have not been investigated. Concerning with anesthetic effects, it has been suggested that isoflurane may provide protection against brain ischemia compared with halothane, although the protective effects of isoflurane have recently been disputed by others. The purpose of the present study is to evaluate the neurologic outcome for 7 day survival, histopathological damage, and the extent of disruption of blood-brain barrier (BBB) after subdural hematoma, especially focusing on whether the difference in anesthesia, halothane or isoflurane, used during the production of subdural hematoma may affect outcome. We also examined the effect of cerebral perfusion pressure during the insults on the outcome.

MATERIALS AND METHODS

Thirty-three male Wistar rats weighing 350-450 g were anesthetized with either halotane or isoflurane and the lung was ventilated after tracheal intubation. Thereafter, the animals were divided into three groups: the halothane (n=11) and halothane + dopamine (n=11) groups received 1.3 MAC halothane, and the isoflurane (n=12) group received 1.3MAC isoflurane. Mean arterial blood pressure (MABP) in the halothane + dopamine group was maintained above 90 mmHg by intravenous infusion of dopamine (10-30 μg/kg/min) during the production of subdural hematoma and the following 30 min, while in the halothane and isoflurane groups no interventions were given to support the blood pressure during the experiment. The hematoma was produced by subdural injection of 150 μl autologous non-heparinized blood over 7.5 min via a left parietal burr hole. The temporal muscle temperature was maintained between 36.8 - 37.2°C. $PaCO_2$ was maintained between 28 - 32 mmHg. Right parietal extradural pressure (EDP) and bilateral fronto-occipital electroencephalograms (EEGs) were monitored. These measurements and monitoring were carried out until 30 min following the production of subdural hematoma. Then, wounds were closed, inhalation of anesthetics was discontinued, and the trachea was extubated when spontaneous respiration was deemed adequate. Rats were evaluated neurologically on 2, 4, and 7 days after the insults. A neurologic deficit score (NDS) of 0 indicates normal, 17 indicates deep coma, and 18 indicates death. After the 7 day period, rats were perfusion-fixed and the brain was removed for subsequent histological examination (H & E stain).
Additional ten rats anesthetized with either halothane or isoflurane were

subjected to acute subdural hematoma and received 1 ml of 2 % Evans blue solution at 12, 16, or 20 h for examination of disruption of BBB.

RESULTS

There were no significant differences in physiological variables among groups except MABP and cerebral perfusion pressure (CPP, CPP=MABP-EDP). During the subdural injection of the blood, EDP increased to 30-60 mmHg and EEGs were progressively slowed in all groups, the EDP and EEG pattern returning to control 30 min and 10 min later, respectively. MABP and CPP in the halothane group were significantly lower than those in the other two groups throughout the experiment (Fig. 1). At 1-6 h

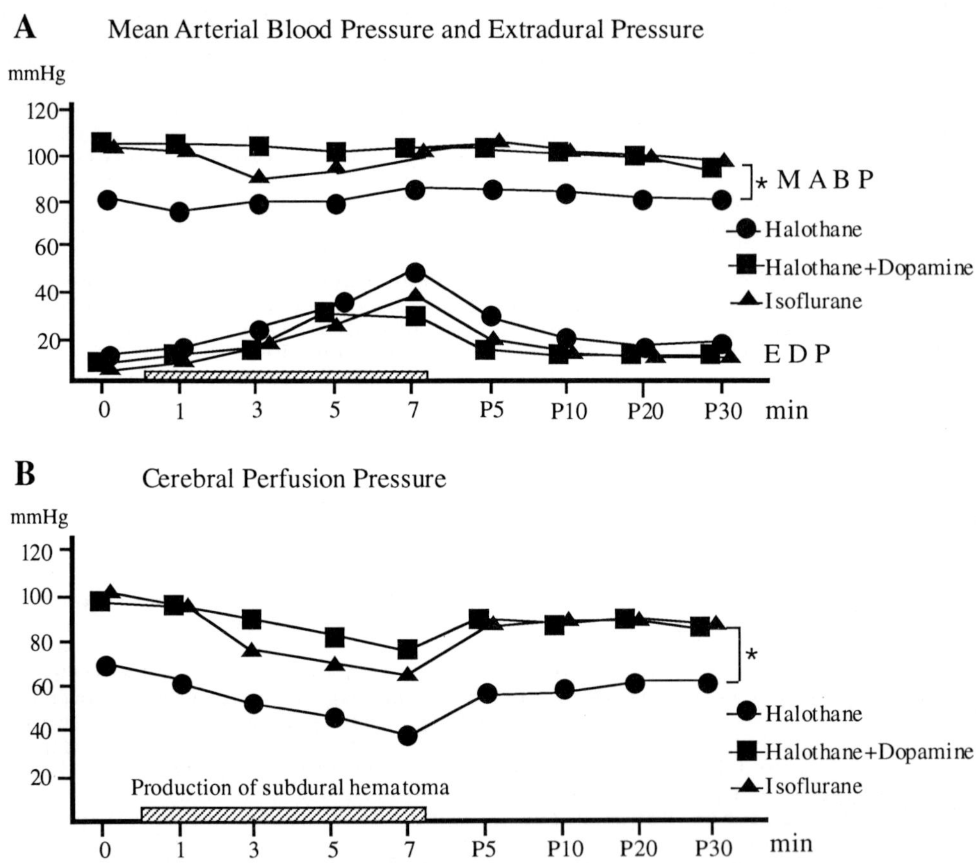

Fig. 1 A: Mean arterial blood pressure (MABP) and extradural pressure (EDP), B: cerebral perfusion pressure (MABP-EDP), during production of subdural hematoma (hatched area) and the following 30 min. P5, P10, P20, and P30 indicate 5, 10, 20, and 30 min post-hematoma, respectively.

after production of subdural hematoma, all rats fed themselves and neurologic deficits were minimum. Thereafter neurological finding became worse. 15 to 50 h after the insult, died 10 of 11 rats in the halothane group, 5 of 11 in the halothane + dopamine group, and 6 of 12 in the isoflurane group. The remaining rats (1 in the halothane, 5 in the halothane + dopamine, and 6 in the isoflurane group) survived for 7 days and the neurologic recovery was almost complete (NDS= 0-3). The mortality in the halothane group was significantly higher than that in the halothane + dopamine and isoflurane group (91% halothane vs. 45% halothane + dopamine and 50% isoflurane). There were no significant differences in mortality or NDS between the halothane and isoflurane groups. Histopathological examination at 7 days after the insults revealed cortical necrosis beneath the hematoma but showed no definite damage in the subcortical regions. Evans blue penetration was mainly observed in the hippocampal CA3 region ipsilateral to the hematoma. The extent of Evans blue staining increased with the elapsed time from 12 to 20 h following hematoma production. There were no apparent differences among groups in the histopathological damage and BBB disruption, though the limited number of rats survived in each group makes conclusive analysis difficult.

DISCUSSION

In the present rat model of acute subdural hematoma, a progression of neurologic deficits after a lucid interval was observed. Higher mortality following acute subdural hematoma in the the halothane group where the insults were produced under halothane anesthesia without blood pressure support can be ascribed to the lower MABP and hence lower CPP during the production of the insults. This may be supported by the fact that the poor outcome was counterbalanced by maintaining MABP and CPP as seen in the improved outcome in the halothane + dopamine group. Although autoregulation of cerebral blood flow (CBF) in this model of acute subdural hematoma has not been examined, it has been reported that autoregulation of CBF is disturbed after acute brain injury such as head trauma and brain ischemia. Towards the end of the period of subdural injection of blood, mean CPP in the halothane group reduced to 50 mmHg probably below the lower limit of autoregulation and the decrease in CBF or brain ischemia may have occurred. In addition, the better outcome in the halothane + dopamine and isoflurane groups where MABP and CPP during production of subdural hematoma were kept at a comparable and supposedly adequate level may indicate an importance of maintaining CPP during neurosurgery such as evacuation of intracranial hematoma, rather than the choice of volatile anesthetics.

REFERENCES

1. Miller JD, Bullock R, Graham DI, Chen M-H, Teasdale GM (1990) Ischemic brain damage in a model of acute subdural hematoma. Neurosurgery 27:433-439

Session XX: Drugs and Anesthetic Agents (2)

Chairmen: G. Teasdale and S. Nagao

THAM Therapy and Traumatic Brain Injury: A Double-Blind, Randomized Study

MICHAEL J. ROSNER and SHEILA D. ROSNER

Division of Neurosurgery, University of Alabama at Birmingham, Birmingham, AL, USA

INTRODUCTION

An early, prospective but non-blinded study suggested that THAM was efficacious in improving mortality after traumatic brain injury [1]. We have subsequently further tested the hypotheses that THAM would be associated with improved intracranial pressure control, reduced mortality, and reduced morbidity when compared with placebo controls.

METHODS

105 patients GCS ≤ 7 were randomized into a double-blind, placebo-controlled study in blocks of ten within 24 hours of injury. THAM was begun at 2 cc/kg x 60 min and continuously infused at 1 cc/kg/hr until ICP was controlled with CSF drainage alone. THAM was then tapered over 72 hours by 25% reductions. Daily records of ICP, CSF output, mannitol and catecholamine dosage used for CPP maintenance [2], along with 100 physiologic variables were recorded daily. A CPP "therapy index" equal to CSF output (cc's) plus catecholamines (mg) plus mannitol (grams) was used to estimate the intensity of CPP therapy. Barbiturate therapy was not used. $PaCO_2$ was maintained at 35 torr.

RESULTS

The groups did not differ in GCS, initial ICP, or CSF lactate. ICP and CPP were maintained in THAM patients. CPP index was 200 ± 7.3 in the treated versus 245 ± 10.6 in the control group ($p < .001$) and this was a function of less CSF drainage (101 ± 4.0 vs. 132 ± 4.1 cc/day), lower catecholamine use (36 ± 3.1 vs. 42 ± 7 mg/day) and less mannitol (51 ± 4.0 vs. 59 ± 4.2 gm/day). Mortality was the same in both groups (21 versus 20). There was little difference in GOS but FIM scores are still being analyzed: ICP was controlled sooner ($6.8 \pm .7$ vs. $8.3 \pm .8$ days) length of ICP monitoring (16.3 ± 10 vs. 22.4 ± 16, $p < .03$) and ICU stay (14 ± 12 vs. 17 ± 15) was also shorter in the THAM group but the latter difference might have occurred by chance. Creatinine averaged 1.7 vs. 1.3 mg% in the controls ($p < .001$)

DISCUSSION

The use of THAM in traumatic brain injury clearly helps reduce intracranial hypertension. The amount of mannitol or other therapies directed at either ICP or CPP is reduced in a statistically reliable and clinically important fashion. The length of ICP monitoring with the THAM patients was 16 days versus 22 days in the control patients. This is very important in economic terms and reducing the length of stay in the ICU ($p < .03$). While the mortality did not differ between the groups, there were significantly fewer deaths due to uncontrolled intracranial hypertension in those patients treated with THAM. The difference, unfortunately, was balanced by an increased number of deaths due to acute renal failure. While the absolute level of creatinine was statistically higher in the THAM treated patients, it was not clinically important (1.7 mg% versus 1.3 mg%, THAM versus control, $p < .001$). However, these results are consistent with THAM having the potential to be nephrotoxic at least in certain individuals under certain circumstances. It is not quite clear what these circumstances might be. However, as experience has been gained with the study, renal failure has been reduced and if control of renal failure in THAM treated patients can be achieved, the expectation is that mortality will also improve.

There is some suggestion that morbidity is improved in THAM treated patients though the numbers are too small to clearly conclude this.

The previous study conducted by this same group suggested that THAM helped control intracranial hypertension and this has been confirmed in this larger double-blind study. The importance of this is that intracranial pressure was controlled sooner in THAM treated patients and with less pharmacologic intervention. The actual effects on mortality were not as great as were hoped. In large part, this was due to the extreme success of better techniques of CPP management employed during this study. All patients were managed using CPP based techniques and this has clearly impacted the overall survival and mortality rates [2].

Gaab et al have demonstrated improved tissue edema, and other work has shown improved survival under laboratory conditions [3,4]. THAM clearly affects cerebral edema and ICP in a beneficial fashion. The exact mechanism for the effect is unclear; suggestions that tissue acidosis is improved [4] or toxic effects of hypocarbia are countered [5,6] or both seem tenable.

CONCLUSION

THAM is effective in ameliorating intracranial hypertension, but used in this protocol has not proven either improved morbidity or mortality. It did shorten the period of ICP monitoring and the ICU stay. It is a worthwhile adjunct in the treatment of increased ICP.

REFERENCES

1. Rosner MJ, Elias KG, Coley I: Prospective, randomized trial of THAM therapy in severe brain injury: Preliminary results. In Hoff JT, Betz AL (eds): Intracranial Pressure VII. Berlin, Springer-Verlag: 611-615, 1989.

2. Rosner MJ, Daughton S: Cerebral perfusion pressure management in head injury. J Trauma 30:933-941, 1990.

3. Gaab MR, Seegers K, Goetz C: THAM (tromethamine, "tris-buffer"): Effective therapy of traumatic brain swelling. In Hoff JT, Betz AL (eds): Intracranial Pressure VII. Berlin, Springer-Verlag: 616-619, 1989.

4. Rosner MJ, Becker DP: Experimental brain injury: Successful therapy with the weak base, Tromethamine (with a review of CNS acidosis). J Neurosurg 60:961-971, 1984.

5. Proctor HJ, Cairns C, Fillipo D, et al: Brain metabolism during increased intracranial pressure as assessed by niroscopy. Surgery 96:273-279, 1984.

6. Muizelaar JP, Marmarou A, Ward JD, et al: Adverse effects of prolonged hyperventilation in patients with severe head injury: A randomized clinical trial. J Neurosurg 75:731-739, 1991.

Effect of VA-045 on Behavioral Outcome Following Rodent Impact Acceleration Injury

T. SHIROTANI, M. FODA, and A. MARMAROU

Division of Neurosurgery, Medical College of Virginia, Richmond, VA, USA

Summary

The effect of VA-045, a novel apovincamic acid derivative, on behavioral outcome following closed head injury (CHI) were examined in rats. The blunt head injury was delivered by dropping a weight (450 g) from the height of 2 m. Seventy one male S-D rats were administered ether 2.5% ascorbic acid or VA-045 (1.0 or 5.0 mg/kg) intraperitoneally (I.P.) 30 sec after CHI. The duration of acute suppression of several reflexes and responses was recorded for up to 60 min after CHI. Long-term motor function (beam balance, beam walking and inclined plane) and body weight were made before CHI to 43 days after CHI. Cognitive outcome was assessed with the Morris water maze on Day 14 to 18 after CHI.

All measurements of the parameters of behavioral outcomes in the CHI group were significantly lower than those in the sham group ($p< 0.01$). VA-045 significantly reduced the duration of transient behavioral suppression, and improved long term motor function, cognitive outcome and body weight loss. VA-045 did not reduce the mortality or incidence of apnea. These results suggest that VA-045 may be useful for treating patients with consciousness disturbance, or motor and cognitive deficits after CHI.

Introduction

VA-045 (Taisho Pharmaceutical Co., Tokyo, Japan) is a new compound to which a nitrooxy moiety has been introduced at position 14 of apovimcaminic acid (1). VA-045 selectively dilated canine cerebral artery (2), and improved age-related functional changes, i.e., impairment of performance of passive avoidance (3), increase in spontaneous spindle burst and the facilitation of the caudate spindle (4). This drug also improved the disturbance in consciousness in several experimental animal models (5, 6). Recently a new model producing diffuse brain injury, without focal brain lesions, has developed in rats (7, 8). The present paper describes the effect of VA-045 on behavioral outcome following closed head injury (CHI) in this model.

Materials and Methods

Subjects and Surgical Preparation

Seventy one male Sprague-Dawley rats (Hilltop Lab Animals, Inc., Scottsdale, PA) weighing between 350-375 gram were used. Experiments were performed as described previously(7). Briefly, all animals were initially anesthetized with halothane, then intubated and artificially ventilated with a gas mixture containing nitrous oxide (67%), oxygen (33%), and 1% halothane. A stainless steel disc (10 mm in diameter × 3 mm thick) was placed on the midsagittal suture between bregma and lambda and glued in place with dental acrylic. A traumatic severe head injury was delivered by dropping a weight (450 g) from two meters above the steel helmet. VA-045 (Taisho Pharmaceutical Company) was dissolved in 2.5% ascorbic acid solution. Rats were administered either 2.5% ascorbic acid (vehicle) or VA-045 (1.0 or 5.0 mg/kg) intraperitoneally (I.P.) 30 sec after injury. The helmet was then removed, and the wound was sutured. After the acute neurological assessments were scored, the rats were returned to their cages with free access to food and water. Animals were randomized into the following six groups; 1) sham group, untreated (2.5% ascorbic acid, i.p.; n=10), 2) sham group, treated (1.0 mg/kg VA-045 i.p.; n=11), 3) sham group, treated (5 mg/kg VA-045 i.p.; n=10), 4) 2m injury group, untreated (2.5%

ascorbic acid, i.p.; n=15), 5) 2m injury group, treated (1.0 mg/kg VA-045 i.p.; n=13), 6) 2m injury group, treated (5 mg/kg VA-045 i.p.; n=12).

The Acute Neurological Assessments

Immediately after trauma the rats were removed from the injury device and placed on a table for acute neurological assessments. Following injury, ventilatory support was provided for three minutes. When spontaneous respiration was not recovered, continued ventilatory support was provided maximally for 30 minutes. The duration of convulsive episodes and suppression time of pupillary reflex were recorded. Motor functions were assessed by recording the duration of suppression of pinna reflex, corneal reflex, hind paw reflex, tail movement, head support response, righting, and escape behavior. A battery of behavioral tests used previously to assess outcome following brain injury was used(9, 10).

The Chronic Neurological Assessment

The assessment of locomotor function was conducted by employing the following behavioral tasks. Animals were tested on the beam-balance task, beam-walking task and inclined plane test for two days before injury, every day for ten days after injury and then every three days up to 43 days post-injury. Body weight was also recorded. A battery of behavioral tests used previously to assess outcome following brain injury was used(9, 10).

To assess cognitive performance of the rats after injury, the Morris water maze was used (11, 12). The task employs a metal pool 180 cm in diameter and 60 cm high. This pool was filled with water to a depth of 28 cm. A platform 10 cm in diameter and 26 cm height was used as the hidden goal platform. Rats were given 4 trials per day for 5 consecutive days (Days 14-18 after injury).

Statistical Analysis

The data of mortality and complications were analyzed by a Chi-squared test. Student's t-tests were used to analyze the acute neurological variables. Data from the chronic neurological variables and body weight changes were analyzed by analysis of variance (ANOVA), and significant differences between groups were determined using Scheffe's test or Dunnett's t test. For a difference to be considered statistically significant, a minimum value of $p<0.05$ was required.

Results

Mortality and Complications

The mortality of CHI was 10.0% and the incidence of skull fracture was 12.5%. There was no significant differences between vehicle and treated groups (Table 1). After injury, two rats needed ventilatory support for more than three minutes. But spontaneous respiration was not recovered in all of them even 30 minutes after CHI. These rats were excluded in all neurobehavioral study.

Neurological Assessment

All measurements of the parameters of behavioral outcomes in the CHI group were significantly lower than those in the sham group ($p< 0.01$). The 5.0 mg/kg dose of VA-045 produced significantly shorter durations of suppression ($p<0.01$) than the vehicle treated group on the following measures: pinna, hind paw, tail movement, tonic tail, head supporting, righting and escape responses (Table 1). These animals also had shorter durations of suppression than vehicle treated group on pupillary reflex and corneal reflex, although these differences did not reach statistical significance. The 1.0 mg/kg dose of VA-045 also produced significantly shorter durations of suppression than vehicle treated group on the pinna, righting, escape responses ($p<0.05$), hind paw reflex and head supporting response ($p<0.01$). The duration of convulsion and suppression of pupillary and corneal reflex were not statistically different between groups.

Treatment with 5.0 mg/kg VA-045 significantly ($p<0.01$) attenuated all long-term behavioral deficits and body weight loss. The 1.0 mg/kg dosage was sufficient to reduce behavioral deficits and body weight loss except of inclined plane (Table 1).

When beam-walking, beam-balance and inclined plane tasks were assessed following injury, there were no significant performance differences between the injured and sham animals by 9 days after head injury. To ensure that the assessment of cognitive function was not confounded by motor deficits, testing of Morris water maze started at day 14 after injury. The injured animals took significantly ($p<0.01$) longer than sham-injured animals to find the hidden platform. Rats treated with 5.0 mg/kg VA-

045 took a significantly (p<0.01) shorter time than vehicle-treated rats. Rats treated with 1.0 mg/kg VA-045 also took a significantly (p<0.05) shorter time to find the platform.

Table 1 Neurobehavioral outcome of closed head injury (CHI) and effect of VA-045

	vehicle-treated CHI group vs. sham group	VA-045 1 mg/kg vs. vehicle-treated CHI group	5 mg/kg vs. vehicle-treated CHI group	analysis
mortality	6.7%, $p < 0.01$	15.3%, N.S.	8.3%, N.S.	Chi-square
fracture	13.3%, $p < 0.01$	15.3%, N.S.	8.3%, N.S.	Chi-square
apnea	6.7%, $p < 0.01$	0%, N.S.	8.3%, N.S.	Chi-square
body weight loss	$p < 0.01$	$p < 0.01$	$p < 0.01$	Student's t-test
convulsion	$p < 0.01$	N.S.	N.S.	Student's t-test
pupillary reflex	$p < 0.01$	N.S.	N.S.	Student's t-test
pinna reflex	$p < 0.01$	$p < 0.05$	$p < 0.01$	Student's t-test
corneal reflex	$p < 0.01$	N.S.	N.S.	Student's t-test
hindpaw reflex	$p < 0.01$	$p < 0.01$	$p < 0.01$	Student's t-test
tail movement	$p < 0.01$	N.S.	$p < 0.01$	Student's t-test
tonic tail reflex	$p < 0.01$	N.S.	$p < 0.01$	Student's t-test
head supporting	$p < 0.01$	$p < 0.01$	$p < 0.01$	Student's t-test
righting reflex	$p < 0.01$	$p < 0.05$	$p < 0.01$	Student's t-test
escape reflex	$p < 0.01$	$p < 0.05$	$p < 0.01$	Student's t-test
Morris water maze	$p < 0.01$	$p < 0.05$	$p < 0.01$	ANOVA
beam walking	$p < 0.01$	$p < 0.01$	$p < 0.01$	ANOVA
beam balance (score)	$p < 0.01$	$p < 0.01$	$p < 0.01$	ANOVA
beam balance (latency)	$p < 0.01$	$p < 0.01$	$p < 0.01$	ANOVA
inclined plane	$p < 0.01$	N.S.	$p < 0.01$	ANOVA

NS; not significant, ANOVA; analysis of variance

Discussion

This study demonstrated that VA-045 improved the transient and long-term neurological deficits in a dose-dependent manner. The effect of VA-045 on transient neurological behavioral, such as loss of the righting reflex and the disruption of spontaneous movement, caused by CHI had previously reported (6). VA-045 shortens pentobarbital-induced sleeping time (5), and also ameliorates the disturbed behavior in the head impact models in mice (5).VA-045 recovers CHI-induced reduction of the amplitude of somatosensory evoked potentials (SEP) because of improved effect on CHI-induced failure or malfunction of synaptic transmission within the somatosensory pathway (6). Because injured animals received ventilatory support during the apneic period, it is unlikely that reduced oxygen availability contributed to the behavioral deficits in both vehicle and VA-045 treated animals. Concussive head trauma disturbs the central catecholamine system, cholinergic system, amino acids and energy-related metabolites (13), so these may be involved in the recovery action of VA-045 (5,6). The suspected mechanism of the effect of VA-045 on the transient neurological behavior may be a block of the inhibitory striato-thalamo-cortical system (4), whereas TRH exerts an excitation action on the nerve cells of the brain stem reticular formation (14). Although moderate levels of fluid percussion produce much less axonal injury (15), closed head injury causes more axonal damage (8). We estimate that this axonal damage may produce some of the long-term behavioral deficits in this model. If the hypothesis is correct, VA-045 may reduce axonal injury in this model. A morphological investigation of the effects of VA-045 after closed head injury is now in progress in our laboratory.

VA-045 also reduced cognitive deficits in a dose-dependent manner. There is no evidence of pathological changes in the hyppocampus of this model (8). VA-045 may stabilize neurochemical disruption of the brain's normal neurotransmission. Okuyama et al found that post traumatic administration of VA-045 attenuated the CHI-induced decreased step through latency (STL) in passive avoidance task, and suggested that the ameliorating effects of VA-045 may result from an improvement of the head injury-induced disturbance of cognitive dysfunction (6).

References

1 Kawashima Y, Ikemoto T, Horiguchi A, Hayashi M, Matsumoto K, Kawarasaki K, Yamazaki R, Okuyama S, Hatayama K (1993) Synthesis and pharmacological evaluation of (nitrooxy) alkylapovincaminates. J. Med. Chem. 36:815-819

2 Miyata N, Yamaura H, Tanaka M, Muramatsu M, Tsuchida K, Okuyama S, Otomo S (1993) Effects of VA-045, a novel apovincaminic acid derivative, on isolated blood vessels: cerebroarterial selectivity. Life Sci. 52 PL181-186

3 Ogawa S, Okuyama S, Otomo S (1992) Effects of VA-045, a novel apovincaminic acid derivate, improved cholinergic deficits-induced amnesia in rats. Clin. Neuropharmocol. 15 suppl. 1 Pt. B 563B

4. Okuyama S, Kawashima K, Hashimoto-Kitsukawa S, Ogawa S, Otomo S (1992) Effects of VA-045, a novel apovincaminic acid derivatie, on the age-related impairment of the EEG, caudate spindle and passive avoidance performance deficits in rats. Clin. Neuropharmacol. 15 suppl. 1 Pt. B 460B

5 Okuyama S, Imagawa Y, Ogawa S, Saito Y, Araki H, Otomo S, Sakagawa T, Yamada S. Shima K (1993) The effect of VA-045 on disturbance in consciousness in experimental animal models. Res Comm Chem Parm 82:91-100

6 Okuyama S, Imagawa Y, Ogawa S, Araki H, Otomo S, Sakagawa T, Yamada T, Shima K (1993) Effect of VA-045 on a closed head injury model in rats. Life Sci. 53 PL273-278

7 Marmarou A, Foda MA, van den Brink, Campbell J, Kita H and Demetriadou K (1994) A new model of diffuse brain injury in rats part 1: pathophysiology and biomechanics. J Neurosurg. 80:291-300

8 Foda MA and Marmarou A (1994) A new model of diffuse brain injury in rats part 2: morphological characterization. J Neurosurg. 80:301-313

9 Dixon CE, Lyeth BG, Povlishock JT, Findling RL, Hamm RJ, Marmarou A, Young HF, Hayes RL (1987) A fluid percussion model of experimental brain injury in the rat, J. Neurosurg 67:110-119

10 Lyeth BG, Dixon CE, Hamm RJ, Jenkins LW, Young HF, Stonnington HH and Hayes RL (1988) Effects of anticholinergic treatment on transient behavioral suppression and physiological responses following concussive brain injury in the rat. Brain Res 448:88-97

11 Morris RGM (1981) Spatial localization does not require the presence of local cues. Learn Motivat 12:239-260

12 Hamm RJ, Dixon CE, Gbadebo DM, Singha AK, Jenkins LW, Lyeth BG and Hayes RL (1992) Cognitive deficits following traumatic brain injury produced by controlled cortical impact. J Neurotrauma 9:11-20

13 Nilsson P, Hillered L, Ponten U, Ungersteadt U (1990) Changes in cortical extracellular levels of energy-related metabolites and amino acids following concussive brain injury in rats.J Cereb Blood flow Metab 10:631-637

14 Yasuhara M, Naito N (1983) Effects of TRH-T and DN-1417 on the central nervous system: an electrophysiological study of arousal reaction and evoked muscular discharges. Intern J Neurosci 21:197-224

15 Yaghmai A, Povlishock J (1992) Traumatically induced reactive change as visualized through the use of monoclonal antibodies targeted to neurofilament subunits. J Neuropathol Exp Neurol 51:158-176

Corticotropin Releasing Factor as an Alternative Treatment of Peritumoral Brain Edema

JURI TJUVAJEV[1], HISAO UEHARA[1], REVATHI DESAI[1], CORNELIA MATEI[2], BRADLEY BEATTIE[1], JASON KOUTCHER[2], and RONALD BLASBERG[1]

Departments of [1] Neurology and [2] Radiology, Memorial Sloan-Kettering Cancer Center, 1275 York Avenue, New York, NY 10021, USA

INTRODUCTION.

Peritumoral brain edema significantly contributes to the morbidity and mortality in patients with brain tumors [1]. Corticosteroids have been used in the treatment of brain tumors and associated peritumoral brain edema for over 30 years. Although corticosteroid treatment of brain edema can result in dramatic clinical improvement, their long-term use is often associated with detrimental side effects, especially at high doses [2]. Therefore, it is important to continue to search for anti-edematous agents with similar or even greater potency and lesser toxicity. Recently, human corticotropin releasing factor (hCRF) and other peptides of the corticoliberin superfamily have been shown to inhibit vascular leakage of plasma constituents and tissue swelling in response to injury or injection of vasoactive compounds. We report a series of animal studies that evaluate the anti-edematous potential of hCRF in a well established animal model of peritumoral vasogenic brain edema. hCRF-treated animals were compared to similar groups of Dexamethasone-treated and saline-treated control animals. Treatment response was monitored by magnetic resonance imaging (MRI), by direct measurements of tumor and peritumoral brain water content, and by measuring ICP and volume-buffering capacity of the craniospinal system.

MATERIALS AND METHODS.

Peritumoral Edema Model. Walker 256 (W256) rat carcinoma cell line was grown as monolayers in MEM with 10% fetal calf serum and non-essential amino acids in 5% CO_2, 80% humidity and 37°C. Cells were used for implantation after having become 70% or more confluent. A single-cell suspension of W256 cells was obtained for inoculations by trypsinisation of cell culture monolayers. Sprague-Dawley rats weighing 200-250g were anesthetized with a gas mixture containing 1.5% Fluorothane, 70% nitrous oxide and 30% oxygen. The skull was exposed by a midline scalp incision, and a 2 mm burr hole was made 3 mm to the right side of the sagittal suture and 1 mm posterior to bregma; a 26-gauge short-bevel needle was inserted to a depth of 6 mm under stereotactic control and aseptic conditions. A sterile 10 µl suspension containing $1x10^5$ viable W256 tumor cells was slowly inoculated. The animals were returned to their cages, observed and weighed daily for signs and symptoms of intracranial tumor growth.

MRI Studies. The intensity of blood brain barrier (BBB) breakdown in the i.c. W256 tumors and the extent of peritumoral edema was assessed by MR imaging. MRI was performed on a General Electric CSI system with a 4.7 Tesla 33 cm bore magnet, equiped with shielded gradients. Standard imaging coil was used. The i.c. tumor bearing rats were anesthetized as described above. Rats were placed in a special holder to stabilize the head in the midpoint of the imaging coil and to guarantee the reproducibility of the positioning between imaging sessions. Anesthetic gas mixture was constantly supplied to the animal throughout the imaging session via the tubing hermetically attached to the holder system. Subsequently, Proton Density pre- and T_1-weighted post-contrast enhanced (Gd-DTPA; 0.2 mmol/kg i.v.) images were obtained. Coronal slices were obtained through the area of the i.c. tumor (3 mm thick plus 1 mm gap between slices) using a 256 x 256 matrix, 60 mm field of view. Areas of BTB disruption were detected as the contrast-enhancing regions on T_1-weighted images [TR = 300 msec, TE = 10 msec]. Tumor and edematous brain tissue were detected as the areas of hyperintense signal on Proton Density images [TR = 3000 msec, TE = 10 msec].

Tissue Water Content. Tumor, peritumoral edematous brain, and other stuctures of the brain were sampled, dried at 90° C in a constant temperature oven and reweighed daily until a constant dry weight was achieved (usually 3 to 4 days). Tissue water content in the tumor, peritumoral brain (ipsilateral hemisphere), contralateral hemisphere, cerebellum and medulla was calculated as described elsewhere: % Tissue Water = 100 - [(Wet weight - Dry weight)/Wet weight] x 100].

Measurement of ICP and PVI. Tumor-bearing rats were lightly anesthetized with a gas mixture containing 1 % Fluorothane and 30% oxygen. Animal body temperature was maintained at 37° C with an infrared heat lamp. A 2% Lidocaine gel was applied to the ears and the head fixed in a stereotaxic apparatus. The cisterna magna was stereotactically canulated. After ICP stabilization and measurement of P_o, a 0.05 ml bolus of saline was injected through the stopcock into the cisterna magna and peak ICP (P_p) was measured. Pressure was recorded until ICP reached the baseline P_o level. Pressure-volume index (PVI) was calculated according to Marmarou, et al. (1978) [3]: **PVI = V/log (P_p/P_o),** where V is the volume of saline injected; P_o is the initial or baseline ICP; P_p is the peak ICP after saline injection.

Statistics. Simple statistics of data in groups was done using univariate analysis. The group data were compared using ANOVA analysis and Student t-test; a value of $p < 0.05$ was considered significant.

RESULTS.

Vascular Permeability And Tissue Water Content. To compare the effects of hCRF and Dexamethasone on permeability of the BBB and on water content of tumor and peritumoral brain tissue, rats bearing W256 i.c. tumors were divided into three groups (18 rats/group). Each group received treatment with either hCRF (100 µg/kg s.c. BID), Dexamethasone (1 mg/kg i.m. BID), or Saline (0.1 ml i.m. BID). Therapy was initiated on day 7 after tumor inoculation and it was continued for 3 days. Two sequential MR studies were performed on each animal: the first on day 7 after tumor inoculation, before treatment; the second on day 10 after tumor inoculation, following 3 days of treatment. T1-weighted Gd-DTPA contrast enhanced MR images were used to monitor qualitative changes in BBB permeability. Proton density MR images were used to monitor changes in tissue water content. Changes in ICP and PVI of the cranio-spinal system associated with tumor and peritumoral edema were measured before and after treatment in the same animals. Tumor, peritumoral brain tissue, and other brain structures were assayed directly for tissue water content after 3 days of treatment.

Treatment with hCRF resulted in a reduction in the intensity of contrast enhancement of i.c. W256 tumors on T1 weighted MR images (**Fig. 1 A, B**). A reduction of contrast enhancement reflects a decrease in the permeability of tumor capillaries. The effect of hCRF on the BBB was similar to that obtained with Dexamethasone treatment (**Fig. 1 C, D**). In contrast, there was an increase in the intensity of contrast enhancement of i.c. W256 tumors in control animals (**Fig. 1 E, F**). Increased contrast enhancement of the tumor is associated with an increase in the permeability of tumor vasculature. Both, hCRF and Dexamethasone treatments decreased the proton density signal of tumor and peritumoral brain (**Fig. 2 A, B; C,D**). A decrease in tissue proton density reflects a decrease in tissue water content. In contrast there was an increase in proton density of tumor and peritumoral brain in control animals with i.c. W256 tumors (**Fig. 2 E, F**). An increase in proton density of tumor and peritumoral brain is usually associated with an increase of tumor and peritumoral brain edema. Direct measurements of tissue water content in tumor and peritumoral brain using wet/dry weight measurements confirmed the anti-edematous effects of hCRF and Dexamethasone observed on MRI (**Fig. 3**). Tissue water content in the i.c. W256 tumor and ipsilateral hemisphere was significantly lower in the Dexamethasone and hCRF treated groups compared to saline-treated control animals.

Effects on ICP and PVI. Intracranial pressure (ICP) was not elevated before treatment in all groups of tumor bearing rats, and there were no significant changes in ICP as a result of hCRF or Dexamethasone threatment (data not presented). In contrast, the baseline pressure-volume index (PVI) was reduced before treatment in all W256 tumor bearing animals (**Fig. 4**). PVI increased significantly ($p<0.05$) towards normal after 3 days of hCRF or Dexamethasone treatment. The increase in volume-buffering capacity of the craniospinal system reflects some resolution of peritumoral edema and an overall decrease in volume of the space-occupying lesion. PVI decreased further below baseline values in saline-treated control animals, reflecting a further decrease in the volume-buffering capacity of the craniospinal system as the result of increasing peritumoral brain edema (**Fig. 4**).

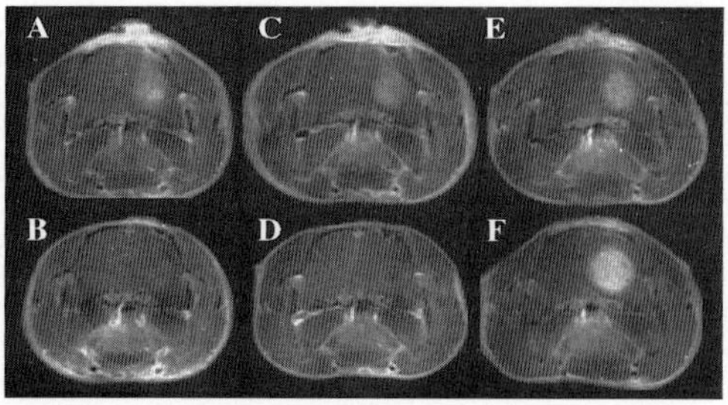

Figure 1. Effects of hCRF and Dexamethasone on the vascular permeability (BBB) of intracerebral W256 carcinomas. T1-weighted Gd-DTPA contrast enhanced MR images of the rat heads are shown in the coronal plane. Pre-treatment and post-treatment images of the same animal are arranged vertically in pairs. Treatment groups included: hCRF (A and B); Dexamethasone (C and D); saline-treated control (E and F).

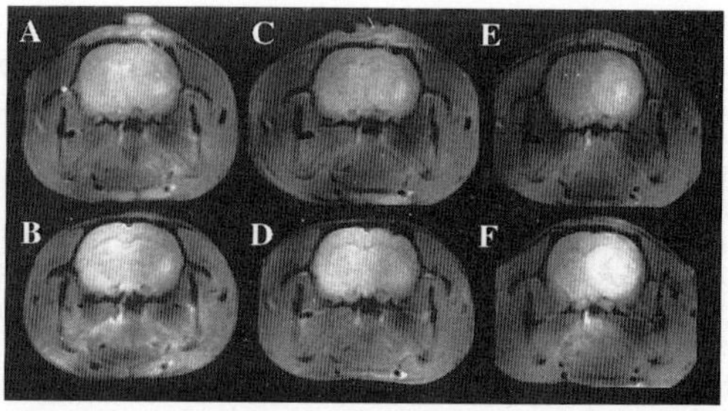

Figure 2. Effects of hCRF and Dexamethasone on the water content of intracerebral W256 carcinomas and peritumoral brain. Proton density MR images of the rat heads in the same coronal planes, obtained during the same imaging session as those in Figure 1. Pre-treatment and post-treatment images of the same animal are arranged vertically in pairs. Treatment groups included: hCRF (A and B); Dexamethasone (C and D); saline-treated control (E and F).

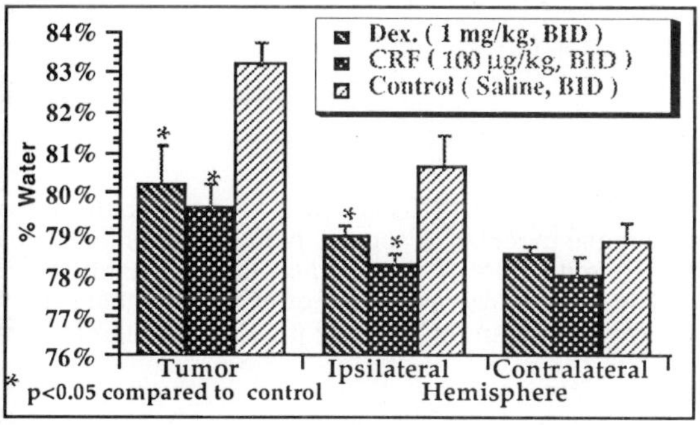

Fig. 3. Tissue Water Content. Mean±SD values of % tissue water content in treatment groups are presented.

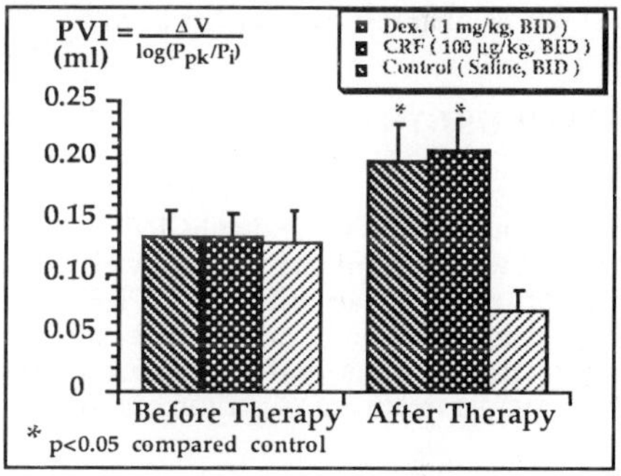

Fig. 4. Pressure-Volume Index. Mean±SD values of PVI in treatment groups are presented.

DISCUSSION

Corticotropin Releasing Factor. Human corticotropin-releasing factor (hCRF) is a naturally occuring 41 residue neuropeptide with a molecular weight of 4.7 kDa. This neurohormone is produced in the hypothalamus and is mainly responsible for stimulating the hypothalamic-pituitary-adrenal axis [4]. It was shown that hCRF inhibits the flare response to intradermal histamine [5] and prevents the vascular leakage induced by a variety of inflamatory mediators which selectively act on postcapillary venules [6]. hCRF also inhibits leakage from cerebral microvessels [7] and lung alveolar capillaries [8]. These latter observations indicate that hCRF acts widely throughout the microcirculation to preserve endothelial cell integrity. It was suggested that anti-edematous action of hCRF appears to result from direct action on blood vessels independent of endocrine function [9].

Effects on Peritumoral Brain Edema. To better differentiate the intracrerbral tumor margin from peritumoral edema, an "early" contrast-enhanced (Gd-DTPA) T1 weighted images were obtained. The contrast-enhanced image predominantly reflects the areas BBB disruption of the tumor provided that imaging is performed early enough after contrast injection [10]. Early imaging limits the extent of diffusion and bulk flow of the contrast agent into areas of peritumoral edema. A comparison of contrast-enhanced T1 and proton density images resulted in a better differentiation of tumor and brain edema.

A substantial reduction in vascular permeability and tissue water content of the tumor and peritumoral brain was observed on MR images after 3 days of treatment with hCRF (100 μg/kg BID) or with Dexamethasone (1 mg/kg BID). In contrast, there was an increase in vascular permeability and tissue water content in the tumor and peritumoral brain of saline-treated control animals. These changes in tumor and peritumoral brain water content were confirmed by direct measurements measurements of tissue water content using wet-dry weight method. Most importantly, the anti-edematous effect of hCRF treatment was comparable to that observed with Dexamethasone. We hypothesize, that hCRF restores vascular permeability by interfering into the cascade of pathological changes in the endothelium induced by various tumor growth and angiogenesis factors (such as PDGF, VEGF, TNF, etc.).

Effects on Viscoelastic Properties of the Brain. Peritumoral edema can dramatically increase the volume of a space-occupying lesion. Increasing volume and stiffness of both the tumor and peritumoral brain tissue depleates the volme-buffering capacity of the cranio-spinal system. If the volume-pressure compensatory mechanisms of craniospinal system fail to keep ICP within the physiological range and intracranial hypertension developes.

Quantitation of volume-buffering capacity of the cranio-spinal system was done by measuring intracranial pressure changes in response to the intrathecal injection of a defined volume of saline. A pressure volume index (PVI) was calculated from these meassurements. Although tumored animals did not demonstrate an increase of baseline ICP in this study, we found that the volume-buffering capacity of the craniospinal system was compromised (decreased PVI). hCRF and Dexamethasone treatment over 3 days were equally effective in reversing this process towards normal, as observed by the increased PVI. In saline-treated control animals the volume-buffering capacity of the cranio-spinal system was reduced over 3 days of study, as manifest by a further decrease in PVI.

CONCLUSIONS.

Our findings demonstrate that hCRF has substantial anti-edematous effects which are comparable to that obtained with Dexamethasone in a well established animal model of vasogenic peritumoral brain edema. The anti-edematouse effect of hCRF is based on a reduction of tumor vascular permeability and subsequent reduction of peritumoral brain edema. The anti-edematouse action of hCRF is potent enough to normalize volume-buffering capacity of cranio-spinal system. hCRF may provide an alternative to corticosteroid treatment of peritumoral brain edema.

REFERENCES

1. Baethman, A. (1978) Pathophysiological and pathochemical aspects of cerebral edema. Neurosurg. Rev., 1: p. 85-100.
2. Weissman, D.E., Dufer, D., Vogel, V, et al (1987): Corticosteroid toxicity in neuro-oncology patients. J Neurooncol, 5: p. 125-128.
3. Marmarou, A., Shulman, K., Rosende, R.M. (1978) A nonlinear analysis of the cerebrospinal fluid system and intracranial pressure dynamics. J Neurosurg, 48: p. 332-344.
4. Vale, W., Spiess, J., Rivier, C., et al. (1981): Characterisation of 41-residue ovine hypothalamic peptide that stimulates secretion of corticotropin and ß-endorphin. Science, 213: p. 1394-1397.
5. Wei, E.T., Gao, G.C., Sessler, D.I. (1990) CRF inhibits the flare response to intradermal histamine in man. Clin Pharmacol Therapeut, 47: p. 192 (Abstract).
6. Kiang, J.G., Poree, L., Wei, E.T. (1987) Anti-inflamatory activity of corticotropin-releasing factor. II. Mechanisms of action. Proc Western Pharmacol Soc, 30: p. 63-65.
7. Wei, E.T., Gao, G.C. (1991) Corticotropin-releasing factor: An inhibitor of vascular leakage in skeletal muscle and brain cortex after injury. Regul Peptides, 33: p. 93-104.
8. Serda, S.M., Wei, E.T. (1992) Epinephrine-induced pulmonary edema in rats is inhibited by corticotropin-releasing factor. Parmacological Research, 26: p. 85-91.
9. Gao, G.C., Dashwood, M.R., Wei, E.T. (1991) Corticotropin-releasing factor inhibition of substance P-induced vascular leakage in rats: possible sites of action. Peptides, 12: p. 639-644.
10. Kenney, J., Schmiedl, U., Maravilla, K., et al, (1992) Measurement of blood-brain barrier permeability in a tumor model using magnetic resonance imaging with gadolinium-DTPA. Magn Res In Med, 27: p. 68-75.

The Effect of U-74389G on Cerebral Edema and ICP in a Cryogenic Injury Model

G. Gambardella, D. d'Avella, S. Toscano, D. Collufio, G.na Caruso, and F. Tomasello

Neurosurgical Clinic, University of Messina School of Medicine, Messina, Italy

INTRODUCTION

The development of brain edema and blood-brain barrier disruption concomitant to traumatic brain injury has been well established in the experimental setting [1], and occurs most predictably in humans in tissue surrounding cerebral contusions [2]. This vasogenic type of brain edema may strongly influence the clinical course of head-injury patients, in whom brain edema elevates intracranial pressure, causes an increase in regional tissue pressure [3], a decrease in regional cerebral blood flow and, in more severe cases, a shift of brain structures causing brain herniation. The goals of head injury experimental investigations include testing of potentially therapeutic drugs that may influence the secondary events that occur in the injured brain. The 21-aminosteroids are a class of compounds that inhibit lipid peroxidation, possess strong cerebral-protective properties efficacious in attenuating damage to the CNS imparted by trauma, ischemia, and subarachnoid hemorrhage, and are devoid of the classical glucocorticoid activity. This study investigates the effect of U-74389G, a novel 21-aminosteroid, on the development of experimental brain edema. The tested compound is very similar to the clinical candidate Tirilazad (U-74006F): the two compounds possess similar pharmacodynamic and pharmacokinetic profiles. We used the cryogenic brain injury rabbit model, the wet/dry weight ratio method to determine brain edema, Evans blue injection to assess blood-brain barrier dysfunction, and an intraparenchymal fiberoptic ministransducer to monitor brain tissue pressure.

MATERIALS AND METHODS

Animals Preparation

Adult male New Zealand albino rabbits (1.5 kg b.w.) were used in this study. Under ketamine and xylazine anesthesia the cryogenic injury was inflicted by applying a 5 mm. diameter freezing probe cooled to -80 °C for 90 sec directly on the dura over the right parietal cortex. The bone was then reimplanted and the cranial window was closed with dental cement. Temperature, arterial pressure, heart rate, and arterial blood gases were monitored and recorded.
Details of the procedure have been reported elsewhere [4].

Treatments

Cold-injured animals were divided into three treatment groups of 5 rabbits each: I) no treatment; II vehicle, and III) treated with U-74389G. Group III rabbits were injected i.v. with 3 mg/kg of U-74389G dissolved in CS-4 vehicle (2 mg/ml), immediately after the lesion and 8 hours thereafter. Group II rabbits received the same amount of vehicle.Drugs were administered through a cannulated femoral vein.

Edema, BBB, and Brain Tissue Pressure Studies

A Camino intracranial pressure probe was introduced through a right fronto-parietal burr hole and inserted intraparenchimally. Brain tissue pressure was recorded until sacrifice. Evans blue (2 ml/kg), an indicator of BBB dysfunction, was administered intravenously 30 minutes prior to sacrifice in all animals. Twenty-four hours after the injury the animals were decapitated and the brains removed. Brain water content was measured in 6 regions, including the lesional and perilesional areas and the contralateral hemisphere. The percent water content of the samples was determined using the wet/dry weight ratio method. An independent Student's *t* test was used to compare results betweeen treatment groups. The blue staining of the brain samples by Evans blue was observed macroscopically.

RESULTS

BBB and Brain Edema Studies

In Group I and II animals, staining by Evans blue was consistently observed 24 hours after injury. An area of dark staining corresponded to the cold lesion site, and light staining was seen in the perilesional areas. Only faint staining was seen in the lesional area in animals treted with U-74389G. In these rabbits no staining was seen in the perilesional areas.
The percent water content measured 24 hours following cryogenic injury in the different cortical areas is summarized as follows and in Figure I:

Cerebral areas	Group I	Group II	Group III
Frontal, ipsilateral	79,19 ±1,7	79,59 ±1,2	78,17 ±1,4 *
Fronto-parietal (lesion), ipsilateral	81,69 ±1,3	80,58 ±1	78,64 ±1,3 *
Parieto-occipital, ipsilateral	79,99 ±3,7	80,44 ±2,5	79,43 ±1,5 *
Frontal, contralateral	77,40 ±0,7	76,10 ±1,3	76,84 ±2,1
Fronto-parietal, contralateral	75,59 ±1,1	75,66 ±1,1	76,84 ±1,7
Parieto-occipital, contralateral	76,38 ±1,2	76,48 ±0,8	76,94 ±0,9

(*Student *t* test statistics: U-74389G statistically significant ($p < 0.05$) from no-treatment and vehicle groups)

Brain Tissue Pressure Studies

Brain tissue pressure recording showed in Group I and II animals a progressive increase after injury up to a peak of 12 ± 3 mmHg 24 hours following injury. Tracings displayed pressure waves alterations indicative of a reduced intracranial compliance. Treatment with U-74389G consistently prevented the occurrence of brain tissue pressure elevations.

DISCUSSION

Lazaroids, 21-aminosteroids, have an amino-group substituted on the 21 carbon of the steroid molecule. This substitution makes the compounds devoid of the classical glucocorticoid activity; this would obviate the significant morbidity associated with the chronic administration of currently used antiedema agents. The compound tested in the present investigation, U-74389G, is a novel 21-aminosteroid very similar to the clinical candidate Tirilazad (U-74006F): infact, the two compounds possess similar pharmacodynamic and pharmacokinetic profiles. This class of molecules is specifically designed to localize within cell membranes and potently functions as oxygen-free radical scavengers and

inhibitors of iron-dependent lipid peroxidation. These drugs display low toxicity and penetrate into the CNS [5]. Efficacy has been demonstrated for these compounds in experimental models of CNS injury from trauma [2,6,7,8,9], ischemia [10], subarachnoid hemorrhage [11], and cryogenic injury [12].
The present study was designed to evaluate the effect of the novel 21-aminosteroid, U-74389G, on the acute pathophysiology of experimental brain injury involving unilateral cold lesion in rabbits. The parameters tested included BBB dysfunction, brain edema and brain tissue pressure. The results reported here show that the treatment with U-74389G significantly prevented the BBB dysfunction and the increase in water content after cryogenic injury observed in no-treatment and vehicle-treated animals, as well as the concurrent increase in brain tissue pressure. This effect on brain tissue pressure was attributed to decrease of vasogenic edema obtained by reducing BBB increased permeability.
In conclusion, the findings in these experiments confirm that U-74389G is effective in reducing some of the acute pathophysiological responses to cryogenic injury. The cold injury model for vasogenic brain edema is presumed to model vascular damage of cerebral contusion.This study supports the beneficial effect of 21-aminosteroids in the treatment of post-traumatic vasogenic brain edema.

Figure I: Percent water content in the lesioned hemisphere 24 hours after injury

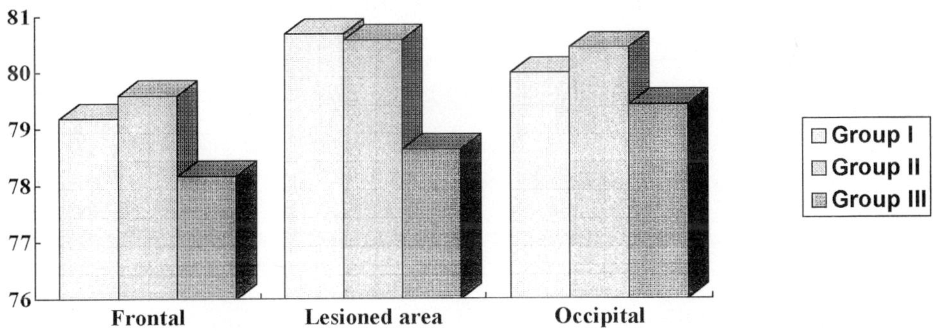

Student *t* test statistics: Group III (U-74389G) statistically significant ($p < 0.05$) from Group I (no-treatment) and Group II (vehicle)

Aknowledgements: U-74389G was a gift from Upjhon Co.

REFERENCES

1. Marmarou A, Shima K (1990): Comparative studies of edema produced by fluid percussion injury with lateral and central modes of injury in cats. In: Long D (ed) Advances in Neurology, Raven Press, Ltd., New York, pp 233-236
2. Dimlich RVW, Tornheim PA, Kindel RM, Hall ED, Braughler JM, McCall JM (1990): Effects of a 21-aminosteroid (U-74006F) on cerebral metabolites and edema after severe experimental head trauma. Adv Neurol 52: 365-375
3. Gambardella G, d'Avella D, Tomasello F (1992): Monitoring of brain tissue pressure with a fiberoptic device. Neurosurgery 31: 918-922
4. Gambardella G, Germanà G, Ciriaco E, Iacopino DG, Muglia U, Tomasello F (1987): Experimental investigations on a model of cryogenic edema. J Neurosurg Sci 31: 133-139
5. Braughler JM, Hall ED, Jacobsen EJ, McCall JM, Means ED (1989): The 21-aminosteroids: potent inhibitors of lipid peroxidation for the treatment of central nervous system trauma and ischemia. Drugs Future 14: 143-152

6. Hall ED, Braughler JM, McCall JM (1988): New pharmacological treatment of acute spinal cord trauma. J Neurotrauma 5: 81-89
7. Hall ED, Yonkers PA, McCall JM, Braughler JM (1988): Effects of the 21-aminosteroid U-74006F on experimental head injury in mice. J Neurosurg 68: 456-461
8. McIntosh TK, Thomas M, Smith D, Banbury M (1992): The novel 21-aminosteroid U-74006F attenuates cerebral edema and improves survival after brain injury in the rat. J Neurotrauma 9: 33-468
9. Sanada T, Nakamura T, Nishimura MC, Isayama K, Pitts LH (1993): Effect of U-74006F on neurologic function and brain edema after fluid percussion injury in rats. J Neurotrauma 10: 65-71
10. Hall ED, Pazara KE, Braughler JM (1988): 21 Aminosteroid lipid peroxidation inhibitor U-74006F protects against cerebral ischemia in gerbils. Stroke 19: 997-1002
11. d'Avella D, Zuccarello M, Tomasello F (1993): Protective effect of U-78517G on local cerebral glucose utilization in the acute stage following subarachnoid hemorrhage. In: Findlay JM (ed) Cerebral Vasospasm, Elsevier, Amsterdam, pp 427-430
12. Arbit E, DiResta GR, Wronski M, Lee J, Galicich JH (1993): The effect of lazaroid on cerebral elastance and edema in a cryogenic injury model. In Avezaat CJJ, van Eijndhoven JHM, Maas AIR, Tans JTJ (eds.) Intracranial Pressure VIII, Springer-Verlag Berlin Heidelberg New York, pp 108-111

The Effect of THAM on Experimental Focal Cerebral Ischemia and Clinical Outcome in Severe Head Injury

T. Kitaoka, S. Nagao, H. Kuyama, K. Fujita, and T. Ogawa

Department of Neurological Surgery, Kagawa Medical School, Miki-cho, Kita-gun, Kagawa, 761-07 Japan

【Introduction】

Cerebral acidosis in focal ischemia or injury is one of the important factors producing brain edema and considered deleterious to cell function and neurologic recovery (7). Amelioration of systemic and focal cerebral acidosis by an alkalizing agents may reduce ischemic brain damage. Tris (hydroxymethyl) aminomethane (THAM) and $NaHCO_3$ have been used to titrate acid. We investigated the effect of THAM and $NaHCO_3$ on focal cerebral ischemia and also the effect of THAM on clinical outcome in severe head injury.

【Materials and methods】

<Animal Experiments> Sixty adult cats were anesthetized with ketamine hydrochloride (30mg/kg) and artificially ventilated. Muscle paralysis was then obtained with intravenous pancuronium bromide (2mg/kg). Catheters were placed in the femoral artery for pressure monitoring and blood sample withdrawal and in the femoral vein for drug infusion. Focal cerebral ischemia was produced by coagulation of the left middle cerebral artery (MCA) using the transorbital approach. Local cerebral blood flow (lCBF) was measured by hydrogen clearance method. Extracellular pH was measured by glass electrode (Kemikarukiki Co. CM-151) on the cerebral cortex. Intracellular pH was calculated with chemical shift of inorganic phosphate measured by magnetic resonance spectroscopy (^{31}P-MRS) using BEM-250/80 NMR system 2 Tesla (Otsuka Electronics, Japan). Six hours after focal ischemia the animals were sacrificed and the brains were coronally sectioned with 5mm-thick slices. The samples of gray and white matter were taken from ectosylvian, suprasylvian and marginal gyri for the measurement of water and lactate contents. Water and lactate contents were measured by specific gravimetric method and enzyme assay respectively. The coronal slices of the brain were immersed in a 2% solution of 2,3,5-triphenyltetrazolium chloride (TTC). The surface of the non TTC-stained area was measured and expressed as percent of the whole coronal section. The animals were divided into three groups. In the control group, physiological saline was continuously infused (2.0ml/kg/hour). The THAM group received continuous administration of 0.3mol THAM (2.0ml/kg/hour). In $NaHCO_3$ group, 7% $NaHCO_3$ (0.7ml/kg/hour) and physiological saline (1.3ml/kg/hour) were infused continuously.

<Clinical Investigation > THAM was administered intravenously as a 0.3-M solution in 7 patients with severe head injury (Table 1). The doses of THAM were calculated depending on the amount of base required to raise pH to 7.6 (4). The calculated loading dose was given over 2 hours, followed by a constant infusion of 1ml/kg/hr for 5 days. All patients were intubated and artificially ventilated. Cerebrospinal fluid (CSF) and arterial blood lactate concentration and acid-base balance were measured repeatedly.

【Results】

<Animal Experiments> In the THAM and $NaHCO_3$ groups, arterial pH was maintained within the normal range, whereas in the control group, arterial pH gradually decreased from 7.42±0.04 to 7.30±0.09 in 6 hours after the MCA occlusion. lCBF measured in the marginal and suprasylvian gyri showed a prompt decrease below 30ml/100g/min after the MCA occlusion and there were no significant differences

among the three groups (Fig.1). Extracellular pH of the marginal gyrus decreased from 7.21±0.11 to 6.86 ±0.10 with 6 hour-ischemia in the control group. However in the THAM and $NaHCO_3$ groups it did no show significant changes (Fig.2). Intracellular pH over the ischemic brain gradually decreased from 7.2 ±0.06 to 6.13±0.61 by the MCA occlusion. Intracellular pH in the THAM and $NaHCO_3$ groups wa 6.23±0.68 and 6.16±0.53 respectively in 6 hours after the MCA occlusion. Although these values were not significantly different, THAM has a tendency to normalize intracellular pH (Fig.2). In the THAM group, water content of the gray matter in the marginal gyrus significantly decreased compared with that in the control and $NaHCO_3$ groups (Fig.3). Tissue lactate content of the marginal gyrus significantly decreased in the THAM group. $NaHCO_3$ significantly increased lactate content of the marginal gyrus (Fig.4). The size of the infarct area in the THAM group was 16.6±10.0%, which was significantly decreased compared with that in control group (25.6±8.4%) (Fig.4).

<Clinical Investigation> Although 4 patients with acute subdural hematoma showed an initial GCS score of 5 or less and 3 of them had hematoma of larger than 120g, 2 patients made a good recovery and the other two were moderately disabled. Three patients with diffuse axonal injury and cerebral contusion made a good recovery (Table 1). The mean value of CSF lactate was 37.2 mg/dl before the treatment. CSF lactate decreased to 11.6 mg/dl in 3 days after THAM infusion.

Table 1 Summary of cases

Case No.	Age	Sex	Type of Trauma	GCS	GOS
1	51	M	acute subdural hematoma	4	MD
2	43	M	acute subdural hematoma	5	GR
3	14	F	diffuse axonal injury	5	GR
4	31	M	contusion	4	GR
5	16	M	acute subdural hematoma	5	GR
6	16	M	diffuse axonal injury	5	GR
7	73	F	acute subdural hematoma	4	MD

【Discussion】

In cerebral ischemia, there is an increased intracellular hydrogen ion concentration because of th excessive lactate accumulation, resulting in intracellular acidosis. Staub et al. (7) reported that acidificatio below pH 6.8 led to an immediate swelling of glial cells. Cell viability decreased in relation to the severit of acidosis at pH 5.6 and below. They also proposed the mechanism of the acidosis induced glial swelling H^+-ions which are accumulating in the extracellular compartment are buffered by bicarbonate resulting i the formation of CO_2 and water. CO_2 diffuses into the intracellular compartment resulting in intracellula acidification by formation of H_2CO_3. The H^+ and HCO_3^- ions are exchanged against extracellular Na^+ an Cl^- ions. Consequently Na^+ and Cl^- accumulate in the cell. In addition, protonated lactic acid can freel penetrate the cell membrane due to its lipophilicity, which raise the intracellular osmotic load. Hillered et a (3) reported that mitochondrial respiration was inhibited by a decrease in pH which may lead to permanent suppression of ATP production. Therefore amelioration of cerebral acidosis may reduc ischemic brain damage.

Ischemia due to the MCA occlusion encompasses a densely ischemic core and a less densely ischemi penumbral zone. The gyral topography of the ischemia following the MCA occlusion in cats was reporte that ectosylvian and marginal gyri were ischemic core and penumbral zone respectively (8). In this stud THAM significantly decreased water content of the gray matter in the marginal gyrus, which suggeste THAM can effect in the area of peri-infarct penumbra, but not in the ischemic core. It was supposed that i the ischemic core irreversible cell damage occurred and the effective dosage of THAM did not reach due t the markedly decreased lCBF.

In this study, there were no significant differences in lCBF among the three groups. Extracellular pH di not change significantly in the THAM and $NaHCO_3$ groups, whereas that in the control group decrease These data suggest that alkalizing agents improve extracellular pH, however have no effect on cerebr

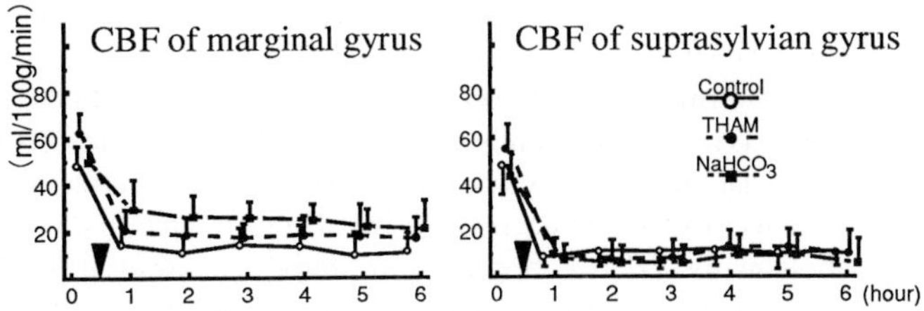

Fig.1

Figure 1
lCBF measured in the marginal gyrus (left) and suprasylvian gyrus (right) showed a prompt decrease after the MCA occlusion and there were no significant differences among the three groups.

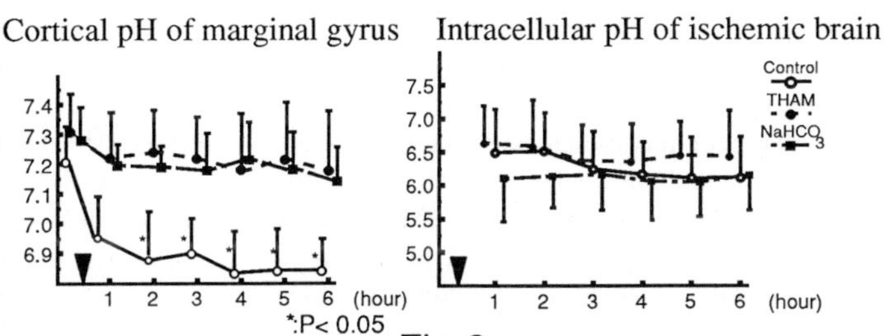

Fig.2

Figure 2
Left :Extracellular pH of the marginal gyrus decreased in the control group. However in the THAM and $NaHCO_3$ groups extracellular pH did not show significant changes.
Right :THAM has a tendency to normalize intracellular pH.

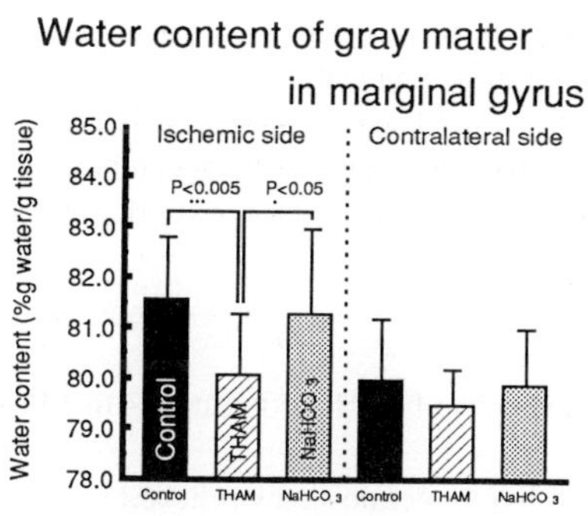

Fig.3

Figure 3
In the marginal gyrus, water content of the gray matter in the THAM group significantly decreased compared with that in the control and $NaHCO_3$ groups. *: p<0.05,
***: P<0 .005

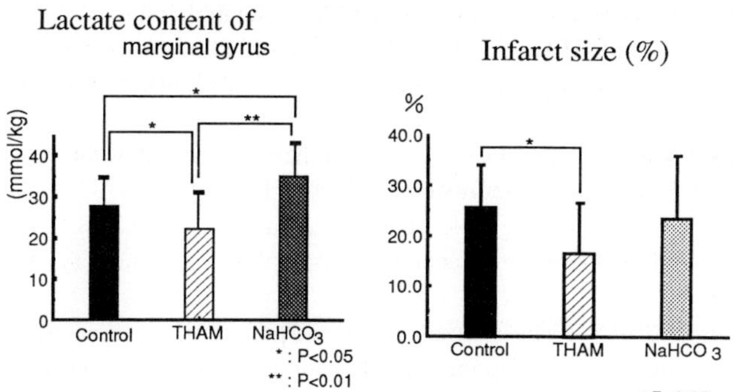

Fig.4

Figure 4
Left :Tissue lactate content of the marginal gyrus significantly decreased in the THAM group. $NaHCO_3$ significantly increased lactate content of the marginal gyrus.
Right : The size of infarct area in the THAM group significantly decreased compared with that in the control group.
*: P<0.05

circulation in cerebral ischemia. THAM has a tendency to normalize intracellular pH and significantly decreased water content of the gray matter and the infarct size.

Thirty percent of THAM is the non-ionized form (5), which can cross the plasmatic membrane and directly effect intracellular acidosis. Moreover THAM acts partially as an osmotic diuretics, since THAM is eliminated in its ionized form with an equimolar amount of bicarbonate (2). Thus THAM is effective for reducing brain edema and infarct size. It is also likely that decrease in the size of infarct area may be resulted from improved cerebral metabolism by THAM, because our study also showed THAM significantly decreased lactate content of the marginal gyrus. On the other hand, $NaHCO_3$ significantly increased lactate content of the marginal gyrus. This result suggests that $NaHCO_3$ infusion may be harmful and contribute to brain tissue swelling and dysfunction. $NaHCO_3$ infusion was reported to cause paradoxical intracellular acidosis, which is attributed to increased intracellular CO_2 (1). This may account for ineffectiveness of $NaHCO_3$ for focal ischemia.

Yoshida et al. (9) showed that administration of THAM minimized oxidative energy store depletion and decreased production of brain lactate in experimentally injured brain. They also found that THAM treatment decreased brain edema, which is consist with our result.

In head injury patients, hyperventilation has been recommended as a useful therapeutic method. However, Muizelaar et al. (4) reported hyperventilation could not sustain alkalinization in the CSF, where as THAM could in patients with traumatic brain injury. In the present study, THAM decreased CSF lactate and 5 of 7 patients made a good recovery, although all patients showed an initial GCS score of 5 or less. These results suggested that THAM ameliorated brain lactate production and resulted in reduced brain edema, which might lead to improving the clinical outcome. The loading dose of THAM varied between patients in this study. The loading dose was calculated as in the literature (4). However, it was usually less than the total recommended dose, because the total volume of intravenously infused solutions was enhanced by hyperosmotic agent, fluid and electrolytes, which tended to overload. Additional studies are needed in terms of the dosage of THAM to be used and the timing of its application.

In conclusion normalization of systemic and perifocal acidosis with THAM is effective in reducing cortical edema, lactate accumulation and infarct size in the early stage of focal cerebral ischemia probably due to the improvement of intracellular acidosis. Clinical study also suggests that THAM ameliorates cerebral lactic acidosis and improve the outcome in severe head injury.

<References>

1. Arieff AI, Leach W, Park R, et al. (1982) Systemic effects of $NaHC0_3$ in dogs. Am J Physio 242: F586- F591
2. Goetz RH, Selmonosky A, State D (1961) Anuria of hypovolemic shock relieved by tris(hydroxymethyl) aminomethane (THAM). Surg Gynecol Obstet 112:724-728
3. Hillered L, Ernster L, Siesjo BK (1984) Influence of in vitro lactic acidosis and hypercapnia on respiratory activity of isolated rat brain mitochondria. J Cereb Blood Flow Metabol 4: 430-437
4. Muizelaar JP, Marmarou A, Ward JD, Kontos HA, et al. (1991) Adverse effect of prolonged hyperventilation in patients with severe head injury: a randomized clinical trial . J Neurosurg 75: 731-739
5. Rosner MJ, Becker DP (1984) Experimental brain in jury: Successful therapy with the weak base, tromethamine with an overview of CNS acidosis . J Neurosurg 60: 961-971
6. Siesjo BK (1988) Acidosis and ischemic brain damage. Neurochemical Pathology 9: 31-88
7. Staub F, Baethmann A, Peters J, et al. (1990) Effects of lactacidosis on volume and viability of glial cells. Acta Neurochi r Suppl 51: 3- 6
8. Strong AJ, Venables GS, Gibson G (1983) The cortical ischemic penumbra associated with occlusion of the middle cerebral artery in the cat: 1. Topography of changes in blood flow, potassium ion activity, and EEG. J Cereb Blood Flow Metabol 3: 86-96
9. Yoshida K, Marmarou A (1991) Effects of tromethamine and hyperventilation on brain injury in the cat. J Neurosurg 74:87-96

Poster I: Methodology

Chairman: M. Maeda

Infections Complications of Intracranial Pressure Monitoring

R. ALBERTI[2], A. BIESTRO[1], M. CANCELA[1], P. MESA[1], A. CORDOBA[2], and B. BOROVICH[2]

[1] Intensive Care Unit, [2] Department of Neurosurgery, Hospital de Clínicas, Montevideo, Uruguay

INTRODUCTION.

Traumatism is the main cause of death in our country for patients aged between 0 and 30 years. Head injury prevails in the pathology.
Controlling the increase of ICP plays a fundamental role in the terapeutical handling of such patients as well as knowing the CPP. There fore the PIC monitoring technique is essential in Intensive Care Units. An infections complication is one of the greatest risks.

OBJETIVE.

The purpose is to show the incidence of such complication and its relationship with variables resulting from applying such technique.

MATERIALS AND METHODS.

47 patients that had entered the ICU between 1989 and 1993 were studied. A 48% incidence of nosocomial infection was found (with a mean of 1.2). Ages varied from 10 to 58 years (a mean of 25). Patients stayed in the Unit from 3 to 101 days (a mean of 11) and the ICP monitoring took from 1 to 11 days (a mean of 3.5). The GSC on entering hospital was from 3 to 15, with a mean of 6.
ICP was monitored by means of:

- Subdural screw bolt (Richmond/Mac Graw) in 34 patients (72.3%)
- Subdural catheter in 9 patients (19.1%)
- Subdural screw bolt plus subdural catheter in 3 patients (6.3%)
- Intraparenquimal catheter in 1 patient (2.1%)

Inmediately after the monitor was withdrawn a bacteriological culture of the remaining liquid of the screw and the tip of the subdural catheter was performed. The test was positive when nosocomial germs were present. The diagnosis of infection in the Central Nervous System (CNS) was made by means of clinical testing, laboratory data and CT scanning.
The following variables were analyzed:

- Device used vs. positive cultures (Table 1)
- Monitoring time vs. positive cultures (Tables 2 and 3)
- Surgery vs. positive cultures (Table 4)
- Device used vs. Infection (Table 5)
- Monitoring time vs. Infection (Table 6)
- Duration of the stay in ICU vs. Infection (Table 7)
- Surgey vs. Infection (Table 8)
- Positive cultures vs. Infection (Table 9)

RESULTS

Device used vs. postive cultures

Table 1	CULTURES+	CULTURES-
Sudural Screw	6	10
Subdural catheter	1	5
Subd C.+Screw	1	1
Intraparenq. C.	1	0

Fisher's Proof = 0.28
Fisher's Proof = 0.41
Test of x^2 = 2.93 (N/S)

Monitoring time vs. Positives cultures

Table 2	CULTURES+	CULTURES-
> 4 days	7	5
≤ 4 days	2	11

Fisher's Proof : p=0.035 (S)
Relative Risk : 3.79 - 1.17 (S)

Monitoring times vs. Positive cultures

Table 3	CULTURE +	CULTURE -
2 days	0	5
4 days	2	6
6 days	5	0
8 days	2	3
10 dias	0	2

Fisher's Proof = 0.01 X^2 = 13.28 (S)
Fisher's Proof = 0.51

Neurosurgery vs. Positives Cultures

Table 4	CULTURE+	CULTURE -
C/ intervention	5	9
S/ intervention	4	7

Fisher's Proof : p=0.64 (N/S)
Relative Risk : 0.98 - 0.34 (N/S)

Device used vs. Infection

Table 5	YES INFECTION	NO INFECTION
Subdural Screw	1	33
Suodural Catheter	0	9
Subd. C.+ Screw	0	3
Intraparenq. C.	1	---

Test of x^2 = 23.17 (Significant)
Fisher's Proof = 0.02 (S)

Monitoring time vs. Infection

Table 6	YES INFECTION	NO INFECTION
> 4 days	2	18
≤ 4 days	0	29

Fisher's Proof : p=0.16 (N/S)

Duration in ICU vs. Infection

Table 7	YES INFECTION	NO INFECTION
> 10 days	2	27
≤ 10 days	0	17

Fisher's Proof : p=0.392 (N/S)

Neurosurgery vs. Infection

Table 8	YES INFECTION	NO INFECTION
C/ intervention	2	20
S/ intervention	0	25

Fisher's Proof : p=0.213 (N/S)

Positive cultures vs. Infection

Table 9	YES INFECTION	NO INFECTION
Patients c/cult. +	2	7
Patients c/cult. —	0	38

Fisher's Proof : p=0.033 (S)

DISCUSSION.

Nosocomial germs were found regardless of the device used for monitoring ICP (Table 1). Their presence, conversely, was related to the monitoring time (Tables 2 and 3). Even though, infection was indeed associated with the device used, it was no because of the device itself, but by virtue of penetration through biological barriers (Table 5). The subdural area did not appear as a favorables medium for the development of infection. Therefore the performance of the Subdural Screw bolt/Catheter proved to be excellent with respect to infection, all the more considering that the rate of nosocomial infection in our Unit amournts to 48%.

REFERENCES.

Rosner, M. J.; Becker D. P.:ICP monitoring: Complications and associated factors. Clin. Neurosurg. 23: 494-519, 1976.

A New Ventricular Catheter with an Integrated Pieco-Resistive Sensor at Its Tip—First Experiences

J. Piek[1] and P. Raes[2]

[1] Neurochirurgische Universitätsklinik, Moorenstr. 5, 40225 Düsseldorf, Germany
[2] Draeger Medical Electronics, IBC weg 1, 5680 Best, The Netherlands

INTRODUCTION

Monitoring of ventricular fluid pressure is indicated in various clinical situations and is estimated as the "gold standard" of ICP monitoring [1]. In cases of elevated ICP - like in patients with head injuries - its main advantage is discontinuous drainage of CSF to control ICP. Dislocation or occlusion of the ventricular catheter however may occur frequently during the monitoring period.
In patients with spontaneous intraventricular haemorrhages continuous drainage of CSF may be desirable. Overdrainage or occlusion of the system is a problem in this patient group.
In patients with suspected normal pressure hydrocephalus long-term monitoring of ICP may be indicated combined with bolus injections to determine intracranial compliance or resistance. Continuous ICP monitoring during bolus injections of fluid to the intracranial compartment cannot be done with most of the devices available.

ICP DEVICE

To overcome these problems we designed a combination of a "classic" ventricular catheter combined with a pieco-resistive transducer at its tip (Fig. 1) using the same transducer which has already proven clinical reliability in more than 200 patients used for cerebral tissue pressure recordings [2-6]. The device allows:

* to record VFP simultaneously via chip (in the ventricle itself) and via the fluid-filled system;
* to withdraw or drain CSF from or to inject fluid into the ventricle while ICP is simultaneously monitored via the chip in the ventricle;
* still to record brain tissue pressure in cases of misplacement or dislocation of the ventricular catheter or in cases of progressively narrowing ventricles due to brain edema.

RESULTS

Up to now we have used this system in 11 patients (4 SAH, 3 head injuries, 3 normal pressure hydrocephalus, 1 tumour) with a total monitoring time of 1239 hours (max. 372 hours).
No additional complications (e.g. haemorrhages, infections) were observed. Parallel recordings gave excellent correlations of pressures monitored via chip or by the fluid-filled system.
Besides the advantages already mentioned the system does not require additional equipment (except one zero-point simulator per ICU at costs of approximately 300 $ US) and will be prized in the 400 - 500 $ range when on the market in late autumn 1994.
Currently tests in larger patient groups are running in Germany and different countries in Europe to improve the final design.

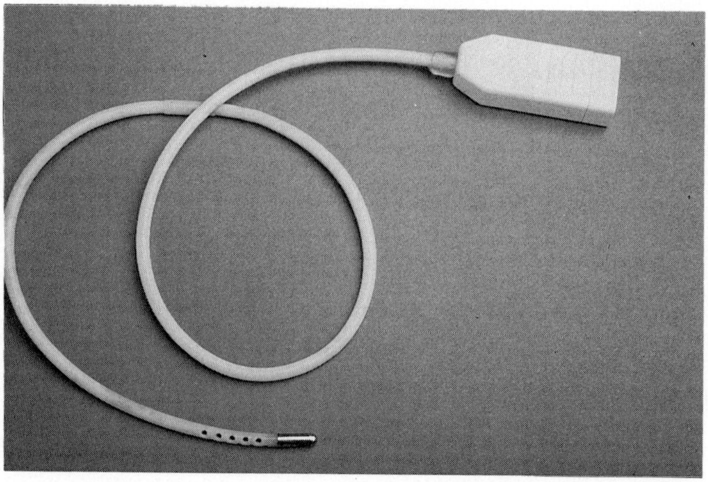

Fig. 1: New ventricular catheter with sensor and drainage holes at its tip

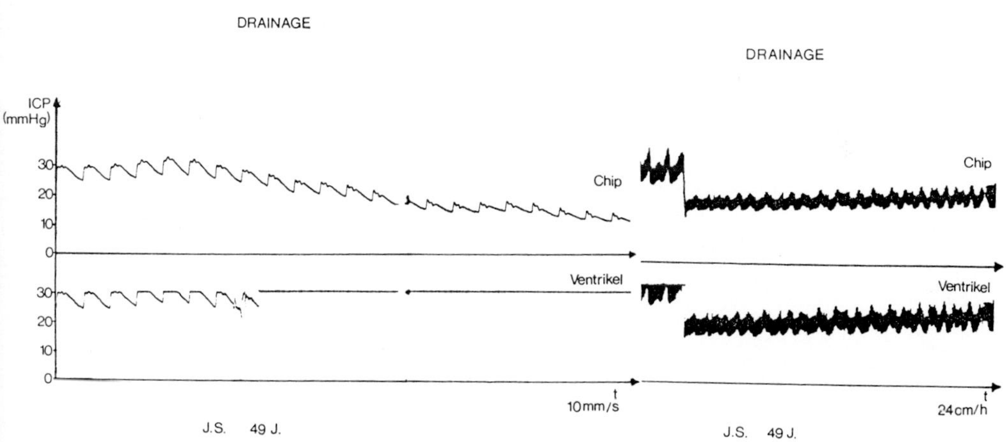

Fig. 2 a, b: Examples of simultaneous recordings of VFP via chip (upper curve) and via the fluid-filled system (lower curve) during CSF drainage in a patient with head injury. Note: VFP is continuously recorded in the ventricle while draining CSF.

REFERENCES

1. Miller JD (1989) Measuring ICP in patients - Its value now and in the future? In: Hoff JT, Betz AL (eds.) ICP VII. Springer, Berlin, Heidelberg, New York, pp 5 - 15
2. Piek J, Kosub B, Küch F, Bock WJ (1987) A practical technique for continuous monitoring of brain tissue pressure in neurosurgical patients. Preliminary results. Acta Neurochir 87: 144 - 149
3. Piek J, Plewe P, Bock WJ (1988) Intrahemispheric gradients of brain tissue pressure in patients with brain tumours. Acta Neurochir 93: 129 - 132
4. Piek J, Bock WJ (1990) Continuous monitoring of cerebral tissue pressure in neurosurgery (experience with 100 patients). Intensive Care Med 16: 184 - 188
5. Piek J, Bock WJ (1993) Continuous monitoring of supratentorial tissue pressure in neurosurgical routine. Experience with 125 patients. In: Avezaat CJJ, van Eiyndhoven JHM, Maas AIR, Tans JTJ (eds.): ICP VIII. Springer, Berlin, Heidelberg, Tokyo, New York, pp 11 - 16
6. Piek J, Ern G, Messing (1993) Continuous monitoring of infratentorial tissue pressure following elective tumour surgery. In: Avezaat CJJ, van Eiyndhoven JHM, Maas AIR, Tans JTJ (eds.): ICP VIII, Springer, Berlin, Heidelberg, Tokyo, New York, pp 17 - 19

A Trial of Intracranial Pressure Measurement from External Auditory Canal—Clinical Analysis

Y. Doumoto[1], T. Oizumi[1], K. Mizoi[2], M. Matsuyama[3], T. Ohira[3], and S. Toya[3]

[1] Department of Neurosurgery, Keio University Ise Keio Hospital, Tokiwa, Ise, Mie, 516 Japan
[2] Department of Medical Electronics, Ise Keio Hospital, Tokiwa, Ise, Mie, 516 Japan
[3] Department of Neurosurgery, Keio University, Shinjuku-ku, Tokyo, 160 Japan

INTRODUCTION

The ICP is measured directly from within the intracranial space. There is, however, a significant risk of infection, and it is necessary to violate the brain in order to insert the cannula. Capacity of external auditory canal (EAC) was reported to be diminished in the rised ICP patients on the elevation of ICP by Marchbanks in 1987 [1]. His report suggested the canal pressure changes could be a clue to catch the ICP quantitatively. On this hypothesis we started to measure the pressure changes in the EAC for seeking for a non-invasive and reliable method, by which a time serial information of the ICP change would be available in clinical practice. Our observations which suggest a close relationship between the EACP and the ICP will be presented.

METHODS AND CASES

The tiny pressure sensor (Electric Condenser type) was embedded in a ear-piece of several sizes, of which tip was designed to fit the EAC orifice suitaly for detecting pressure changes in the EAC. These ear-pieces were kept firmly in position with head-band, in fashion of head -phone, for stable recording of long time. The pressure picked up was recorded through band pass filter after adequate amplication. Electrocardiogram and pulsation of the cartid artery were also recorded simultanously. Measuremets were made on 11 normal adults and many clinical cases.

RESULTS

We called this wave "external auditory canal pressure wave (EACPW)". As shown in Fig. 1, the normal EACP changes show rhythmic cycles, beeing synchronized with electrocardiogram. The waves are basically biphasic; the first compinent is a deep and sharp negative deflection following cardiac ejection, and the second is a lower positive shoot followed by a rather gentle trail to the next cycle. In patients with rised ICP, the first negative wave tends to become shallow, and the second wave shows flattened pattern in Fig. 2. The abnormal EACPW in a patient with subdural hematoma turned towards normal pattern in pace with the convalescence after surgery.

DISCUSSION

The pressure of the cerebro-spinal fluid is transmitted to the inner ear via both the cochlear aqueduct and the endolymphatic duct. External ear pressure is transmitted more via the round window through the middle ear cavity than via the ossicular chain [2]. And further, Suzuki et al. have demonstrateed that an increment in CSF pressure was completely transmitted to the endolymphatic space without any time lag or gradient [3]. Our data show clearly that the EACP reflects the ICP changes. These results suspected that this procedure is being considered as a possible non-invasive method of serial ICP measurements.

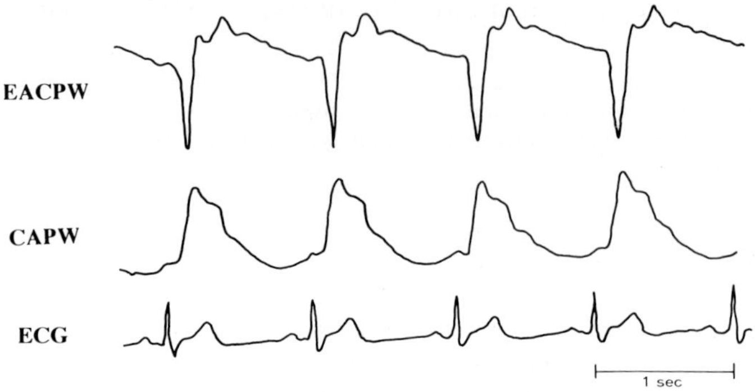

Fig. 1 Simultaneous recording of EACPW, CAPW, and ECG.
(EACP : External Auditory Canal Pressure Wave, CAPW : Carotid Arterial Pressure Wave)

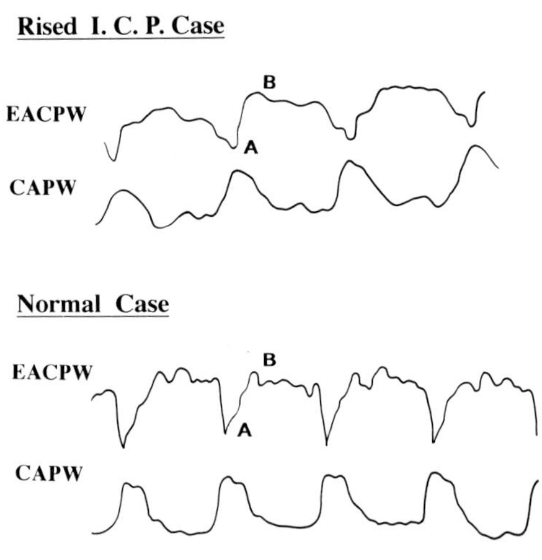

Fig. 2 Comparison between rised ICP case and normal case .

REFERENCES

1. R. J. Marchbanks, A. Reid (1987) The effect of raised intracranial pressure on intracochlear fluid pressure : three case studies. British Journal of Audiology 21 : 127 - 130
2. S. Nishihara (1990) Pressure Transmission to the Inner Ear. Jibi Rinshou 83 : 449 - 456
3. T. Suzuki, T. Nakashima (1993) Effects of increased cerebrospinal fluid pressure on cochlear and cerebral blood flow. Eur Arch Otorhinolaryngol 250 : 332 - 336

Transcranial and Extracranial Doppler Ultrasonography in Raised Intracranial Pressure: Clinical Study

A. Mangiola[1], C. Anile[1], D. Catapano[1], and G. Maira[2]

[1] Institute of Neurosurgery, Catholic University, Rome, Italy
[2] University of Perugia, Italy

INTRODUCTION

The optimal treatment of patients with intracranial hypertension demands an understanding of cerebral blood flow (CBF) and, as a consequence, also an understanding of cerebral perfusion pressure (CPP). As reported by Hassler et al. [1], a correlation exists between CPP and the transcranial doppler (TCD) waveform during intracranial hypertension up to brain circulatory arrest. In the past, however, the doppler blood flow velocity measurement of the internal carotid artery (ICA) at the neck proved to allow a rapid and accurate assessment of the so-called "brain tamponade" [2]. The main purpose of this study is to compare the relationship between CPP variations and CBF velocity modifications evaluated by means both of the transcranial and extracranial doppler ultrasonography in patients suffering from intracranial hypertension due to different causes.

MATERIALS AND METHODS

Our series consists of 33 patients in coma for cerebral causes, who underwent a monitoring of intracranial pressure (ICP) by means of a catheter inserted into a lateral ventricle. The CBF velocity variations were evaluated monitoring the blood flow velocity at the intracranial level (middle cerebral artery insonated by TCD), and extracranial level (ICA insonated by traditional continuous wave doppler). Two parameters have been mainly taken into consideration: the diastolic blood flow velocity and the resistance index (RI = systolic - diastolic / systolic velocity). The CBF velocity variations were considered during spontaneous and/or therapeutical ICP modifications induced by CSF withdrawal and/or decompressive craniectomy.

RESULTS

In all the patients a progressive ICP increase was associated to CBF velocity variations. Such modifications measured by TCD were characterized by a progressive reduction in the diastolic blood flow velocity and RI increase; this trend was evident when the ICP rose above 20 mmHg (Fig. 1). At the extracranial level the same CBF variations appeared later, when ICP increased above 35 mmHg. Over this value we observed a rapid decrease of diastolic blood flow velocity associated to a very important RI increase (Table 1). In 9 patients who underwent a decompressive craniectomy, a prompt ICP reduction and a CBF velocity increase appeared immediately after the surgical procedure. Nevertheless, in all the patients with a RI value > 0.7 at the extracranial level, we always documented a further progressive ICP increase leading to intracranial circulatory arrest, independently of the therapeutic procedures adopted.

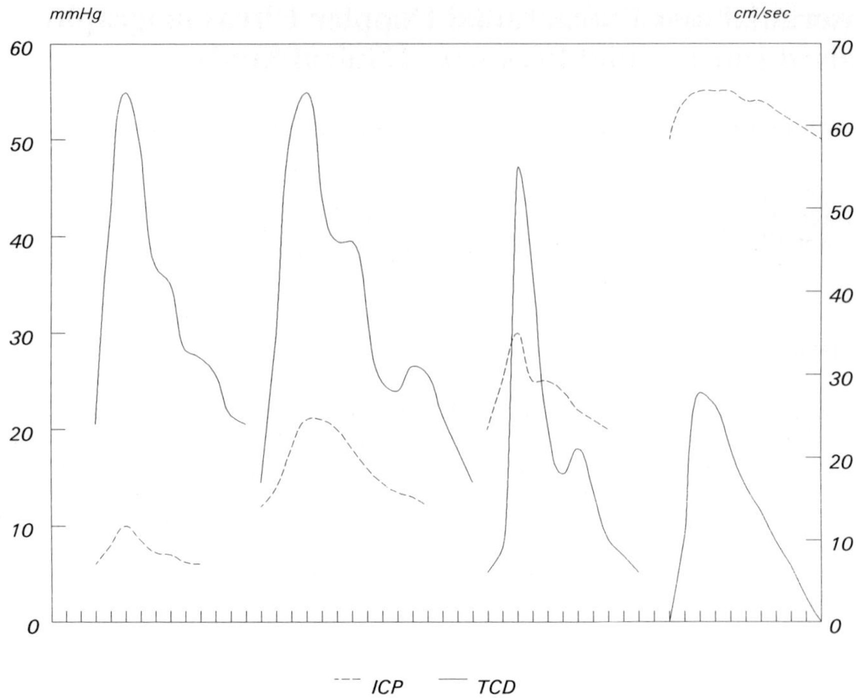

Fig. 1: Relationship between progressive ICP increase and CBF velocity variations evaluated by TCD

Table 1: Relationships between diastolic ICP and RI at extracranial internal carotid artery level

ICP	RI
< 35 mmHg	.523 ± .07
> 35 mmHg	.958 ± .07

DISCUSSION

Our findings suggest a major sensitivity of the TCD in comparison with the extracranial one in order to evaluate CBF velocity variations during intracranial hypertension. The appearance of blood flow velocity modifications at the extracranial level seems to express a more severe impediment in the mechanisms regulating the CBF. The opening of the intracranial system to the atmosphere, obtained by the decompressive craniectomy, seems to be a procedure able to restore an adequate CBF.

REFERENCES

1. Hassler W, Steinmetz H, Gawlowski J (1988) Transcranial doppler ultrasonography in raised intracranial pressure and in intracranial circulatory arrest. J Neurosurg 68:745-751.
2. Lindegaard K-F, Grip A, Nornes H (1980) Precerebral haemodynamics in brain tamponade. Part 1: Clinical studies on blood flow velocity. Neurochirurgia 23:133-142.

A Trial of Intracranial Pressure Measurement from External Auditory Canal—Experimental Analysis

M. MATSUYAMA[1], T. OHIRA[1], Y. DOUMOTO[2], K. MIZOI[3], and S. TOYA[1]

[1] Department of Neurosurgery, Keio University Shinjuku-ku, Tokyo, 160 Japan
[2] Department of Neurosurgery, Keio University Ise Keio Hospital, Ise, Mie, 516 Japan
[2] Department of Medical Electronics, Keio University Ise Keio Hospital, Ise, Mie, 516 Japan

INTRODUCTION

Intracranial pressure consists of two components; the one is static pressure of the intracranial fluid, and the other is cyclic fluctuations given rise to superimposedly by cardiac ejection and respiratory movement. Little attention, however, has been paid to the later wave component in clinical practice, though this component is known to be notably deformed in response to the elevation of intracranial pressure.

It has been strongly suggested by us that the measurement of intracranial pressure, non-invasive, could take place of the invasive measurement of intracranial pressure, as far as the cyclic component is concerned.

The benefit and limitations of the external auditory canal pressure measurement were investigated experimentally on cats, in comparison with conventional invasive procedures.

MATERIALS AND METHODS

Adult cats weighing 2.0 to 4.0 kg were anesthetized with 30mg/kg ketamine administered intramuscularly, and 40mg/kg pentobarbital sodium intraperitoneally. Respiration was supported by respirator during experiment. The intracranial pressure was measured simultaneously with the external auditory canal and also blood pressure: the intracranial pressure was transmitted by a catheter indwelled in citerna magna, the external auditory canal pressure was picked up by a tiny microphone embedded in the canal orifice, and blood pressure was recorded with a catheter inserted into carotid artery.

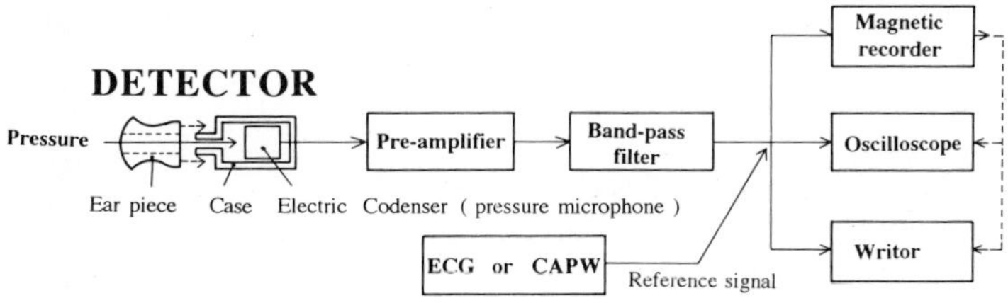

Fig. 1 Detection System of EACP
EACP: External Auditor Canal Pressure
CAPW: Carotid Arterial Pressure Wave

RESULTS

The detected pressure wave had a certain pattern and it altered simultaneously with heart beat. The wave had also different pattern from BP wave, and ICP pulse wave. When ICP was elevated, the pressure wave increased in amplitude and the pattern changed to multi-peak shape. Under the investigation of correlation, external auditory canal pressure showed higher coefficient with ICP than BP.

Table 1 EACP showed higher coefficient to ICP than BP.

Cat No.	EACP-ICP coefficient	EACP-BP coefficient
#1	0.67	0.45
#2	0.86	0.81
#3	0.77	0.41
#4	0.79	0.62
#5	0.66	0.87
mean	0.75	0.63

DISCUSSION

Relationship between cerebrospinal fluid pressure and the inner ear fluid pressure has been studied, and transmission of CSF pressure changes to the inner ear has been demonstrated in humans and animals.[1,2]

The EACP is mainly derived from carotid artery pressure(blood pressure) wave and intracranial pressure. It is strongly suggested that external auditory pressure wave includes informations of ICP.

REFERENCES

1. Carlborg B, Farmer JC(1983) Transmission of cerebrospinal fluid pressure via the cochlea aqueduct and endolymphatetic sac. Am J Otolaryngol 4:273-282

2. Feldman RM, Allen GW(1966) Effects of cerebrospinal fluid pressure on the cat cochlea. Arch Otolaryngol 84:86-89

Non-Invasive ICP Monitoring in Infants—The Rotterdam Teletransducer Revisited

R.J.A. PETERS[2], P.W. HANLO[1], R.H.J.M. GOOSKENS[3], K.P.J. BRAUN[3], C.A.F. TULLEKEN[1], and J. WILLEMSE[3]

Departments of [1] Neurosurgery and [3] ChildNeurology, University Hospital Utrecht, Box 85500, 3508 GA Utrecht, The Netherlands
[2] Department of Biomedical Engineering, Free University Hospital, Amsterdam, The Netherlands

INTRODUCTION

Intracranial pressure (ICP) monitoring in young infants can be useful in a variety of neurological conditions, such as hydrocephalus. ICP monitoring, however, is only of clinical importance when the measurement equipment is accurate and completely reliable. Measurements should show a high correlation with the actual ICP. Although several studies have suggested a close relation with simultaneously measured intraventricular pressure, a serious criticism of fontanometers has been that these non-invasive ICP measurements are not sufficiently reliable for use in clinical practice.
The literature contains little information on the accuracy or validation of the anterior fontanelle pressure (AFP) measurements using the Rotterdam Teletransducer (RTT).
The aim of the present study was to reassess the physical qualities of the RTT and to evaluate its validation by relating the measured AFP to the actual ICP, represented by the intraventricular pressure (IVP).

MATERIALS AND METHODS

Rotterdam Teletransducer.
The RTT, an applanation technique, is composed of a resonator and an electromagnetic coupled impedance measurement device. The resonator comprises a passive coil capacitor system enclosed within a piston. The location of the capacitor is such that one of the plates forms the flat top of the piston. Changes in pressure applied to the top of the piston influence the value of the capacitor and thus the resonance frequency. Accurate depth positioning of the piston is essential. The Pressure Depth Curve is used to adjust the piston to the fontanelle.

To assess the most important physical modalities of the RTT, in-vitro and in-vivo experiments were performed.

- In vitro, the RTT is tested using a specially developed calibration device.
  Firstly, the performance of the RTT was examined under ideal laboratory conditions, and secondly, bearing in mind that clinical factors may have a negative effect on the accuracy of the calibration, these were then investigated in simulated conditions.
- To validate the RTT in vivo, several longterm AFP and IVP measurements were performed simultaneously in hydrocephalic patients, in order to verify the relationship between the pressure measured by the RTT and the actual IVP.

RESULTS

- In Vitro Measurements.
  During the first hour the results show a rapid drop in measurement output, following switch-on. After three hours, there is no significant output drift.

The results of 90 calibration measurements at two points (0 and 40 mmHg) show a largest pressure deviation between 10 and 20 mmhg with maximum deviation limits ranging from -1.4 up to 1.0 mmhg (Fig. 1).
The difference between measured pressure, after switching on, and three hours later is at least 3 mmhg. Furthermore, the manipulation of the piston and subsequent zerodrift apparently effects the accuracy of the measurement, revealing deviation limits ranging from -2.6 up to 1.3 mmhg.
- In Vivo computerized Measurements.
These measurements show a high correlation (r: 0.96 - r: 0.98) between the AFP measured with the RTT and the IVP values. The difference between AFP and IVP increases with increasing pressure (Fig. 2).

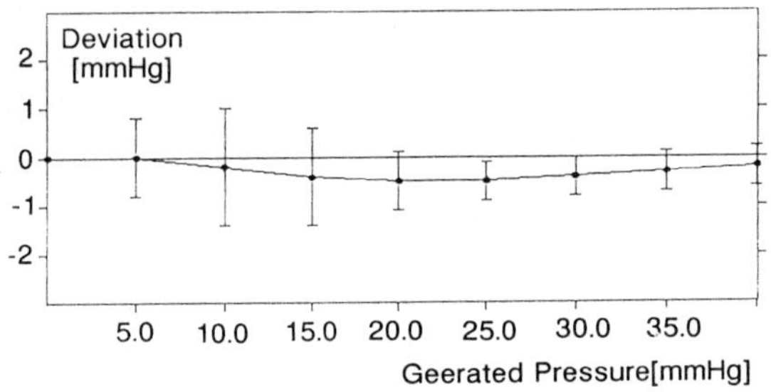

Fig. 1 RTT Calibration Measurements

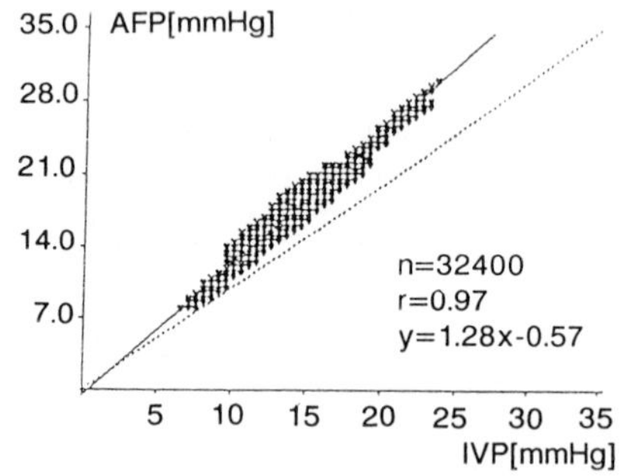

Fig. 2 The relationship between AFP and IVP

CONCLUSIONS

The relationship between AFP, measured by the RTT, and IVP, as documented in our study, has not been established previously.
The RTT has been proved to be an accurate and reliable device for determining the ICP by measuring the AFP, if extended operating procedures are taken into account. Firstly, a stabilization period of at least 3 hours should be allowed. The piston should then be adjusted to the calibration device on the plateau of the pressure depth curve, followed by calibration at two points (0 and 40 mmhg) on the calibration device. Finally, the piston should be moved from the calibration device to the fontanelle and the offset (zero) adjusted, just prior to the moment at which the piston touches the skin. We concluded that hardware improvements to reduce thermal stabilization time and to improve the gain and offset adjustment procedures might increase the reliability of the RTT even further.

REFERENCES

1. Maas AIR, Jong DA de (1986) The Rotterdam Teletransducer: state of the device. Acta Neurochir (Wien) 79: 5-12
2. Overweg-Plandsoen WCG (1990) The Rotterdam Teletransducer. Anterior fontanelle pressure monitoring in infants. Thesis Rotterdam pp 28-37
3. Schettini A, McKay L, Majors R, Mahig I, Nevis A (1971) Experimental approach for monitoring surface brain pressure. J. Neurosurg 34: 38-47

Software for Intracranial Pressure Recording and Waveform Analysis

W. Zabolotny[1,2], M. Czosnyka[1,2], and P. Smielewski[1,2]

[1] Warsaw University of Technology, Nowowiejska 15/19, 00-665 Warsaw, Poland
[2] MRC Cambridge Centre for Brain Repair and Academic Neurosurgical Unit, Addenbrooke's Hospital, P.O. Box 167, Cambridge CB2 2QQ, UK

SUMMARY

Reliable data recording is essential in clinical and experimental studies on cerebrospinal dynamics. In clinical work however it is important to provide on-line signal analysis of acquired data to estimate the clinical state of the patient. Our programs allow simultaneous recording and analysis of data, working on single IBM PC compatible (even laptop) computer, equipped with a low cost analog-to-digital board. In many applications computers may replace expensive and inconvenient magnetic data recorders, reducing numbers of equipment needed beside patient's bed. Recorded data are stored on computer's disc, allowing easy access, off-line analysis and archivisation. The off-line data analysis can be performed using our off-line analysing software, or using algorithms written in MATLAB-386TM (by The Math Works Inc.) package. A well-defined communication protocol allows the user to create his own data analysing software.

DATA ACQUISITION SYSTEM

The main component of the data acquisition system is an analog-to-digital converter driver library (ADCONV), working with a digital data recorder (WREC). This program allows recording of up to 8 biological signals with 12-bit resolution and maximum sampling frequency 200 Hz or more (depending on the speed of the computer). This software, working in Microsoft Windows 3.1TM environment makes full use of its graphics user interface and multitasking capabilities. Up to 32 programs (including user written software) can run simultaneously, recording and analysing in different ways data provided by ADCONV converter driver. Because of the well-defined communication protocol the user can easily add to the system his own analysing or recording programs (processing acquired data on-line, or even in real-time). The trend monitor program allows screen presentation of trends of measured signals allowing assessment of the state of the patient.

OFF LINE DATA ANALYSIS

The recorded data can be browsed sample by sample or in a condensed way using another program (WINVIEW - recorded data viewer). The user can select parts of data containing especially interesting events and copy them into another file. There is also possibility to analyse selected data using user written analysis procedure.

The recorded data can be analysed off-line using another program (ICMR). This software permits the multichannel spectral processing of the data recorded previously, analysis of the signals' correlations and the event detection. Original sampling frequency can be changed to observe fast or slow signal fluctuations; data are stored on the computer disk and can be transferred to the ASCII format.

For more sophisticated signal analysis there is a possibility of importing recorded by WREC data into the MATLAB-386TM package. With this feature user can implement his off-line data analysing algorithms in a very simple way, writing them in a Pascal-like programming language. This feature is particularly convenient for testing new methods of data analysis or implementing algorithms requiring very sophisticated signal processing.

APPLICATION OF SOFTWARE

The program proved to be very useful in both clinical and laboratory practice. One of its most important applications was a comparison between the pulse waveform of ICP and Intracranial flow velocity (FV) to distinguish between the vasogenic oscillations (B waves) and high rises in ICP having characteristics of plateau waves or being caused by an expansion of intracerebral mass.

Material

Data was recorded in Addenbrooke's Hospital in head injured ventilated patients (25) exhibiting pattern of B waves and elevations of ICP not related to repetitive cerebral blood volume oscillations. Intracranial pressure (ICP) and flow velocity maximal (FVx) signals were recorded with sampling rate 40Hz-80Hz (depending on case).

Method

The recorded data were browsed using WINVIEW data viewer and segments containing B-waves were extracted as a group of files. The segments containing plateau waves were further extracted as another group of files. Data from both groups of files were analysed using algorithms written using MATLAB-386TM package. The analysis algorithm calculated mean value of intracranial pressure (ICP mean), mean value of flow velocity maximal (FVx mean), pulse wave amplitude of flow velocity maximal (FVx amp) and pulsatility index of flow velocity maximal (FVx PI). In group of files containing plateau waves, values corresponding to the plateau have been grouped together, for each patient, and compared with those corresponding to lower pressure values. In group of files containing B-waves, for each patient, values corresponding to the higher ICP values have been compared with values obtained for lower ICP values.

Results and Discussion

Results of comparison showed that increase of ICP during B-waves was correlated with increase of blood flow velocity ($p < 0.001$), and increase of blood flow velocity's pulse amplitude ($p < 0.0004$). There was no significant change in pulsatility index of flow velocity during the B-wave. Increase of ICP during plateau waves was well correlated with decrease of blood flow velocity ($p < 0.002$) and less so with simultaneous increase of blood flow velocity's pulse amplitude ($p < 0.112$). This resulted in a significant increase of pulsatility index of blood flow velocity ($p < 0.019$).

Decrease of mean value of blood flow velocity maximal combined with simultaneous increase of pulse wave amplitude of this signal seems to be a good indicator of critical ICP fluctuations. Pulsatility index of flow velocity maximal seems to be a good parameter for detection of such fluctuations.

REFERENCES

1. Czosnyka M.,Zaworski W.,Laniewski P. et.al. :A system for intracranial pressure processing and interpretation in intensive care, Advances in Biomedical Measurement, Ed.:E. Carson et.al., Plenum Press, 1988, pp.101-110.

2. M.Czosnyka , L.Batorski, P.Laniewski et.al.:A computer system for the identification of the cerebrospinal compensatory model. Acta Neurochirurgica, (1990) 105: pp. 112-116.

3. M. Czosnyka, P. Wollk Laniewski, P. Darwaj, M. Duda, L. Batorski, W. Zaworski, Software for Neurosurgery Intensive Care, Intracranial Pressure VII, Springer-Verlag Berlin Heidelberg 1989, pp 84-87.

Comparison of Telemetric Epidural and Intraventricular Pressures

M.A. Williams[1], G.S.F. Ling[1], M.S. Schnitzer[1], A.Y. Razumovsky[1], M. Longerbeam[2], J.G. Chubbuck[3], and D.F. Hanley[1]

[1] Departments of Neurology and Neurosurgery, Johns Hopkins Medical Institutions, 600 N. Wolfe Street, Meyer 8-140, Baltimore, MD 21287-7840, USA
[2] BME Systems, Inc., 2340 Monumental Avenue, Baltimore, MD 21227, USA
[3] LifeSensors, Inc., 5741 Maguire Road, Noble, OK 73068, USA

INTRODUCTION

We previously developed and tested a telemetered ICP (T-ICP) sensor in animals and humans, including implantation in human subjects for as long as 10 years [1-4]. The sensor reliably produced a T-ICP measurement, but measurement accuracy deteriorated with time due to baseline drift, causing the apparent T-ICP to increase compared to lumbar CSF pressure in all sensors [4]. A subgroup of sensors subsequently displayed a declining apparent T-ICP due to loss of integrity of the sensor case closure. These early T-ICP sensors were interrogated using electronic laboratory test equipment, which required the operator to have engineering expertise.

We have re-engineered and reconstructed the T-ICP sensor to correct the problems with baseline drift and hermeticity. We also have incorporated microcomputer control and analysis of sensor interrogation into the design for on-line pressure recording. The purpose of this study was to define the accuracy of the redesigned T-ICP device during experimental acute intracranial hypertension.

METHODS

Six male beagle dogs were anesthetized with 35 mg/kg pentobarbital i.v., intubated, and ventilated. An 18-mm burr hole was created over the right hemisphere. A threaded collar was affixed to the skull overlying the burr hole and the T-ICP sensor was threaded into the collar to an appropriate depth determined by measuring the change in T-ICP with depth [5]. A ventricular catheter was inserted in the opposite hemisphere for ventricular fluid pressure (VFP) measurement and artificial CSF infusion.

T-ICP Data Acquisition System

The T-ICP sensor data acquisition system consists of 1) a 50 MHz 486 computer that runs custom software for data acquisition and on-line display, 2) a separately housed interrogation circuit and barometer, and 3) an interrogation coil. The interrogation hardware contains circuitry to 1) generate a radiofrequency (RF) excitation signal from 25 to 50 MHz transmitted by the interrogation coil, and 2) determine the frequency at which the RF signal resonates with the sensor [1-4]. The system samples and processes the resonant frequency and barometric pressure data to compute T-ICP in real time. The resonant frequency correlates with the absolute pressure within the sensor, and T-ICP is computed by subtracting the barometric pressure from the absolute sensor pressure.

Experimental Protocol

VFP was elevated from 15 to 95 mm Hg in 10 mm Hg increments by raising a reservoir of artificial CSF. At the end of the protocol VFP and T-ICP were recorded as VFP returned to normal. VFP and T-ICP were collected simultaneously at 50 points per second on the T-ICP data acquisition system. For each dog, simultaneous data points for VFP and T-ICP at each VFP were compared by linear regression.

RESULTS AND DISCUSSION

The linear regression results for each dog are presented in Table 1. Data from one experiment are shown in Figure 1. Our results demonstrate that the re-engineered telemetric epidural pressure sensor is accurate over a range of 15-95 mm Hg in experimental acute intracranial hypertension in dogs. The small pressure difference between VFP and epidural T-ICP is consistent with previous comparisons of VFP and epidural pressure. Maximum variance between VFP and T-ICP occurs at higher pressures (50-90 mm Hg), where such variance is physiologically less important than it is a lower pressures (0-30 mm Hg).

Table 1 Slope, intercept, and correlation coefficient of T-ICP as a function of VFP for each dog.

Dog	Slope	Y-intercept	r^2
1	0.86	-0.5	0.98
2	0.92	6.9	0.98
3	1.33	2.5	0.98
4	1.06	6.1	1.00
5	0.97	-5.7	0.98
6	0.97	-5.1	0.99
Mean ± SEM	1.02 ± 0.03	0.7 ± 1.1	

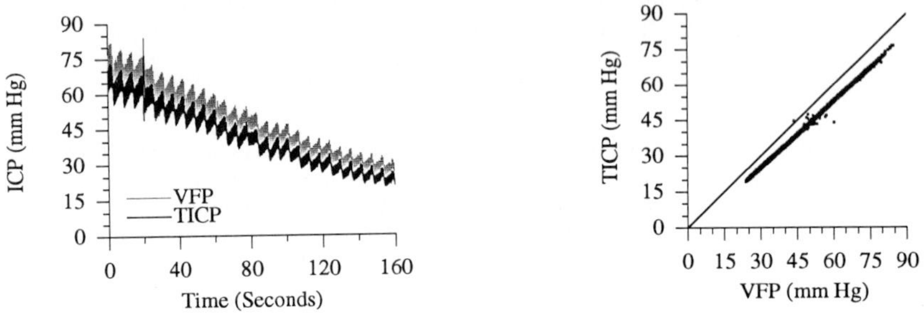

Figure 1 (Left) Dynamic wave form comparison of VFP (top) and T-ICP in one animal. (Right) Scatter plot of 8170 points. Regression line: T-ICP = 0.93xVFP - 3.3, (r^2 = 1.0). Line of identity is shown for comparison.

We have improved the accuracy and feasibility of an implantable T-ICP sensor with potential for clinica use. The application of microcomputer control to the T-ICP device permits easily obtained, automatic on-line display of T-ICP wave form and numerical value. Because ICP and absolute T-ICP senso pressure are equally affected by barometric pressure, T-ICP can be recorded regardless of patient positio relative to an external reference, which makes T-ICP recording during complex awake behavior possible.

The following factors remain to be evaluated in our T-ICP sensor: 1) Baseline drift in comparison to VF over a period of months; 2) interrogation reliability through tissue; 3) MRI safety, compatibility, and imag disruption; 4) biocompatibility and tissue reaction after prolonged implantation; and 5) placement in huma subjects, including depth, apposition pressure and applanation tolerance.

There are numerous potential uses for a practical T-ICP system. ICP is chronically disordered in hea injury, subarachnoid or intracerebral hemorrhage, meningitis, encephalitis, brain tumor, pseudotumo cerebri, and hydrocephalus. Because ICP cannot be measured for long periods with contemporar devices, the effect of prolonged ICP elevation on these diseases is unknown. Further development o T-ICP sensing technology is warranted for clinical use and research.

REFERENCES

1. Walker AE, Viernstein LJ, Chubbuck JG (1977) Intracranial pressure monitoring in neurosurgery. In Fleming DG, Ko WH, Neuman MR (Eds) Indwelling and implantable pressure transducers. CR Press, Cleveland, pp 69-77
2. Gucer G, Viernstein LJ (1979) Intracranial pressure in the normal monkey while awake and aslee J Neurosurg 51:206-210
3. Gucer G, Viernstein LJ, Chubbuck JG, Walker AE (1979) Clinical evaluation of long-term epidura monitoring of intracranial pressure. Surg Neurol 12:373-377
4. Gucer G, Viernstein L, Wang A, Szymanski R (1988) Ten-year follow-up on the performance of telemetric intracranial pressure sensor. Neurosurg 22:892-895
5. Schettini A, Walsh EK (1974) Experimental identification of the subarachnoid and subpi compartments by intracranial pressure measurements. J Neurosurg 40:609-616

Supported by NS 27795-03 and the Brain Trauma Foundation Fellowship in Neurotrauma and Critical Care

Clinical Evaluation of Hydrocephalus Using an Osaka Telesensor

Hiroji Miyake, Tomio Ohta, Yoshinaga Kajimoto, Jun Deguchi, Motohiro Arai, and Masanori Matsukawa

Department of Neurosurgery, Osaka Medical College, 2-7 Daigakucho, Takatsuki, Osaka, 569 Japan

INTRODUCTION

We consider various factors such as clinical triad,PVL on CT,reflux and delayed clearance on cisternography,and pressure waves on continuous ICP monitoring, to determine the indications for shunt procedure in hydrocephalic patients. However, these factors are still not definitive. We report the usefulness of responses on ICP and CBF by Diamox® as an indicator for shunt. We also report postural ICP difference, which has not previously been reported precisely.

MATERIALS AND METHODS

We investigated thirty-two hydrocephalic patients (SAH:16, idiopathic NPH:9, others:7) who were treated at Osaka Medical College between October 1991 and March 1994. All of these patient underwent V-P shunt using an Osaka telesensor, a Sophy programmable valve and an On-Off flushing reservoir. Postural ICP difference were measured by the Osaka telesensor. The relationship between the appearance of B waves on the pre-operative (pre-op) ICP recordings and prognosis was investigated. In the recent six cases, XeCT with intravenous administration of Diamox®(1000mg) was used in pre-op examination, with simultaneous recording of the ICP. Pre-op condition was simulated by closing the shunt for 1 day. The efficacy of the V-P shunt was evaluated by improvements in consciousness level, mental activity, gait disturbance and urinary incontinence.

RESULTS

Twenty-two patients showed clinical improvement after V-P shunt. B waves were observed in nineteen cases during continuous recording in the pre-op condition. However, there were no B waves seen in ten cases who showed no clinical improvement after shunt. ICP in the upright position after the clinical condition stabilized following, shunt showed a negative value (-16.0±5mmHg). Postural ICP difference between supine and upright was about 20 mmHg. ICP differences between the sitting and upright positions were not remarkable. Diamox® administration caused 17 to 54% (average 34.4%) increase in CBF on XeCT. The ICP response to Diamox® was divided into two groups. Group A, which showed remarkable ICP increase(77 to 146%) included four cases. All cases in group A showed B waves on pre-op ICP recording and clinical improvement after shunt. Group B, which showed slight ICP increase(22,24%) and no B waves,did not improve clinically.

Table 1 Summary of recent 6 clinical cases

Case	Etiology	B wave	Response to Diamox® ICP(%)	Response to Diamox® CBF(%)	Prognosis
1.M.T*	SAH	+/-	133%↑	37%↑	Improved
2.T.K	Idopathic	+	146%↑	/	Improved
3.K.Y	Idiopathic	-	24%↑	17%↑	Unchanged
4.H.O	Head injury	+	120%↑	28%↑	Improved
5.K.N	SAH	-	97%↑	54%↑	Improved
6.S.Y	Idiopathic	-	22%↑	36%↑	Unchanged

* a case of external decompression

DISCUSSION

Our fully implantable Osaka telesensor is very useful in monitoring ICP especially in daily activity[1,2]. ICP in an upright position proved to be negative. The postural ICP difference between supine and upright positions was about 19 mmHg, while there was no difference between sitting and upright positions.

The increase in CBF after rapid intravenous administration of Diamox® was proven in all five cases by XeCT. This increase in CBF was thought to be caused by vasodilatation due to the inhibition of carbonic anhydrase. Although statistically unproven, there seems to be no remarkable difference in the degree of CBF increase between groups A and B, while ICP responses were quite different. This fact indicates that the ICP response to Diamox® represents the buffering ability of CSF space. The increase in CBF caused marked ICP elevation in group A, which have some CSF circulatory disturbances, while the same degree of CBF increase did not cause ICP elevation in group B, in which the CSF compensation mechanism was thought to be normal.The appearance of B waves on the continuous ICP recording in pre-op conditon correlated well with clinical improvements after shunt, as already reported. However, this necessitates overnight ICP recording, which is very inconvenient for patients. The marked ICP increase caused by Diamox® coincides with the apperance of B waves and the combination of CBF and ICP responses to Diamox® is a good indicator for shunt operation[3].

REFERENCES

1.Miyake H,Ohta T,Nagasawa S,Takatsuka H,Yamashita M,Osaka K (1991) Clinical Experience with a New Ventriculo-Peritoneal Shunt Using a Telemetric Intraventricular Pressure Sensor,an On-Off Flushing Reservoir and a Sophy's Programmable Hydrostatic PressureValve.Current Tr Hyd (Tokyo)1:79-84

2.Ohta T,Miyake H,Nagasawa S,Nagano Y,Tanabe H(1993) Chronologic Changes in Intraventricular Pressure and Ventricular size After Ventriculo-Peritoneal Shunt-Telemetric Measurement Using Osaka Telesensor(NS-20). In:Avezaat CJJ,van Eijndhoven JHM,Maas AIR,Tans JTJ(eds) Intracranial Pressure VIII.Springer-Verlag,Berllin,Heidelberg,pp889-895

3.Yoshida S,Yonekawa Y,Kawano T,Miyake H,Goto Y,Yamashita K,Kaku Y(1991) Changes of CSF Pressure Induced by Acetazolamide Administration Test-As an Indicator of Shunt Operation for So-Called Normal Pressure Hydrocephalus-Brain and Nerve 43:43-48

Poster II: Monitoring

Chairman: J. Goffin

Intracranial Pressure Monitoring of Meningeal Carcinomatosis

Y. Takeda[1], T. Onitsuka[2], T. Koba[1], T. Miki[2], J. Haraoka[2], and H. Ito[2]

[1] Department of Neurosurgery, Social Health Insurance Medical Center, Shinjuku-ku, Tokyo, 169 Japan
[2] Department of Neurosurgery, Tokyo Medical College, Shinjuku-ku, Tokyo, 160 Japan

SUMMARY

Two groups of patients, the first with pathognomonic findings of meningeal carcinomatosis (MC) on computed tomography (CT), the second without those have been investigated by intracranial pressure monitoring, CBF study and RI cisternography. MC is presumed to be tight brain characterized by the raised ICP, the freqent pressure waves, and the impaired CPP. Even in the patients without the pathognomonic findings, it is not at all uncommon that MC has already developed to a critical condition with disorder of CBF and CSF flow dynamics. Our results suggest that a serious threat to neurosurgical practice is also presented in such patients.

INTRODUCTION

In meningeal carcinomatosis (MC), the diagnosis and the treatment may be delayed, because the pathognomonic findings on computed neuroimaging are not always obtained in its earlier stage. This study was designed to clarify the clinicopathophysiology of MC with special reference to the CT scan and ICP monitoring.

MATERIALS AND METHODS

Twelve patients with MC were divided into two groups : group Ⅰ, seven patients with characteristic CT findings of MC such as ventriculomegaly, cisternal, sulcal and ependymal enhancement ; group Ⅱ, the remaining five without those. In all 12 patients, ventricular fluid pressure (VFP), arterial blood pressure, and cerebral perfusion pressure (CPP) were polygraphically measured and analyzed with a data-recorder. The time from the onset of MC to the monitoring averaged 3.1±2.1 months. CBF study by ^{133}Xe method of 5 cases and RI cisternography of 9 cases were carried out as simultaneously as possible.

RESULTS

Analysis of ICP : A waves were observed in 5 cases of group Ⅰ and in 3 cases of group Ⅱ. B waves were observed in all cases of both groups. In all cases, the occurrence rate of both A and B waves (OR_A, OR_B) averaged 2.34±0.54times/hour, 74.0±16.6%time, respectively. Mean resting pressure (R) and Mean peak pressure (P) averaged 28.8± 12.2mmHg, 58.9± 13.7mmHg, respectively. Mean CPP corresponding with R and P (CPP_R, CPP_P) markedly reduced, averaging 79.1± 15.9mmHg, 50.9± 12.7mmHg, respectively. Both OR_A and OR_B in group Ⅰ were higher, and both CPP_R and CPP_P in group Ⅰ were lower, than in group Ⅱ. Statistically, these are significant. Although R and P in group Ⅰ tended to be higher than in group Ⅱ, this has no statistical significance (Table 1).

CBF and RI study : CBF in all 5 cases averaged 34.8± 8.4ml/100g/min. There was no significant difference in the impaired CBF between the groups. RI cisternography showed delayed clearance in all 9 cases. The impaired CSF absorption in RI study was especially evident in group Ⅰ.

Clinical aspect : Although the neurological symptoms appeared earlier, and were more various in group Ⅰ than in group Ⅱ, the difference in the clinical aspects between the groups was scarcely significant. Hydrocephalus was uncommon even in group Ⅰ(Table 2). The patients were followed by CT and 2 out of 5 patients of group Ⅱ became compatible with group Ⅰ.

Table 1 Comparison on the analyzed factors between the groups

	Pressure waves		Factors analyzed (mmHg)			
	OR_A (times/hr)	OR_B (%time)	R	P	CPP_R	CPP_P
Group Ⅰ	2.52±0.61	77.5±15.4	30.0±14.2	59.8±10.4	75.0±18.3	47.3±11.4
Group Ⅱ	2.03±0.25	68.7±19.3	27.0±10.3	57.5±6.50	85.8±17.7	56.3±14.4
p value	p<0.02	p<0.05	NS	NS	p<0.02	p<0.01

Table 2 Clinical Aspects

	the onset〜 ICPmonitoring (month)	CSF-protein content (ventricle) (mg/dl)	ventricular dilatation (Evans' index)	survival time (month)
Group Ⅰ	3.4±1.9	133.0± 34.3	0.32±0.07	5.5±2.8
Group Ⅱ	2.2±0.8	151.0±125.3	0.27±0.02	5.3±2.5

DISCUSSION

It is especially noteworthy that despite absence of hydrocephalus, MC potentially develops severe intracranial hypertension with pressure waves. The pathophysiology of group Ⅰ appear to be more advanced than that of group Ⅱ. But only the difference in the stage of MC can hardly explain this phenomenon, because no ventriculomegaly was found even in group Ⅰ. Hansen et al. [1] have reported similar patients with some etiologies such as spinal tumor and Guillian-Barré syndrome. The reason for this phenomenon is not well understood. Decreased conductance to CSF outflow, increased venous pressure, decreased cerebtral tissue compliance, and increased elastance of the CSF space were proposed by previous investigators [1][2][3]. Especially in MC, mechanical and functional obstruction of the arachnoid villi appears to be responsible for these factors. MC is characterized by the elevation of resting pressure, the frequent pressure waves, and the reduction of CPP. Our results demonstrated that a critical condition was also presented in the cses of group Ⅱ. The degree of progression on CT findings does not always parallel the change of impaired ICP and CBF. Great care should be recommended to have an accurate diagnosis and appropriate treatments in the management of MC.

REFERENCES

1. Hansen K, Gjerris F, Sørensen PS (1987) Absence of hydrocephalus in spite of impaired cerebrospinal fluid absorption and severe intracranial hypertension. Acta Neurochir(Wien) 86: 93-97
2. Gjerris F, Sørensen PS, Vorstrup S, Poulson OB (1985) Intracranial pressure, conductance to cerebrospinal outflow and cerebral blood flow in patients with benign intracranial hypertension (pseudotumor cerebri). Ann Neurol 17:158-162
3. Donaldson JO (1981) Pathogenesis of pseudotumor cerebri syndromes. Neurology (Ny) 31:877-880

Lumbar CSF Pressure Measurement in Idiopathic Normal Pressure Hydrocephalus in the Aged

MASATSUNE ISHIKAWA and HARUHIKO KIKUCHI

Department of Neurosurgery, Kyoto University, 54 Kawaharacho, Shogoin, Sakyoku, Kyoto, 606 Japan

SUMMARY

Continuous lumbar cerebrospinal fluid pressure (CSF) measurement was done in twenty patients who were suspected of idiopathic normal pressure hydrocephalus (NPH) in the aged. Based on this, they were divided into a high pressure group (12 cases) and normal pressure group (8 cases). The mean pressure was 16.5 mmHg in the former and 9.6mmHg in the latter, and the difference was statistically significant. Clinical symptoms and CT findings were not different between both groups, except for CSF removal test. Shunt surgery was performed in the high pressure group with 75 percent improvement. Thus, continuous lumbar CSF pressure measurement and CSF removal test were useful for selection of idiopathic NPH in the aged.

INTRODUCTION

Normal pressure hydrocephalus (NPH) is commonly developed after subarachnoid hemorrhage. However, it can also develope in the aged without clear etiology. This idiopathic type of NPH is difficult to differentiate from other forms of senile dementia and one might miss an oppotunity for surgical treatment. In this paper, we will report our experience of 20 cases who were suspected of idiopathic NPH.

MATERIALS AND METHODS

Twent patients, ranging from age 55 to 79 years, were studied. They were suspected of idiopathic NPH, because they had not any history of stroke or trauma and had at least one of the classical triads for NPH: dementia, gait disturbance and urinary incontinence.

Continuous lumbar CSF pressure measurement was done in 20 cases by means of thin polyethylene catheter. The measurement was carried out over night for more than 8 hours. Based on this, they can be divided into a high pressure group (H group; >13mmH of baseline pressure or >15% of pressure waves /hour) and a normal pressure group (N group). Shunt surgery was done for patients in H group. Clinical features in both groups were compared. Statistical analyses were done with the significant difference at $p<0.05$.

RESULTS

The baseline pressure in the H group (12 cases) was 16.5±3.1 mmHg and that in the N group(8 cases) was 9.6±1.7 mmHg and the difference was statistically significant. Baseline pressure and the frequency of pressure waves were significantly high in the H group. There were no significant differences in clinical symptoms and CT findings between the two groups, except for clinical improvement after CSF removal, which was noted in all 7 cases subjected to spinal tap in the H group. No difference was noted on C cisternography and cerebral blood flow measurements between them. Shunt surgery was done in cases of H group and it was effective in 9 of 12 cases (75%).

DISCUSSION

In the aged, gait disturbances or dementia are relatively common symptoms, so that one may miss the oppotunity to perform a shunt, which provides improvement of symptoms in case of idiopathic NPH. Clinical sypmptoms and CT or MRI failed to make the diagnosis. On the continuous CSF measurement, high baseline pressure and frequent pressure waves could be shown even in a case of brain atrophy. Shunt surgery was indicated for patients in the high pressure group with a fairly high success rate. Although it may be effective on CT even in patients in the normal pressure group, no good reason for surgery could be determined only by the continuous measurement of CSF pressure.

The present study also shows the importance of CSF removal test by spinal tap. In the high pressure group, symptoms were improved within several days, regardless of the volume removed. This is the easiest way to select patients for shunt surgery. although there may be false negative cases.

The idiopathic NPH is a surgically treatable condition, so that it is important to be alert to the presence of this disorder in the aged, even in case of brain atropy. Continuous CSF pressure measurement and CSF removal test were useful in the diffential diagnosis.

	High pressure group	Normal pressure group
Cases	12	8
Age	66.5(55-79)	66.9(58–73)
Dementia		
none	2	0
mild	2	2
moderate	2	2
severe	6	4
Gait disturbance		
none	0	0
mild	2	2
moderate	8	5
severe	2	3
Urinary disturbance		
none	6	3
mild	1	3
moderate	5	2
severe	0	0
Ventricular dilatation		
mild	1	1
moderate	9	5
severe	2	2
Periventricular low density		
mild	6	3
moderate	4	4
severe	2	1
Widening of cerebral sluci		
mild	5	2
moderate	6	5
severe	1	1
nproved after CSF removal	7/7	0/3
aseline CSF pressure(mmHg)	16.5±4.0	9.6±1.7
T cisternography	7	3
BF measurement	4	3

able 1. Summary of 20 cases suspected of idiopathic normal pressure ydrocephalus.

Cerebral Perfusion Pressure in Head Injured Children

A.D. Mendelow[1], I.R. Chambers[2], P.J. Kane[1], L. Treadwell[1], A. Jenkins[1], R.E. Bullock[1], and P.J. Crawford[1]

[1] Department of Surgery (Neurosurgery), University of Newcastle upon Tyne, UK
[2] Regional Medical Physics Department, Newcastle General Hospital, UK

INTRODUCTION

McGraw's [1] observation that the survival of patients with a severe head injury is improved by maintaining cerebral perfusion pressure (CPP) above 80 mmHg has been supported by studies in several other centres [2,3]. We have shown that CPP averaged over an hour was the best predictor of outcome from severe head injury [2] and Contant et al.[3] also pointed to the duration of low CPP as being important. In each of these studies no attempt was made to stratify the patient group according to age and presumably children (patients aged ≤ 16 years) were included within the study groups. The aim of this study was to investigate the relationship of CPP and outcome in severely head injured childrenwho are known to have a lower mean blood pressure than adults.

METHODS

All children studied were admitted to Newcastle General Hospital in the time period August 1988-April 1993. All had a severe head injury (Glasgow Coma Scale on admission to the neurosurgical unit ≤ 8) and required intracranial pressure (ICP) monitoring as a routine part of their management. ICP was measured continuously with the Camino™ subdural screw (n=23) or by ventriculostomy connected to an external pressure transducer (n=6) over periods ranging from 6.4 to 127.8 hours. Blood pressure was measured continuously via a cannula in a radial artery. ICP, Mean arterial blood pressure (MABP) and CPP data were monitored continuously as described previously [4] and the data collected on a Psion Organiser for later analysis. In the data analysis "average minimum CPP" is defined as the minimum CPP calculated over any one hour period of monitoring and outcome was determined at six months using the Glasgow Outcome Scale [5]. "Independent" outcome is defined as those children who made a good recovery or were moderately disabled; "poor" outcome describes those children who were severely disabled, vegetative or dead.

RESULTS

Twenty nine children were studied (age range 7 months to 16 years, mean 9.2 ± 0.76). Eight patients died. In survivors the outcome scores at six months post injury were: 4 severely disabled; 5 moderately disabled; 12 good recoveries. There were no vegetative survivors.
Average minimum CPP for each group is shown in Figure 1. Higher values of average minimum CPP are associated with better outcome with the threshold for poor and independent outcome lying between 41 and 57 mmHg. Assuming a threshold value of 50 mmHg a comparison of poor and independent groups is shown in Table 1. Chi squared analysis supports the observed improved outcome in children with average minimum CPP greater than 50 mmHg (Table 1, $p < 0.01$)

CONCLUSION

We have previously shown that average minimum CPP is an important predictor of outcome following severe head injury [2]. This study supports this observation and points to the importance of maintaining CPP in the management of paediatric head injury. Although the number of patients in this study is small it is interesting to note that the mean values of CPP in each outcome group in children are lower than those we reported in a larger group of adults and children [6]. This may reflect fundamental differences in cerebral vascular physiology between adults and children and merits further investigation.

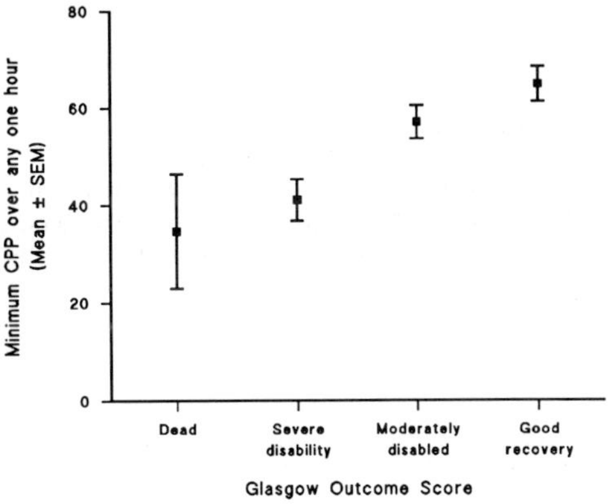

Figure 1 Minimum CPP and outcome

Table 1

	Outcome		
CPP	Independent	Poor	Total
> 50mmHg	14	3	17
≤ 50mmHg	3	9	12

REFERENCES

1. McGraw CP (1989) A cerebral perfusion pressure greater than 80mmHg is more beneficial. In: Hoff JT, Betz AL (eds) Intracranial Pressure VII. Springer-Verlag, Berlin, Heidleberg, pp 839-841.
2. Mendelow AD, Allcutt DA, Chambers IR, Jenkins A, Crawford PJ, Sultan H. Intracranial and cerebral perfusion pressure in the head injured patient: Which index? (1993) In: Avezaat CJJ, Eijndhoven JHMv, Maas AIR, Tans JTJ (eds) Intracranial Pressure VIII, Springer-Verlag, Berlin, Heidleberg, pp 544-548.
3. Contant CF, Robertson CS, Gopinath SG, Narayan RK, Grossman RG (1993) Determination of clinically important thresholds in continuously monitored patients with head injury. J. Neurotrauma 10, Suppl 1, S57.
4. Chambers IR, Clark A, Kane PJ, Allcutt DA, Mendelow AD (1993) Continuous monitoring and recording of cerebral perfusion pressure. In: Avezaat CJJ, Eijndhoven JHMv, Maas AIR, Tans JTJ (eds) Intracranial Pressure VIII, Springer-Verlag, Berlin, Heidleberg, pp 544-548.
5. Jennet B, Bond M (1975) Assesssment of outcome after severe brain damage. Lancet i: 480
6. Mendelow AD. Chambers IR, Clark A, Kane PJ, Allcutt DA, Jenkins A, Crawford PJ, Bullock RE (1993) Cerebral perfusion pressure: the 60 minute average minimum value and outcome from severe head injury. J. Neurotrauma 10, Suppl 1, S213.

Intracranial Pressure Monitoring in the Posterior Fossa

W.S. Poon

Neurosurgical Unit, Department of Surgery, Prince of Wales Hospital, The Chinese University of Hong Kong, Shatin, New Territories, Hong Kong

SUMMARY

Simultaneous monitoring of direct posterior fossa pressure (PFP) and intraventricular pressure (IVP) was carried out in 25 patients with posterior fossa pathology. In a closed fluid system, PFP and IVP correlated well. In patients with raised pressure, those with hydrocephalus without a mass lesion (n=4) exhibited no differential pressure between PFP and IVP, whereas those with obstructive hydrocephalus with a posterior fossa mass lesion (n=4) exhibited significant differential pressure at two minutes after CSF drainage.

INTRODUCTION

Direct posterior fossa pressure monitoring (PFP) has been shown to be safe and effective in a prospective study of 20 patients following tumour surgery [1]. However, its potential role and clinical significance have not been explored.

MATERIALS AND METHODS

Between April 1991 and March 1993, 25 patients after removal of a mass lesion in the posterior fossa had simultaneous measurements of PFP and IVP. Direct PFP measurement was obtained using the Camino subdural fiberoptic transducer and IVP via a standard ventricular catheter through a pre-coronal burr hole. All patients were managed in the Intensive Care Unit, fully sedated and ventilated with 30° head elevation. The zero level of the IVP was taken at the projected site of the PFP transducer. Simultaneous mean PFP and IVP measurements were compared in a closed fluid system. When raised intracranial pressure occurred (>30mmHg), repeat CT brain scan was performed immediately to differentiate two groups of patients: (1) post-operative haematoma in the posterior fossa with obstructive hydrocephalus, and (2) hydrocephalus without a mass lesion. The differential pressure between PFP and IVP at two minutes after CSF drainage in these two groups of patients was compared.

RESULTS

In a closed fluid system, PFP and IVP correlated well in the pressure range -2 to 105 mm Hg:

$$[PFP] = 1.1\ [IVP] + 0.1 \text{ mm Hg, where, } r^2 = 0.96,\ p < 10^{-6}.$$

In the group of patients with hydrocephalus without a mass lesion (n=4), no significant differential pressure existed between PFP and IVP at 2 minutes after CSF drainage (15.5 ± 2.1 *vs* 17.5 ± 2.6 mm Hg, $p>0.1$), whereas in patients with obstructive hydrocephalus and a posterior fossa mass lesion (n=4), a significant differential pressure was demonstrated (20.1 mm Hg, 35.3 ± 2.8 *vs* 15.2 ± 3.6 mm Hg, $p<0.001$) (fig. 1). In the 17 patients without raised intracranial pressure, CSF drainage was not required.

Table 1. Demographic and clinical data of the 25 patients

No. of Patients	Age (years)	Pathology	Patients complicated by raised ICP	Outcome of patients with raised ICP
16	2-63	Tumour	Hydrocephalus Hydrocephalus	VP shunt; good recovery VP shunt; good recovery
5	53-70	Primary post fossa haematoma	Post-operative haematoma Post-operative haematoma Hydrocephalus	Re-opening; disabled Re-opening; died VP shunt; disabled
4	19-28	Head injury	Cerebellar contusion Cerebellar contusion	Brain dead Resolved; good recovery

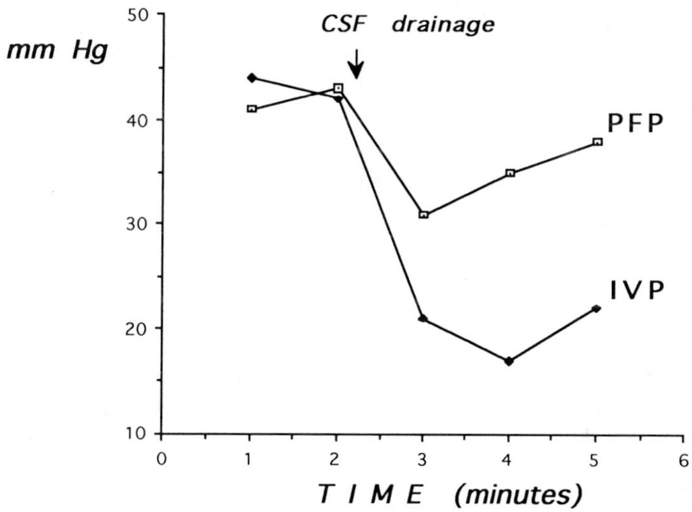

Fig. 1 In the 4 patients with obstructive hydrocephalus and a posterior fossa mass lesion, a significant differential pressure was demonstrated between PFP and IVP.

DISCUSSION

In a closed fluid system over the pressure range of -2 and 105 mm Hg, PFP and IVP correlated well, with an 82% corresponding rate within 5 mm Hg (71/85 data pairs). A significant differential pressure (20.1 mm Hg) was demonstrated between PFP and IVP in a small group of patients who developed a posterior fossa mass lesion causing obstructive hydrocephalus when CSF drainage was established. This may be of clinical importance in the early detection of post-operative haematoma in the posterior fossa.

REFERENCES

1. Rosenwasser RH, Kleiner LI, Krzeminski JP, Buchheit WA (1989) Intracranial pressure monitoring in the posterior fossa: a preliminary report. J Neurosurg 71: 503-505.

Anterior Fontanelle Pressure Monitoring in Hydrocephalic and Normal Infants

J.-L. WAYENBERG[1], N. MASSAGER[2], F. VALENTE[3], D. VERMEYLEN[4], C. RAFTOPOULOS[5], P. FRANCO[4], and D. DETEMMERMAN[6]

[1] Department of Paediatrics, Hôpital Français-Reine Elisabeth, 180 av. J Goffin, B-1080 Brussels, Belgium
[2] Faculty of Medicine, [3] Laboratory of Medical Statistics, Public Health School, [4] Neonatal Intensive Care Unit, [5] Department of Neurosurgery, [6] Department of Paediatric Surgery, Hôpital Erasme, Université Libre de Bruxelles, route de Lennik, B-1070 Brussels, Belgium

SUMMARY

In order to test the value of ICP monitoring for the assessment of hydrocephalus and shunt system in infants, we compared sleep anterior fontanelle pressure (AFP) recordings obtained in 17 normal infants, 16 patients with hydrocephalus and 11 patients with shunted hydrocephalus. Both basal AFP and pressure waves were analysed. In progressive hydrocephalus the AFP recordings were never normal, even in the absence of increased mean AFP. Plateau wave rate was the most sensitive and specific variable for the diagnosis of progressive hydrocephalus. The occurrence of pressure waves in shunt dysfunction contrasted with the relatively flat aspect of the AFP recordings of infants with well-functioning shunts. We conclude that, if the age of the patients is taken into account for the interpretation of the recordings, AFP monitoring is an useful tool for the evaluation of ventricular dilatation and shunt function in infants.

INTRODUCTION

In infants, it may be difficult to differentiate progressive from *a vacuo* hydrocephalus and well-functioning from dysfunctioning ventriculo-peritoneal derivation (VPD). Several studies pointed out the usefulness of ICP monitoring in these conditions [1]. Our aim was to compare the ICP patterns obtained by means of a non invasive technique in normal infants and in patients with hydrocephalus.

MATERIAL and METHODS

We studied 17 normal infants and 27 patients with hydrocephalus. According to their clinical condition and cerebral imaging results, the hydrocephalic patients were divided into four groups: *a vacuo* hydrocephalus (AV, n=8), progressive hydrocephalus (PR, n=8), well functioning VPD (SF, n=7) and VPD dysfunction (SD, n=4). The fontanelle pressure (AFP) was continuously recorded by means of the Rotterdam Teletransducer [2]. We studied both basal AFP (expressed as mean AFP and mean pulse pressure amplitude) and pressure waves (noted as plateau waves (PW) and B-like waves (BW). We measured the duration and the amplitude of each PW, the mean AFP occurring during PW and the PW rate. We measured the maximal amplitude of BW and the BW rate.

RESULTS

All variables but one (mean AFP between normal infants, SF and SD groups) were significantly different between the groups (Table I). In group PR mean AFP was normal in 4 out of 8 patients but an increased pulse pressure amplitude (PPA) and/or increased pressure wave amplitude and/or duration were observed in all cases. The frequent occurrence of pressure waves with an amplitude higher than 4 mmHg in SD recordings contrasted with the relatively flat aspect of the SF recordings. PW activity rate (> 25%) was the most sensitive and specific variable for the diagnosis of progressive hydrocephalus (respectively 88% and 100%). BW activity rate (> 25%) was the best variable for the assessment of VPD function.

Table I: some of the AFP variables in the five groups (mean ± SD, in mm Hg)

groups	age	basal AFP variables		Plateau waves variables			B-like waves variable	
		mean AFP	mean PP	PW rate	PW max	maximal AFP	BW rate	BW max
	(months)			(%)	amplitude	during PW	(%)	amplitude
normal infants	4.6 ± 3.6	7.5 ± 2.6	3.2 ± 1.4	10.7 ± 9.3	8.8 ± 6.5	21.5 ± 10.5	7.2 ± 5.6	5.0 ± 3.2
group AV	5.4 ± 2.3	6.2 ± 3.0	2.4 ±1.1	8.3 ± 15.7	7.8 ± 3.3	16.2 ± 3.4	12.6 ± 6.3	3.5 ± 1.8
group PR	6.7 ± 3.8	10.9 ± 3.7	4.5 ± 1.6	28.2 ±16.9	12.7 ± 6.9	27.9 ± 13.2	37.8 ± 28.5	10.1 ± 5.5
p values [1]	NS	**	**	**	*	*	**	*
group SF	3.9 ± 2.4	5.6 ± 1.8	1.9 ± 0.5	0.8 ± 1.9	4.0 ± 0.5	11.0 ± 1.5	4.0 ± 2.3	2.6 ± 1.2
group SD	8.1 ± 4.3	10.4 ± 3.5	4.6 ± 1.8	18.6 ± 16.8	11.8 ± 7.3	29.7 ± 8.4	43.4 ± 14.3	8.9 ± 1.7
p values [2]	NS	NS	*	**	*	*	**	*

Kruskal-Wallis test for statistical significance: NS not significant * $p<0.05$ ** $p<0.01$

[1] between normal infants and infants with *a vacuo* and progressive hydrocephalus

[2] between normal infants and infants with well-functioning and dysfunctioning VPD

DISCUSSION

Our study is based on a reliable transfontanellar device [3]. Our data confirmed previous studies which reported that ICP monitoring may provide helpful information for the differentiation of progressive and *a vacuo* hydrocephalus [1] and for the evaluation of the VPD function [4]. As reported increased ICP is inconstant in progressive hydrocephalus. Many neurosurgeons based their intervention on the occurrence of "high" amplitude pressure waves. Because of the increasing values of the AFP variables with age and the physiological occurrence of both PW and BW [3], interpretation of the recordings must take into account the age of the patient and the characteristics of PW and BW in normal infants. Nevertheless AFP monitoring is in our experience a valuable technique for the evaluation of hydrocephalus and VPD function.

Acknowledgement: This work was supported by a grant of the Foundation Lekime Ropsy

REFERENCES

1. Gaab M, Koos Th (1984) Hydrocephalus in infancy and childhood: diagnosis and indication for operation: Neuropediatr 15;173-179

2. de Jong DA, Maas A, van de Voort E (1984) Non-invasive intracranial pressure monitoring. A technique for reproducible fontanelle pressure measurements. Z Kinderchir 39:274-276

3. Wayenberg JL, Raftopoulos C, Vermeylen D, Pardou A (1993) Non invasive intracranial pressure monitoring in neonates and infants: the Rotterdam Teletransducer. Arch Dis Child 69:493-497

4. Longatti P, Scanarini M, Gerosa M, Ori C, Carteri A (1982) ICP monitoring and function of CSF shunts. In: Paraicz E (ed) ICP in infancy and childhood. Karger. Basel, pp 144-146 (Monographs in Paediatrics vol 15)

Anterior Fontanelle Pressure Variations During Sleep in Healthy Infants

J.-L. Wayenberg[1], D. Hasaerts[1], P. Franco[2], F. Valente[3], and N. Massager[4]

[1] Department of Paediatrics, Hôpital Français-Reine Elisabeth, 180 av. JJ Goffin, B-1080 Brussels, Belgium
[2] Neonatal Intensive Care Unit, Hôpital Universitaire Erasme, 808 route de Lennik, B-1070 Brussels, Belgium
[3] Laboratory of Medical Statistics, Public Health School, [4] Faculty of Medicine, Université Libre de Bruxelles, route de Lennik, B-1070 Brussels, Belgium

SUMMARY

Our aim was to study the intracranial pressure (ICP) variations during sleep in normal infants. Using a non invasive method ICP was measured continuously during polysomnography in twelve healthy infants. We analysed the variations of mean basal ICP, mean basal pulse pressure amplitude and maximal amplitude of both plateau and B-like waves between quiet sleep 1-3 and rapid eye movement (REM) stages. Mean ICP, mean pulse pressure amplitude and B-like waves amplitude increased significantly during stage 1 and REM sleep. Plateau waves occurred exclusively during quiet 1 and REM sleep. These physiological features must be known in order to allow a correct interpretation of continuous ICP measurements in infants.

INTRODUCTION

There are very few studies of ICP patterns in normal individuals because they required invasive procedures. In the young infant non invasive ICP monitoring is now possible throughout the open fontanelle [1]. Such methods permit a new approach of the physiology of the ICP in the young infant. Our aim was to study the variations of non invasive ICP between the sleep stages in normal infants.

PATIENTS and METHODS

Twelve healthy infants aged from 1 to 12 months (median 4.5 months) were studied during a 10 hours night monitoring session of a research program on infant's sleep [2]. Six-channels electroencephalogram, right and left electro-oculograms, thoracic ampliation, electrocardiogram and anterior fontanelle pressure (AFP) were simultaneously recorded. AFP was measured by means of the Rotterdam transducer [1], a device that give reliable results and high quality charts [3]. The recordings were classified into awakening, quiet sleep 1 to 4, rapid eye movement (REM) sleep, movements and undetermined sleep according to the data of the literature [4]. We calculated mean AFP and mean cerebral pulse amplitude (CPA) during each sleep stage and noted the maximal diastolo-diastolic pressure wave amplitude of both plateau waves and B-like waves. Using Friedman's test we compared these variables between quiet 1-3 and REM stages.

RESULTS

73.6 hours were available for the study (mean 368 min per infant, extremes 228-583 min). All AFP variables increased significantly in quiet sleep 1 and REM sleep (Fig. 1). Plateau waves and sharp-pointed B-like waves were observed during quiet sleep 1, especially when the infant was falling asleep, and during REM sleep. Plateau waves occuped frequently the whole REM periods. During quiet sleep stages 2 and 3 the AFP traces were relatively flat, showing only small rounded pressure waves.

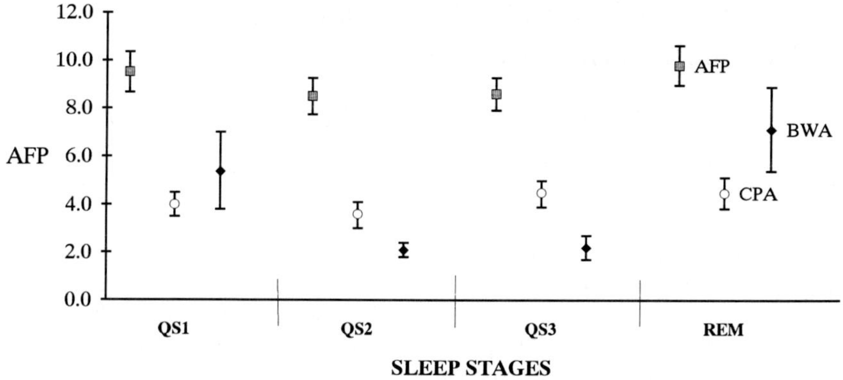

Fig. 1: mean AFP, mean CPA and maximal B-like wave amplitude (BWA) during quiet (QS) and REM sleep (mean ± standard error, in mm Hg)

DISCUSSION

This study confirms in healthy infants the presence of the sleep AFP variations previously observed in infants with hydrocephalus [5]. These variations may be explained by cerebral metabolism and blood flow variations between the sleep stages [6]. Plateau waves have been demonstrated to be related with cerebral blood volume increases in hydrocephalic infants [7] and doppler studies in adults with head trauma demonstrated the association between B waves and variations of the cerebral blood flow [8]. The same pattern of cerebral blood flow velocity variations was observed in healthy adults, suggesting the physiological occurrence of B waves [9]. In contrast plateau waves were never reported before in normal individuals. Our data may have important clinical implications: the normal occurrence of pressure waves must be kept in mind during the interpretation of ICP traces in infants and, in order to provide helpful information, a continuous sleep recording is needed in clinical practice.

Acknowledgement: This work was supported by a grant of the Foundation Lekime Ropsy

REFERENCES

1. de Jong DA, Maas A, van de Voort E (1984) Non-invasive intracranial pressure monitoring. A technique for reproducible fontanelle pressure measurements. Z Kinderchir 39:274-276

2. Kahn A, Grosswasser J, Rebuffat E, Sottiaux M, Blum D, Foerster M, Franco P, Bochner A, Alexander M, Bachy A, Richard P, Verghote M, Le Polain D, Wayenberg J-L (1992) Sleep and cardiorespiratory characteristics of infants victims of sudden death. Sleep 15:287-292

3. Wayenberg JL, Raftopoulos C, Vermeylen D, Pardou A (1993) Non invasive ICP monitoring in neonates and infants: the Rotterdam Teletransducer. Arch Dis Child 69:493-497

4. Tharp B (1984) Neonatal and pediatric EEG. In: Aminoff M (ed) Electrodiagnosis in clinical neurology. Churchill. New-York. pp 101-105

5. Pierre-Kahn A, Gabersek V, Hirsch J-F (1976) ICP and REM sleep in hydrocephalus. Child's Brain 2:156-166

6. Mises J, Gabersek V, Lacombe J (1979) Polygraphie du sommeil avec enregistrement de la PIC et mesure du volume sanguin cérébral chez le nourrisson hydrocéphale. Rev EEG Neurophysiol 9:228-235

7. Madsen PL, Schmidt JF, Wildschiodz G, Friberg L, Holm S, Vorstrup S, Lassen NA (1991) Cerebral O2 metabolism and cerebral blood flow in humans during deep and REM sleep. J Appl Physiol 70:2597-2601

8. Newell DW, Aaslid R, Stoos R, Reulen HJ (1992) The relationship of blood flow velocity fluctuations to intracranial pressure B waves. J Neurosurg 76:415-421

9. Mautner-Huppert D, Haberl R, Dirnagl U, Villringer A, Schmiedek P, Einhaupl K (1989) B- waves in healthy persons. Neurol Res 11:194-196

Changes in EDP, EEG and rCBF Following Cerebral Embolism in Rats

Yoshikazu Okada, Takeshi Shima, Tetsuji Takeda, and Kanji Yamane

Department of Neurosurgery, Chugoku Rousai Hospital, Japan

Introduction: Intracranial main cerebral artery embolism has been known to deliver serious ischemic brain damage with massive brain swelling (1,2), and has been required to clarify the relationships between the increase in intracranial pressure, the decrease in regional cerebral blood flow (rCBF) and the impairement of cerebral functions. While intracranial pressure monitoring should be prerequisite for these studies, lately the small animal models have been required to make experimental studies. We have developed the rat main cerebral artery embolization model whose clinicopathological findings closely resemble those in human (3), and have designed microballoon system to measure changes in epidural pressure (EDP) (4). The purpose of this study is to investigate relationships between epidural pressure (EDP), electrocorticography (ECoG) and (rCBF in our rat embolization model.

Material and Method: Embolization model was made by a silicone cylinder (400 or 500 μ m in diameter and 1 mm in length) injection into the rat internal carotid artery. The head was fixed in a stereotaxic apparatus to apply ECoG electrodes, rCBF sensors and an apparatus for EDP measurement. EDP was recorded with our specially designed microballoon system, which was demonstrated to be closely related with the intracranial pressure rainging 0 to 70 mmHg (4). A small burr hole was made at the parietal region of the embolized side and a microballoon was placed on the dura with a stereotaxic apparatus, and the system was opened to the air to establish the zero point. Embolization was performed after obtaining stable EDP recording of the zero point. The rCBF was measured at the bilateral basal ganglias with hydrogen clearance method, in which hydorgen gas was generated electrolytically. Two channels of raw ECoG were recorded from cortical electrodes symmetrically placed on the dura at the parietal regions. Variables were monitored within 5 hours after embolization and then the brains were removed to ascertain the embolized sites. Data were analyzed from the animals embolized at the intracranial internal carotid artery.

Results: Microballoon system could be used to monitor EDP for 5 hours following embolization. EDP, systemic arterial blood pressure (SABP) and ECoG demonstrated variable changes such as rapid increase in EDP with progressively flattening of ECoG (Fig. 1).

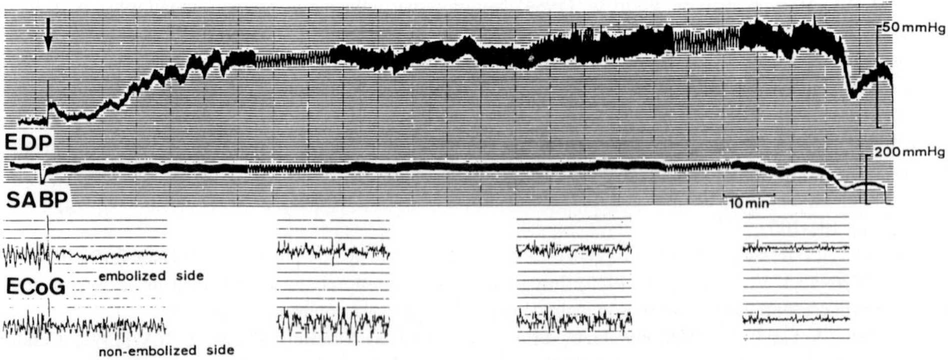

Fig. 1: A representative recording of ICP, SABP and ECoG following embolization. EDP rapidly increases after embolization (arrow) and drastically decreases at 3 hours with changes in ECoG into flat pattern. suggesting cerebral herniation.

Relationship between EDP and ECoG: In 400 μ m embolus group, EDP was measured in 10 animals and the mean EDP rose 12.3 ± 6.3 (± SD), 17.9 12.4, 20.4 ± 15.2 mmHg at 30 min, 1, 2 and 3 hours embolization, respectively. ECoG changes into the flat pattern, defined as the ECoG amplitude declined to less than 30% of the control ECoG amplitude, could be seen in the 2 rats after 3 hours embolization. In 500 μ m embolus group, EDP was measured in 13 rats. The rats demonstrated serious increase in EDP and mean EDP was 28.5 ± 10.4, 38.0 ± 8.0 and 47.4 ± 9.7 mmHg at 30 min, 1 and 2 hours embolization, respectively. ECoG changed into the flat pattern in 10 of 12 rats with prominent increases in EDP, which suggested cerebral hermination. The mean EDP value in the rats presenting with the flat pattern of ECoG was 51.2 ± 9.1 mmHg.

Relationship between rCBF and ECoG (Fig.2): In the 9 rats embolized within 400 μ m embolus, rCBF value at the control state, 49.1 ± 4.0 ml/100g/min, decreased significantly to 28.0 ± 3.6 ml/100g/min at 30 min which was kept constantly by 5 hours. In the 8 rats embolized with 500 μ m embolus, rCBF decreased from 47.5 ± 7.0 to 26.5 ± 4.2 ml/100g/min at 30 min which continued to decline within 3 hours. Mean rCBF value in the rats showing the flat pattern of ECoG was 18.3 ± 2.8 ml/100g/min.

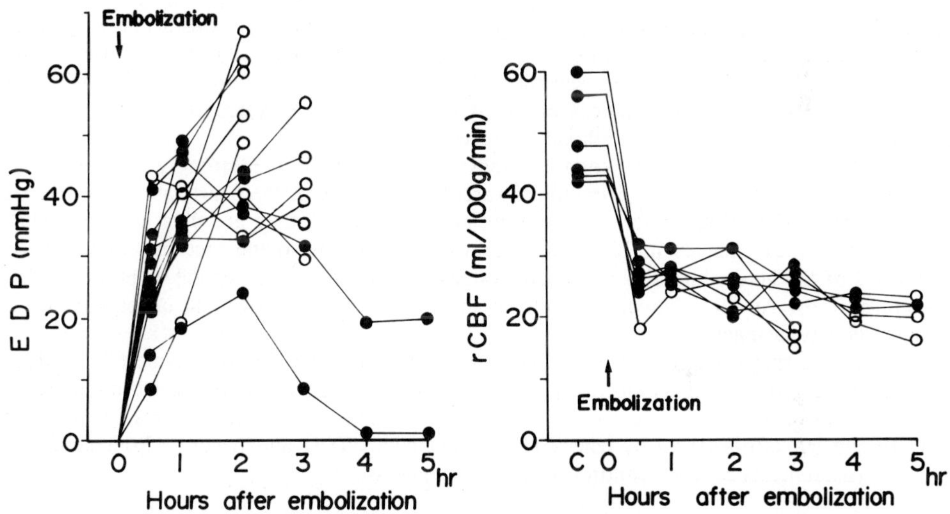

Fig 2: Changes in EDP, rCBF by hydrogen clearance and ECoG following embolization with 500 μ m embolus. Open circles indicate ECoG changes into flat pattern.

Conclusion: The rat embolization model demonstrated drastic changes in EDP, rCBF and ECoG following main cerebral artery occlusion. In the rats showing flat pattern of ECoG, EDP progressively rose to 51 mmHg and mean rCBF decreased to 18 ml/100g/min within 1-3 hours embolization. These data suggested that our rat embolization model and microballoon system would be available to clarify critical values of pathophysiological parameters in acute brain swelling due to cerebral embolism.

References

1. Shaw CM, Alvord ECJr, Berry RG (1959) Arch Neurol 1: 161-177
2. Okada Y, Shima T, Yamamoto M, et al (1983) J. Neurosurg 58: 500-507
3. Okada Y, SHima T, Ohta K, et al (1987) in J. Cerebos-Navarro and R. Ferszt (eds), Raven Press PP 101-105
4. Yamane K, Shima T, Okada Y, et al (1994) Surg Neurol 41: -in press-

Monitoring Intracranial Dynamics by Transcranial Doppler. A New Doppler Index: Trans Systolic Time

P.W. Hanlo[1], R.J.A. Peters[2], R.H.J.M. Gooskens[3], R.M. Heethaar[4], R.W.M. Keunen[5], A.C. van Huffelen[6], C.A.F. Tulleken[1], and J. Willemse[3]

[1] Departments of Neurosurgery, [3] ChildNeurology, [6] Clinical Neurophysiology, University Hospital Utrecht, Box 85500, 3508 GA Utrecht, The Netherlands
[2] Departments of Biomedical Engineering, [4] Medical Physics, Free University Hospital, Amsterdam, The Netherlands
[5] Department of Neurology and Clinical Neurophysiology, Leyenburg Hospital, The Hague, The Netherlands

INTRODUCTION

Since the introduction of Transcranial Doppler sonography (TCD), several investigators have described the relationship between raised intracranial pressure (ICP) and Doppler waveform. This waveform has been expressed in several indices, such as the Pulsatility Index (PI) and the Resistance Index (RI). These indices are used to demonstrate elevated ICP and to indicate the need for shunt-implantation in childhood hydrocephalus.
PI and RI, however, do have certain disadvantages as both are strongly influenced by the hemodynamic properties of the extracranial vascular system, e.g. the heart rate. Both indices also have a broad range of reference values, especially in children, they are thus not very reliable in detecting insidious changes in ICP. These drawbacks are due to the fact that these indices are composed of the actual blood flow velocity values and do not encounter the slope of the Doppler waveform itself. An ideal Doppler waveform analysis should be performed in respect of the time related velocity changes.
The aim of the study is to define a new Doppler index, the Trans Systolic Time (TST), through a hydrodynamic model, and its electrical analogon. The TST should reflect specific changes in the TCD waveform induced by changes in the mean ICP. The applicability of this index, compared with PI and RI, is illustrated by consecutive simultaneous TCD and Anterior Fontanelle Pressure (AFP) measurements in three children with hydrocephalus.

MATERIALS AND METHODS

Using the information obtained from a hydrodynamic model of the intracranial system and its electrical analogon, a mathematical description of the TST envelope, which formed the basis of the TST, was derived.
To investigate the applicability of the TST in clinical practice, pre- and postoperative TCD recordings in hydrocephalic patients were analyzed. All of the TCD recordings were carried out over a period of at least one hour, using a 2 Mhz pulsed Doppler instrument (TC-2-64B, EME, Germany). The middle cerebral artery, opposite to the side of the shunt was chosen and insonated according to the Aaslid technique. The TST for each single measurement was calculated, measuring the width of the systolic peak at the level of Vtst (Vtst= Vpeaksystolic + Venddiastolic/2) (Fig 1).

Non-invasive AFP measurements, using the Rotterdam teletransducer, were carried out simultaneously. The TCD and AFP measurements were averaged over the measurement. The mean Doppler indices and AFP values were subjected to pre- and postshunt comparison.

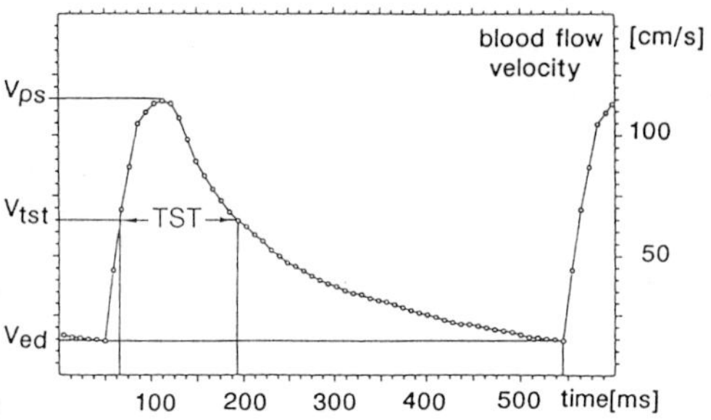

Fig. 1 Single Measurement of TST

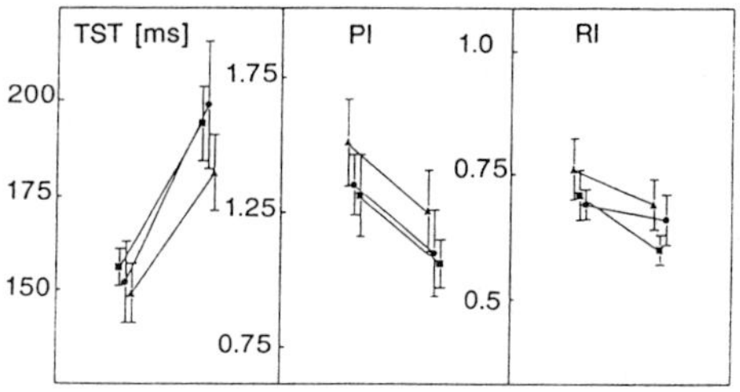

Fig.2 Three pre- and postoperative TCD and AFP measurements

RESULTS

Three pre- and postoperative TCD and AFP measurements were analyzed, covering a total of 819 pre-operative and 804 post-operative cardiac cycles, respectively. There was a significant decrease in AFP (respectively 54%, 48% and 67%) after shunt implantation. Post-operatively, the TST increased by 31%, 21% and 24% respectively; PI decreased by 18%, 17% and 18%, and RI decreased by 4%, 9% and 15% (Fig 2).

CONCLUSIONS

The present study focuses on the use of TCD in evaluating the effect of elevated ICP on cerebral hemodynamics in childhood hydrocephalus. Several methods for interpreting the Doppler signal are described, the ones most commonly used being PI and RI. There is, as yet, no consensus concerning these Doppler indices in relation to intracranial pressure. Variations in PI and RI occur as a result of the different states of the infant during measurements. These effects on the Doppler waveform, induced by both intracranial and extracranial factors, alter the actual values of the blood flow velocities. For these reasons, therefore, a new Doppler index has been developed, namely the Trans Systolic Time (TST). Because this TST is a time-related index, it provides a simple method of waveform analysis.

The TST value is strongly related to the Doppler envelope, the down-stroke changes in particular. Mathematically, it can be concluded that the shape of the down-stroke curve is mainly determined by the cerebrovascular resistance. Compression of the venous vascular system, induced by increased ICP, results in a decrease of TST. This is illustrated by clinical observations in hydrocephalic children. TST increases significantly with a decrease in ICP after shunting. The TST was also found to be less influenced by incidental pressure fluctuations than PI and RI within a single measurement.

Compared with PI and RI, therefore the TST provides a more specific reflection of the physical properties of the intracranial system.

Does ICP Monitoring Indicate the Delayed Appearance of Traumatic Intracerebral Hematoma?

S. Kobayashi[1], H. Yokota[2], and S. Nakazawa[1]

[1] Department of Neurosurgery, Nippon Medical School, Tokyo, 113 Japan
[2] Department of Critical Care Medicine, Nippon Medical School, Tokyo, 113 Japan

INTRODUCTION

Defining intracerebral hematomas which can be confirmed by serial CT scanning (SCT) after head injury as CT diagnosed traumatic intracerebral hematomas (CTD. DTICH) [1, 2], we have conducted extensive studies on the condition. The value intracranial pressure (ICP) in predicting the development of CTD. DTICH was evaluated in patients having impaired consciousness following severe head injury.

MATERIALS AND METHODS

Of patients admitted with severe head injury to our hospital during the past 4 years, included in this study were 17 in whom the diagnosis of CTD. DTICH was established by SCT and data from the first CT study performed within 24 hours injury and ICP monitoring were available. In all patients in whom ICP was monitored an endotracheal tube was introduced and hyperventilated by a controlled amount to achieve a blood $PaCO_2$ of approximately 25 to 30mmHg at the onset of the monitoring. The outcome was determined based on Glasgow Outcome Scale at discharge.

RESULTS AND DISCUSSION

The ICP upon admission was divided into 4 types as follows; ICP 0–10mmHg (4 cases), ICP 11–20mmHg (5 cases), ICP 21–40mmHg (5 cases) and ICP over 41 mmHg (3 cases). The patients were classified by ICP monitoring (Fig. 1).

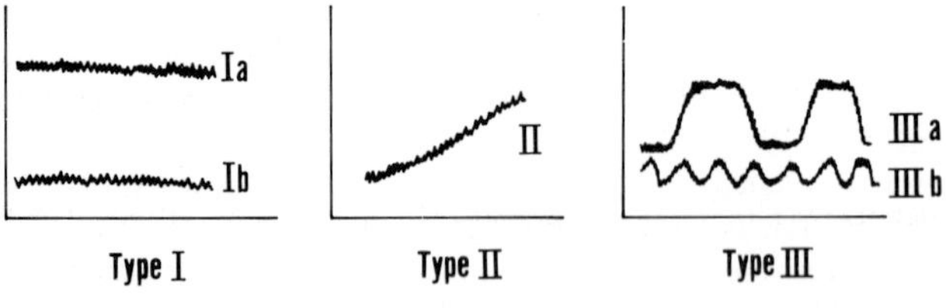

Fig. 1 The ICP course in CT diagnosed delayed traumatic intracerebral hematoma.

Namely, ICP remained practically unchanged at the level around as high as 50mmHg in 3 (Type Ia) and around 20mmHg in 2 (Type Ib). ICP showed gradual elevation in 3 (Type II) . ICP monitoring revealed pressure A wave in 6 (Type IIIa) and B wave in 3 (Type IIIb) (Fig. 2).

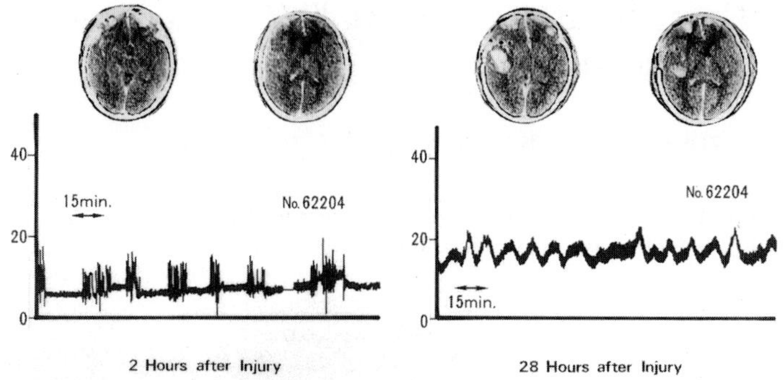

Fig. 2 54-year-old male. The ICP showing B wave 28 hrs after injury. At that time, serial CT scanning indicating development of CTD. DTICH in left temporal region.

The outcome was as follows : Type Ia (dead=3) , Type Ib (dead=1, GR=1) , Type II (dead=1, PVS=1, GR=1) , Type IIIa (dead=3, MD=1, GR=2) , and Type IIIb (dead=3).

The value of monitoring intracranial pressure in patients with severe head injuries has been well demonstrated [3, 4]. It indicates when serial CT scanning is necessary. A further CT scan made when the baseline of intracranial pressure rose and/or some kind of pressure wave appeared; in the present series, several delayed traumatic intracerebral hematomas were indicated with serial CT scanning at this time.

We conclude that the ICP type of CTD. DTICH after severe head injury was diverse, and the outcome of CTD. DTICH was not predictable by ICP types.

REFERENCES

1. Diaz FG, Yock DH Jr, Larson D, Rockswald GL (1979) Early diagnosis of delayed posttraumatic intracerebral hematomas. J Neurosurg 50 : 217-223

2. Stecen KG, Kishore PRS, Miller JD, Girevendlis AK, Maurice H, Lipper MB, Becker DP (1979) The genesis and significance of delayed traumatic intracerebral hematoma. Neurosurgery 5 : 309-313

3. Kobayashi, S, Nakazawa S, Yano Y, Otsuka T (1983) The value of intracranial pressure (ICP) measurement in scute severe head injury showing diffuse cerebral. In : Ishii S, Nagai H, Brock M (eds) Intracranial Pressure V. Springer-Verlag, Berlin, pp527-531

4. Dearden NM, Miller JD (1989) Paired comparison of hypnotic and osmotic therapy in the reduction of intracranial hypertension after severe head injury, In : Hoff JT, Betz AL (eds) Intracranial Pressure VII. Springer-Verlag, Berlin, pp474-481

Improving Compensatory Reserve by Craniectomy and Dural Scarification

D.J. Price[1], Z. Czosnyka[2], G. Kotas[1], and M. Czosnyka[2]

[1] Neurosurgical Department, Pinderfields Hospital, Wakefield, UK
[2] Neurosurgery Unit, Addenbrooke's Hospital, Cambridge, UK

INTRODUCTION

Over the years, decompressive craniotomy for refractory post-traumatic intracranial hypertension has been controversial. Removal of a large bone flap is often insufficient to be effective and opening the dura results in cerebral herniation with infarction of potentially viable brain tissue.

In the last year, five patients with severe head injured had developed persistent falls in cerebral perfusion pressure below 50mmHg despite ventricular drainage, mild hypocapnoea, Mannitol, Propofol and arterial pressure support. In desperation, large unilateral or bilateral craniotomy flaps were turned. In the first 2 patients, the intracranial pressure remained high and dural compliance was increased by superficial scarification of the outer layer of the dura in a criss-cross fashion to release the fibrous lattice and allow the dura to herniate further under pressure. Following this procedure in the other three patients, perfusion pressures of above 70mmHg were easily achieved. All 5 patients recovered and 4 had only minimal residual disabilities. It is naive to presume that this simple surgical procedure contributed to their good recovery but the dramatic effect on the mean ICP and CPP warranted further investigation.

METHOD

The opening of a fluid filled vessel was occluded with human dura and an underlying layer of clingfilm was necessary to ensure that the system was watertight. A wave-form generator, infusion pump transducer and a thin needle to create a constant outflow resistance were connected (Fig. 1). A series of infusions at 0.2, 0.3 and 0.5 mls per minute were made and the signal from the pressure transducer was processed in a microcomputer. A Fast Fourier Transform was used to measure the amplitude of the wave-form.

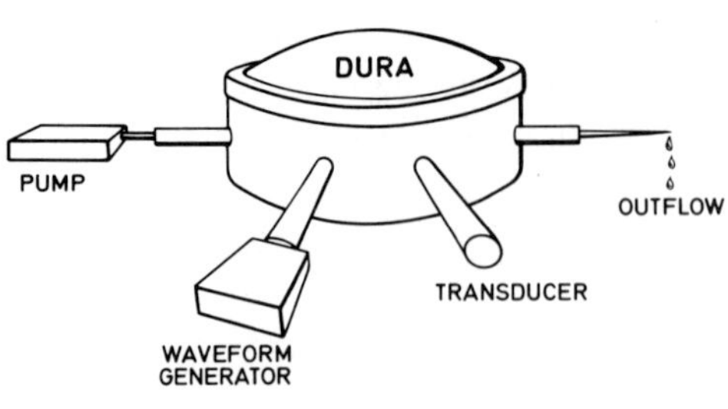

Fig. 1 Diagram of the experimental model to measure Pressure Volume Index

RESULTS

When the dura was covered with a tin lid to simulate an intact cranium, the amplitude was high at approximately 20mmHg. The pressure rose rapidly with each infusion and the pressure-volume index proved to be as expected low (0.2 ml). When the lid was removed, the amplitude fell to 10mmHg and the rise with each infusion was slower and the PVI was 0.46 mls. After scarification, the amplitude fell below 10mmHg and the rise in ICP in each infusion was more sluggish with the PVI rising to 0.7 ml. The results are summarised in figs. 2 and 3.

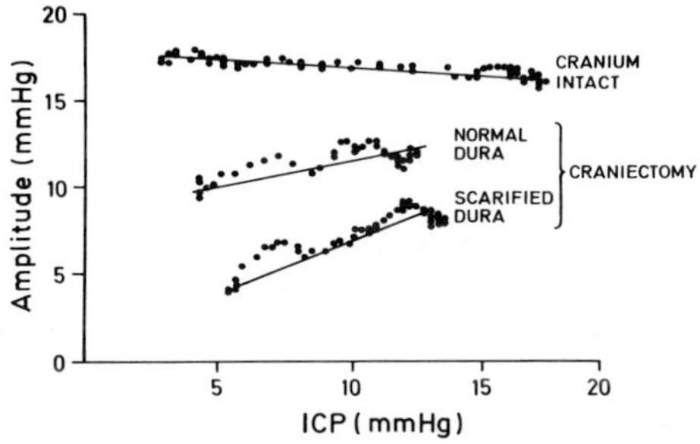

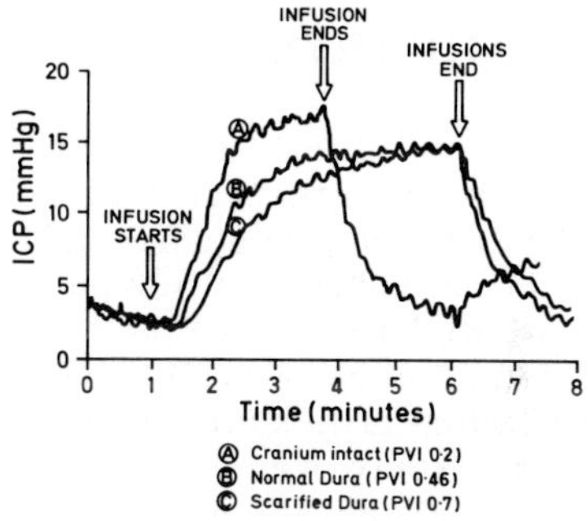

Figs. 2 and 3 Changes in Pulse Wave Amplitude and Pressure Volume Index with surgical modification of the dura.

DISCUSSION

When Yamaura reviewed retrospectively a series of 207 patients who were treated with a large craniectomy over the maximal cerebral contusion, he came to the conclusion that this method of decompression is indispensable provided it is carried out promptly. The dura was opened widely but some critics were concerned about the infarction of potentially viable brain tissue at the dural opening. Enthusiasm for craniectomy has more recently been revived with the life saving effects for patients with cerebral and cerebellar infarcts. At the last intracranial pressure symposium, Anile presented a small retrospective series of head injuries. All those with an ICP above 40 mmHg within the first 24 hours who did not have a decompressive craniotomy perished but in the group with the same severity of intracranial hypertension and an external decompression, 35% survived and of these, 67% made a good recovery.

CONCLUSIONS

For those patients with severe post traumatic hypertension with compromised cerebral perfusion, craniectomy may well be beneficial. Scarification of the dura appears to enhance the decompression.

Changes and Pathological Significance of Early Responses of Direct Cortical Response (DCR) in Brain Injury

M. NISHIKATA[1], S. ENDO[1], N. HAYASHI[1], K. YAMATANI[2], and A. TAKAKU[1]

[1] Department of Neurosurgery, Toyama Medical and Pharmaceutical University, Sugitani, Toyama, Toyama, 930-01 Japan
[2] Department of Neurosurgery, Toyama Red Cross Hospital, Higashidenjigata-cho, Toyama, Toyama, 930 Japan

INTRODUCTION

Since Adrian et al. reported the direct cortical responses(DCR) in 1936, DCR have been used to study the cortical function. Four typical waves of DCR are recognized,P1,N1, P2, and N2. In the past studies, a N2 component recorded at about 10 msec after stimulation, called as dendritic potential (DP), mainly has been investigated. On the other side, we have noticed the earlier components of P1 and P2 which have the latency range within 5 msec (we call them as the early potentials : EPs). Recording and characterization of EPs are difficult, because they are largely influenced by DP. In this experimental study, we examined the proper condition to record EPs without influence of DP. The pathophysiological analysis of EPs under the local brain compression are also investigated.

MATERIALS AND METHODS

Six adult dogs, weighted about 10 kg, were premedicated with atropine (0.03mg/kg) and ketamine (25-35mg/kg) IM. Femoral venous and arterial catheters were placed and blood pressure was continuously monitored with intermittent analysis of arterial blood gases. Body temperature was measured with a rectal probe and kept near 37℃ with a warming pad. Endotracheal intubation was performed and thiopental sodium (2-5mg/kg) and pancronium bromide (0.05mg/kg) as required. Respiration was regulated to maintain a $PaCO_2$ of 35-40 torr.

After craniotomy, a silastic leaflet embedded 1mm gold ball electrode was placed over the post crucinate gyrus. This leaflet is constructed such that two stimulating electrodes are placed 1 mm apart and the recording electrode is placed 3 mm distant on the isoelectric line. A platinum disk electrode was placed in the ipsilateral temporalis muscle to serve as a reference. To record the DCR, stimuli were given as 5-8mAmp square waves pulses of 0. 1 msec duration.

Experimental I : Recording of EPs; To eliminate the DP, the conditions associated with recording EPs were examined, changing the time constant. Further more, the polarity of stimuli was changed every 10 times, and EPs were added 20 times in total. For the purpose of reproduction of EPs, each recording was repeated 5 times, and the values were averaged.

Experimental II : Change of EPs under the local cerebral compression; Local cerebral compression was done by the glass column with a weight of 50g/cm^2 (36.2mmHg) and 100g/cm^2(72.5mmHg), and serial change of EPs was compared with the pathological findings. The period of brain compression was 1 hour, and after decompression, the DCR was recorded until 2 hours. Just before the end of each study, evans blue was injected intravenously, and the pathological study of brain damage were performed.

RESULTS

Experimental I. Recording of EPs; Each component of DCR changed according to the different time constant from 0.3 sec to 0.8 msec (low cut filter change 0.5-200Hz). When the time constant was 0.8 msec (low cut filter 200Hz), the DP disappeared, and the EPs could be recorded obviously. Under this recording condition, the EPs were divided into two components : P1 with about 1.8 msec latency and P2 with about 3.0 msec latency. The following examinations were performed under this condition.

Experimental II. Change of EPs under the local cerebral compression; The 6 cases were divided into two groups according to the pathological findings : 4 cases of macroscopically no damage of the brain (3 cases of 50g compression and 1 case of 100g compression), and 2 cases of subcortical bleeding (100g compression)

In the group with no pathological findings, the EPs changes showed various patterns during local cerebral compression;1) both P1 and P2 did not disappear, 2) only P1 remained and P2 disappeared, 3) both P1 and P2 disappeared. Howevere all of them recovered immediately after decompression .

In the two cases with subcortical bleeding, the EPs changes showed the different patterns;1)both waves disappeared,2) P1 remained but amplitude decresed and P2 disappeared. After decompression, changes of P1 recovered immediately, but that of P2 did not.

CONCLUSION

We established the recording condition of ERs without influence of DP. We also found that disappearance of P2 of ERs was related to the subcortical damages under local brain compression. P2 may indicate the subcortical function and be one of the intraoperative monitoring of subcortical damages.

REFERENCES

1. Adrian ED (1936) The spread of activity in the cerebral cortex. J.Physiol 88:127-167
2. Chang HT (1951) Dendritic potential of cortical neurons produced by direct electrical stimulation of the cerebral cortex. J.Neurophysiol 14:1-21
3. Eisenberg HM, Turner JW, Teasdale G, Rowan J, Feinstein R, Grossman RG (1979) Monitoring of cortical excitability during induced hypotention in aneurysm operation. J.Neurosurg 50:592-602

Complications of Ventricular Fluid Pressure Monitoring—A 2 Year Prospective Study

J. PIEK

Neurochirurgische Universitätsklinik, Moorenstr. 5, 40225 Düsseldorf, Germany

INTRODUCTION

Following the fundamental work of Adson and Lillie [1], Guillaume and Janny [2], and Lundberg [3] continuous monitoring of intracranial pressure (ICP) has become a routine method in most neurosurgical units. Numerous epidural, subdural, and intraparenchymatous [Literature in 4] devices have been developed, but monitoring of ventricular fluid pressure (VFP) still remains the "gold standard" [5] of ICP recording.
To evaluate the complications of VFP monitoring we prospectively studied all patients with spontaneous intracranial haemorrhages and head injuries who underwent VFP monitoring during a period of 2 years (1991 - 1992).

PATIENT GROUP

53 of total 237 patients with head injuries and 68 of total 185 patients with spontaneous haemorrhages of different severity were studied (patient data in Tabel 1).

Table 1: Patient data

	Spontaneous Haemorrhage	Head Injury
Patient Number	68	53
Age, mean (years)	49.1 (8.7 - 74.9)	38.5 (2.2 - 75.3)
med. (years)	49.0	37.8
Sex (male/female)	48/20	27/26
Recording time, mean (days)	7.57 (1 - 27)	6.16 (1-21)
med. (days)	5.5	5.0
Ventilated	65 patients	52 patients
Mannitol therapy	47.05 %	67.92 %
THAM therapy	29.41 %	49.05 %
High-dose barbiturate therapy	48.52%	81.13 %
Etiology/Pathology	42 aneurysms	4 3 haematomas
	2 angiomas	10 2 haematomas
	2 coagulopathy	2 epidural haematoma
	4 hypertension	9 subdural haematoma
	18 other/unknown	3 intracerebral haematoma evacuated

PROTOCOL AND DEFINITIONS

In the O.R. VFP monitoring was installed via a routine right frontal burr-hole. The disposible monitoring and drainage system was connected under sterile conditions. In the ICU it was only opened once daily to withdraw CSF for cell count or bacteriological analysis. No routine antibiotics were used. Each day a wound dressing was performed without the use of antiseptics. From day 3 on daily analysis of CSF protein and cell count was performed. In cases of CSF cell count > 100/3 cells additional bacteriological examination of CSF was done. At the end of the monitoring period all ventricular catheters were examinated for bacteriological contamination.

RESULTS AND DISCUSSION

Monitoring time varied from 1 - 27 days with a mean of 7.57 days (haemorrhage group), and from 1 - 21 days (mean 6.16 days) in the trauma group respectively.

A detailed information of all complications is given in *Table 2*. 4.9% of all patients showed intracerebral haemorrhages (< 0.5 cm in diameter) in the routine control CT scan, but only 1 patient developed a large haematoma due to pneumonia, sepsis and consecutive coagulopathy on the 7th day of monitoring (initial CT scan without haematoma). Although 98.34% of all patients had CSF cell counts > 100/3 cells, and another 14,05% had bacterial contamination of the ventricular catheter at the end of the monitoring period, only 2 patients developed clinical signs of meningitis as defined by Mc Gee and Kaiser [6]. These patients had pre-existing traumatic rhinoliquorrhoea.

Table 2: Summary of all complications

Complication	Spontaneous haemorrhage	Head Injury
Subcortical haemorrhage (CT: < 0.5 cm diameter)	2	4
Haemorrhage (letal)	1 (patient with coagulopathy)	0
Meningitis	0	2 (both patients with CSF leak)
Contamination of catheter	9	7
CSF cell count > 100/3 cells	63	46
Catheter dislocation	4	3
Occlusion	4	2

Compared to other groups with long-time experiences in VFP monitoring (4% in Lund [7] and 4.23 % in Stochietti´s group (4.23 % [8]) the infection rate in the study group was remarkably low (1.65%). This was true although we examined each catheter removed from a patient as a routine test and bacteriological contamination was not an indication for antibiotic treatment in our patients. There was no correlation between high-dose thiopentone therapy and infection and/or contamination in the study group.

We did not find a correlation between underlying disease and infection rate like Sundbärg [7], but a correlation between bacteriological contamination and duration of monitoring was obvious: contamination was observed only in patients with recording times longer than 7 days.

Other complications were extremely rare: only 6 patients showed small (< 0.5 cm diameter) subcortical haemorrhages in the CT scan around the catheter inserted Only 1 massive bleeding was observed in a patient with initially normal CT scan who developed septicemia and disseminated intravascular coagulopathy 7 days after insertion of the ventricular bolt. Narrayan and coworkers [9] observed 1.4% haemorrhages in a group of 225 patients with head injuries and VFP monitoring, but 61 of their patients had initially normal CT scans.

Monitoring of VFP is cheap and reliable. Its further advantage is the possibility of draining CSF to control ICP. Compared to these advantages the low rate of complications (0.8% mortality, 1.65% infections, 4.9% small haematomas) is acceptable. The study shows that sterile handling of the systems and a strict protocol for inserting and maintaining VFP recordings can even further reduce infection rates without prophylactic use of antibiotics and antiseptics. VFP recordings longer than 7 days however should be avoided not to increase the rate of bacteriological contamination.

REFERENCES

1. Adson AW, Lillie WL (1927) The relationship of intracerebral pressure, choked disc, and intra-ocular tension. Trans Amer Acad Ophth Otolaryng 30: 138 - 154
2. Guillaume J, Janny P (1951) Manometrie intracranienne continue: interet de la methode et premiers resultats. Rev Neurol 84: 131 - 142
3. Lundberg N (1960) Continuous recording and control of ventricular fluid pressure in neurosurgical practice. Acta Psychiat Scand (Suppl 149) 36: 1 - 193
4. Gaab M (1980) Die Registrierung des intrakraniellen Druckes. Habilitationsschrift, Universität Würzburg
5. Miller JD (1989) Measuring ICP in patients - Its value now and in the future? In: Hoff JT, Betz AL (eds.) Intracranial Pressure VII. Springer, Berlin, Heidelberg, New York, pp 5 - 15
6. Mc Gee ZA, Kaiser AB (1985) Acute menigitis. In: Principles and practice of infectious diseases. J. Wiley and Sons, New York, pp 561 - 573
7. Sundbärg, G, Messeter K, Nordström CH (1986) Intracerebral versus intraventricular pressure recording. In: Miller JD, Teasdale GM, Rowan JO, Galbraith SL, Mendelow AD (eds) Intracranial Pressure VI. Springer, Berlin, Heidelberg, New York, pp 187 - 192
8. Stochetti N, Serioli T, Mergioni M (1989) Rate of infection and cost containment in intracranial pressure recording. In: Hoff JT, Betz AL (eds.) Intracranial Pressure VII. Springer, Berlin, Heidelberg, New York, pp 98 - 100
9. Narayan RK, Kishore PRS, Becker DP (1987) Intracranial pressure: to monitor or not to monitor? J Neurosurg 87: 144 - 149

Poster III: Biophysics I

Chairman: S. Kobayashi

Epidural Measurement of Intracranial Compliance by Means of High Frequency Centroid: Comparison to Intraventricular or Intraparenchymal Recordings

A. RAABE and J. SCHÖCHE

Neurosurgical Clinic, Flemmingstraße 2, 09116 Chemnitz, Germany

INTRODUCTION

Intracranial compliance is widely accepted as an earlier and more sensitive indicator of impending neurological deterioration due to cerebral edema or mass lesion than intracranial pressure (ICP) alone [1, 2, 3, 4].

Pressure volume index (PVI) with constant term (Po) correction is at present the most useful test for intracranial compliance assessment [5]. However, PVI measurement requires volumetric manipulation, increases the risk of infection and does not allow continuous monitoring. Moreover, epidural pressure measurement is preferred in many hospitals because of the fewer and less severe complications, which makes PVI assessment impossible.

In 1986 Bray et al. introduced the concept of estimating PVI by the high frequency centroid (HFC) and demonstrated a good correlation with PVI [6]. By Robertson et al. HFC was shown to be related to the outcome after severe head injury [7].

Although also HFC has several limitations, it would be attractive to test the reliability of the same technique in epidural pressure (EDP) measurement. Before useing HFC in epidural pressure measurement two questions should be answered:

1. is there a reliable linear correlation between epidural HFC (eHFC) and intraventricular or intraparenchymal HFC (iv/ipHFC)?
2. what happens to eHFC in case of faulty and thus misleading epidural pressure data, i.e. considerable differences between mean EDP and intraventricular (IVP) or intraparenchymal pressure (IPP), which might result in erroneous management decisions?

MATERIALS AND METHODS

Twenty patients of different intracranial pathology, admitted to the Neurosurgical Intensive Care Unit between March 1, 1993 and March 30, 1994 were included in this study. All fulfilled the following criteria:

1. simultaneous recordings of EDP and IVP or IPP,
2. to reduce the influence of physiological pressure gradients both sensors were placed supratentorial unilateral with a maximum distance of 6 cm ,
3. only monitoring systems with a flat frequency response up to 60 Hz were used.

After filtering at 25 Hz and analog to digital conversion wave form sampling was performed routinely at 60 Hz. Continuous pressure recordings were obtained by bedside computer systems creating one file every minute for signal analysis. As two pressures were measured simultaneously every minute one data pair of EDP and IVP or IPP was acquired. 1024 point FFT was used for transformation into the frequency domain and HFC calculation. HFC was calculated for each data pair as the amplitude weighted average frequency between 4 and 15 Hz [6, 8]. No HFC correction factor for the heart rate was applied.

In twenty patients a total of 490 hours of simultaneous EDP and IVP or IPP recordings were obtained. Duration varied from 1 hour to 6 days with a mean of 24,5 hours per patient. From this 29400 data pairs 2308 representative data pairs were used for analysis.

RESULTS

As demonstrated in fig. 1, regression analysis of the 2308 data pairs showed a linear correlation between EDP and IVP or IPP ($r=0.85$; $p<0.0001$), however, the slope of the regression line disclosed proportionallly higher EDP values (EDP=1.48 IVP/IPP - 8.90). Below 25 mm Hg, the relationship between EDP and IVP or IPP seems to be flatter and pressure values are more comparable (EDP=1.17 IVP/IPP - 4.17). At higher pressure values (>25 mm Hg) the slope is getting steeper (EDP=1.96 IVP/IPP - 23.35). This is a well known and reported phenomena in EDP measurement.
Regression analysis of eHFC and iv/ipHFC revealed a strong linear correlation ($r=0.95$; $p<0.00001$) even at pressures higher than 25 mm Hg, i.e. independent of the breakpoint in EDP-IVP/IPP relationship mentioned above (fig. 2).
65% of the values outside the 95% confidence interval of the eHFC-iv/ipHFC regression line came from only one patient. In this patient we observed periods of poor correlation between EDP and IPP (EDP=0.53 IPP + 1.40) with conspicuous overdamping of EDP waves. In those periods, eHFC was statistically significant lower than iv/ipHFC ($p<0.05$). 20% of the values outside the 95% confidence interval were observed at EDP values of less than 5 mm Hg, and the remaining 15% were seen during the first hour after implantation of the epidural pressure measuring device.

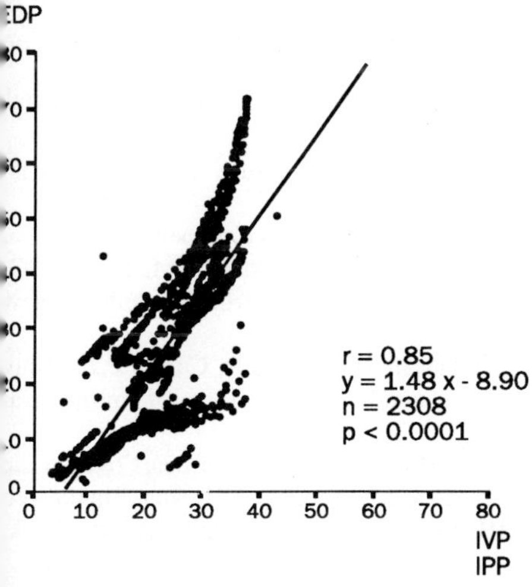

Fig. 1 Correlation of EDP and IVP or IPP

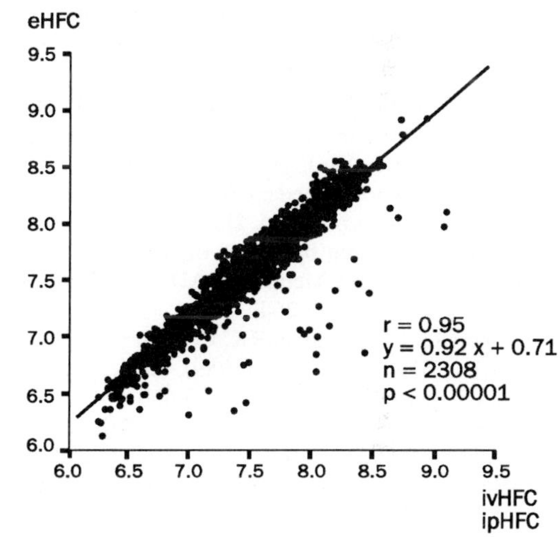

Fig. 2 Correlation of eHFC and iv/ipHFC

DISCUSSION

Despite of faulty EDP measurements defined as differences of more than 10 mm Hg between EDP and IVP or IPP there was a strong linear correlation of eHFC and iv/ipHFC. As HFC is calculated from the frequency domain it is expected to remain unaffected as long as only mean pressure variations occur. The same holds true in symmetrically pressure wave amplitude increase, which theoretically do not affect the amplitude weighted average frequency as the increase in power of the frequencies is proportional at the whole frequency domain. Signal independent mean pressure variations and symmetrically pressure wave amplitude increase could be expected in case of pressure offsets and/or vector forces.
In one patient, overdamping in EDP signal was observed. The statistically significant lower eHFC could be explained by disproportional larger decrease in the higher harmonics, that causes a shifting of the amplitude weighted average frequency to lower values.
The findings mentioned above support the hypothesis, that faulty epidural pressure recordings that might result in erroneous management decisions are probably due to:

1. offset pressures
2. vector forces
3. signal overdamping

From the data of this study we conclude, that epidural HFC measurement is as reliable as intraventricular or intraparenchymal HFC measurement. Only in overdamped signals, the epidural HFC is expected to be lower than the intraventricular or intraparenchymal HFC. We did not investigate, whether in fact the HFC could replace the PVI in early detection of reduced volume buffering capacity to identify those patients at risk for development of fulminant ICP increase. There should be more clinical studies to provide evidence of a correlation between HFC and PVI as well as HFC and the outcome in severe head injury. So we can confirm the reliability but not the validity of the concept of HFC in EDP measurement.

REFERENCES

1. Miller JD, Leech P (1975) Effects of mannitol and steroid therapy on intracranial volume-pressure relationships in patients. J Neurosurg 42:274-281
2. Shapiro K, Marmarou A (1982) Clinical applications of the pressure-volume index in treatment of pediatric head injuries. J Neurosurg 56:819-825
3. Sullivan HG, Miller JD, Becker DP, Flora RE, Allen GA (1977) The physiological basis of intracranial pressure change with progressive epidural brain compression. An experimental evaluation in cats. J Neurosurg 47:532-550
4. Tans JT, Poortvliet DC (1983) Intracranial volume-pressure relationship in man. Part 2: Clinical significance of the pressure-volume index. J Neurosurg 59:810-816
5. Avezaat CJJ, van-Eijndhoven JH (1984) Cerebrospinal fluid pulse pressure and craniospinal dynamics. A Jongbloed en Zoon, The Hague
6. Bray RS, Sherwood AM, Halter JA, Robertson C, Grossman RG (1986) Development of a clinical monitoring system by means of ICP wave form analysis. In: Miller JD, Teasdale GM, Rowan JO, Galbraith SL and Mendelow AD (eds) Intracranial Pressure VI. Springer. Berlin Heidelberg New York Tokyo. pp 260-264.
7. Robertson CS, Narayan RK, Contant CF, Grossman RG, Gokaslan ZL, Pahwa R, Caram P,Jr., Bray RS,Jr., Sherwood AM (1989) Clinical experience with a continuous monitor of intracranial compliance. J Neurosurg 71:673-680
8. Contant CF, Robertson CS, Narayan RK, Hayes C, Grossman RG (1993) Effects of heart rate on the shape of the intracranial pressure wave and related parameters. In: Avezaat CJJ, van Eijndhoven JHM, Maas AIR, Tans JTJ (eds) Intracranial pressure VIII. Springer. Berlin Heidelberg New York. pp 356-362

Fuzzy-Logic Based Pattern Classification for Identification of Potentially Misleading Data in Epidural Pressure Measurement

A. RAABE[1], N. BITTERLICH[2], R. TOTZAUER[2], S.F. BOCKLISCH[2], and J. SCHÖCHE[1]

[1] Neurosurgical Clinic, Flemmingstraße 2, 09116 Chemnitz, Germany
[2] Department of System Theory and Fuzzy Systems, Technical University Chemnitz, Reichenhainer Str. 70, 09126 Chemnitz, Germany

INTRODUCTION

Epidural pressure (EDP) measurement has always been an attractive alternative for pressure monitoring, because complications are much less severe than those of intraventricular (IVP) or intraparenchymal pressure (IPP) measurement. However this technique has not been universally accepted because it is often affected by unacceptable large differences between EDP and IVP or IPP [1, 2, 3]. So misleading EDP readings represents the main side effect with EDP measurement, because they may result in erroneous management decisions [4].
Until this time, efforts have concentrated in improving the transducer hardware, however the rate of faulty EDP measurements remains high. In a recent study, Aschoff et al. [5] investigated several highly sophisticated sensors and found faulty EDP recordings in 37% of all trials.
In this study we investigated the possibility of identifying faulty EDP readings by means of advanced forms of signal analysis of the epidural pulse pressure wave (EDPPW) and fuzzy pattern classification. Our hypothesis was that any disturbance leading to a deviation from the correct EDP does also cause changes in the signal of EDPPW. Thus the signal of a correct EDP recording (no difference to a reference pressure) was assumed to be different from the signal of a EDP recording with a remarkable (arbitrary defined) difference to a reference pressure. If that would be true, one could become suspicious of inaccurate EDP data without simultaneous measurement of any intradural pressure.

MATERIALS AND METHODS

Twenty-five patients of different intracranial pathology were included in this study. All fulfilled the following criteria:

1. simultaneous recordings of EDP and IVP or IPP,
2. to reduce the influence of physiological pressure gradients both sensors were placed supratentorial unilateral with a maximum distance of 6 cm,
3. only monitoring systems with a flat frequency response up to 60 Hz were used
4. to classify patterns of different quality of EDP measurement and not different patients at least 50% of all entered patients must be present for classification with periods of both correct and faulty EDP recordings.

After filtering at 25 Hz and analog to digital conversion wave form sampling was performed routinely at 60 Hz. In twenty-five patients a total of 490 hours of simultaneous EDP and IVP or IPP recordings were obtained. Duration varied from 5 minutes to 6 days with a mean of 21 hours per patient. 136 periods of EDP recording representative for steady state periods of one minute to twelve hours were chosen for signal analysis. 89 descriptors of the EDPPW were calculated, 66 from frequency domain and 23 from time domain. Thus every period of EDP measurement was characterized by a set of descriptors of the EDPPW and by the difference to IVP or IPP. Group definition was based on the difference between EDP and IVP or IPP. EDP periods of less than 10 mm Hg difference to IVP or IPP were assigned to the "CORRECT" group and EDP periods of 10 mm Hg or more than 10 mm Hg difference to IVP or IPP were assigned to the "FAULTY" group. We tested fuzzy-logic based pattern classification program FUCS [6, new version 1992] and discriminant analysis. After constructing classificator by learning by doing, we reclassified all periods of EDP measurement without knowing the difference pressure between EDP and IVP or IPP, i.e. without group assignment. It should be tested, if it is possible to identify faulty EDP recordings without simultaneous measurement of IVP or IPP. It must be emphasized, that no EDP pulse wave and no period of EDP recording could be classified by the eye.

RESULTS

Figure 1 shows the mean EDP and IVP or IPP values of the 136 recorded periods. 31 periods of EDP situated outside the 10 mm Hg difference lines were assigned to the group "FAULTY". 105 periods of EDP inside the 10 mm Hg difference lines were assigned to the group "CORRECT". 10 additional periods of simulated dislocation of the epidural sensor below the galea aponeurotica or into the burr hole with loss of dural touch but striking "reliable" EDP pulse wave were assigned to a third group labelled "DISLOCATION".

Without knowing pressure difference between EDP and IVP or IPP, fuzzy pattern classification of EDP wave form descriptors was able to identify 143 (98%) of all entered EDP periods correctly. All periods with less than 10 mm Hg difference to IVP or IPP were identified as "CORRECT". All periods of dislocation were identified as "DISLOCATION". 28 of 31 periods of EDP with more than 10 mm Hg difference to IVP or IPP were identified as "FAULTY". Classification failure was seen in 3 periods of the group "FAULTY" which were identified as "DISLOCATION".

Discriminant analysis was able to identify 133 (92%) of all EDP periods. Classification failure was seen in 13 (8%) cases.

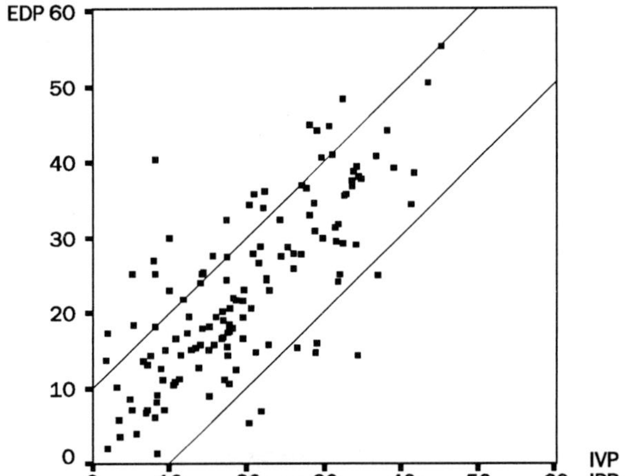

Fig. 1. Results of 136 periods of simultaneous EDP and IVP or IPP measurement. Lines represent the 10 mm Hg pressure difference zones.

DISCUSSION

In this study, a classification software tool was able to identify inaccurate EDP recordings without any reference pressure measurement. This is of importance, because faulty EDP readings are a serious and generally underestimated problem, even in the scientific literature. Our results confirm the data of Aschoff et al. [5] even with sensors of the new generation. In clinical practice we learned to verify high EDP values by IPP measurement before starting potentially dangerous therapeutic steps (barbiturate coma, hypothermia).

It appears to be very difficult for any new EDP measuring device to exclude error source caused by the biological system, but it might be possible to recognize it. Improved hardware with integrated signal analysis software tools establishing the "intelligent" ICP monitoring are still the future. However, a clinical software system in EDP monitoring able to identify implausible EDP readings would be useful for any clinician.
The results of this study encourage to further investigations. Signal analysis of EDPPW and fuzzy pattern classification might be an approach to the problem of misleading EDP recordings.

REFERENCES

1. Jorgesen PB, Riishede J (1972) Comparative clinical studies of epidural and ventricular pressure. In: Brock M, Dietz H (eds) Intracranial pressure. Springer. Berlin Heidelberg New York. p 41
2. Sundbarg G, Nornes H (1972) Simultaneous recording of the epidural and ventricular pressure. In: Brock M, Dietz H (eds) Intracranial pressure. Springer. Berlin Heidelberg New York. p 46
3. Zierski J (1980) Extradural, ventricular and subdural pressure recording comparative clinical study. In: Shulman K, Marmarou A, Miller JD, Becker DP, Hochwald GM, Brock M (eds) Intracranial pressure IV. Springer. Berlin Heidelberg New York. pp 371-376
4. Powell MP, Crockard HA (1985) Behavior of an extradural pressure monitor in clinical use. J Neurosurg 63:745-749
5. Aschoff A, Betsch M, Albert F, Hund E, Hampl J, Tronnier V (1991) Fehlerquellen und Komplikationen epiduraler und ventrikulärer Hirndruckmessungen. In: Druschky KF, Erbguth F and Neundörfer B (eds.) Schwerpunkte neurologischer Intensivmedizin. Perimed. Erlangen. pp 218-222
6. Bocklisch SF (1986) A diagnosis system based on fuzzy classification. Computers in Industry 7:73-82

Idiopathic Normo-Pressure Hydrocephalus: A Prospective Study in 23 Consecutive Patients

C. Raftopoulos[1], J. Deleval[2], C. Chaskis[1], A. Leonard[2], F. Cantraine[3], F. Desmyttere[1], S. Clarysse[4], and J. Brotchi[1]

[1] Department of Neurosurgery, 'Erasme' Hospital, Université Libre de Bruxelles, Bruxelles, Belgium
[2] Department of Neurology, 'Erasme' Hospital, Université Libre de Bruxelles, Bruxelles, Belgium
[3] Department of Computer Science, Faculty of Medicine, Université Libre de Bruxelles, Bruxelles, Belgium
[4] Harvey Cushing Center, 'Erasme' Hospital, Université Libre de Bruxelles, Bruxelles, Belgium

Introduction

Idiopathic normo-pressure hydrocephalus (INPH) remains a difficult entity to deal with. Controversy exists as to whether or not shunting can really improve mental function and on the ability of a quantified intracranial pressure monitoring (ICP-Mo) to predict postoperative improvement rates [1,2]. Different studies have pointed to the lack of a prospective study concerning the surgical outcome of this condition [2,5]. We have performed such a study on INPH patients shunted on basis of ICP-Mo [4].

Population and Method

Shunting was recommended when *'high'* waves (amplitude > 9 mmHg; three types: great symmetrical wave, intermediate wave and plateau wave) were present [3]. Forty-two patients were submitted to an ICP-Mo. Twenty-four showed high waves. Twenty-three patients were operated on (Pudenz-Schulte medium valve; P-S Medical, 928 Garden Street, Santa Barbara, California 93101, 805-968-1546, USA). The pre and postoperative clinical states (gait and neuropsychology) were assessed by a quantitative procedure. The neuropsychologists were not informed of the other results and particularly of the ICP-Mo.

Results

A clear post-shunting improvement was seen in 96% of the patients at one year with a statistically significant correlation between the sum of *'high'* wave relative frequencies (High wave relative frequency) and the grade of improvement ($P < 0.05$). At the same time, 67% of shunted patients showed a significant improvement in mental function. Only one patient was not improved postoperatively. This patient has the lowest high wave relative frequency (0.7%). No residual deficit was observed in this series.

Discussion

Considering the *chronological appearance of postoperative improvement*, we observe that the majority of bladder improvement appears during the first postoperative week, the majority of gait improvement appears during the first two postoperative months and that the major increase in cognitive functions is at two months postoperatively with the visuoconstructive skills improving essentially between two months and one year.

If we consider *the grade of improvement*, urinary dysfunction and gait apraxia are the two problems most improved by the shunting procedure. However the 67% of neuropsychological improvement with five patients (24%) greatly improved emphasizes the plasticity of the aging brain.

In our series, *no residual deficit* could be observed. Such a fact could be related to close follow-up allowing us to rapidly treat complications and to the use of a medium pressure valve.

FORECASTING THE IMPROVEMENT GRADE ON BASIS OF THE GREAT SYMMETRICAL WAVE RELATIVE FREQUENCY: A NEW OPPORTUNITY

For the Great Symmetrical wave relative frequency(GSRF) and the High wave relative frequency (HRF), regression analysis has clearly demonstrated a statistically significant correlation ($P < 0.05$) between their logarithms and the grade of improvement. One can remark that HRF ($P = 0.024$) although being the sum of high waves relative frequencies has not a greater correlation with the improvement grade than GSRF ($P = 0.013$). This correlation between *GSRF, HRF and improvement grade*, in contradiction to previous literature [1], allows us to give prognostic information regarding surgery to the family and the referring doctor.

CONCLUSIONS

We recommend the use of quantitative ICP-Mo as a criterion for surgery (*HRF > 1%*) and to predict the improvement rate (*GSRF and HRF*). An increase in the mental functions is often demonstrated (67%) one year after surgery and a high rate of clinical improvement (96%) with no residual deficit is possible even when dealing with INPH.

REFERENCES

1. Cardoso ER, Piatek D, Del Bigio MR, Stambrook M, Sutherland JB (1989) Quantification of abnormal intracranial pressure waves and isotope cisternography for diagnosis of occult communicating hydrocephalus. Surg Neurol 31: 20-27

2. Clarfield AM (1989) Normal-pressure hydrocephalus: saga or swamp. JAMA 262: 2592-2593

3. Raftopoulos C, Chaskis C, Delecluse F, Cantraine F, Bidaut L, Brotchi J (1992) Morphological quantitative analysis of intracranial pressure waves in normal pressure hydrocephalus. Neurol Res 14: 389-396

4. Raftopoulos C, Deleval J, Chaskis C, Leonard A, Cantraine F, Desmyttere F, Clarysse S, Brotchi J (1994) Cognitive recovery in idiopathic normal pressure hydrocephalus. A prospective study. Neurosurgery (In Press)

5. Vanneste J, Augustijn P, Dirven C, Tan WF, Goedhart ZD (1992) Sunting normal-pressure hydrocephalus: do the benefits outweigh the risks? A multicenter study and literature review. Neurology 42: 54-59

Computer Simulation Study of Intracranial Hemodynamics and ICP Pulse Wave Form

M. HASHIMOTO and K. TOKUDA

Department of Neurosurgery, Noto General Hospital, Nanao, Ishikawa, Japan

INTRODUCTION

It is generally accepted that the configuration of intracranial pressure pulse wave form (ICP PWF) is influenced by intracranial hemodynamics, compliance, cerebral vasotonicity, and venous drainage[1,4]. The configuration of the ICP PWF represents three fairly consistent components (P1, P2 and P3)[2,4]. In the present study, we construct flow simulation model of intracranial hemodynamics, and simulate ICP PWF closely simillar to clinical analysis[1]. In this model, we investigate the relation between the change of ICP PWF and the venous outflow system under the different intracranial circulation time.

METHODS

Computer simulation model of intracranial hemodynamics is constructed by i think^{TM} (High Performance SYSTEMS inc.). We construct this model by six basic building blocks (1. Cardiac output 2. Resistant artery, 3. Vascular bed, 4. Venous pool, 5. Sinus, 6. Cardiac return.) (Fig.1-A). Cardiac output as normal carotid arterial flow is inputted to this model. ICP PWF is calculated by algebraic relationship [ICP = GRAPH(Volume of Resistant artery + Vascular bed + Venous pool)]. In this software, the intracranial blood volume is converted automatically to pressure value by pressure volume relationship courve (GRAPH). Cardiac return is defined as jugular venous flow. In this model, circulation time on each building blocks is able to control as transit time. So, we estimate the one cardiac cycle configulation of ICP PWF(Fig.1-B) in the continuous changes of transit time in Vascular ved. The transit time shows how long flow the vascular bed.

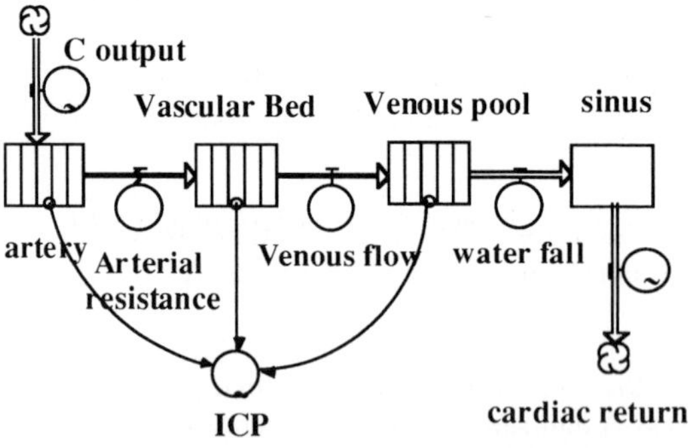

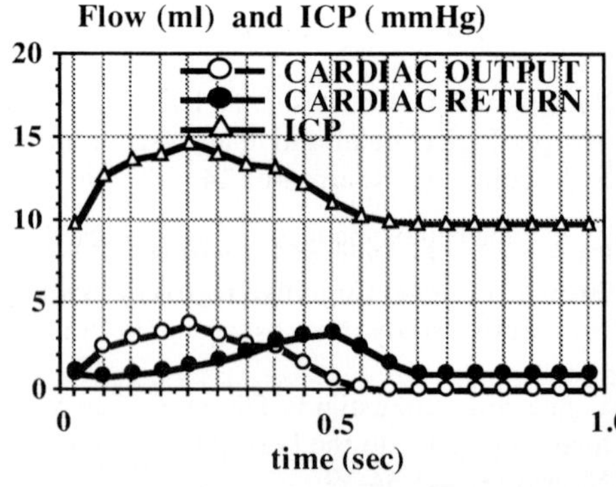

Fig.1-A) Intracranial Hemodynamic model is constructed by some building blocks. Cardiac output and Cardiac return data that are shown in Fig.1-B) is inputted into this simulation model. In this model, ICP PWF is calculated automatically as pressure volume relationship.

RESULTS AND DISCUSSION

Ihe changes of ICP PWF (Fig.2-a) is divided into 4 phases in these condition. In the First phase, with an ıncrease of transit time, each P1,P2 and P3 amplitude gradually augmented its amplitude. In the second ›hase, P1 is disappeared in the ICP-PWF and then in the third phase, P2 amplitude is augumented more ·apidly and ICP-PWF changes its configuration to monotonous one. In the last 4th phase, the increase of ICP amplitude was not observed no more. These continuous changes of ICP PWF is closely simillar to :linical analysis[1].

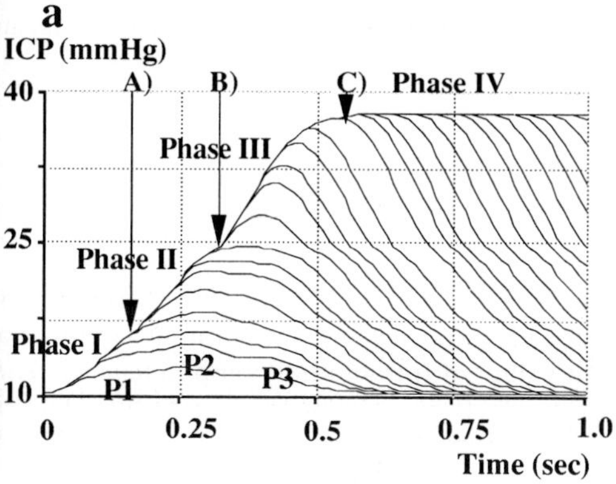

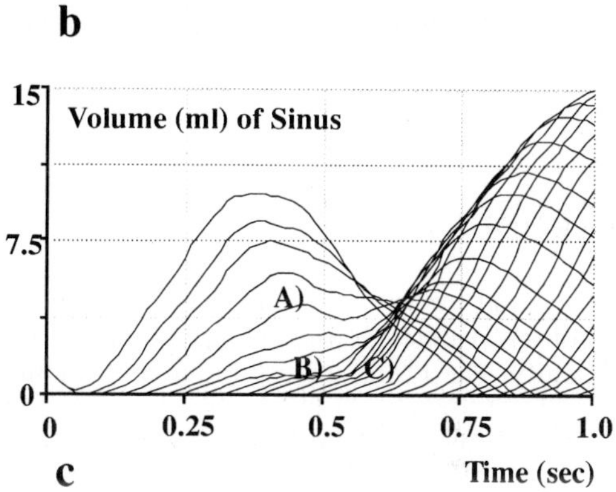

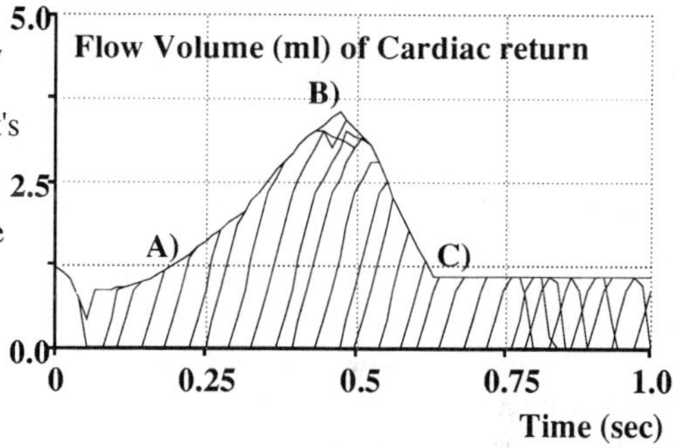

'ig. 2-a. ICP PWF changes is traced simulteniously n the continuous changes of transit time of vascular ›ed. In these simulated ICP PWF, four phases and it's norphological changing points (A, B,C) are clearly dentified. The sinus volume(Fig.2-b) and the flow 'olume of cardiac return (Fig.2-c) is simulated on the ame condition. Each point of A, B, C in Fig.2-a is een on the changing points of the venous outflow ondition.

n the simulation of Sinus volume and Cardiac return flow (Fig.2-b and c), each 4 phase is related to enous drainage condition. In the first phase (Fig.2-b), sinus flow is decreased gradually. In the second 'hase, sinus systolic flow is decreased more than sinus diastolic flow (Fig 2-b, B) and then in the 3rd hase, sinus systolic flow is not observed(Fig.2-b, B~C). In the 4th phase, because of the delay of blood irculation, cardiac return flow is disappeared (Fig.2-c, C). It has been suggested that ICP PWF are nfluenced by intracranial venous drainage and intrathoracic pressure variations[1,3,4]. In this study, the ıorphological changing points of ICP PWF and its amplitude coincide with the venous outflow condition vhich modulate directly to the intracranial compliance. The result suggests that the ICP-PWF reflects the ıtracranial hemodynamic condition include the venous drainage system. The computer simulation model f intracranial hemodynamics is useful for the theoretical investigation of the the genesis of ICP-PWF.

.EFERENCES

. Hashimoto M.(1989) Intracranial Pressure Pulse Wave Form and Its dp/dt Analysis of Plateau Waves. ICP VII : 225-227.

. Cardoso ER. (1983) Analysis of the cerebrospinal fluid pulse wave in intracranial pressure. J Neurosurg 59 : 817-821.

. Harmer J, Alberti E et al. (1977) Influence of systemic and cerebral factors on the cerebrospinal fluid pulse waves. J Neurosurg 46: 36-45.

. Hashimoto M. (1993) Changes of intracranial pressure and pulse wave form induced by various mechanical stresses upon intracranial hemodynamics. ICP VIII : 367-371.

A New Method of Measuring Intracranial Compliance— An Experimental Study

T. Ohta, M. Matsukawa, H. Miyake, and Y. Kajimoto

Department of Neurosurgery, Osaka Medical College, 2-7 Daigaku-machi, Takatsuki, Osaka, 569 Japan

INTRODUCTION

Intracranial compliance has been reported to be a more sensitive indicator of impendin neurological deterioration [1,2]. However, it is not easy to measure intracranial complianc clinically. Therefore, we tried to determine the equivalent of intracranial compliance (C) usin an epidural pressure (EDP) sensor produced by Spiegelberg Co. (Germany), and compared th C values between two different models of intracranial hypertension.

MATERIALS AND METHODS

Nine adult dogs weighing 8 to 12 kg were used. Dogs were ventilated mechanically with roon air under general anesthesia with intraperitoneal injection of Nembutal (25 mg/kg). EDP wa recorded continuously by the Spiegelberg EDP sensor, placing the air pouch epidurally throug a right frontal burr hole. **Experiment 1**(n=6): we produced acute intracranial hypertension b intermittent expansion (0.3 ml at a time) of an epidural balloon placed in the left tempora region during normocapnia. When EDP was stable, additional 0.1 ml of air was loade automatically at each intermittent increment (Fig.1), and the resulting pressure change (dP) b the loading air was recorded. The change in the volume of the air pouch (dV) after loading (0. ml) could be calculated, and then the C value was calculated by dV/dP. The clinical status c the dogs was estimated by pupillary size and ABR. **Experiment 2** (n=3): we produced anothe intracranial hypertension with hypercapnia induced by the decreasing respiration rate. The C value was obtained by the same manner. After recovering pCO_2, we completed experiment using the same dogs during normocapnia and compared the C values obtained from tw different models of intracranial hypertension.

RESULTS

The relationship between balloon volume and EDP demonstrated a classic exponential curve EDP was markedly raised when the balloon volume reached more than 2.5-3.5 ml, and a abnormal ABR was observed (Fig.2). The C value remained stable until balloon volum reached 2.0 ml, and then it decreased relative to further inflation (Fig.3). The C value change more during lower level of EDP (Fig.4). During EDP exceeding 40 mmHg, the C value in th hypercapnia group was greater than that of the epidural balloon groups even the same level c EDP (Fig.5).

DISCUSSION

Measurement of Pressure Volume Index (PVI) or Volume Pressure Response (VPR) with bolus manipulation methods provides useful information about the intracranial environment [1,2]. However, it is difficult to implant the catheter into the collapsed ventricle, while implantation of an EDP sensor is easy and safe. We, therefore, tried to measure intracranial compliance by loading air into the air pouch of the Spiegelberg EDP sensor. Since air is compressible, the resulting volume expansion of the air pouch after loading (0.1 ml) depends upon ICP. In other words, the degree of air pouch dilatation is thought to reflect the intracranial stiffness. The C value was well correlated to clinical exacerbation and thought to be an excellent indicator of intracranial compliance for the following two reasons; the change in the C value was more sensitive under lower level of EDP, and different C values were obtained even in the same level of EDP during EDP exceeding 40 mmHg in different intracranial hypertension models.

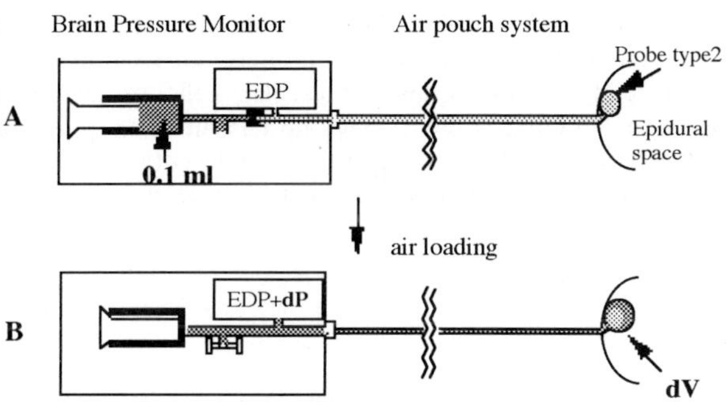

Fig.1 The shematic drawing of the Spiegelberg EDP sensor
(A: EDP measurement stage, B: after air loading)

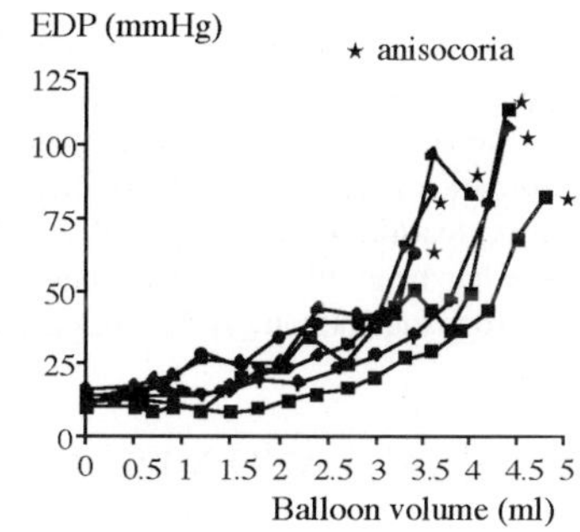

Fig.2 Relationship between balloon volume and EDP. (n=6)

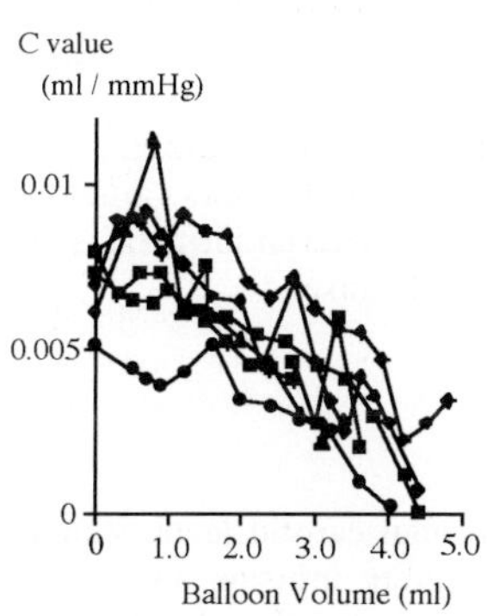

Fig.3 The relationship between balloon volume and the C value. (n=6)

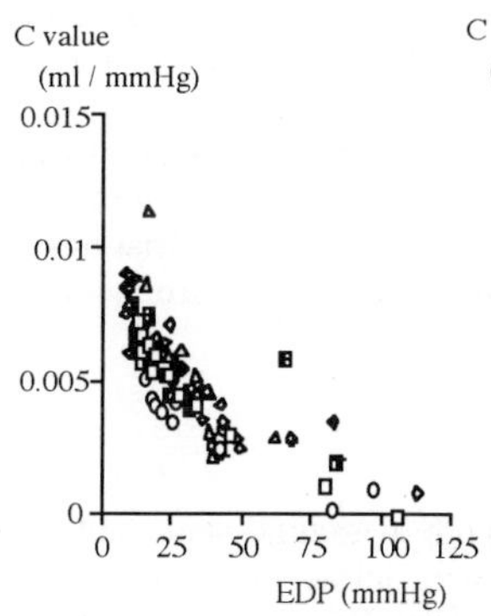

Fig.4 The relationship between EDP and the C value. (n=6)

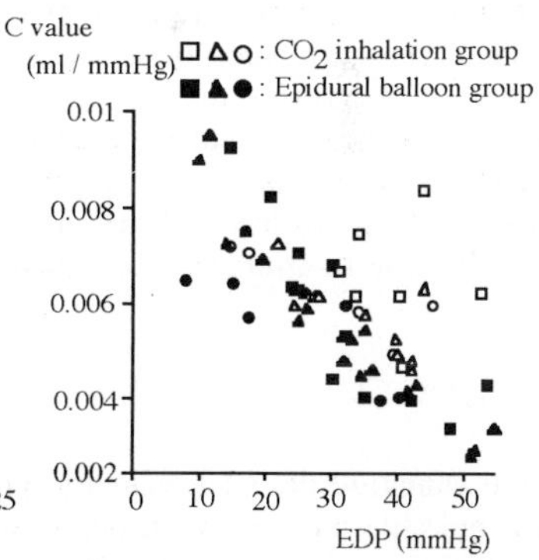

Fig.5 Relationship between EDP and the C value in differnt two groups. (n=3)

REFERENCES

1. Miller JD, Garibi J, Pickard JD (1973) Induced changes of cerebrospinal fluid volume. Effects during continuous monitoring of ventricular fluid pressure. Arch Neurol 28:265-269.

2. Marmarou A, Shulman K, LaMorgese J (1975) Compartmental analysis of compliance and outflow resistance of the cerebrospinal fluid system. J Neurosurg 43:523-534.

CBF Velocity and Intracranial Hypertension. An Experimental Study

C. ANILE[1], A. MANGIOLA[1], R. GASPARI[2], F. DELLA CORTE[2], D. CATAPANO[1], F.F. ANGILERI[1], P. SANTINI[1], and G. MAIRA[3]

Institutes of [1] Neurosurgery and [2] Anesthesiology, Catholic University, Rome, Italy
[3] University of Perugia, Italy

INTRODUCTION

It is a well known fact that the cerebral blood flow (CBF) remains relatively constant within a large range of variations in the cerebral perfusion pressure (CPP). To explain this property different theories have been advanced. Among these, the capability of the smooth muscular cells of adapting "automatically" the vascular diameter in relation to variations in the trans-mural pressure (the so-called "autoregulation"), has acquired a greater importance [1]. Recently, however, some criticism to this theory has been advanced by some authors [2]. This study was planned in order to investigate the CBF regulatory mechanism(s) during intracranial hypertension.

MATERIALS AND METHODS

In 8 pigs a reversible intracranial hypertension was produced by infusing saline into a cerebral ventricle to obtain a condition of so-called "brain tamponade" for a period of 15 to 60 minutes. The intracranial pressure was measured through the same needle utilized for the infusion; arterial blood pressure through a catheter inserted in the common carotid artery. CBF variations were analyzed by evaluating blood flow velocity intracranially at the sagittal sinus and at the internal carotid level by doppler technique. The correlation between flow and flow velocity in a vessel of a known diameter gives the possibility of measuring the flow variations provided that the vessel diameter remains constant. This condition is satisfied, in our experimental model, at least as far as the CBF velocity measurement from the sagittal sinus is concerned; in fact, the anatomical structure of the sinus strongly limits variations in its cross section. On the contrary, blood flow velocity variations recorded at arterial intracranial level may be due also to arterial vascular diameter variations produced by different causes.

RESULTS

In basal condition the CBF velocity, both at sagittal sinus and at intracranial carotid level, showed a typical pulsatile pattern synchronous with intracranial pulsation. Both during infusion and recovery phase, the reduction in CPP to about 40 mmHg was instantaneously associated with a decrease in the diastolic and systolic values at carotid level, while at sinus level no CBF velocity modification was observed. When CPP was below this limit, while at carotid level the systolic CBF velocity remained stable and the diastolic value became negative (Fig. 1), at sinus level the CBF velocity reduced until reverberating waves were observed simultaneously at arterial and venous level (Fig. 2).

DISCUSSION

The instantaneous changes in the intracranial carotid CBF velocity following CPP changes and the synchronism between arterial and venous pulsatile CBF velocities suggest the occurrence of an hydraulic "autoregolatory" mechanism duc to the passive distension of the arterial walls caused by an increased down-stream outflow resistance at Starling's resistor level [3].

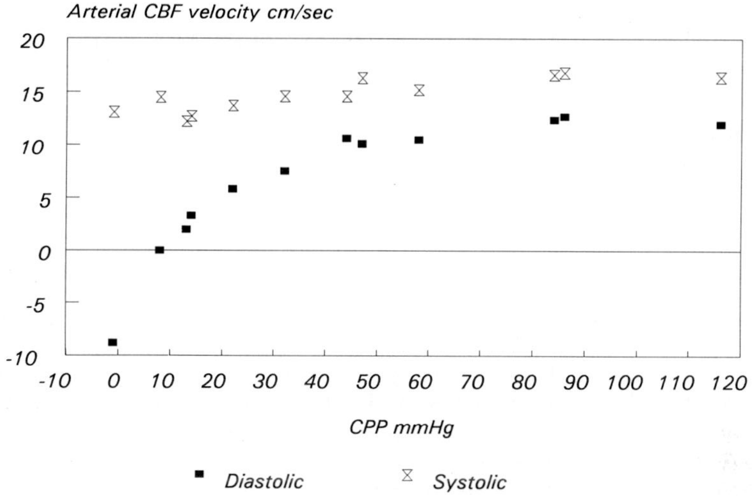

Fig. 1: Example of arterial CBF velocity variations during intracranial hypertension produced by saline infusion.

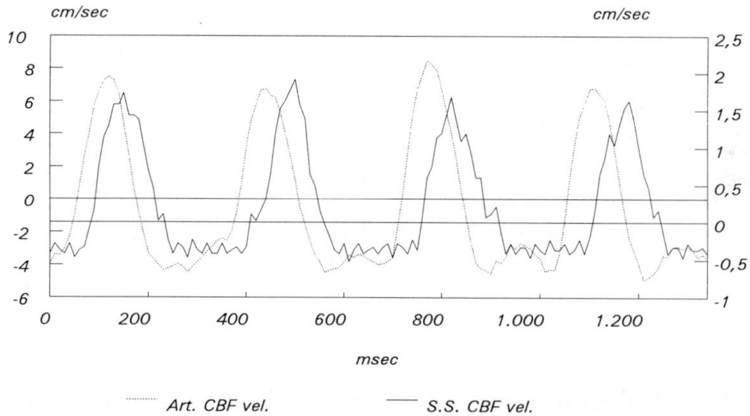

Fig. 2: Arterial and sagittal sinus CBF velocity reverberating waves in brain tamponade.

REFERENCES

1. Portnoy HD, Chopp M, Branch C, Shannon M (1982) Cerebrospinal fluid pulse waveform as an indicator of cerebral autoregulation. J Neurosurg 56:666-678.
2. Aaslid R, Newell DW, Stooss R, Sorteberg W, Lindegaard K-F (1991) Assessment of cerebral autoregulation dynamics from simultaneous arterial and venous transcranial doppler recordings in humans. Stroke 22:1148-1154.
3. Chopp M, Portnoy HD, Branch G (1983) Hydraulic model of the cerebrovascular bed: an aid to understanding the volume-pressure test. Neurosurgery 13:5-11.

CSF Pulse Pressure and CBF Velocity Transmission in Experimental Intracranial Hypertension

C. ANILE[1], A. MANGIOLA[1], R. GASPARI[2], F. DELLA CORTE[2], D. CATAPANO[1], F.F. ANGILERI[1], P. SANTINI[1], and G. MAIRA[3]

Institutes of [1] Neurosurgery and [2] Anesthesiology, Catholic University, Rome, Italy
[3] University of Perugia, Italy

INTRODUCTION

Different opinions have been expressed about the source and propagation of the pulse pressure originating within the intracranial system. The major part of the authors think it originates from the arterial tree or from capillaries; Portnoy in his papers stressed the idea that it comes from venous pulsation because of the strict similarity between CSF and venous pulse pressure. The understanding of the origin of the intracranial pulsation is essential in order to formulate a reasonable model of the intracranial system mainly regarding the correlations between ICP, CBF and intracranial buffering capacity. In a rigid skull, in fact, a pulsatile arterial inflow needs to be matched with a synchronous pulsatile venous outflow to maintain a constant volume, as stated by the Monro-Kellie doctrine. In this study we will report the data regarding the morphology and the transmission of the cerebral arterial and venous flow velocity correlated to the arterial and intracranial pulse pressure.

MATERIALS AND METHODS

In 8 pigs a reversible condition of intracranial hypertension was produced by infusing saline into a lateral ventricle. The following parameters were simultaneously measured: arterial blood pressure (ABP) by a catheter inserted into the right common carotid artery, ICP by the same needle utilized for the infusion, arterial and venous blood flow velocity by two ultrasound probes located intracranially, respectively, at internal carotid artery (ICA) and sagittal sinus (SS) level through two appropriated skull windows. All the signals were stored in a magnetic tape for delayed computerized processing based on Fourier's spectral analysis in order to recognize both the typical morphological features and the temporal correlations of the different parameters recorded.

RESULTS

In all the animals the ABP signal precedes all the other signals; the blood flow velocity wave at ICA level starts 40 ms after the onset of the ABP, immediately followed by the ICP wave onset. These three signals are very similar in shape and their spectral composition shows a clear predominance of the first harmonic (Fig. 1). The onset of the blood flow velocity wave at SS level is synchronous with that of the ICA wave; on the contrary, its shape is quite different in basal condition and until CPP remains in the autoregulatory range (> 40 mmHg), showing a bicuspidate contour (Fig. 2a) with a predominance of the second harmonic. This typical shape changes below the autoregulatory limit when it becomes more similar to the arterial one (Fig. 2b and c).

DISCUSSION

These findings confirm what Aaslid et al. have already described in humans [1] regarding the synchronism between the pulsatile arterial and venous in/outflow in the intracranial system; this mechanism of balance, compensating the variations in the cerebral arterial blood volume following the autoregulatory response, is able to maintain a constant CBF until the buffering capacity of the venous bed is exhausted. Our findings also suggest that the venous pulsation is the consequence of a vascular compression, probably at Starling's resistor level, due to the arterial pulsation immediately propagating through the CSF spaces.

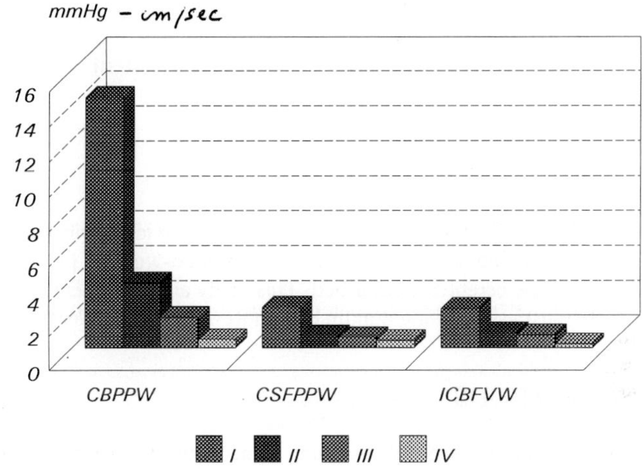

Fig. 1: I, II, II and IV harmonics of the simultaneously recorded carotid (CBPPW), CSF pulse pressure (CSFPPW) and intracranial carotid blood flow velocity waveforms (ICBFVW).

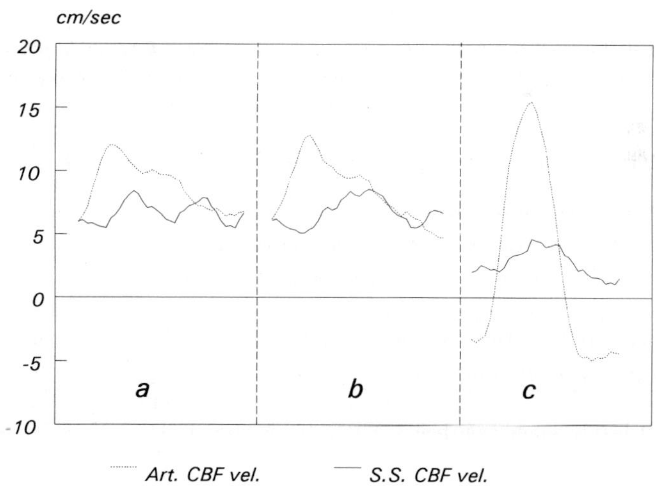

Fig. 2: Simultaneously recordings of arterial and sagittal sinus CBF velocity in the "autoregulatory" range (a) and during progressive intracranial hypertension (b, c).

REFERENCES

1. Aaslid R, Newell DW, Stooss R, Sorteberg W, Lindegaard K-F (1991) Assessment of cerebral autoregulation dynamics from simultaneous arterial and venous transcranial doppler recordings in humans. Stroke 22:1148-1154.

Analysis of Cerebrovascular Pressure Transmission in Severe Head Injury

S.B. Lewis[1], I.R. Piper[2], and P.L. Reilly[1]

[1] Department of Neurosurgery, Royal Adelaide Hospital, North Terrace, Adelaide, South Australia 5000, Australia
[2] Department of Clinical Neurosciences, University of Edinburgh, Western General Hospital, Crewe Road, Edinburgh, EH4 2XU, UK

INTRODUCTION

Intracranial pressure (ICP) waveform has been analysed as a way of identifying the underlying mechanisms responsible for raised ICP following head injury [1,2]. Piper and co-workers [3] described 4 patterns of pressure transmission across the cerebrovascular bed. This study aimed to identify these patterns of cerebrovascular pressure transmission using minute by minute waveform collection and analysis.

MATERIALS AND METHODS

20 patients with severe head injury (GCS < 9 following resuscitation) were studied. Patients with a bone flap removed or severe chest trauma were excluded. Arterial blood pressure (BP) was monitored via an optimally damped fluid filled arterial catheter-transducer system. ICP was monitored by a fibre optic pressure tip transducer (Camino) placed intraparenchymally. End-tidal carbon dioxide (ETCO2), jugular bulb oxygen saturation (SjO2) and pulse oximetry were monitored and recorded continuously. Waveform data was collected using the Edinburgh waveform analysis system [3] permitting minute by minute sampling of BP and ICP waveforms with online analysis and calculation of amplitude and phase components of the transfer function. Waveform samples were selected in 20 minute segments for analysis. Samples rejected if they occured 1) within 45 minutes following orotracheal suctioning and physiotherapy, 2) within 90 minutes following therapy for raised intracranial pressure or 3) during periods of overdamping or monitor malfunction. Prospective coding of waveforms was based on the criteria of Piper et al [3],

Table1. Amplitude transfer function classification [3]

Type 1:	All harmonics within 100% of the amplitude of the third harmonic.
Type 2:	The first harmonic is greater than twice the amplitude of the third harmonic.
Type 3:	One or more harmonics above the third harmonic are greater than twice the amplitude of the third harmonic, with the first and second harmonics within 100% of the amplitude of the third harmonic.
Type 4:	Waveforms not fulfilling the above criteria.

Table 1. The first six harmonics and the phase shift of the fundamental or first harmonic was analysed.

RESULTS

15 males and 5 females with a mean age of 28 years (14 to 65) were monitored for 76 +/- 50 hours. Median GCS following resuscitation was 6 (3 to 8). 5,944 waveforms were analysed. Curve type 1 was the most frequent comprising 43% (2,568) of analysed waveforms. Curve type 2 comprised 22% (1330), curve type 3 comprised 15% (898) and curve type 4 comprised 20% (1148).

For curve type 1 and 4 a negative fundamental phase shift was observed. For curve types 2 and 3 a positive phase shift was observed (see fig. 1). Further examination of curve type 2 phase shift revealed two subclasses of amplitude transfer function curve type. A subpopulation of 658 waveforms (curve type

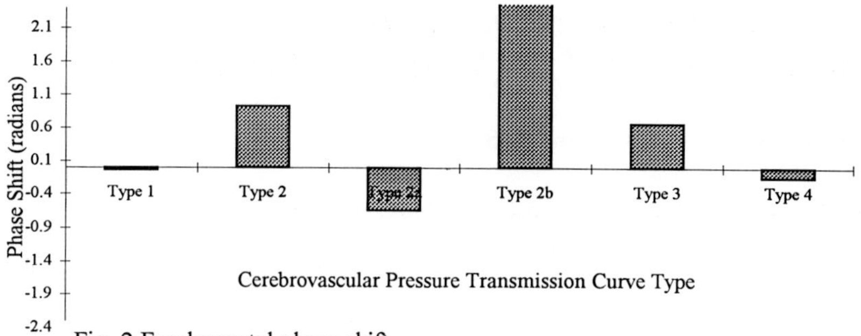

Fig. 2 Fundamental phase shift

2a) was associated with a markedly negative phase shift (mean -0.6 +/- 0.20), while the remaining 672 waveforms (curve type 2b) were associated with a markedly positive phase shift (mean 2.47 +/- 0.34). Curve type 2a and 2b were associated with an signifiicant elevation ($p < 0.05$) in ICP (20 mmHg) compared to the other curve types which were associated with an ICP of less than 15 mmHg. Mean jugular bulb oxygen saturation was significantly higher (73%) in subtype 2b (associated with a positive phase shift) compared to type 1 and type 3 ($p < 0.5$). The remainder were associated with a jugular bulb oxygen saturation of less than 67% and were not significantly different between types. There were no significant differences in any of the other monitored parameters.

DISCUSSION

This study confirms the presence of cerebrovascular pressure transmission patterns in acute closed head injury as described by Piper et al [3]. Consistent with their study was the finding of an association between curve type 2 and a higher ICP than that associated with curve type 1 and 3. Of particular interest in this study was the identification of two subtypes for curve type 2 based on differing phase shift characteristics. A wide standard deviation for positive phase shift for the combined type 2 group (+/- 1.57) prompted further analysis of this group to examine the distribution of phase shifts within the group. A clear division into two subgroups was evident with group 2a displaying a markedly negative phase shift compared to groups 1 and 4, while group 2b had a markedly positive phase shift compared to curve type 3. It was also interesting to note that curve 2b was associated with a significantly higher SjO2. than any of the other curve types suggesting increased global cerebral blood flow. Recent work by Piper and coworkers [4] demonstrated that elevated fundamental amplitude transfer function was associated with an increased negative phase shift under conditions of active arteriolar vasodilation. When autoregulation was impaired an increased fundamental amplitude frequency was associated with a positive phase shift.
The findings of this current study suggest that an elevated transmission of the first harmonic between BP and ICP waveforms may be associated with either a negative phase shift, perhaps indicating intact autoregulation or a positive phase shift which may indicate loss of autoregulation and passive vasodilatation.

REFERENCES

1. Chopp M, Portnoy HD (1980) Systems analysis of intracranial pressure. Comparison with volume-pressure test and CSF pulse amplitude analysis. J Neurosurgery 53: 516-527.
2. Robertson CS, Narayan RK, Contant CF, Grossman RG, Gokaslan ZL, Pahwa R, Caram P, Bray RS, Sherwood AM (1989). Clinical experience with a continuous monitor of intracranial compliance. J Neurosurgery 71:673-680 .
3. Piper IR, Miller JD, Dearden NM, Leggate JRS, Robertson I (1990) Systems analysis of cerebrovascular pressure transmission: an observational study in head injured patients. J Neurosurg 73:871-880.
4. Piper IR, Chan KH, Whittle IR Miller JD (1993) An experimental study of cerebrovascular resistance, pressure transmission, and craniospinal compliance. Neurosurgery 32:805-815.

Towards the Mechanism of Development "B"— And "Plateau-Waves" of the Ventricle Fluid Pressure

E. Sirovskiy, V. Amcheslavski, and I. Savin

N.N. Burdenko Research Institute of Neurosurgery, Moscow, Russia

INTRODUCTIUN

Untill recently there has not been a universal point of view concerning the causes and mechanism of the occurence of the spontaneous VFP fluctuation. The purpose of the present investigation was to study the regularities and features of the development "B" – and "plateau – waves" of the VFP depending on the location of the tumor, the severity of the clinical state of the patient and bioelectrical brain activity.

MATERIAL AND METHODS

The monitoring of the VFP was performed in 169 neurosurgical patients after the removal of intracerebral gliomas (67), of subtentorial tumors (45) and the tumor of basal extracerebral location (57). The severity of the clinical state was assessed by standard methods used in neurosurgery and by means of the Glasgow Coma Scale (GCS). According to severity, patients were divided into 3 groups. Patients of the 1st group were in a state of compensation or subcompensation (GCS 15–13). Those of the 2nd group were in a state of moderate decompensation or in the critical state (GCS 12–8). The 3d group consisted of patients in a moderate, deep or unlimited comatose state (GCS 7–4). Bioelectrical brain activity was assessed by the EEG and for continuous EEG assessment a "Berg–Fourier" analyzer was used.

RESULTS AND DISCUSSION

<u>1. Tumor location.</u> In group of patients after removal of hemispheric gliomas (the mean VFP – 27.1±0.4 mm Hg) "B" – and "plateau – waves" of VFP were most after obvious. The deeper and more medial the tumors is localized the more often spontaneous undulating VFP changes appear and the more are they expressed. In a group of patients operated for basal tumors (the mean VFP – 12.1±2,9 mm Hg) "B –waves" were seen significantly seldom and their amplitudes did not exceed 20 mm Hg. In this group "plateau–waves" were seen in only 1 case. In some cases of VFP hypo– or hypertension between "palisade" consisting of "B–waves" had observe a special section of VFP which is typical of the "plateau–waves" but without the VFP increase (unrealized "plateau–waves") (Fig.1).Thus, there is a marked dependence of the frequency of the developing spontaneous VFP changes of the tumor location. Most frequently "B"– and "plateau – waves" were registered in those cases when the tumor affected diencephalic structures.

<u>2. EEG.</u> In all patients during the VFP "plateau–waves" increase had observed strictly outlined EEG changes. In the majority of cases with "plateau–waves" there was revealed a reduction of the bioelectrical activity. (Fig.2). There was established a strong negative correlation between fluctuation of the VFP and the EEG total power ($r = -0.812$; $P<0.01$). In cases when we reduce the VFP hypertension artificially (with the help of the drainage or drug therapy), the EEG picture was practically unchanged, that is the EEG changes on the "plateau" remained. (Fig.3).The obtained data allow to suggest that in a cause–effect relation between the VFP changes and EEG dynamics by the occurrence time the changes of the bioelectrical activity are considered the primary ones.

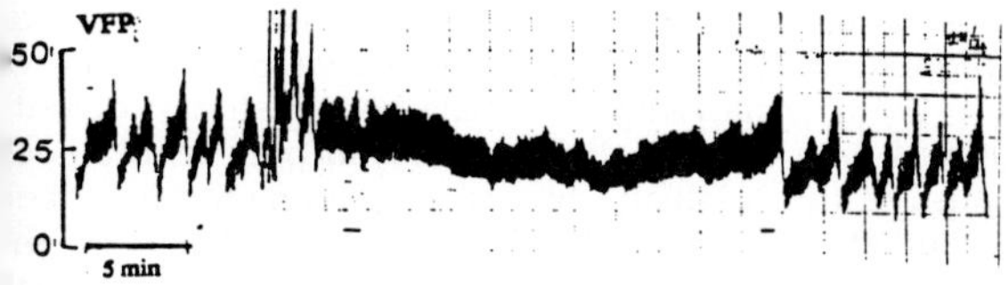

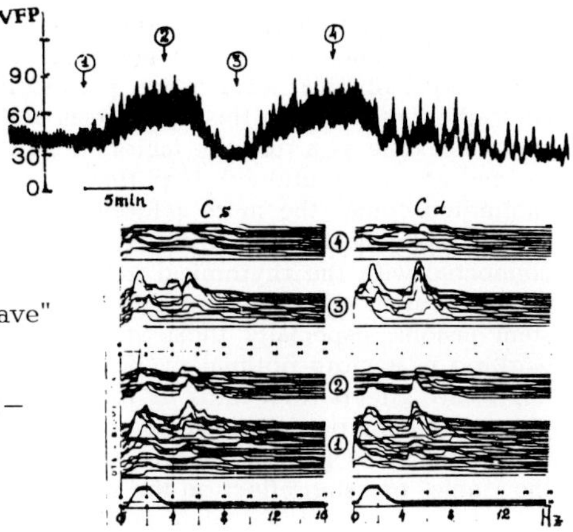

Fig. 1 (right) VFP hypertension."Unrealized plateau—wave" between "palisade" of "B—waves".

Fig. 2 (left) The reduction of bioelectrical activity (Berg—Fourier analyses of EEG) during "plateau—waves" (1,2,3,4 — the moments of synchronization).

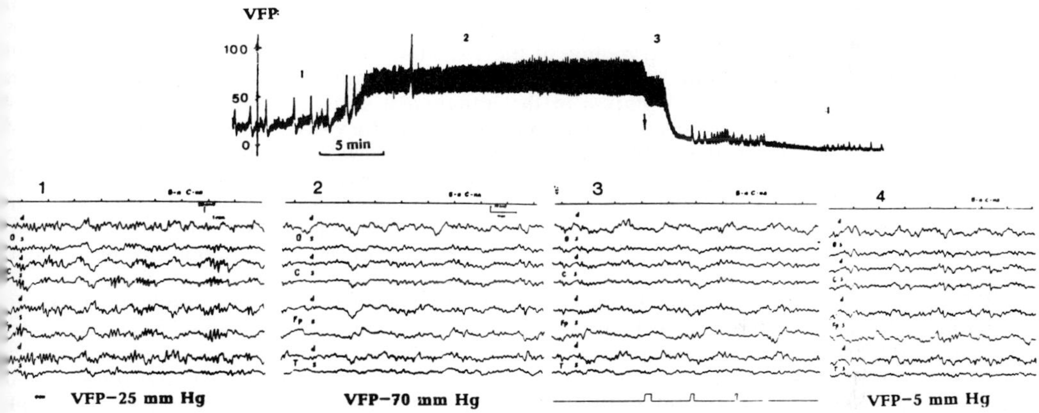

Fig. 3. EEG during "plateau — wave". The EEG picture was practically unchanged after decrease of VFP with help of drainage (arrow) (1,2,3,4 —the moments of synchronization).

3. Clinical condition. In patient 1st group "B—waves" were obviously less frequent (their amplitude did not exceed 20 mm Hg). "plateau—waves" were not registered at all. In 3 cases "unrealized plateau — waves" were registrated.In patients of 2nd group (GCS 12—8) "B—waves" were registered more often and its amplitude reached to 50 mm Hg. The following fact is worthy of attention. In patients without "B—waves" or when these fluctuation were irregular or of a very low amplitude the course of disease was much more severe and signs of brain hypoxia were present. In patients in 3d group (GCS 7—4) the "B—waves" were registrated not so often then 2nd group and its amplitude didn't exceed 20 mm Hg; "Plateau—waves" occurred also more seldom, and sometimes their duration increasing up to 15—25 min. (Fig.3). Thus, there is a strict and clear dependence of the development of VFP spontaneous fluctuations on severity of clinical state. "B" — and "plateau — waves" most often occurred and were revealed in patients in critical state (GCS 12—8). It is important to stress that in patients in a terminal state or brain death "B"—and "plateau — waves" disappeared completely.

According to the modern hypothesis the causes of the occurrence of the "plateau—waves" consis of the disturbance of pre— or post capillary regulation; the disturbances of the venous outflow, o a decrease of the brain stem perfusion (1, 2, 3). Analyzing the obtained material definit contradictions between this hypothesis and clinical date are revealed. Namely: in patient in a dee comatose state as a rule the factors are the cause of the "plateau—waves" development (accordin to the above mentioned hypothesis) are retained or increased. However, the closer to th "unlimited coma" the more seldom "B" — and "plateau — waves" appear and before the deat they completely disappear. It is suggested that the mechanism of "B" — and "plateau — waves" i connected with the rhythmical activity typical of the medullar centers free from the influence c the brain stem vasomotor centers. We suggest(4) that in the patients with diencephalic and brai stem lesions, especially those in a critical state, hypothalamic—bulbar vasomotor centers sta working in a more optimal cyclic regime, thus providing a rhythmical alteration of pressure an depressive effects (that finds its form in "B—waves" of the VFP). In cases when after the dilatatio phase the constriction phase is not present "plateau — waves" are developed. Consequently, th reason that the "plateau—waves" appearance is always connected with the periodical stopping c the "tonic" pressing effect on the vessels. This effect make take place during its refractors period c its exhaustion. In cases when the vasomotor center exerts not a cyclical but a continuos "tonic effect, "plateau—waves" are formed periodically exhausting the centers' power resources withou accompanying "B—waves". The period of power resources restoration is accompanied by th vessels dilatation phase and corresponds to the "plateau—waves" duration. The absence of "B"- and "plateau—waves" in patients in the coma state may be explained by the fact that th vasomotor center can't produce a vasopressor effect. Thus the "starting" factor of "B" an "plateau—waves" is a cyclic working regime of the vasomotor centers. However, the degree of th VFP increase will depend on the venous outflow, capillary regulation, reabsorption of CSF an other mechanism physiological adaptation of the intracranial system (P—V dependence). If thes mechanism are preserved, the transition to a cyclic regime of the vasomotor center will lead only t a characteristic change of the VFP curve form without developing hypertension (unrealize "plateau—waves" (Fig.1). As the physiological adaptation is exhausted, the VFP is increased. Th "B—waves" reflect neurogenic rhythmic changes in vascular tone that appear in case of th diencephalic brain stem structures functional overexertion. The aim of such a cyclic effect on th brain arterial vessels, probably, is to facilitate and to accelerate the blood supply to the damage structures (hypoxia). It's carried out by the "pumping" effect through the blood vessels—"th peripheral heart effect". So the "B—waves" may be considered as the result of maximu mobilization of the CNS reserve mechanisms aimed at preserving brain function. This suggestion proved by the fact that in critical patients with "B—waves" the clinical and laboratory signs brain hypoxia are less prominent, and postoperative course of the disease and the prognosis a more favorable then in cases without "B—waves". The appearance of "plateau—waves" is a sign of the compensatory mechanisms failure and from of this point of view they are diagnostically ar prognosticate important.

REFERENCES

1. Matsuda M., Yoneda S., Handa H. (1979) Cerebral hemodynamic changes during plateau—wav in brain tumor patients. J.Neurosurgery, 50, N.4,:483—488.
2. Rosner M.J., Becker D.P. (1982) The Ethiology of plateau—waves: A Theoretical model wi experimental validation. In: ntracranial pressure V (Tokyo) Ed.by S.Ishii,H.Nagai and M.Bro Springer—Verlag Berlin—Heidelberg 1983. pp.301—306.
3. Searle J.R., Sullivan H.G. Plateau waves ethiology. In:Intracranial pressure V (Tokyo). Ed.b S.Ishii, H.Nagai and M.Brock Springer—Verlag Berlin—Heidelberg 1983. pp.297—300
4. Sirovskiy E.B. (1991) On the mechanisms of the development of CSF pressure spontaneo fluctuation. J.Voprosi Neirochirurgii, 3: 18—23.

Poster IV: Biophysics II

Chairman: K. Shima

Computerised Lumbar Infusion Test—Multicentre Experience in Clinical Studies in Hydrocephalus

M. Czosnyka[1], F. Gjerris[2], W. Maksymowicz[3], D. Price[4], M. Roszkowski[5], H. Whitehouse[1], and J.D. Pickard[1]

[1] MRC Cambridge Centre for Brain Repair and Academic Neurosurgical Unit, Addenbrooke's Hospital, P.O. Box 167, Cambridge CB2 2QQ, UK
[2] Department of Neurosurgery, University Hospital, Copenhagen, Denmark
[3] Department of Neurosurgery, Medical Academy, Warsaw, Poland
[4] Pinderfield's Hospital, Wakefield, West Yorkshire, UK
[5] Neurosurgery, Child's Health Centre, Warsaw-Miedzylesie, Poland

The Computerised Infusion Test is a method for accurate computer analysis of the traditional constant rate infusion. It is worthwhile to stress that this method allows the infusion to be made into any accessible fluid compartments. Lumbar infusion, even if it has understandable limitations, is the least invasive and therefore, the most often performed. The next most frequent approach is an intraventricular infusion via Ommaya Reservoir. Hydrocephalus is more complex than a simple disorder of CSF circulation. However, because the CSF shunting is purely a mechanistic way of treatment, the biomechanics of the pressure volume compensation should be examined before a shunt is implanted. The physical effect of a shunt is to reduce the so called resistance to CSF outflow to about 6-8 mmHg/ml/min - which is the typical hydrodynamic resistance of most of shunts. If a patient's own resistance is normal, around 8 mmHg/ml/min [1], a shunt cannot help, because there is nothing to reduce. The authors accept that the safe limit of normal resistance is around 12 or 13 mmHg/ml/min [2]. Our common experience suggests that not only resistance, but other compensatory parameters are helpful in the diagnosis of hydrocephalus. Therefore, the main problem is how to distinguish between different types of disorders presenting with ventricular dilatation from specific patterns of the cerebrospinal fluid pressure recorded during infusion test.

MATERIAL AND METHOD

Three hundred and fifty infusion tests were performed in five different centres (136 in children). There were no serious complications after the test. The most important clinical findings will be briefly summarised in the next section. The model of the cerebrospinal volume compensation estimated during the test has been described by Marmarou [3] and only slightly supplemented later. Apart from opening pressure and resistance to CSF outflow the pressure-volume index (PVI), system compliance, estimated CSF formation rate and pulse wave amplitude are measured. During infusion the computer calculates mean pressure and pulse amplitude and presents both variables with time on the x axis. The resistance to CSF outflow can be calculated using even a pocket calculator as the difference of the plateau pressure during infusion minus resting pressure, divided by the infusion rate. However, in the majority of cases strong vasogenic waves or excessive elevation of pressure does not allow the precise measurement of the final pressure plateau. The computer calculates the compensatory parameters even in difficult cases by examination of amplitude-pressure relationship, volume-pressure curve retrieval or the least mean square model fitting [4].

RESULTS AND DISCUSSION

The natural question is whether the lumbar infusion gives such precise measurement of outflow resistance as lumbo-ventricular perfusion described by Borgensen and Gjerris [5]. This method gives a very accurate estimate of the resistance, assessed on multiple intraventricular pressure levels. The method is more invasive in comparison to lumbar infusion. Both tests were compared in a heterogeneous group of patients presenting with a ventricular dilatation. An excellent correlation ($r=0.98$; $p<0.001$) between the results of

the tests was found. A conclusion has been made that computerised lumbar infusion is an accurate method for measurement of the conductance of CSF outflow.
However, the main aim of infusion test is not only to measure the resistance to CSF outflow, but generally to predict which cases may improve with shunting. Therefore, the recognition of different types of disorders presenting with ventricular dilatation is crucial.
Patients suffering from brain atrophy have, in contrary to hydrocephalic patients, normal conditions for CSF circulation. Typically the opening pressure, resistance to CSF outflow and pulse amplitude are low. The pressure volume index is high, reflecting very low elasticity of atrophic brain. Also, very specifically, there are no vasogenic waves seen in the pressure recording. System is being inflated and deflated passively, like a balloon.
Normal pressure hydrocephalus (NPH) presents with the normal opening pressure, low pulse amplitude and high PVI. Again, as in the brain atrophy, the CSF system is very compliant [6]. The increased resistance to CSF outflow (>12 mmHg/ml/min) and B waves allow NPH to be distinguished from atrophy.
Lumbar infusion is not recommended in "non communicating hydrocephalus". However, this type of hydrocephalus sometimes gives a very unspecified pattern in CT. In those rare cases when lumbar infusion is performed the resistance to CSF outflow is normal, because the lumbar infusion is not able to detect the proximal narrowing in CSF circulatory pathways. The resting pressure, pulse amplitude, and paradoxically, PVI are high.
Finally in acute hydrocephalus the resting pressure and the resistance to CSF outflow are high. The PVI is low and the pulse amplitude is high indicating a poor compensatory reserve. Non communicating hydrocephalus investigated using an intraventricular approach gives the same pattern of parameters.
Another application of Computerised Infusion Test is the assessment of shunt functioning in vivo. If a shunt is functioning properly, the resistance to CSF outflow never exceeds 10 mmHg/ml/min, an exception being the flow-regulating Orbis-Sigma valve [7].
The resting pressure should be around or below the shunt's opening pressure. Tests repeated after shunting should always be compared to the test performed before surgery. Commonly, a sharp plateau of the pressure trend is seen about 2-4 mmHg above the level of shunt opening [7].
Three points were discussed: the test's accuracy, sensitivity to reveal different types of disordered CSF circulation and the ability to assess the shunt functioning in vivo. Computerised lumbar infusion test is a low invasive, fast and reliable method of investigation in hydrocephalus. This form of examination is particularly helpful to avoid unnecessary shunting.

REFERENCES

1. Albeck MJ, Borgesen SE, Gjerris F, Schmidt JF, Sorensen PS (1991) Intracranial pressure and cerebrospinal fluid outflow conductance in healthy subjects. J.Neurosurg 74: 597-600
2. Borgesen SE, Gjerris F (1982) The predictive value of coductance to outflow of CSF in normal pressure hydrocephalus. Brain 105: 65-86
3. Marmarou A, Shulman K, Rosende RM (1978) A nonlinear analysis of cerebrospinal fluid system and intracranial pressure dynamics . J.Neurosurg 48: 332-344
4. Czosnyka M, Batorski L, Laniewski P, Zaworski W (1990) A computer system for the identification of the cerebrospinal compensatory model. Acta Neurochirurgica 105: 112-116
5. Borgesen SE, Gjerris F, Sorensen SC (1978) The resistance to cerebrospinal fluid absorption in hymans. A method of evaluation by lumbo-ventricular perfusion , with particular reference to normal pressure hydrocephalus. Acta Neurol Scand 57: 88-96
6. Czosnyka M, Batorski L, Roszkowski M, Tomaszewski J, Wocjan J, Walencik A, Zabolotny W (1993): Cerebrospinal compensation in hydrocephalic children. Child's Nerv. System 9:17-22
7. Czosnyka M, Maksymowicz W, Batorski L, Koszewski W (1990) Comparison between classic-differential and automatic shunt functioning on the basis of infusion tests. Acta Neurochirurgica 106: 1-8

Effects of Decreasing Cerebral Perfusion Pressure on Pulsatility of Cerebral Blood Flow Velocity—A Modelling Study

S. Piechnik[1], M. Czosnyka[1,2], H. Richards[2], P. Kirkpatrick[2], P. Smielewski[1,2], and J.D. Pickard[2]

[1] Institute of Electronics Fundamentals, Warsaw University of Technology, Nowowiejska 15/19, 00-665 Warsaw, Poland
[2] MRC Cambridge Centre for Brain Repair and Academic Neurosurgical Unit, Addenbrooke's Hospital, P.O. Box 167, Cambridge CB2 2QQ, UK

INTRODUCTION

Mathematical modelling and computerised simulation of cerebral dynamics may help the understanding of complex mechanisms that regulate cerebral blood flow and cerebrospinal fluid circulation. Some simplification of the model is required for better control of the computer process, and this has to be balanced against restrictions in the final accuracy of the calculations. However the use of even a restricted set of model parameters may provide the possibility of accurate on line assessment of the neurosurgical patient. Already, some of the model parameters, like resistance of reabsorption of cerebrospinal fluid and compliance of cerebrospinal compartment, are widely used for this purpose. Every newly created model must prove its precision in a number of simulations of clinical tests. Comparison of the results to different phenomena observed "in-vivo" gives an important feedback that can clarify the interpretation of different mechanisms, thus enabling more accurate understanding of physiology and better modelling.

In this study, the original model of cerebrospinal dynamics was utilised to examine the changes in pattern of cerebral blood flow velocity (FV) in cerebral arteries measured using Transcranial Doppler flowmetry. The investigations concern possible reasons for observed rise in pulsatility of FV in area of lower limit of autoregulation.

MATERIAL

The analysis of intracranial hypertension caused by ICP plateau waves was performed on a basis of computer monitoring of head injured patients in Addenbrooke's Hospital in Cambridge, UK. The patients were sedated, paralysed and ventilated with $PaCO_2$ level between 25 and 35 mmHg. Up to four signals were monitored in a patient. ABP was recorded using an arterial line. ICP was monitored either using a Camino transducer (Model V420, Camino Laboratories) placed subdurally or by subdural drain connected to an external pressure transducer. Flow velocity mean and maximum values were measured in Middle Cerebral Artery (MCA) using TCD ultrasonograph (PcDop 842, SciMed, Bristol, UK).

In a study of systemic hypotension waveforms of Arterial Blood Pressure (ABP) and Flow Velocity recorded during experimental gradual haemorrhage in 10 New Zealand rabbits were used. Animals were studied under licence of the UK Animals Act., Scientific Procedures, 1986. ABP was recorded from the common carotid artery using a fibre-optic catheter connected to a direct pressure monitor. Flow velocity was recorded from the basiliar artery using 8 MHz pulsing Doppler ultrasound probe and Transcranial Doppler sonograph (model as above). The probe was positioned over the dura exposed by a posterior frontal burr hole. The analogue signals were digitised using 12-bit analogue-to-digital converter (DT2814, Data Translations, USA) with a sampling frequency of 50 Hz (150 Hz in rabbits). Data were read from the converter and stored in IBM compatible computer memory using specialised recorder program (WREC) written by W. Zabolotny, Warsaw University of Technology, Poland [3].

METHOD

To complete our investigations we created two models suitable to use authentic data as an input for computer simulation. The first model can accept as an excitation ABP and venous pressure in saggital sinuses, the other one is adapted for ABP and ICP input. Both models simulate pressure and flow conditions in two major pathways of fluids transported in intracranial space: blood and CSF. Hydrodynamic structures representing both models were represented by equivalent electrical circuits. The electrical circuits are described by a specific set of non-linear differential equations, which are subject of computer evaluation in special simulating software running on IBM-PC compatible computers. The differential equations are solved using the Rung-Kutta IV method with manual step size correction. The model was previously checked for most of clinical and experimental situations using artificially generated input signals, and proved to be a useful and reliable method for signal prediction and analysis[2]. The new, enhanced version of the software gives an opportunity to read directly computer disk files with real, clinically and experimentally recorded signals instead of working with pure artificially simulated arterial and venous or intracranial pressures. Furthermore, we can use the real signals as an excitation for the model and produce corresponding output. Using this method the simulated and real outputs were compared and visible discrepancies were minimised by appropriate trimming of model parameters (compartmental resistances and compliances).

RESULTS & DISCUSSION

Clinical data including computer records of monitoring 5 head injured patients revealed that above a certain ICP level, corresponding to averaged CPP 35 mmHg (range from 30 to 43 mmHg), flow velocity diastolic started to decrease, thus decreasing mean FV and increasing its pulsatility. When the recorded ICP and ABP waveform were substituted as an input to the model the same divergent behaviour of simulated systolic and diastolic values of simulated blood flow through basal arteries was reconstructed. The changes of systolic and diastolic flow velocity recorded during experimental arterial hypotension showed a similar pattern. Below averaged ABP diastolic of 55 mmHg (range from 65 to 44 mmHg) flow velocity started to decrease and flow velocity was stable. Flow velocity started to decrease when ABP systolic fell below 53 mmHg. Again the simulation showed a good convergence with the recorded signals when the threshold of autoregulation was set for values corresponding to the threshold observed on FV diastolic.

The high level of the accuracy of the simulation was obtained only after the additional introduction to the normal, slow autoregulatory mechanism, an independent mechanism of temporary closing of arteriolar vessels for low transmural pressures, i.e. for low CPP. This mechanism is dependent on actual values of CPP, instead on CPP time average. Therefore, in both cases, the divergent behaviour of systolic and diastolic FV was caused by wide gap between CPP diastolic and systolic. When CPP diastolic decreases below the level of CPP_{close}, set as a threshold of the described phenomenon, FV diastolic decreases, FV mean also starts to smoothly decline but FV systolic is stable. When CPP systolic falls below the lower limit of autoregulation, the decrease in autoregulatory reserve is complete. This transient zone characterised by gradual divergence between systolic and diastolic FV, increase in FV pulsatility and slow decrease in FV time average, is theoretically equal to peak-to-peak CPP pulsations.

REFERENCES

1. Aaslid R: Cerebral Haemodynamics, Transcranial Doppler, Ed. by DW Newell and A Aaslid, Raven Press, New York 1992
2. Czosnyka M, Piechnik S., at al: The Dynamics of cerebral Blood Flow, Perfusion pressure and CSF Circulation - A Modelling Study. Intracranial Pressure VIII, Springer-Verlag Berlin Heidelberg 1993.
3. Zabolotny W, Czosnyka M, Smielewski P. Portable Software for Intracranial Pressure Recording and Waveform Analysis. Intracranial Pressure IX, Springer-Verlag Tokyo.

Effects of Acute Compliance Fluctuation on Slow ICP Waves: Frequential Aspects

J.-J. LEMAIRE[1], J. CHAZAL[1], J.-L. GUTKNECHT[1], P. PICARD[1], B. IRTHUM[1], and J.-Y. BOIRE[2]

[1] Service of Neurosurgery, University Hospital, Clermont-Ferrand, France
[2] Laboratory of Biomathematics, Statistics and Medical Computing, Faculty of Medicine, Clermont-Ferrand, France

SUMMARY

Thirty three ICP curves extracted from daily recordings were analysed. ICP data were collected from 19 patients who suffered from different hydrocephalic conditions, and treated with discontinuous CSF ventricular drainage. We explored the frequential effects on slow ICP waves of an acute compliance increasing induced by the drainage opening (Opd). The study in the frequential domain consisted of an analysis of the power spectrum of which were noted the frequency (F, Hz) of the most important spike of power (P, arbitrary unit, a.u.). This was done for the frequency bands of B waves (BW, from $8 * 10^{-3}$ Hz to $50 * 10^{-3}$ Hz) and infra B waves (IB, below $8 * 10^{-3}$ Hz) which included the A waves: FBW and PBW, FIB and PIB, respectively. We found that the Opd induced a reduction of PBW ($P<0.01$) and PIB ($P<0.05$), an inversion of the ratio of PIB over PBW, and an alteration of FBW which tended to a mean value of $13.36 * 10^{-3}$ Hz (0.8 wave/min). We found a decreasing exponential relation between the mean ICP (MeP) and the FBW before the Opd ($p<0.05$). We also found increasing linear relations between, MeP and PBW (only for the Opd, $P<0.01$), and MeP and PIB (for both Opd and closed drainage, $P<0.05$). Pathophysiological considerations are discussed.

INTRODUCTION

About forty years after the first main descriptions of the slow ICP waves [1] [2], few works have studied the fluctuations of their frequential aspects [3]. The purpose of this study was to explore the frequential effects on these waves (A and B types) of an acute compliance increase, induced by the opening of a CSF ventricular drainage. Previous studies [4] [5] have already shown the relationship between the craniospinal enclosure (CSE) compliance and B wave amplitude.

MATERIALS

Nineteen patients suspected of raised ICP were included: 10 male and 9 female with a mean age of 51 ranging from 6 to 77. The clinical circumstances were: 16 acute hydrocephalus (13 subarachnoid haemorrhages secondary to an arterial aneurysm rupture, 1 ventricular and 2 cerebro-ventricular spontaneous haemorrhages), 1 post infectious hydrocephalus, 2 chronic obstructive hydrocephalus (1 arachnoid cyst and 1 posterior fossa tumour). ICP was monitored (P10EZ* transducer, Gould Medical, U.S.A.; CM 130* monitor, PPG Hellige, France), recorded (sampling:$166.6 * 10^{-3}$ Hz, PICSOFT*, Sophysa, France), and controlled by intermittent CSF drainage (Heyer-Schulte External CSF drainage system, Baxter*, U.S.A.).

Thirty-three daily ICP recordings were analysed. For each recording, we selected two 25min-periods: the first immediately before a CSF drainage opening (closed drainage, Cld), and the second just after the opening (open drainage, Opd). The opening pressure of the drainage device was adjusted from 7 to 15 mmHg. The mean MeP (MeP = mean ICP during the 25-min period) Cld was 25 mmHg (mean SD_{MeP}=3.8 mmHg) and the mean MeP Opd was 5.9 mmHg (mean SD_{MeP}=1.44 mmHg).

Because of the short duration of recording, it was impossible in clinical routine to measure the quantity of CSF subtracted.

METHOD

1°) ICP Data Analysis:

The frequential analysis of each 25min-period of ICP data consisted in a fast Fourier transform which provided the power spectrum. We noted the frequency (F, Hz) of the most important spike of power (P, arbitrary unit: a.u.) and this was done only (because of the Shannon theorem) for the frequency bands of B waves (BW, from $8 * 10^{-3}$ Hz to $50 * 10^{-3}$ Hz) and infra B waves (IB, below $8 * 10^{-3}$ Hz) which included the A waves: FBW and PBW, FIB and PIB, respectively [3]. We also analysed the ratio of PIB over PBW (R) which represented the power predominance of the two frequency bands.

2°) Global Data Analysis:

We compared the distributions of PBW, PIB and R in the Cld and Opd conditions (χ^2 test): 1°) for PIB we distinguished high ($>250*10^{-3}$ a.u.) and low ($\leq 250*10^{-3}$ a.u.) values; 2°) for PBW we distinguished high ($>100*10^{-3}$ a.u.) and low ($\leq 100*10^{-3}$ a.u.) values.
We also correlated the MeP to the frequential parameters (F, P), and this for the two conditions of drainage (Opd, Cld).

RESULTS

1°) Effects of the OpD on Frequential Parameters

Independently of clinical circumstances, we found that the OpD was associated with a reduction of PIB and PBW (χ^2 test: PIB, $P<0.05$; PBW, $P<0.001$).
The observation of the R distribution (fig 1) showed when R Cld < 10-20 (high BW power tendency), then R Opd increased (high IB power tendency), and inversely if R Cld > 10-20.

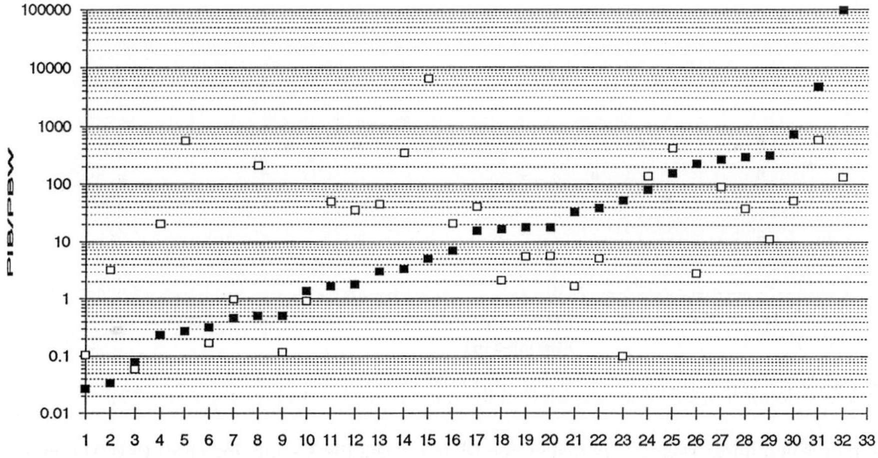

Fig 1 Distribution of the ratio PIB over PBW, before (solid square) and after (empty square) the CSF drainage opening. Data before the drainage opening have been put in increasing order on the X axe (n=33).

We also noted that the OpD induced an alteration of FBW (fig 2) which tended toward a mean value of 13.36 * 10^{-3} Hz or 0.8 wave/min (SD= 5.9 * 10^{-3} Hz).

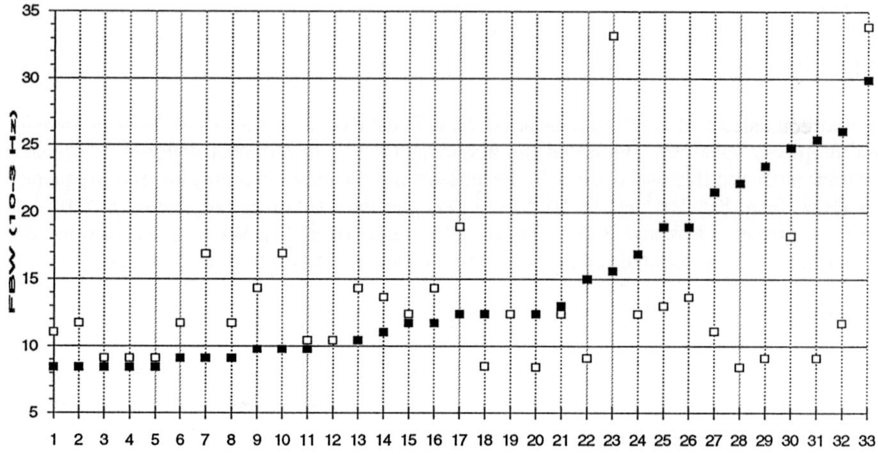

Fig 2 Distribution of FBW, before (solid square) and after (empty square) the CSF drainage opening. Data before the drainage opening have been put in increasing order on the X axe (n=33).

2°) Relationships between Frequential Parameters and MeP

We found a decreasing exponential relation (P<0.05) between the MeP and the FBW in case of Cld (fig 3).

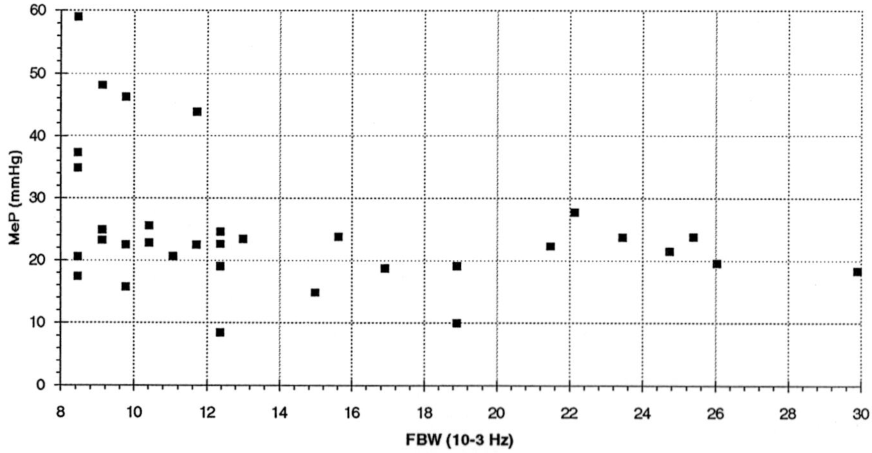

Fig 3 Distribution of FBW versus MeP in the condition of closed drainage (n= 33).

We also found increasing linear relations between, the MeP and the PBW (only for Opd, P<0.01), and the MeP and the PIB (for both Opd and Cld, 0.02<P<0.05).

DISCUSSION

It seemed logical, in view of routine bedside observations, to find a reduction of the wave power after the drainage opening. But it must be considered that this was slightly overestimated because of the buffer effect of the pipe drainage device on the pressure (extracranial transducer).

However the frequential response was not influenced by this phenomena because of the slow frequencies studied.

The frequential alterations of slow ICP waves induced by the increase of CSE compliance (the "equilibrium frequency" of $13.36 * 10^{-3}$ Hz and the alteration of the distribution of wave power between the BW and IB frequency bands) existed regardless of the initial (MeP_{Cld}) and final (MeP_{Opd}) ICP levels. This fact and the quickness of the frequential response suggest the presence of sensor(s?) inside the CSE which may be sensitive to the compliance.

The ICP level also seems able to modulate the frequential characteristics of the slow waves. In the BW frequency band: 1°) the FBW is lower when MeP tends toward higher values, in conditions of low compliance (Cld); 2°) when the compliance is higher (Opd) the PBW seems correlated to MeP. In the IB frequency band, the PIB is correlated to the ICP whatever the compliance conditions.

REFERENCES

1. JANNY P (1950) La pression intracrânienne chez l'homme. Thesis. Paris. 80 pages.

2. LUNDBERG N (1960) Continuous recording and control of ventricular fluid pressure in neurosurgical practice, Acta Psy and Neurol Scand 36 (suppl.149).

3. LEMAIRE J-J, BOIRE J-Y, CHAZAL J, IRTHUM B (1994) A computer software for frequential analysis of slow ICP waves. Comput Methods Programs Biomed 42 : 1-14.

4. DINARGL U, GARNER C, HABERL R, MAUTNER D, SCHMIEDEK P, EINHAUPL KM (1989) Correlation between B-Waves and intracranial pressure - volume relationships. In: Hoff JT, Betz AL (eds) ICP VII. Springer. Berlin, Heidelberg, pp 213-216.

5. NEWELL D W, AASLID R, STOOSS R, REULEN HJ (1991) Spontaneous fluctuations in cerebral blood flow as a cause of B waves. In: Avezaat CJJ, Van Eijndhoven JHM, Maas AIR, Tans JTJ (eds) ICP VIII. Springer-Verlag. Berlin, Heidelberg, New York, pp 424- 428.

CSF Dynamics Modeling in Man

H. FRIDÉN and J. EKSTEDT

Department of Neurology, University Hospital, S-901 85 Umeå, Sweden

INTRODUCTION

There is still no agreement about how to model the volume/pressure relationship of the CSF space. We present a five parameter mathematical model that well approximates the relationship in its full physiological volume range.

MATERIALS AND METHODS

Our method of accessing the CSF system is by two puncture needles, inserted into the lumbar subarachnoidal space of the patient (1). One needle is used only for pressure measurement, the other also for infusion and drainage of CSF. By using our volume accounting method (2), which takes into account both external and internal gains and losses, it was possible to obtain net CSF volume/pressure curves from the recorded data.

Out of a stock of about 300 investigations of CSF hydrodynamics that included the volume/pressure relationship, 31 were selected for this presentation. These were the cases with technically successful recordings and with V/p curves of different shapes over large volume and pressure ranges. No consideration was taken to diagnosis.

RESULTS AND DISCUSSION

The obtained CSF volume/pressure (V/p) relationships of the patients were modeled using an elementary mathematical model. The model considers both that the V/p-curve bends downwards as CSF is withdrawn at pressures below venous blood pressure and that it bends upwards as CSF is infused at pressures above resting pressure, Fig. 1. The model has three terms and five parameters and expresses the CSF pressure (pc) at any time as a function of the CSF volume (Vc):

$$p_c(t) = p_{offset} + \frac{A_{\min}}{(V_{\min} - V_c(t))} + \frac{A_{\max}}{(V_{\max} - V_c(t))} \qquad (V_{\min} < V_c(t) < V_{\max})$$

The first term is an offset term, mainly related to venous blood pressure. The second and third terms describe the relationship as CSF volume approaches its minimum and maximum dynamic levels, respectively. $A_{\min}$ and $A_{\max}$ define the bending of the function at its extremes and is related to the work needed to respectively "fully" drain or fill the CSF system. The suitability of the model is demonstrated by its application on data obtained from investigations on 31 patients with different pathologies. A summary of the obtained model parameters is shown in Talbe 1.

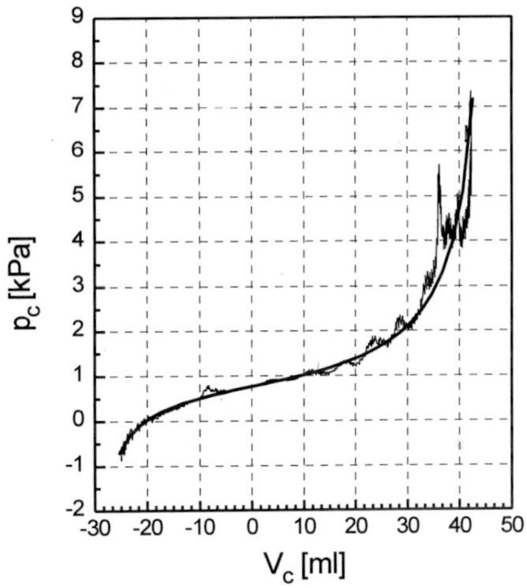

Fig. 1: The calculated V/p relationship and the fitted model for one of the patients. The recording is made during a phase of constant flow infusion at about 3 ml/min from low pressure to high pressure. The volume accounting method is used to calculate the net volume change from the recorded gross volume change.

Table 1: Summary of estimated model parameters for 31 patients with different pathologies. V_{range} is the dynamic CSF volume range ($=V_{max} - V_{min}$).

	P_{offset}	A_{min}	V_{min}	A_{max}	V_{max}	V_{range}
Unit	[kPa]	[kPa*ml]	[ml]	[kPa*ml]	[ml]	[ml]
Mean	0.72	8.2	-27	20	40	67
S.D.	0.48	8.4	11	8.4	7.1	14
Median	0.73	5.0	-26	18	39	67
Min	-0.26	0.3	-58	9	30	39
Max	2.08	33.4	-8	51	54	110

REFERENCES

1. Ekstedt J (1977) CSF hydrodynamic studies in man 1. Method of constant pressure CSF infusion. J Neurol Neurosurg Psychiatry 40: pp 105-119
2. Fridén H, Ekstedt J (1986) Volume accounting: A method for the study of CSF-hydrodynamics. An aid for parameter estimation and validation of pressure/flow models. In: Miller D, Teasdale GM, Rowan JO (eds) Intracranial Pressure VI. Springer-Verlag, Berlin Heidelberg: pp 54-61.

The Effect of Nimodipine on Cerebral Elastance and Edema in a Cryogenic Injury Model

E. Arbit, G.R. DiResta, J. Lee, R. Volkert-Fatzinger, and P. Bral

Neurosurgery Research Laboratory, Memorial Sloan-Kettering Cancer Center, New York, NY 10021, USA

SUMMARY

Nimodipine (N) produced a shift of the volume-pressure curve to the left with a simultaneous decrease in cerebral edema in a cryogenic injury rat model. The decrease in elastance may be due to a decrease in cerebrovascular resistance and an increase in cerebral blood volume. The known cerebroprotective benefits of N may well outweigh the risks of decreased elastance particularly if the latter is due to an increase in cerebral blood flow.

INTRODUCTION

Nimodipine, a dihydropyridine calcium channel blocker, has been reported to possess anti-ischemic effects, reduce neurological deficit in various models of focal and global cerebral ischemia, and has a preferential vasodilatory effect on CNS blood vessels. The effect of N on ICP are variable with studies showing both an increase and decrease in ICP. The effect of N on ICP, cererbral elastance and compliance is particularly pertinent, given the fact that N is currently and is planned to be more widely used in clinical situations often associated with abnormal ICP elevations. This study was undertaken to examine the effects of N on cerebral elastance and edema in a cryogenic injury model.

METHODS

A slow-release pellet impregnated with N (Innovative Research of America, Toledo, Ohio) was used to administer N to the animals. This approach was used to minimize the hypotensive effects normally observed when N is infusion. These pellets were prepared to achieve circulating N concentration of 10-20 ng/ml plasma shortly after implantation and maintain the level for at least 24 hours. Circulating plasma levels of N were measured using the Nifedipine enzyme immunoassay (EIA) plate kit by STC Corp. (Bethlehem, Pa). Nimodipine has a 96.5% cross reactivity with this EIA kit and therefore could be reliably measured.

Male, Sprague-Dawley rats were divided into 3 groups. Two groups received a cyrogenic lesion while the third served as the normal control. The two lesion groups were divided as follows: Nimodipine Pellet and Pellet matrix (drug control). The pellets were administered using a double-blind protocol. Under general anesthesia, a right parietal craniectomy and a cryogenic lesion were performed (Wallach Surgical Devices, CN). A N pellet or a placebo were implanted into the neck of the animal using a trochar. Blood samples were taken at 0,3, 6,24 and 48 hours post pellet implantation from a cannula inserted to the right femoral artery. Each sample was centrifuged and the plasma was withdrawn and rapidly frozen. EIA analysis was performed by STC, Inc. after all samples were obtained.

The pressure-volume measurements were peformed using a grease infusion technique 24 hours after the cryogenic lesion. Each animal was induced and anesthetized as above. The left femoral artery and vein were exposed and catheterized for measurement of systemic blood pressure, and infusion of fluids, respectively. Two craniotomies were performed next. The first was made over the left temporal cortex (dura intact) for fluid infusion. The second was made over the right occipital cortex (dura opened), to measure intracranial pressure using a Camino pressure transducer. Following the surgery, and prior to fluid infusion, a femoral arterial blood sample was taken to ensure that pH, p02 and pCO2 were within normal limits. A continuous slow fluid infusion (8 mcg/min) was started 15 minutes later and continued until the Cushing response was observed. At this point infusion was stopped, and the animal was euthanized by infusion of saturated KCl solution into the femoral vein, and decapitated. The brain was removed from the skull and divided into small sections for determination of % water content.

RESULTS

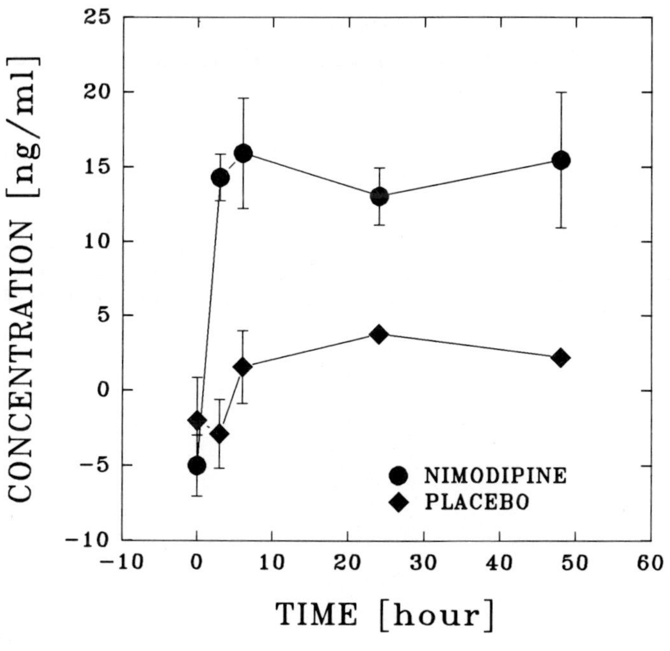

Fig. 1 plots the temporal concentration of circulating N in the animals. N concentration plateaued to 15 ng/ml, 3 hours post-implantation and remained at that level throughout the duration of the study

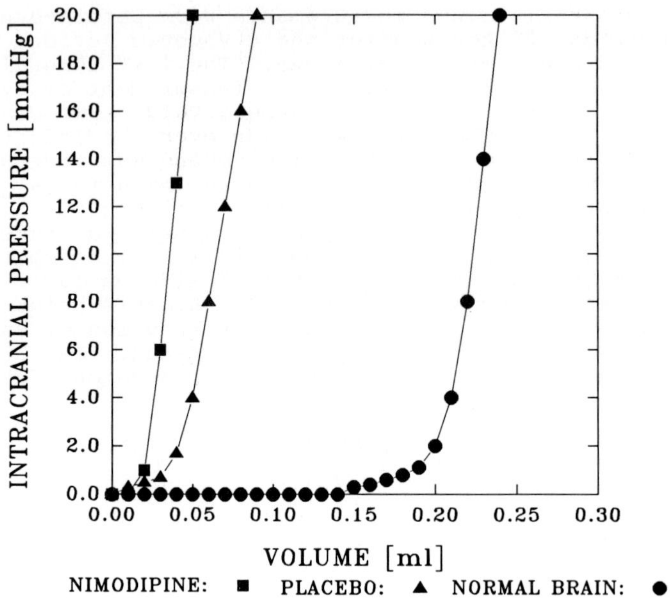

Fig. 2 plots the pressure-volume relationship obtained from the continuous slow infusion measurements. Analysis of the curves reveals that the slope of the rising portion of each groups' curve were not significantly different. A significant difference, however, was observed between the two lesion groups and control at the volume where pressure began to rise. Both cryogenic lesion groups shift the curve to the left of control; the N group shifts the curve furthest away from control

NIMODIPINE IN PERIREG.	NIMODIPINE IN CONTRA.	PLACEBO IN PERIREG.	PLACEBO IN CONTRA.	CONTROL NO INJURY
85.772 ±2.207	80.676 ±1.721	84.766 ±2.849	81.826 ±1.113	86.852 ±1.836

Table 1 - presents the brain % water content data for the four groups

DISCUSSION

Several beneficial physiological effects of Nimodipine on ischemia and stroke have been observed and put to use in clinical settings. These include the ability to increase CBF selectively, to inhibit constriction of cerebral vessels in response to a number of vasoactive agents and to block postischemic hypoperfusion. While these findings have been repeatedly confirmed, the effect of N on ICP has been variable. The effects of N on ICP is of concern given the fact that increase in CBF may result in increased cerebral blood volume and an increase in fluid and protein extravasation (edema) to result in increased ICP. Bedford reported a roughly 30% increase in ICP in patients with supratentorial lesions treated with a calcium channel blocker. It was speculated that this effect was secondary to a reduction in cerebrovascular resistance and an increase in cerebral blood volume (1). Tatehishi et al reported a consistent increase in ICP in patients with cerebrovascular disease and trauma given N for control of arterial hypertension (2). A CSF pressure increase ranging from 50%-90% was observed in patients with no neurological disorders given nicradepine (3). In cats with and without elevated ICP, ICP is increased by 20% and 30% respectively during nifedipine-induced hypotension (4). Contrary to studies showing an increase in ICP as a result of calcium channel blockers administration several studies showed either no effect or decrease in ICP. Hadley found that N caused a sustained decrease in ICP and shift of the volume-pressure curves down and to the right in a baboon stroke model. The mechanism responsible for ICP reduction could not be attributed to a temporary drop in mean arterial pressure seen with the infusion of N and the authors speculated that the effect was due to a global reduction in cerebrovascular volume (5). Gaab et al reported no effect on ICP by infusion of nimodipine in head injured patients, although the ICP pulse amplitude increased significantly (6). Our study, addressing specifically the effect of nimodipine on the volume-pressure curve and brain edema in a cryogenic injury model, demonstrated a shift of the curve to the left as compared to placebo and control (no injury) treatment groups. There was a small but significant decrease in edema between perilesional regions and contralateral parenchyma in both placebo and nimodipine treated animals but not in comparison to non-injured parenchyma. From these observations it is suggested that the decrease in brain elastance reflects the increase in cerebral blood volume due to decrease in cerebrovascular resistance rather than increase in edema. The increase in CBF that is associated with N administration did not increase edema, as can occur in some experimental paradigms (7) but rather attenuated the extent of perilesional edema as has been observed previously, perhaps by a direct cytoprotective effect on neural tissue (8).

CONCLUSION

In a cryogenic injury rat model Nimodipine showed a shift of the volume-pressure curve to the left with a simultaneous decrease in cerebral edema. It is suggested that the decrease in elastance was due to a decrease in cerebrovascular resistance and increase in cerebral blood volume. The known cerebroprotective benefits of N outweigh the risks of decreased elastance particularly if the latter is due to an increase in cerebral blood flow.

BIBLIOGRAPHY

1. Bedford RF, Dacey R, Winn HR, Lynch C: Adverse impact of a calcium entry-blocker (verapamil) on intracranial pressure in patients with brain tumors. J Neurosurg 59:800-802, 1983

2. Tateishi A, Takanobu S, Takeshita H, Suzuki T, Tokuno H: Effects of nifedipine on intracranial pressure in neurosurgical patients with arterial hypertension. J Neurosurg 69:213-215, 198

3. Nishikawa T, Omote K, Namiki A: The effects of nicradipine on cerebrospinal fluid pressure in humans. Anesth Analg 65:507-510, 1986

4. Giffin JP, Cotrell JE, Hartung: Intracranial pressure during nifedipine-induced hypotension. Anesth Analg 62:1078-1080, 1983

5. Hadley MN, Spetzler RF, Fifield MS, Bichard WD, Hodak JA: The effect of nimodipine on intracranial pressure. Volume-pressure studies in a primate model. J Neurosurg 66:387-393, 198

6. Gaab MR, Haubitz I, Brawanski A: Acute effects of nimodipine on cerebral blood flow and intracranial pressure. Neurochirurgia (suppl 1):93-99, 1985

7. Harris RJ, Branston NM, Symon L, Bayhan M, Watson A: The effect of a calcium antagonist, nimodipine, upon physiological response of the cerebral vasculature and its possible influence upon focal cerebral ischemia. Stroke 13:759-766, 1982

8. Jacewicz M, Brint S, Tanabe J, Pulsinelli WA: Nimodipine pre-treatment improves cerebral blood flow and reduces brain edema in conscious rats subjected to focal cerebral ischemia. J Cereb Blood Flow Metab 10:903-913, 1990

Paradoxical Responses to Pressure Volume Tests: Analysis with a Mathematical Model

M. URSINO[1], S. ROSSI[2], and N. STOCCHETTI[2]

[1] Department of Electronics and Automatics, University of Ancona, via Brecce, I60131 Bianche, Italy
[2] First Department of Anaesthesia and Intensive Care, Hospital of Parma, via Abbeveratoia, I43100 Parma, Italy

INTRODUCTION

Fluid injection or withdrawal tests are often used to derive information on the status of cerebrospinal fluid (CSF) dynamics and intracranial elasticity in patients with severe neurosurgical disorders. Traditional models impute the intracranial pressure (ICP) response to these tests to a balance between CSF production rate, CSF reabsorption rate and the craniospinal storage capacity [1]. However, much evidence has been gathered in recent years, showing that ICP time pattern during clinical tests may be significantly affected by cerebral blood volume changes too, and by the status of brain hemodynamics [2]. Aim of this work is to propose a more complete description of clinical ICP responses in head-injured patients with the aid of a mathematical model. The latter includes not only CSF circulation and craniospinal elasticity, but also autoregulation adjustments in cerebrovascular caliber.

MATERIALS AND METHODS

Intracranial pressure monitoring was instituted in comatose trauma patients admitted to an intensive care unit. The measurement was done through a system composed of a ventricular catheter inserted into the frontal horn of a lateral ventricle then tunnelled for about 5 cm under the scalp. Arterial pressure was simultaneously measured through a catheter inserted into the radial artery. Arterial CO_2 and arterial oxygen content were carefully controlled in each patient. The pressure-volume maneuvers consisted in the injection or withdrawal of 1 to 4 ml of saline according to the bolus technique described by Marmarou et al. [1]. ICP and arterial pressure data were sampled at a rate of 20 Hz and stored in the hard disk of a personal computer. Both signals were numerically low-pass filtered in order to eliminate respiratory and cardiac pulsating waves.

Data concerning 18 patients were then analyzed using an original mathematical model of craniospinal dynamics [3]. Description of the craniospinal dynamics includes CSF circulation, the craniospinal pressure-volume characteristic, the hemodynamic properties (hydraulic resistance and elasticity) of cerebral vessels at the level of major intracranial arteries, pial arterioles and cerebral veins, the collapsibility of the terminal venous cerebrovascular bed (bridge veins and lateral lakes) and the action of feedback mechanisms regulating cerebral blood flow. The latter have been assumed to work mainly on pial arteries and arterioles.

A best fitting between model simulation curves and clinical tracings has been achieved individually for each patient using an automatic minimisation algorithm, and modifying just four model parameters, each with a clear clinical and physiological significance. They are, the CSF outflow conductance, the intracranial elastance coefficient (analogous to the PVI by Marmarou) and the strength and time constant of cerebral blood flow autoregulatory mechanisms.

RESULTS

The 18 examined patients can be roughly subdivided into 2 classes. In a first group of patients (8 on 18) ICP exhibited quite a traditional pattern, characterized by a monotonic return toward baseline following the maneuver. These patients are classified by the minimisation algorithm as having defective autoregulation (in fact, the algorithm provides a value for the autoregulation strength lower than 1/3 the normal one). An example of the ICP response to a 2 ml injection in a patient of the first class is shown in Fig. 1a together with model simulation of the same maneuver.

In a second and more numerous group of patients (10 on 18) we observed a paradoxical response, i.e. a delayed ICP increase following saline injection and a delayed ICP decrease following withdrawal. The model imputes these responses to active cerebral blood volume changes caused by autoregulation mechanisms. In fact, the minimisation algorithm always predicts a value for the autoregulation strength in these patients close to normal. An example of paradoxical response in a patient of the second group is shown in Figs. 1b, with reference to 2 ml injection maneuver.

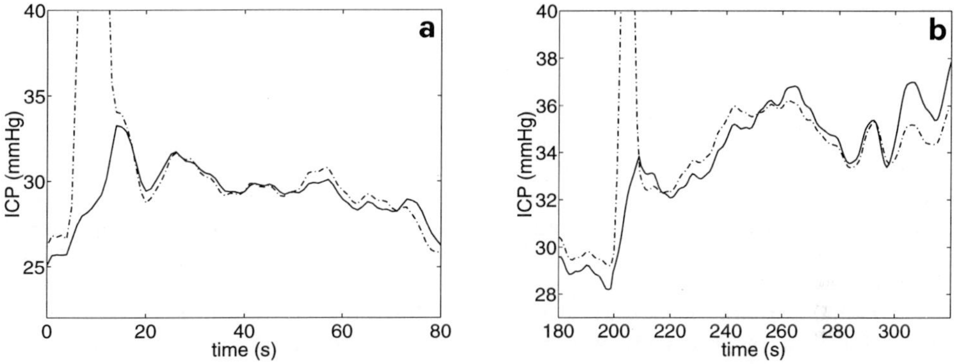

Fig. 1 - ICP response to a 2 ml injection maneuver in two different patients, with "traditional" and "paradoxical" response, respectively. Dotted lines are clinical tracings, while continuous lines were obtained via mathematical simulation. Peaks in clinical curves are artefacts produced by the injection maneuver.

DISCUSSION

As in most "traditional" ICP models, the clinical tracings observed in the first class of patients (Fig. 1a) can be explained as the result of an altered balance between CSF production rate, CSF reabsorption rate, and intracranial storage capacity. However, the traditional concepts of intracranial dynamics are unable to explain paradoxical responses as the one shown in Fig. 1b. In our opinion, interpretation of these responses requires the role of cerebral hemodynamics and autoregulation to be taken into account.

The proposed model is able to explain paradoxical responses quite well, imputing them mainly to active cerebral blood volume changes caused, at the arteriolar level, by feedback mechanisms regulating cerebral blood flow. Following an ICP increase (injection maneuver) in patients with preserved autoregulation, these mechanisms elicit arteriolar vasodilation and an increase in cerebral blood volume which, in turn, is responsible for the secondary delayed ICP rise. The opposite paradoxical effect (vasoconstriction with a delayed reduction in cerebral blood volume and ICP) is evident in the same patients following saline withdrawal.

Results of the present study suggest that analysis of ICP dynamics in patients with severe brain damage might provide information as to the status of mechanisms regulating cerebral blood flow, and this information might be quantitatively extracted through the use of non-linear mathematical models and automatic identification procedures. The effect of autoregulation on ICP should be recognized to avoid misinterpretation of clinical tracings, and to design an adequate treatment for intracranial hypertension.

REFERENCES

1. Marmarou A, Schulman K, La Morgese J (1975) Compartmental analysis of compliance and outflow resistance of the cerebrospinal fluid system. J. Neurosurg. 43: 523-534.
2. Rosner MJ (1987) Cerebral perfusion pressure: link between intracranial pressure and systemic circulation. In: Wood JH (ed.) Cerebral blood flow. McGraw Hill, NewYork, pp 425-448.
3. Ursino M, DiGiammarco P (1991) A mathematical model of the relationship between cerebral blood volume and intracranial pressure changes: the generation of plateau waves. Ann. Biomed. Eng. 19: 15-42.

Blood Flow Velocity in the Middle Cerebral Artery During Lumbar CSF Infusion Tests in Patients with Ventricular Dilatation

H. WHITEHOUSE, M. CZOSNYKA, P. SMIELEWSKI, and J.D. PICKARD

MRC Cambridge Centre for Brain Repair and Academic Neurosurgery Unit, Addenbrooke's Hospital, P.O. Box 167, Cambridge, CB2 2QQ, UK

The diagnostic criteria for so called normal pressure or symptomatic hydrocephalus remains controversial but should include cerebrospinal fluid (CSF) pressure and CSF outflow resistance (Rcsf) measurements [1]. Although this test is used routinely in the diagnosis of hydrocephalus and the assessment of shunt function it is invasive, and therefore unsuitable for initial screening procedures and sequential testing over prolonged periods. A less invasive technique for the assessment of CSF hydrodynamics would be of great benefit in these cases. Transcranial Doppler (TCD), a non-invasive ultrasound technique, has been used to explore the inter-relationship between CSF and haemodynamics in patients with shunt malfunction and raised intracranial pressure (ICP)[2,3].The aim of this study was to determine whether TCD can replace direct ICP measurement when CSF volume is increased during the assessment of cerebrospinal compensatory parameters providing a less invasive, one needle infusion test technique.

MATERIALS AND METHODS

Computerised infusion tests and simultaneous transcranial Doppler studies were performed in 26 patients, 17 males and 9 females with an age range of 6 to 78. The patients had either been previously shunted and were assessed for shunt malfunction (N=5), or they had ventricular enlargement confirmed by computed tomography (CT). **The infusion tests were performed using 2 lumbar needles, one to measure ICP and the other to infuse fluid.** The Computerised Infusion Test software [4] allowed the pressure time trend to be plotted on-line with off-line calculation of Rcsf and other cerebrospinal compensatory parameters.

Blood flow velocity in the middle cerebral artery was measured via the temporal window during the entire infusion test using TCD. The TCD and ICP data were recorded and the following parameters calculated: Flow velocity diastolic (FVd), flow velocity systolic (FVs), flow velocity time averaged (FV), the amplitude of the flow velocity pulse wave (PP=FVs-FVd) Goslings pulsatility index (PP/FV)and mean ICP. These parameters were noted for each patient at baseline pressures and at plateau pressures during infusion.

RESULTS

In all patients an increase in CSF volume during infusion produced a gradual increase in ICP. As ICP increased FV decreased and the amplitude of the flow velocity pulse wave (FVs-FVd) increased. When used to calculate PI a significant increase in PI was seen ($p< 0.0003$). Neither the mean PI nor the percentage change in PI correlated well with baseline ICP ($p<0.64$). Correlation of the percentage change in PI with increased ICP during infusion was better ($p<0.0014$), but still not as significant as the relationship between percentage change in PI and

Rcsf ($p<0.0001$). To determine whether the changes in PI were dependant on Rcsf the patients were divided into 2 groups. Group I with normal Rcsf (Rcsf $<$13mmHg/ml/min) and group II with increased (Rcsf $\geq$13mmHg/ml/min). FV and baseline PI were not significantly different in the 2 groups. If however a typical simultaneously recorded ICP and TCD trace for each group are considered certain trends become apparent:

- group I where Rcsf $<$ 13mmHg/ml/min FVs and FVd are well correlated. As ICP increases FVs and FVd both decrease. Although PP therefore remains constant PI increases due to a decrease in FV.
- group II where Rcsf $\geq$ 13 mmHg/ml/min FVs and FVd are less well correlated. As ICP increases FVs remains almost constant and FVd decreases giving an increase in PP. This coupled with a decrease in FV gives a greater increase in PI than seen in group I.

In both groups there is a significant increase in PI during infusion ($p<0.05$). However there is a significant difference between the 2 groups for both the change in pulsatility and the ratio of PI before and during infusion (PI/PI_b).

DISCUSSION

In this group of patients there was no correlation between PI and baseline ICP contrary to reports in the literature [2,3].This may be attributed to several factors including:

- the majority of patients in this group had normal or moderately increased ICP. Other studies have shown the relationship between PI and ICP is not reliable unless ICP is significantly increased.
- the increases in ICP may not have been reflected in the CPP.

This study has shown that there is a significant correlation between the change in PI during increased ICP and Rcsf. The ratio of PI before and during infusion (PI/PI_b) is therefore considered to be a reliable parameter for the classification of normal and disturbed absorption capacity. This suggests that TCD may replace direct ICP measurement during infusion tests, providing a less invasive technique.

REFERENCES

1. Børgesen SE, Gjerris F(1982) The predictive value of conductance to outflow of CSF in normal pressure hydrocephalus. Brain, 105:65-86
2. Quinn MW, Pople IK (1992) Middle cerebral artery pulsatility in children with blocked cerebrospinal fluid shunts. Jounal of Neurology, Neurosurgery and Psychiatry, 55 :325-327.
3. Chadduck WM, Crabtree HM, Blankenship JB, Adametz J (1991) Transcranial Doppler ultrasonography for the evaluation of shunt malfunction in pediatric patients. Childs Nervous System, 7:27-30.
4. Czosnyka M, Batorski L, Laniewski P (1990) A computer system for the identification of cerebrospinal compensatory model. Acta Neurochirurgica (Wien), 105:112-116.

Changes in Jugular Oxygen Saturation Associated with Intracranial Pressure Waves

KOSAKU KINOSHITA, YOICHI KATAYAMA, TERUYASU HIRAYAMA, SADAHIRO MAEJIMA, and TAKASHI TSUBOKAWA

Department of Neurological Surgery, Nihon University School of Medicine, Itabashi-ku, Tokyo, 173 Japan

SUMMARY

In the present study, SjO_2 was monitored continuously together with ICP in patients with severe traumatic brain injury, and the changes in jugular oxygen saturation (SjO_2) observed in association with pressure waves were analyzed. During B waves, the SjO_2 can be seen to increase and decrease rhythmically either with or between rises in ICP. In contrast, the A wave was commonly associated with a concomitant fall in SjO_2. Other investigators have reported an increase in SjO_2 associated with the A wave, suggesting that hyperemia could be the cause of the A wave. However, the A wave must elicit a decrease in cerebral perfusion pressure and vasodilatation simultaneously, each of which will influence the cerebral blood flow in opposite directions. Such a characteristic of the A wave might explain why SjO_2 does not necessarily increase in association with its occurrence.

INTRODUCTION

While the changes in cerebral circulation caused by an elevated intracranial pressure (ICP) have been examined by investigated with various techniques, the dynamic circulatory changes associated with pressure waves are not yet entirely clear. In the present study, the jugular bulb venous oxygen saturation (SjO_2) was monitored continuously together with ICP in patients with severe traumatic brain injury, and the changes in SjO_2 observed in association with pressure waves were analyzed.

MATERIALS AND METHODS

Continuous monitoring of SjO_2 together with ICP was performed in 68 patients with severe traumatic brain injury, and the changes in SjO_2 associated with 66 episodes of pressure waves in 6 patients were analyzed. The SjO_2 and ICP were monitored in the 68 patients with severe head injury within 24 hours after trauma. The Glasgow Coma Scale scores ranged from 4 to 8 in the first 24 hours after injury. All patients were underwent continuous monitoring of their systemic arterial pressure (SAP), ICP, respiration pattern, oxygen saturation of arterial blood and also SjO_2. The SjO_2 was recorded from a fiberoptic oximetry catheter placed in the right jugular bulb. In vivo calibration was performed every 8 hours and / or after the episodes of pressure waves.

RESULTS

Most of the pressure wave episodes were observed when the patients were released from the initial intensive medical control of ICP with controlled ventilation. Among the waves, 14 were A waves and 52 were B waves (Table 1; Fig. 1). The relatively low incidence of pressure wave episodes in the present series may be related to therapeutic interventionfor an elevated ICP. A decrease in SjO_2 of varying degrees was clearly observed in association with 7 episodes of A waves. SjO_2 progressively decreased (Table 1) and then increased in parallel with a rise and fall in ICP, respectively. In all of these episodes, a typical change in SAP, i.e., a slight but detectable decrease in SAP, was noted during the rising phase of ICP. When the increase in ICP terminated with a sudden increase in SAP, both SjO_2 and ICP rapidly returned to the original levels in parallel. In the remaining 5 episodes of A waves, no clear decrease in SjO_2 was observed and, instead, an increase was sometimes noted. In other episodes with a transient rise in ICP, which usually appeared to be caused by increases in SAP, SjO_2 commonly increased. An increase in SjO_2 synchronous with an increase in ICP was seen in association with episodes of B waves (Table 1) .

DISCUSSION

It has been reported that transient rises in ICP are usually accompanied by an increase in SjO_2, unless the cerebral circulation is critically impaired (1). In agreement with such findings, an increase in SjO_2 was frequently observed in the present study in association with a B wave or transient increase in SAP. Transcranial Doppler monitoring of blood flow velocity has demonstrated velocity fluctuations at frequencies similar to those of B waves. The mechanism responsible for B waves has thus been attributed to cerebral blood flow (CBF) fluctuations (2). In contrast, the present study demonstrated that a decrease in SjO_2 was not uncommon when a typical A wave was observed. This implies different underlying pathophysologies for A waves and other transient rises of ICP, even though vasodilatation is presumably the cause of both events. Since SAP does not increase when typical A waves occur, the A wave must elicit a decrease in cerebral perfusion pressure concurrently with vasodilatation, each of which will influence CBF in opposite directions. Such a characteristic of the A wave may explain why SjO2 does not necessarily increase in association with its occurrence.

Table 1. Transient changes in ICP, with an increase or decrease in SjO_2, were frequently observed in association with pressure waves.

	max. ICP (mmHg)	max. SjO2 (%)	min. SjO2 (%)	Δ SjO2 (%)
A wave	55.3±9.4	78.3±2.7	72.9±2.7*	5.5±2.4 (decrease in SjO2)
B wave	44.5±5.1	75.5±2.6	69.8±3.5**	5.1±2.2 (increase in SjO2)

Mean ± SD, *,** $P < 0.001$ (max. SjO2 vs. min. SjO2), max: maximum, min: minimum
Δ SjO2 : increase or decrease in SjO2 associated with pressure waves.

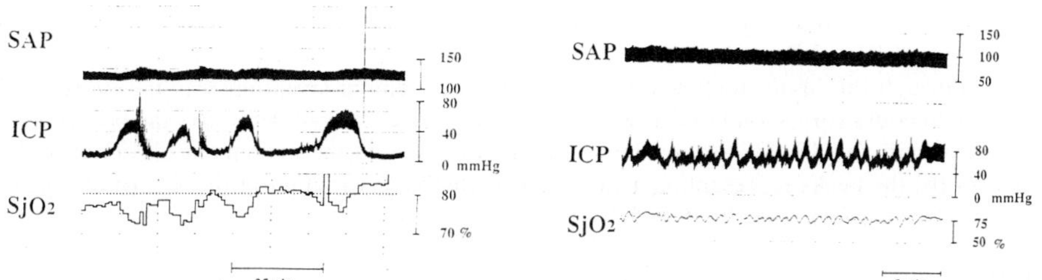

Fig.1 Recording of SjO2 during intracranial pressure wave episodes
Left: SjO2 progerssively decreased in association with A waves.
Right: Increase in SjO2 was observed in the episodes of B waves.
SAP: systemic arterial pressure, ICP: intracranial pressure
SjO2: jugular bulb venous oxygen saturation

REFERENCES

1. Rafferty C., Teasdale G.M., Bullock R., Fitch W., and Farling P. (1993) Changes in jugular bulb oxygen saturation and associated changes in intracranial pressure. Intracranial Pressure VIII : 418-423
2. Newell D.W., Aaslid R., Stooss R., and Reulen H.J. (1993) Spontaneous fluctuations in cerebral blood flow as a cause of B waves. Intracranial Pressure VIII : 424-428

Correlation of Recurring 2-9/min Pressure Wave with Slow Brain Movement and Compliance Observations in the Human

K. Lewer Allen[1] and E.A. Bunt[2]

[1] Formerly Head of Department of Neurosurgery, [2] School of Mechanical Engineering, University of the Witwatersrand, Johannesburg, South Africa

Introduction

A rhythmic oscillatory movement of CSF, of frequency 2-9/min, was early (1947) detected and described by the first author [1]; this was seen especially in the confined Aqueduct of Silvius during open operation, and this visible wave form was then designated a '3rd wave' - as being distinct from the cardiac and respiratory waves. Later (in 1960), Lundberg made his epic statement on pressure waves of 0.5-2/min frequency which he designated ß-waves. Later still Allen & Goldman [2], making measurements using a ventricular, as well as a spinal, volume gauge coupled to the CSF system, showed a rhythmic sinusoidal pressure wave of 2-9/min frequency, and in later papers [3,4] the first author reported on the use of a sensitive telemetry technique to further examine this '3rd (pressure) wave' in the naturally closed system, as seen in Fig. 1 (which occurred in response to a laugh). Also, in 1970 White et al [5], using echographic monitoring of the unvented head, reported a rhythmic centripetal brain movement of similar frequency (2-7/min), which they interpreted as a volumetric flux associated with an alternating downstream displacement of CSF through the ventricles. In personal communication, Prof White confirmed that in his opinion the '3rd wave' and his movement observation represented the same phenomenon.

An analogous density wave of periodicity within the 2-9/min range, as determined by rapid serial scanning, was later reported by the present authors [6] who observed a slow regular vascular energised wave motion (VEW) of periodicities 56, 86, 150, 224 and >224 s which was observed to be rolling physically through the brain. Included in this periodic movement spectrum was the pulse 25-56 s in duration which could correspond to the '3rd wave'. The work described here links the occurrence of this 2-9/min wave with (a) this VEW movement (and indirectly with the movement observed by White et al) and with (b) the peaks representing a slow (300 s) rhythmic variation in the rate of change of brain compliance (CRI), as reported in 1993 [7].

Results

A typical example of a telemetred 2-9/min wave is shown in Fig. 1 [3]. It appeared only in conditions of middle to normal pressure range (not being observed in the low or high pressure extremes). It was prominent in sleep and in the hydrocephalic with slackened ventricles, and we interpreted it as a normally recurring phenomenon. Its characteristic appearance is that of the cardiac wave superimposed upon a 'ground wave' of the characteristic frequencies quoted, with the added feature that the overall wave amplitude is amplified at the peaks of the regular underlying wave, suggesting a resonant coupling. This superimposition further suggests that the system compliance hardens and softens in a regular manner. The 'ground wave' apparently has a harmonic relationship with the cardiac and respiratory waves.

Fig. 2 is a representation of experimental **P** and **T** ordinates in the hyperbolic format discussed in [7],

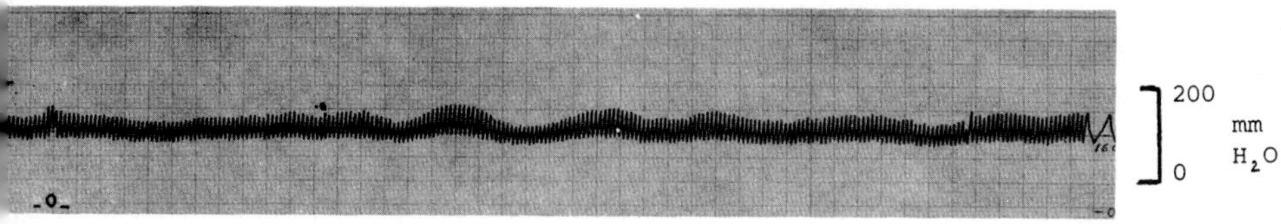

Fig. 1 Typical 2-9/min wave

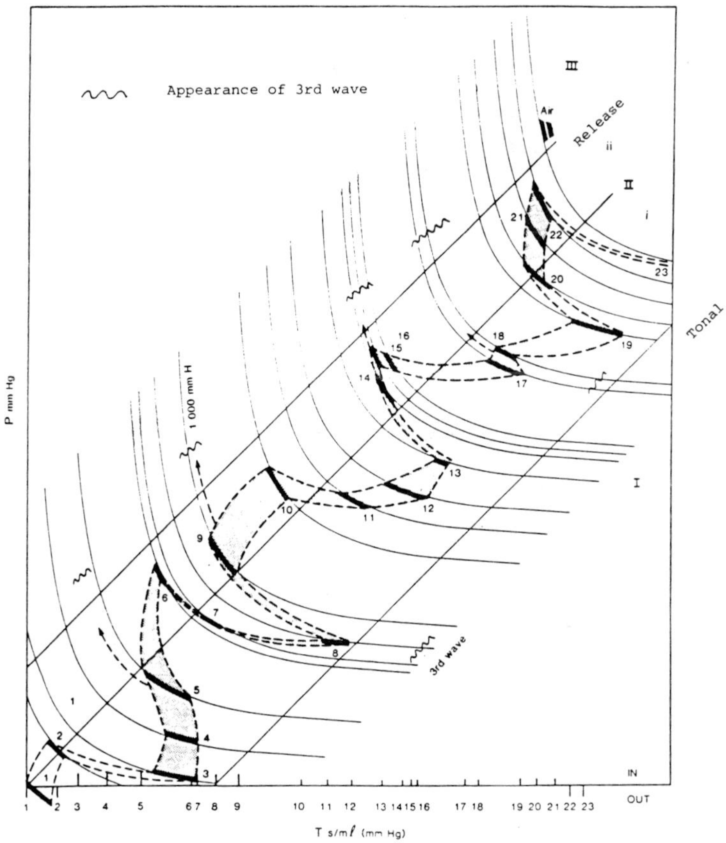

Fig.2 Typical sequential work diagram

on which phenomena such as changing compliance associated with the elapse of time are plotted as spaced hyperbolas. In this form of data plotting, a 'hard' condition is associated with the upper left portion of the hyperbolas, and a 'soft' condition with the lower right, the whole plot representing sequential rate of change of compliance over a stress cycle. The case represented is a clinically near-normal one. The compliance rate pulsation seen is believed to represent the 'ground wave' referred to above, since the 2-9/min wave was found to occur at points of maximum change, namely, at points just preceding and during the peaks and troughs of this wave (of much longer period, namely, ~300 s). Fig. 2 indicates an operating band between limits of a lower ('tonal') and an upper ('release' - observed volume compensation) level of hardness [7]. The 2-9/min wave appeared to trigger a 'trimming' (minor fluid volume change) action on a mechanism of larger volume change (mainly venous), in order to confine compliance within optimal limits - possibly by an autoregulatory response.

Conclusion

The observed pattern of the 2-9/min wave form and its appearance at peaks and troughs of the slow wave representing rate of change of compliance strongly suggests an interdependence between vascular components. It may thus represent the triggering of a trimming (autoregulatory) mechanism superimposed upon the inevitable slow modulated flux brought about by a vascular energised wave as it maintains a flow of the more inert venous and CSF bulk fluids, of which the compliance rate variation is an index. The regular ranging of compliance rate between the limits shown in Fig. 2 strongly suggests a sensing response to change as well as providing an indication that the 2-9/min wave is associated with a normal homoeostasis.

It appears unlikely that the 2-9/min oscillation is synonymous with the ß-wave of Lundberg, since it has its own frequency, sinusoidal shape and purposeful relationship to the CRI *as well as an ability to sustain itself for up to 8 min in resonant response.*

References

1. Allen KL (1947) "The clinical significance of low cerebrospinal fluid pressure". Ch.M. thesis, University of the Witwatersrand, Johannesburg.
2. Allen KL & Goldman HI (1967) "Phasic presssure characteristics of the cerebrospinal system". S.A.J. of Surgery 5(4): 151-8.
3. Allen KL & Sun HA (1971) "A study of the pressure of the cerebrospinal fluid in man by remote monitoring through the skull". Symposium on Telemetry, CSIR, Pretoria.
4. Allen KL (1973) "Telemetric monitoring of CSF pressure". J.Neur., Neurosurgery & Psych. Dec. 922.
5. White DM, Jenkins CO & Campbell JK (1970) "The compensatory mechanism for volume changes in the brain". 23rd Annual Conference on Engineering in Medicine and Biology, Washington, D.C., Nov. 15-19.
6. Allen KL & Bunt EA (1986) "Rhythmic brain movement and density variations shown by rapid sequential CT scanning in the human subject". In Miller JD et al (eds) Intracranial Pressure VI. Springer-Verlag, Berlin Heidelberg, pp 437-40.
7. Allen KL & Bunt EA (1993) "Experimentally derived law governing the time relationship of pressure-volume adjustment to stress in the human craniospinal system for use as a diagnostic and management tool". In Avezaat CJJ et al (eds) Intracranial Pressure VIII. Springer-Verlag, Berlin Heidelberg, pp 720-5.

Poster V:
ICP and Systemic Factors

Chairman: K.S. Choi

Induced Hypotension and Brain Tissue Response

A. SCHETTINI[1], E.K. WALSH[2], and G.J. BOUMA[3]

[1] VA Medical Center, Richmond, VA, USA
[2] University of Florida, Gainesville, FL, USA
[3] University of Amsterdam, Amsterdam, The Netherlands

INTRODUCTION

Controlled hypotension is frequently used in neurosurgery in operations for vascular tumors and aneurysms. There is, however, the possibility of cerebral vascular expansion resulting in intracranial hypertension causing changes in intracranial compliance and possible cerebral ischemia. There is also an effect on the brain tissue mechanical response properties, in particular the elastic response, a measure of the stiffness or softness of the tissue, which could effect surgical procedures. The principal results to be reported here concern the elastic response properties of in vivo brain tissue measured in a series of tests on dogs (n=15) using adenosine triphosphate (ATP)-induced hypotension. At the same time simultaneous measurements of CSF dynamics and cerebral hemodynamics were made and have been described previously [1]. The changes in tissue response are compared to results of earlier studies involving graded bleeding [2,3], sodium nitroferricyanide (SNP) and trimethaphan camsylate (TMP) [3].

METHODS

For the ATP-induced hypotension, tests were made on 15 conditioned male dogs weighing 21±3 kg and prepared for the measurements of CSF dynamics [pressure-volume index (PVI), compliance (C), CSF outflow resistance (R_o)] [1], local cerebral blood flow [1], and brain elastic properties (see, e.g., [3]). The brain elastic response properties were measured with a coplanar pressure-displacement transducer. The elastic response test yields two elastic parameters[1]: a tangent modulus, G_o, which is a direct measure of brain tissue elasticity; and a curvature modulus, $\bar{G}_o$, a quantitative measure of the nonlinearity of the response [3]. Measurements were made under control conditions (MAP≈115 mmHg), then under mild (MAP≈70), moderate (MAP≈50) and marked (MAP≈40 mmHg) hypotension. The stages of ATP dosage, infused through the femoral vein, averaged to 2, 4, and 6 mg/kg/min, respectively. Each stage was held relatively constant for 30 min during which the variables under study were measured. The ATP infusion was then discontinued, the animals allowed to recover, and all measurements repeated at 20 min of recovery.

RESULTS

The results for G_o and $\bar{G}_o$ for successive stages of hypotension are shown in Fig. 1. The brain elastic parameters at control were within the normal range for dogs [3]. At mild hypotension the elastic parameter G_o was unaffected while the nonlinearity, as measured by $\bar{G}_o$ decreased by 51%. At moderate hypotension the elastic response was measurably softened, as reflected by a 23% decrease in G_o and a further linearization of the response in a continued fall in $\bar{G}_o$. At marked hypotension, MAP = 41± 1, there were no further significant changes in the elastic parameters. Mean values at recovery were within baseline values. These results are in contrast to those for hypotension due to graded bleeding, SNP, and TMP, all of which showed a measurable increase in stiffness (G_o) at moderate levels of hypotension.

[1]Although brain tissue exhibits viscoelastic behavior, the present tests identify the elastic response since the time of insertion (loading) was short compared to the relaxation time of the brain tissue.

DISCUSSION

Simultaneous measurements of CSF dynamics showed a measurable decrease in the compliance during the initial stages of ATP-hypotension, indicating an increase in the system elastance (the reciprocal of C) [1]. The decrease in G_o reflects a softening of the tissue. The two together indicate a swollen, congested brain. The change in the character of the response measured by $\bar{G}_o$ is interpreted as a result of a decrease in both wall tension and transmural pressure in the cerebral resistance vessels. It should be of interest that moderate ATP-hypotension caused a decrease in the stiffness of brain tissue while the other three methods caused measurable increases.

REFERENCES

1. Schettini A, Walsh EK (1993) CSF dynamics and cerebral hemodynamics in ATP-induced hypotension. In: Avezaat CJJ, van Eijndhoven JHM, Maas AIR, Tans JTJ (eds) Intracranial pressure VIII. Springer-Verlag. Berlin. pp 738-743

2. Schettini A, Walsh EK (1983) Brain elastic parameters and cerebral hemodynamics in hemorrhagic hypotension. In: Ishii S, Nagai H, Brock M (eds) Intracranial pressure V. Springer-Verlag. Berlin. pp 282-285

3. Walsh EK, Schettini A (1984) Calculation of brain elastic parameters in vivo. Am J Physiol 247: R693-R700

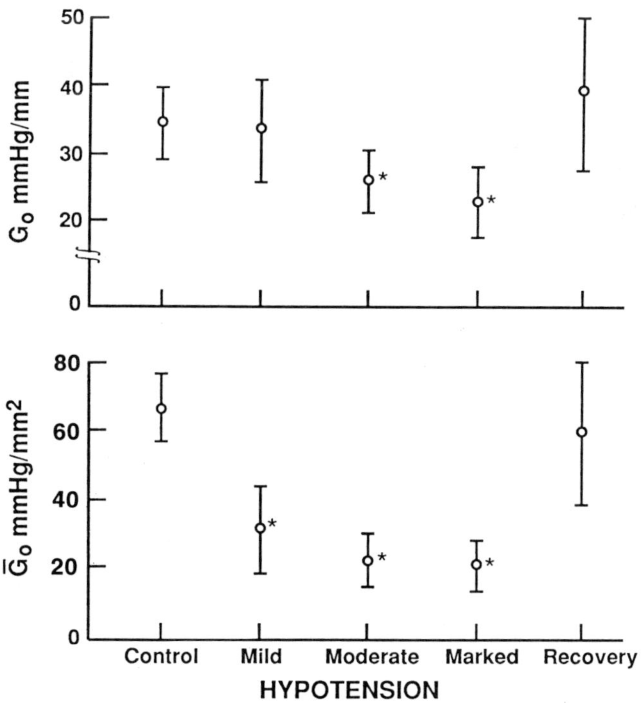

Fig.1. Elastic parameters at increasing stages of hypotension (means ± S.D., n=15,*p<0.05)

Prospective Evaluation of Risk Factors for Development of Acute Traumatic Intracranial Haematoma After Minor Head Injury in Elderly Patients

K.H. Chan, S.C.P. Ng, Y.W. Fan, and C.F. Fung

Division of Neurosurgery, Department of Surgery, The University of Hong Kong, Queen Mary Hos
Hong Kong

INTRODUCTION

The majority of patients who sustain minor head injury will have an uneventful outcome. A small proportion of cases would subsequently develop intracranial haematoma (ICH). Early detection and treatment of ICH would improve mortality. This becomes important especially in patients who are considered to be at low risk. It is well known that mortality and morbidity increase with rising age after traumatic brain injury. The present study aims to define risk factors for development of ICH after minor head injury in elderly patients.

MATERIAL & METHOD

From January 1985 to December 1988, 995 hospitalized patients who were above the age of 60 years and sustained minor head injury, defined as post-resuscitation admission Glasgow Coma Score (GCS) of 13 to 15 points were studied. All patients were admitted directly from the Accident and Emergency Department to the Neurosurgical ward. Patients were managed according to a standard protocol that included hourly neurological observation for 72 hours. Patients discharged would be followed up two weeks after injury. All deaths had post-mortem examination. All cases had skull X-ray performed (anteroposterior, lateral and Towne's view). Computerized tomography (CT) scanning was done when GCS was less than 15 points, presence of skull fracture and whenever clinically indicated. The end-point of the study was development of acute ICH within 72 hours of injury, documented by CT scan, surgery and/or post-mortem.

Thirteen potential risk factors for prediction of ICH were collected prospectively. Univariate analysis was first used to identify significant parameters. Multivariate logistic regression analysis was then used to define factors of independent significance. Significance was taken at 5% level.

RESULTS

Of the 995 patients studied, 408 were male and 587 were female with a mean age of 77 years (range: 60-100 years). Ninety-nine patients had road traffic accident, 34 were assaulted, 159 fell from height, 52 were hit by falling object, 694 had slip and fell and in 43 cases the mode of injury was unknown.

Twenty-three patients (2.3%) developed ICH (1 extradural, 2 subdural, 15 intracerebral and 5 had a combination of ICH). Univariate analysis revealed four significant risk factors (Figure I).

Figure I: Significant risk factors identified by univariate analysis

risk factors	no. of patients	no. of patients with ICH	p value
(1) headache			
present	216	10	0.021
absent	779	13	
(2) post-traumatic amnesia			
present	28	3	0.018
absent	967	20	
(3) Glasgow Coma Score			
13	7	3	
14	44	5	< 0.0001
15	944	15	
(4) Skull fracture			
present	23	15	< 0.0001
absent	972	8	

The following factors were not significant; history of loss of consciousness, vomiting, post-traumatic epilepsy, under the influence of alcohol or drug, associated medical illness, focal neurological signs, long bone fracture, chest or abdominal injury. Multivariate logistic regression showed two factors of independent significance, they included Glasgow Coma Score less than 15 and skull fracture. The logistic model which describes the relationship between the probability of development of ICH and the combination of risk factors is as followed:

$1/\{1 + \text{Exp.}[-1.9374(GCS)-4.4282(SF)+4.6167]\}$, where GCS=Glasgow Coma Score and SF= skull fracture.

The risks of development of ICH with different combination of risk factors were:
(1) no risk factor = 1%, (2) GCS<15 = 6.7%, (3) skull fracture = 46.2% and (4) GCS<15 plus skull fracture = 83.3%.

CONCLUSION

Patients at increased risk of development of ICH after minor head injury can be identified at the time of admission to hospital. This may help in formulating guidelines for admission and early identification and treatment of patients with ICH.

Idiopathic Intracranial Hypertension: Clinical Review of 25 Patients

L. Sipos, P.D. Lees, and N.F. Lawton

Wessex Neurological Centre, Southampton General Hospital, Southampton, UK

Summary

A retrospective study of twenty-five consecutive patients with idiopathic intracranial hypertension (IIH) is presented. All of the patients presented with headache and visual disturbances and all but two showed papilloedema. The CT scan of brain in all but one case showed no intracranial abnormality with small or normal ventricles. Lumbar puncture (LP) and cerebrospinal fluid (CSF) pressure measurement revealed elevated CSF pressure in every case. Two patients required no treatment at all. In 75% medical therapy failed and 16 patients underwent a lumboperitoneal shunt insertion either as a first treatment or following unsuccessful conservative therapy. In 50% of the surgically treated patients at least 1 shunt revision had to be performed due to migration or kinking of the lumbar drain or disconnection.

The clinical course and the therapeutic options in the treatment of idiopathic intracranial hypertension are discussed

Introduction

One of our patients with IIH had a very complicated course of the disease. During her 5-year history -apart from the LP monitoring- she underwent 19 operative procedures. Her case persuaded us to collect patients with IIH to analyse their clinical course.

Although pseudotumour cerebri or benign intracranial hypertension (BIH) is a well known entity it's etiology and management due to the unknown pathophysiology is still controversial.

Pseudotumour cerebri is a syndrome of raised intracranial pressure (ICP) characterized by minor to severe headache (HA) with blurred vision often associated with symptoms of raised intracranial pressure including diplopia. Computer tomography (CT) or magnetic resonance imaging (MRI) of the brain show no evidence of intracranial mass or hydrocephalus. The typical patient is an obese, young female. On neurological investigation papilloedema is found with n focal neurological sign, although abducens and facial nerve palsies have been reported [1,2]. There are several reported factors associated with pseudotumour cerebri but more than 50% of the cases are idiopathic. Although different drugs and surgical procedures -lumbo-peritoneal shunt, subtemporal decompression, optic nerve sheath fenestration- have been used the treatment of IIH is still empirical.

The aim of our retrospective study was to evaluate the clinical course of IIH and the outcome of conservatively and/or surgically treated patients.

Representative case

HM at the age of 18 in November 1988 presented to the Wessex Neurological Centre with a 6 month history of HA with no other clinical signs. General examination of this overweight lady was unremarkable and the neurological examination showed papilloedema with no focal neurological sign. Her visual acuity (VA) was 6/6 bilaterally. CT scan of the head revealed no intracranial abnormality. At LP the opening pressure was 29 and mean pressure during 30 minutes 24 mmHg. Conservative treatment was commenced (acetazolamide and steroids) but acetazolamide was stopped due to side effects. Her HA was well controlled with steroids but returned following their discontinuation. An LP shunt was inserted two months after her initial presentation. During the following 3 years 7 LP shunt revisions were performed due to low pressure HA, disconnection or infection. In December 1992 a stereotactic insertion of a ventriculo-peritoneal (VP) shunt was performed with medium pressure Pudenz valve. Her LP shunt had been removed and repair of a pseudo-meningocele performed next month. Within the next two months her VP shunt had been revised due to recurrent HAs and the Pudenz valve had been removed. An LP shunt was inserted later but despite her functioning shunts her VA deteriorated. She presented with a VA 6/18 on the right and 6/9 on the left with severe HA. In March 1993 bitemporal craniectomy and decompression of the right optic nerve were performed. Following these procedures her VA improved and her HA eased. She was then well for 6 months but due to infection both of her shunt systems were removed. Following that she was well and free from HA .

Clinical material

Between 1982 and 1992 IIH was diagnosed in 25 consecutive patients -including our representative patient- at our unit. The diagnosis was based both on clinical picture and lumbar pressure monitoring. Among the 25 patients 19 were female and 6 male with an age distribution between 11 and 60 years (average 27 years). The duration of symptomatology ranged from a week to 3-years. All of the patients presented with headache and all but 3 had visual symptoms, such as blurred vision, obscuration or diplopia. On examination 23 out of 25 patients were overweight and in all but two patients papilloedema was found. Twelve patients had decreased VA and 6 of them presented VF defect as well. One patient with normal VA showed VF defect. Two of the patients had 6th nerve palsy. One patient beside the classical signs of IIH developed polydipsia and polyuria. The past medical history revealed the following associated factors: use of oral contraceptive in 6, hypertension in 2, remote head injury in 2, asthma in 2 -one of them with ovarian cyst-, endocrine disorder in 1, sterilization in 1, hypochromic anaemia in 1 and menorrhagia in 1 case.

In every case brain CT was performed which showed no space occupying lesion with normal or small ventricles. In one case the CT scan revealed a large arteriovenous malformation (AVM) which later was confirmed by angiography. In other 6 cases on angiography or magnetic resonance angiography (MRA) we could detect no sinus obstruction. In three cases empty sella was found on the CT scan.

All patient underwent lumbar puncture and CSF pressure monitoring for 30 minutes which showed CSF pressures between 18.5 and 58.8 mmHg. The CSF was investigated in all cases and showed slightly elevated protein only in 2 patients.

Two patients with slightly elevated CSF pressure and mild symptoms received no treatment. Thirteen patients were treated with steroids (dexamethasone or prednisolone) either alone or in combination with diuretics and 3 with diuretics (acetazolamide or thiazide) alone. Of the 16 patients treated conservatively on average for 3.9 weeks 10 needed surgical treatment due to persistent headaches and/or visual symptoms. One patient died during steroid therapy due to deep venous thrombosis and pulmonary emboli.

Sixteen patients were treated with lumboperitoneal (LP) shunt. In 9 cases the LP shunt was inserted with and in 7 without lumbar reservoir (Forth Medical). Following operation in 3 cases transient and in 2 permanent low pressure headache developed. In the latter 2 shunt revision was performed with Orbis-Sigma Valve (Cordis) and there was no overdrainage later. In 1 case low back pain developed which resolved a few weeks later.

In those patients with a reservoir at least 1 revision was performed in 3 cases. In one patient the reservoir had been changed to a Sigma-Orbis valve which worked well later. In the rest of the cases 2 revisions each had to be performed due to disconnection and blocked lumbar drain. In those cases without reservoir revision was performed in 4 cases. In 1 case the infected shunt was removed 15 month following the initial operation and the patient remained well. In another case revision was due to migration of the lumbar drain. In 2 patients 4 and 5 revisions, respectively had to be performed due to disconnection or blocked lumbar drain. One patient despite the elevated CSF pressure and deterioration in his VA refused operation. He was followed up for 3 years and since his VA was gradually worsening and had permanent HA an LP shunt was inserted. His HA improved immediately following the operation. In 1 patient a horizontal-vertical (HV) valve (Cordis H-V valve system) was inserted and needed no revision.

In those patients where VA was impaired in all but 1 case improvement was detected either during medical therapy or after LP shunt insertion. There was only 1 patient in whom the VA deteriorated during medical therapy but improved following LP shunt operation (Fig. 1).

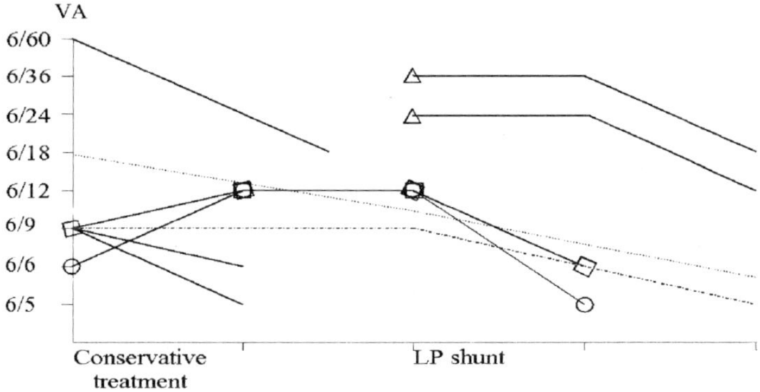

Fig. 1 Changes in VA during conservative treatment and following LP shunt insertion

Discussion

Idiopathic intracranial hypertension, pseudotumour cerebri or benign intracranial hypertension is characterized by increased CSF pressure with no intracranial mass or hydrocephalus. Since the severe papilloedema may threaten visual acuity instead of BIH the term idiopathic intracranial hypertension (IIH) would seem to be more appropriate than benign intracranial hypertension.

The etiology of IIH is unknown and probably multifactorial. The most likely factors leading to elevated CSF pressure are block in CSF absorption, increased resistance to CSF outflow or increased rate in CSF formation or diffuse brain swelling [3,4,5]. Whether these defects should produce IIH or hydrocephalus is still unclear [6].

Other authors have suggested the importance of increased cerebral blood volume, rise of sagittal sinus pressure either due to thrombosis or cranial venous outflow obstruction or brain oedema [4,5,7]. Due to the wide variety of relating and/or precipitating factors in IIH Johnston et al proposed a mechanism-based classification to replace the current concept based on the clinical picture [8].

The annual incidence of pseudotumour cerebri is 0.9/100000 and women are affected 2 to 8 times more than men [9]. The typical clinical picture is HA with papilloedema, although there are reported cases of IIH without papilloedema [10]. Sometimes abducens or facial nerve palsy can be detected. The patients in most of the cases are obese women of child-bearing years. Menstrual irregularities, endocrine or haematologic disorders, hyper or hypovitaminosis A, withdrawal of corticosteroid therapy, use of oral contraceptives, drug reactions (tetracycline, nalidic acid, psychiatric drugs) and head injury have all been included in pathogenesis [8,11].

Similarly to the literature in our material the young, obese female patients were affected more than 3.2 times more than male. All of them presented with headache and all but 3 with associated blurred vision, obscuration or diplopia. The neurological examination showed papilloedema in all but 2 cases. The pastmedical history revealed the frequent associated factors, i.e. use of oral contraceptives, head injury, asthma, endocrinological disorder, hypertension, menorrhagia or hypochromic anaemia.

A wide variety of treatment modalities have been advocated in IIH including diuretics, steroids, serial lumbar punctures, CSF shunting, subtemporal and optic nerve decompression or fenestration. Both diuretics and steroids are widely used as the first treatment, but their effect is frequently temporary.

The possible mechanism of action of these drugs is by decreasing the CSF production [12,13,14] or it may be that the steroids directly influence the conditions of fluid transfer across the arachnoid villi. Although resolution of signs and symptoms can be achieved by prolonged steroid therapy intracranial pressure may remain high and side effects occur in a significant number of patients [15].

Although Johnston et al [15] reported a high success rate with steroids 75% of our patients failed to respond to this therapy. On the other hand symptoms were temporarily eased in those patients where diuretics were given either with steroid or alone.

Different CSF shunting procedures give rapid resolution of intracranial pressure and are widely used. With the use of lumboperitoneal shunt it was possible to overcome the problem of small ventricles [15,16]. In

all of our cases where medical therapy failed or because of the severity of the clinical picture LP shunt insertion was performed either with our without reservoir.

Although the optic nerve decompression improves visual function in vision-threatening papilloedema intracranial pressure may still remain high [17].

Those patients who needed no therapy or responded well to medical therapy might represent a milder clinical course of IIH. The other group of patients suffers from a more severe form of IIH and there was a need to relieve the raised ICP urgently. All of these patients underwent an LP shunt insertion but 50% of them needed at least one revision. Although there was no need for revision when an HV or further revision when a Sigma-Orbis valve was inserted we can not yet recommend the use of either valve due to the small number of cases.

We would recommend no therapy if the CSF pressure is under 20 mmHg and HA resolves with LP. In other cases a combination of dexamethasone and diuretic (acetazolamide or thiazide) would be the next choice for 2 to 4 weeks. If the symptoms still persist or the VA is worsening an LP shunt needs to be inserted. The place of optic nerve decompression isn't yet clear.

A prospective trial might indicate whether the use of an HV or Sigma-Orbis valve reduces the number of LP shunt revisions.

References

1. Chutorian AM, Gold AP, Brown CW (1977) Benign intracranial hypertension and Bell's palsy. N England J Med 296:1214-1215

2. Round R, Keane J (1988) The minor symptoms of increased intracranial pressure: 101 patients with benign intracranial pressure. Neurology 38:1461-1464

3. Gjerris F, Sorensen S, Vorstrup S, Paulson OB (1985) Intracranial pressure conductance to cerebrospinal fluid outflow, and cerebral blood flow in patients with benign intracranial hypertension (pseudotumor cerebri). Ann Neurol 17;158-162

4. Reid AC, Teasdale GM, Matheson MS, Teasdale EM (1981) Serial ventricular volume measurements: further insights into the aetiology and pathogenesis of benign intracranial hypertension. J Neurol Neurosurg Psychiatry 44; 636-640

5. Mathew NT, Meyer JS, Ott EO (1975) Increased cerebral blood volume in benign intracranial hypertension. Neurology 25:646-649

6. Johnston I, Korgan MK (1991) A familial coincidence of pseudotumor cerebri and communicating hydrocephalus. Neurosurgery 28:727-729

7. Malm J, Kristensen B, Markgren P, Ekstedt J (1992) CSF hydrodynamics in idiopathic intracranial hypertension: A long-term study. Neurology 42:851-858

8. Johnston I, Hawke S, Halmagyi M, Teo C (1991) The pseudotumor Syndrome. Disorders of cerebrospinal fluid circulation causing intracranial hypertension without ventriculomegaly. Arch Neurol 48:740-747

9. Durcan FJ, Corbett JJ, Wall M (1988) The incidence of pseudotumor cerebri. Arch Neurol 45:875-877

10. Spence JD, Amacher AL, Willis NR (1980) Benign intracranial hypertension without papilloedema: role of 24-hour cerebrospinal fluid pressure monitoring in diagnosis and management. Neurosurgery 7:326-336

11. Greer M (1990) Pseudotumor cerebri. in Neurological Surgery ed Youmans JR, WB Saunders Company, pp3514-3530

12. Rubin RC, Henderson ES, Walker MO, Rall DD (1966) The production of cerebrospinal fluid in man and its modification by acetazolamide. J Neurosurg 25:430-436

13. Sato O, Hara M, Asai T (1973) The effect of dexamethasone phosphate on the production rate of cerebrospinal fluid in the spinal subarachnoid space of dogs. J Neurosurg 39:480-484

14. Weiss MH, Nulsen FE (1970) The effect of glucocorticoids on CSF flow in dogs. J Neurosurg 32:452-458

15. Johnston I, Paterson A, Besser M (1981) The treatment of benign intracranial hypertension: a review of 134 cases. Surg Neurol 16:218-224

16. Selman WR, Spetzler RF, Wilson CB, Grollmus JW (1980) Percutaneous lumboperitoneal shunt: Review of 130 cases. Neurosurgery 6:255-257

17. Kelman SE, Heaps R, Wolf A, Elman MJ (1992) Optic nerve decompression surgery improves visual function in patients with pseudotumour cerebri. Neurosurgery 30:391-395

*Present address: National Institute of Neurosurgery, Budapest, 1145. Amerikai út 57. Hungary

Hyperchloremia and Severe Head Injury

M. CANCELA[1], A. BIESTRO[1], R. ALBERTI[2], B. BOROVICH[2], A. SOCA[1], J. GALLO[3], and C. SCOTTI[3]

[1] Intensive Care Unit, [2] Department of Neurosurgery, [3] Laboratorio Central, Hospital de Clínicas, Montevideo, Uruguay

INTRODUCTION.

Electrolyte disorders are frequent after severe head, injury. It was demonstrated that they did not alter the outcome, however, nothing has been mentioned about hyperchloremia (1). With the purpose to prevent hypoosmolar hyponatremia, we decided to use normal saline solution (NaCl 0.9 g/l), as initial and basic fluid in stable head injured patients. After this trial, the result was a normonatremic hyperchloremia. The aim of this study was to investigate the mechanism of this disorder.

MATERIAL AND METHODS.

We studied 11 severely head injured patients (Glasgow Coma Scale Score <8) admitted to our Intensive Care Unit (ICU) in 1992 that developed hyperchloremia. Treatment of increased Intracranial Pressure (> 20 mm Hg) consisted of: Surgical removal of mass lesion, sedation, controlled hyperventilation, osmotherapy, and in severe cases indomethacin and barbiturates. All fluids used were without glucose: normal saline solution, colloids and aminoacid solution. The relationship between chloremia (normal 95-105), rate of hiperventilation (paCO2) and intake of chloride were analyzed. A linear regression was performed between these variables.

RESULTS.

Seven patients were identified having a mean chloremia/day of 110 mEq/l, a mean pCO2 of 25.7 mm Hg and a mean chloride intake of 411 mEq/day (24 g/day).

In this group regression analysis between chloremia and paCO2 showed $r=0.437$ ($p = 0.03$) (Figure 1).

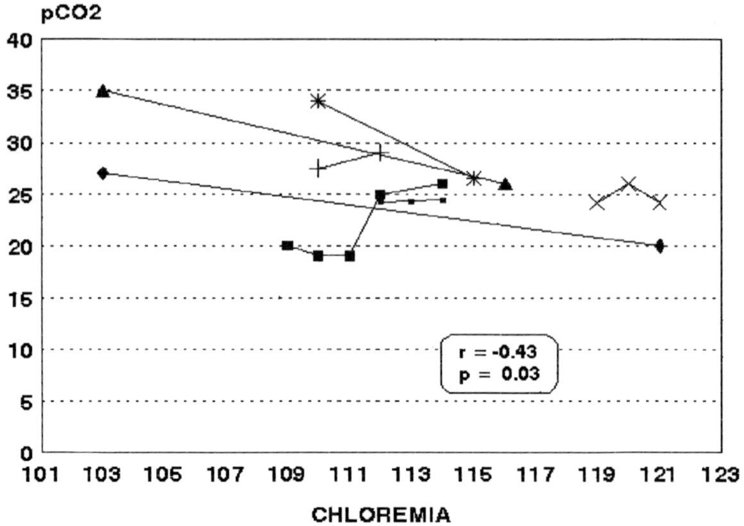

Fig. 1 - Graph showing the relationship between chloremia and rate of hiperventilation in seven patients with great intake of chloride. The tracings represent every one of them.

DISCUSSION.

It is well recognized the propensity of severely head injured patients to undergo hidroelectrolytic disorders during their stay in the ICU. Moreover, it is not clear which is the best fluid to use in hemodynamically stable patients during the initial post-injury phase. Glucose containing solutions may not be convenient because they provide free water that could facilitate hyponatremia. On the other hand it has also been suggested that glucose administration could be detrimental for cerebral metabolism of head injured patients [2]. With normal saline solution, hyponatremia was no longer seen in our ICU as an extracranial complication of severely head injured patients. By contrast, hyperchloremia is increasingly recognized. The most probable explanation of this disorder could be the intake of great amount of chloride in situation of respiratory alkalosis due to controlled hyperventilation, which is being compensated by renal bicarbonate excretion and chloride retention.

It is not known if this disorder may by itself cause brain injury. However, the anion chloride in cerebrospinal fluid (CSF) has an important role in acid-base homeostasis of central nervous system and over the control of ventilation [3]. Although, the chloride concentration in CSF is maintained unchanged despite of marked changes in plasma chloride, this condition could be altered in case of severe head trauma.

We think that this disorder could impair the ventilatory response of patient during weaning of mechanical ventilation. [4].

We conclude that with normal saline solution as basic fluid infusing to head injured patients, hyponatremia is not longer seen but an hyperchloremic state can be produced, particularly if intense hyperventilation is associated.

REFERENCES.

1 - Piek, J.; Chesnut, R; Marshall, L. (1942). Extracranial complications of severe head injury. J Neurosurg 77: 901-907.

2 - Robertson, C.S.; Goodman J.C.; Narayan, R.K. (1991) The effect of glucose administration on carbohydrate metabolism after head injury. J Neurosurg 74: 43-50.

3 - Kazemi, H.; Johnson, D.C. (1986). Regulation of cerebrospinal fluid acid-base balance. Physiol Rev 66: 953-1037.

4 Davidson, T.L.; Sullivan, M.S.; Swanson, K.E.; Adams, J.M. (1993). Cl replacement-alters the ventilatory resonse to central chemoreceptor stimulation. J Appl Physiol 74: 280-285.

A Survivable Closed Head Injury Model in Weanling Rats

BRUCE J. ANDERSEN[1] and SVETLANA V. PRAVDENKOVA[2]

[1] University of Arkansas for Medical Sciences, Little Rock, AR, USA
[2] Sklifosovsky Institute of First Aid, Moscow, Russia

PURPOSE

The development of certain types of neuropathologic changes associated with aging and Alzheimers Disease have been postulated to be accelerated by closed head injury. In an attempt to develop a model to study these changes, we have adapted a closed head injury model for use in weanling Fischer 344 rats, as they are a standard model for age dependent neurologic changes.

METHODS

The weight drop model of closed head injury in rats recently reported by Marmarou [1] was adapted for use in weanling Fischer 344 rats by decreasing the delivered force proportional to the animals' size. This model of consists of a vertical tube though which weights are dropped. The weight drops onto a stainless steel button cemented to the vertex of the animal's skull. This metal button distributes the force evenly, prevents any rotational component, and decreases the incidence of skull fractures. The animal is supported on a contoured foam rest of specific density to allow approximately 2-3 cm of neck flexion upon impact (no additional immobilization is used). This degree of neck flexion has been shown not to produce spinal cord injury or cervical spine fractures, yet allows a small motion component to be a part of the injury model, which more closely approximates the human condition of head injury than a static impact paradigm. The surgical preparation is minimal, requiring only exposure of the vertex and cementing the steel cap to the exposed skull. This incision is easily closed and well tolerated by the animals, making this an ideal model for survivor experiments to examine the long term sequelae of closed head injury. The relationship between impact level, survival rates, skull fracture rate, and neurologic injury in survivors was examined.

RESULTS

Our preliminary data in 100 gram Fischer 344 rats show that an impact of 200 gram meters has 0% mortality, 250 gm/meters has 17% mortality, 313 gm/meters results in a 34% mortality, 338 gram/meters has 80% mortality, and 375 gram/meters results in 100% mortality.

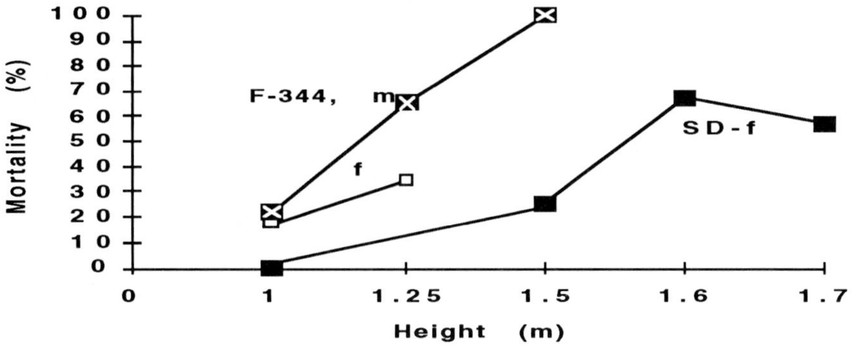

Fracture rates did not correlate with impact level and varied from 0 to 23%

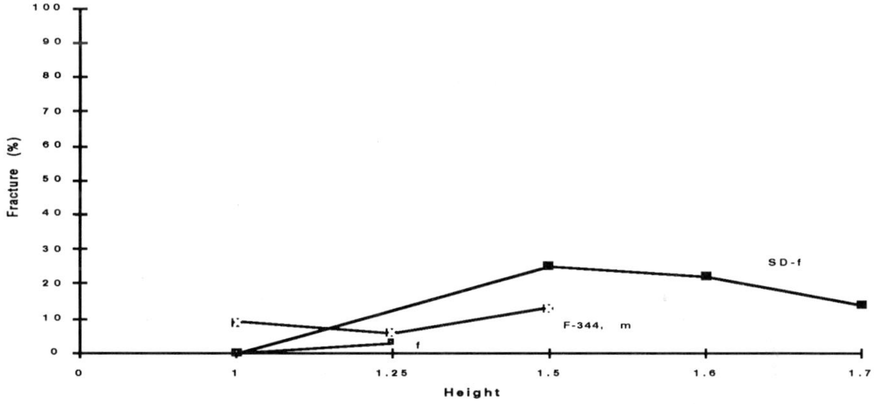

In all impact groups, irrespective of the impact level, survivors without skull fractures show no neurologic deficits after 24 hours that would prevent them from feeding, cleaning, and moving spontaneously. In these animals there is an approximate 48 hour period of zero weight gain, after which they gain weight normally (approximately 10% weight gain/day), leading us to conclude that the establishment of a long term survivor colony is possible if animals with skull fractures are excluded at any impact level.

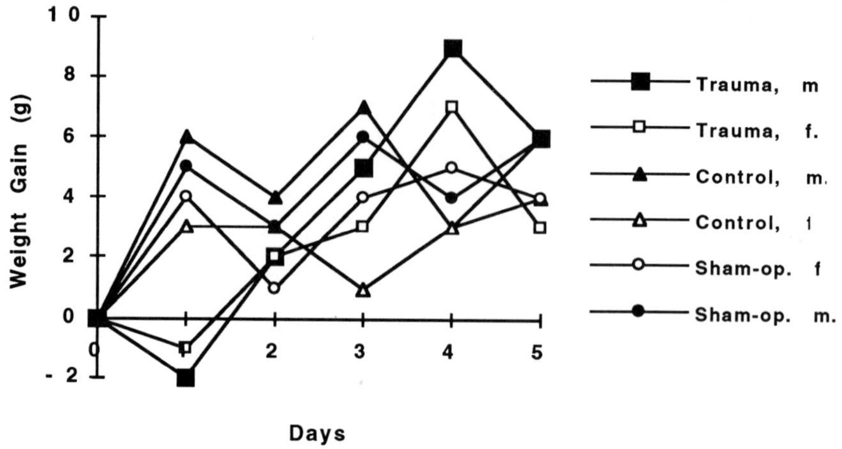

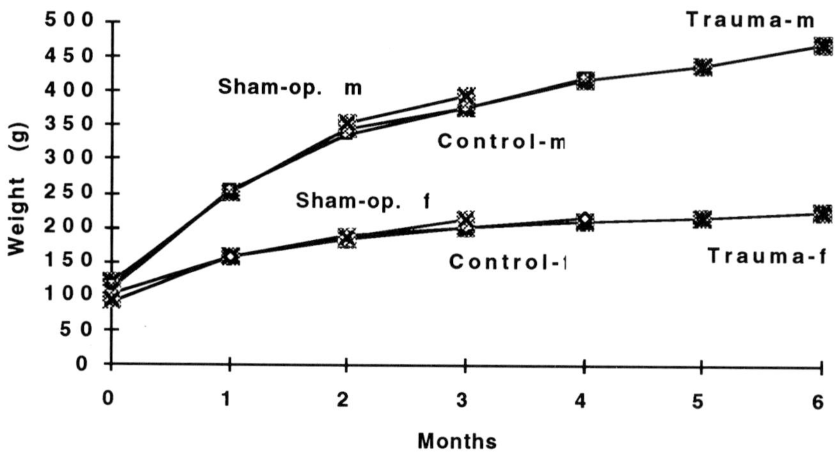

DISCUSSION

The weight drop model of closed head injury in rats recently described by Marmarou is easily adapted to weanling Fischer 344 rats. If animals with skull fractures are excluded, survivors at any injury level appear able to grow and mature normally. Since this rat strain is a standard aging model, the influence that closed head injury has upon the neurobiology of aging (including the histopathology characteristic of Alzheimers Disease) can be studied using a colony of impacted survivors.

REFERENCES

1. Marmarou A, Foda MA, van den Brink W, et al: (1994) A new model of diffuse brain injury in rats part 1: Pathophysiology and biomechanics. **J Neurosurgery 80:** 291-300.

Some Aspects of the Effect of Hyperbaric Oxygenation in Animals with Brain Oedema

P. Belić, V. Borisev, B. Belić, and Lj. Borisev

Clinic for Pediatric Surgery, University of Novi Sad, Yugoslavia

INTRODUCTION

Data attained in medical practice indicate that morbidity and mortality rates resulting from oedema are not decreasing. Etiological factors which cause brain oedema differ depending on which part of the world the material was examined, but not significantly. It is becoming more and more evident that we will soon be able to place an equation sign between the following major causers: pathophysiological changes in the blood vessels of the brain and all types of trauma. Primary damage, followed by secondary disturbances of the neural function are both a clinical and a therapeutic problem. These facts have encouraged the effort to introduce the hyperbaric oxygenation treatment as a choice of treatment of brain oedema in experimental conditions.

MATERIALS AND METHODS

Twenty-two dogs, weighing between 3.5 kg. and 4.5 kg. were anesthetized with Ketamin 25 mg/kg and then artificially underwent the impact of stress. A ramp was specially constructed at a 45 degree angle with a movable chair whose weight could be increased if needed. The intensity of the impact was monitored using an elastic metal plate. TECTRONICS was the type of electronic measuring equipment used and it enabled constant gravity value inspection. The intensity of the impact ranged from 6G to 12G. In each case, there was an RTG confirmation that skull fracture had not occurred. Immediately after the trauma, half of the experimental animals were exposed to 100% oxygen in hyperbaric conditions (Drager types). Animals were sacrificed with an overdose of narcotics (Nembutal). Tissue specimens were taken immediately.

RESULTS AND DISCUSSION

In both parts of the experiment, the following parameters were observed: artery and vein pressure, and glucose and lactate concentration. At the moment fully developed brain oedema was registered, the following changes have been noted: the level of vein blood pressure decreased proportionately to the force of the impact; lactate concentration decreased 5% compared to its normal value; and glucose concentration dropped 50%. Artery blood pressure remained unchanged. After the second treatment in the hyperbaric chamber, vein pressure improved, but glucose concentration did not rise significantly. On the third day of treatment in hyperbaric conditions, a significant decrease of brain oedema has been registered (histologically confirmed - Fig. 1). At this stage, the glucose level increased 85%

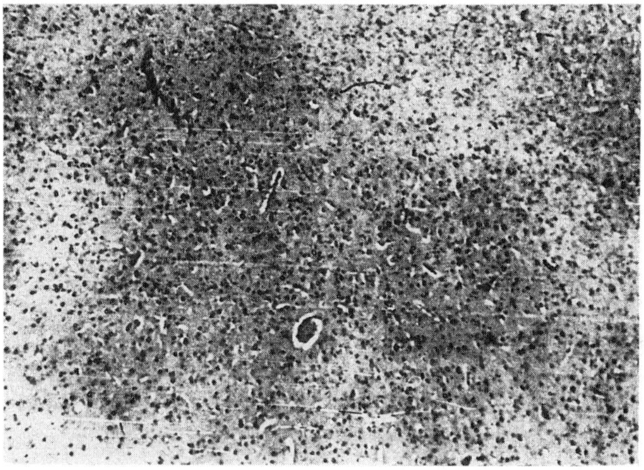

compared to its normal value and vein pressure 94%. It was evident that brain oedema was affected by hyperbaric treatment. Its decrease was followed by an improvement in vein blood pressure. The increase in the glucose level was evident, but it was not as quick as the increase in vein pressure. These results suggest that the effect of hyperoxygenation in hyperbaric conditions causes a decrease of brain oedema and improves neurological disorders linked to it.

REFERENCES

1. Allen JE, Rasmussen H (1971) The effects of oxygen on cellular metabolism. Int. Z Klin. Pharm. Ther Tox. 5:26-33
2. Artru F, Phillipon B, Berger M, Deleuze R (1976) Cerebral blood flow cerebral metabolism and cerebrospinal fluid biochemistry in brain injured patients after exposure to hyperbaric oxygen. Eur Neurol. 14:31-364
3. Balentine JD, Gutsche BB (1966) Central nervous system lesions in rats exposed to oxygen at high pressure. J Am Pathol. 48:107-127
4. Brenk HAS van den, Jemieson D (1962) Potentiation by anesthetics of brain damage due to breathing high pressure oxygen in mammals. Nature 194:777-778
5. Chapman AG, Halsey MJ, Hart GP, Luff NP (1986) Regional amino acid concentration in the brains of rats exposed to high pressures. J Neurochem 47:314-317
6. De La Torre JC, Kawagana HM, Hill PK (1975) Experimental therapy after middle cerebral artery in monkeys. Surg Forum 26:489-492

Does Vasopressin Act to Limit or Reduce Increasing Intracranial Pressure During Experimentally Induced Fever?

T.J. Malkinson[1], J.E. Bruni[2], Q.J. Pittman[1], L.K. Saladin[3], K.E. Cooper[1], and W.L. Veale[1]

[1] Faculty of Medicine, University of Calgary, Calgary, Canada
[2] Faculty of Medicine, University of Manitoba, Winnipeg, Canada
[3] Medical University of South Carolina, Charleston, SC, USA

Experimental evidence indicates that the brain is capable of regulating its fluid and electrolyte balances to maintain homeostasis and that central neuroendocrine systems are involved. Arginine Vasopressin (AVP) and other peptides are known to have specific neurotransmitter and neuromodulatory functions in the brain. AVP has been implicated in the regulation of intracranial pressure (ICP) and brain water balance. There is evidence for an association between changes in cerebrospinal fluid AVP concentrations and disorders associated with raised ICP. Transient intracranial hypertension has been associated with a febrile illness in infants [1].

We have shown that there is a significant increase (13-91 mm saline) in ICP during the initial period of the "chill" phase of an experimentally induced Prostaglandin, Interleukin, or Bacterial Endotoxin fever in the rat, rabbit and cat [2,3,4]. Increases in ICP as measured from the subarachnoid space or the lateral cerebral ventricle in both conscious and anaesthetized animals as well as increases in body temperature are dose-dependent and accompanied by phasic physiological responses characteristic of fever. A complex cascade of events underlies fever [5-review]. The fever however does not progress unchecked. Febrile temperatures rarely exceed 41°C, suggesting a mechanism which acts to limit the maximum temperature reached.

AVP acts centrally as an endogenous antipyretic. Perfusion of the Ventral Septal Area of the rat with a solution containing AVP attenuates a Prostaglandin (PGE1) induced fever [6]. Conversely application of an AVP V1 antagonist enhances the PGE1 fever [7]. Plasma AVP increases after endotoxin administration in the rat [8]. Changes in AVP concentration occur in specific areas of the brain during fever. Plasma and cerebrospinal fluid levels of AVP during fever do not show parallel changes with plasma levels increasing, peaking, and returning to basal levels earlier than cerebrospinal fluid values [9]. This suggests that AVP released into blood and cerebrospinal fluid are regulated independently and originate from different sources.

Saladin and Bruni [10] reported a decrease in ICP (5-26% / 0.2-1.0 mm Hg) with a single injection of AVP (0.125 or 0.5 μg) into the lateral cerebral ventricle. Conversely, the intravenous injection of AVP (4 ng or 0.05 μg produced an increase (5-23%) in ICP. Arterial blood pressure increased in both cases. The opposing ICP response elicited by the two methods of administration suggests that the decrease in ICP following ICV injection is a central effect due possibly to cerebral vasoconstriction and reduced blood volume.

mportant questions remain as to the nature of the relationship between AVP levels ıt various phases of the fever and ICP. Could the rise in ICP be a reflection of ncreasing plasma levels of AVP as shown by Saladin's intravenous administration? Could it be due to the increase in venous pressure which occurs during the "chill" phase of the fever and/or increased cerebral blood volume? Does AVP released during fever from specific brain areas and into the cerebrospinal fluid act in a way o reduce or limit increasing ICP as shown by Saladin when AVP is delivered entrally? Could changing compartmental levels of AVP result in different effects on CP at each phase of the fever? There are several distinct AVP pathways in the entral nervous system and it appears that these may be under separate regulation nd/or subserve different functions. Hariri demonstrated that E. coli endotoxemia n the swine is associated with the development of intracranial hypertension and an ncrease in cerebral blood volume secondary to elevation of cerebrovascular venous olume coupled with reduced oxygen extraction across the brain despite arterial ypotension [11]. In our investigations intraperitoneal administration of 50 μg/kg E. coli endotoxin induces a biphasic fever of 1.01 ± 0.09 °C (n=24) over a period of ight hours in the urethane anesthetized (1.5 gm/kg) rat. A significant rise in ICP 19.38±2.70 mm saline) as measured from the subarachnoid space occurred only uring the initial period of the rising "chill" phase of the fever. Carotid arterial and entral venous blood pressure rise at the start of the fever and heart rate is elevated hroughout the fever. Future investigations involve treatment of the animal with a asopressin antagonist to see how this may affect the ICP response, and ıeasurement of cerebral blood flow and volume.

Experimental evidence supports the conclusion that AVP is an antipyretic modulator ıvolved in limiting increases in body temperature during fever. Perhaps, AVP may lso act as a protective mechanism to reduce or limit increasing ICP during fever.

. Dorfman DH, Vinci RJ (1993) An infant with transient intracranial hypertension associated with a febrile illness. Pediatric Emergency Care 9:92-94
. Malkinson TJ, Cooper KE, Veale WL (1988) Physiological changes during thermoregulation and fever in urethane-anesthetized rats. Am J Physiol 255:R73-R81
Malkinson TJ, Cooper KE, Veale WL (1990) Cerebrospinal fluid pressure in conscious rats during prostaglandin E1 fever. Am J Physiol 258:R783-R787
Malkinson TJ, Veale WL, Cooper KE (1985) Fever and intracranial pressures. Brain Research Bulletin 15:315-319
Moltz H (1993) Fever: Causes and Consequences. Neurosc Biobehav Rev 17:237-269
Ruwe WD, Naylor AM, Veale WL (1985) Perfusion of vasopressin within the rat brain suppresses Prostaglandin-E hyperthermia. Brain Research 338:219-224
Naylor AM, Pittman QJ, Veale WL (1988) Stimulation of vasopressin release in the ventral septum of the rat brain suppresses Prostaglandin E1 fever. J Physiol 399:177-189
Kasting NW, Mazurek MF, Martin JB (1985) Endotoxin increases vasopressin release independently of known physiological stimuli. Am J Physiol 248:E420-E424
Kasting NW, Carr DB, Martin JB, Blume H, Bergland R (1983) Changes in cerebrospinal fluid and plasma vasopressin in the febrile sheep. Can J Physiol Pharm 61:427-431
. Saladin LK, Bruni JE (1993) The effects of intracerebroventricular versus intravenous administration of vasopressin on intracranial pressure in the rat. Neurol Res 15:198-203
. Hariri RJ, Ghajar JBG, Bahramian K, Sharif S, Barie PS (1993) Alterations in intracranial pressure and cerebral blood flow in endotoxemia. Surg Gynecol Obst 176:155-166

Poster VI: CSF Dynamics

Chairman: J.J. Tans

CSF Pressure Parameters and Ventricular Size Dynamics in Aneurysmatic SAH and Head Injured Patients

J. EELMÄE, M. KUKLANE, M. HEINSOO, and A. TIKK

Department of Neurology and Neurosurgery, Tartu University Hospital, 2 L. Puusepp Street, Tartu EE2400, Estonia

SUMMARY

We report that ICP and CSS viscoelastic parameters were more abnormal to the seventh day after aneurysmatic SAH. Patients with a low PVI, compliance and high elastance (independent of their ICP level) should be carefully monitored and these parameters be determined frequently to track intracranial buffering capacity. Enlargement of cerebral ventricles together with the decrease of R to the end of second week after SAH indicates brain tissue damage due to the brain edema and ischaemia. The posttraumatic ventriculomegaly is caused mainly by posttraumatic brain atrophy and the impairment of CSF resorption is not common for patients with severe head injury. The low level of ICP observed in this series is probably the result of an adequate ICP treatment based on monitoring of PVI. Even during low ICP periods there was a fall of PVI in one group of patients. Consequently, the monitoring of PVI might be accepted as a more accurate method for determining of aggressiveness of treatment in severe head injury.

INTRODUCTION

ICP and craniospinal system (CSS) viscoelastic parameters measurements have been considered to be a useful adjunct in the management of patients with aneurysmatic subarachnoid haemorrhage (SAH) and severe head injury. The clinical course over the days following the rupture is of prognostic significance, and several pathological factors can increase the ICP. Obstruction of CSF flow from the basal cisterns due to clot formation [1] or impairment of the absorption of CSF by blockage of the arachnoid villi by red blood cells [2] are responsible for "acute" hydrocephalus [3]. Dilatation of cerebral ventricles and other CSF spaces is common phenomenon after a severe brain injury. The development of ventriculomegaly is detected in up to 90 per cent of survivors of severe craniocerebral trauma [4,5]. However, the mechanism of the development of hydrocephalus is not clearly understood.

The aim of present study was to observe dynamically CSS viscoelastic parameters and on this basis determine the need of ventricular drainage and permanence of ICP recording in patients with aneurysmatic SAH and severe head injury. In addition, dynamical CT investigation were performed to evaluate CSF compartment size and together with CSS viscoelastic parameters decide the indication for shunting operation.

CLINICAL MATERIAL AND METHODS

The series included 13 patients with ruptured saccular aneurysms admitted to the Neurological and Neurosurgical Intensive Care Unit of Tartu University Hospital. The mean age of the patients was 48 years (range 36 to 63 years). Clinical grading of the patients was performed according to the classification of Hunt and Hess. In all cases early diagnostic clarification including CT, cerebral angiography and surgical treatment were performed. The trauma group were performed in a series of 65 consecutive severely head injured patients (Glasgow Coma Score less than 8), who were admitted to the ICU within 1 to 38 hours after injury and who remained comatose at least for 6 hours after the impact. The age range for this group was from 5 to 89 ys., with the mean age of 38 ys.

Ventricular catheter was placed via a right frontal burrhole into the right frontal horn before craniotomy. External transducers Belle-Howell were used for continuous ICP recording. Using the repeated bolus infusion test by Eelmäe [6], following CSS viscoelastic parameters were dynamically calculated after every 2 ml saline boluses: pressure-volume index (PVI), elastance (E), compliance (C) and resistance to CSF resorption (R). Recurrent CT investigations were performed to evaluate ventricular size, periventricular oedema, medline shift and hypodense areas.

RESULTS

In aneurysmatic SAH patients ICP increased during the first seven days, whereupon decreased to the normal level to the end of the second week (Fig. **1**.1.). Elevation of CSS elastance (Fig. **1**.2.) and decrease of compliance were more expressed to the seventh day after SAH. Concomitant changes were observed in PVI and compliance records, however more slight increase in values to the ninth day was admitted (Fig. **1**.3, and **1**.4.). Increased resistance to absorption was detected in the end of the first week (Fig. **1**.5.).

In the trauma group baseline ICP, elastance and resistance to resorption were in normal range (Fig. **2**.1, **2**.2 and **2**.5) during the acute stage and decreased to the end of the first month. The most expressed changes were the decrease of PVI (Fig. **2**.4) in the acute stage and the increase of compliance (Fig. **2**.3) to the end of the study.

During the acute stage Evans index decreased, two months after spontaneous SAH enlarged ventricles were observed (Figure **1**.6.). Similar changes were dedected in the trauma group (Fig. **2**.6).

DISCUSSION

Continuous measurement of ICP in aneurysmatic SAH patients is getting more widely used in neurosurgical intensive care units in order to quarantee reliable monitoring of CSS dynamics. However, still contraverseries exists in the management of these patients postoperatively. Our data shows steadily increasing ICP, being highest to the seventh day. However, only the period between 4 to 7 days abnormal ICP was recorded in this study. More expressed changes were observed in PVI, elastance and compliance dynamics. One must infer from these data that ICP may be lowered by therapeutic interventions, but the effect is transient since the brain remains tight. Thus, with the return of small increment of blood volume or oedema, pressure increases rapidly. This suggest that therapies be directed to increasing PVI as well as reducing ICP [7]. From this point of view, formation of brain oedema of aneurysmatic SAH patients is most expressed to the seventh day after bleeding.

Some investigators have stressed the impaired CSF circulation and resorption as a cause of hydrocephalus [8,9]. Nevertheless, the others have indicated that at least one of the mechanism for the development of hydrocephalus and the dilatation of other CSF containing spaces after the craniocerebral injury is a direct damage to the brain tissue, which leads to ventriculomegaly [10]. In our study enlargement of CSF compartment together with the decrease of resistance to

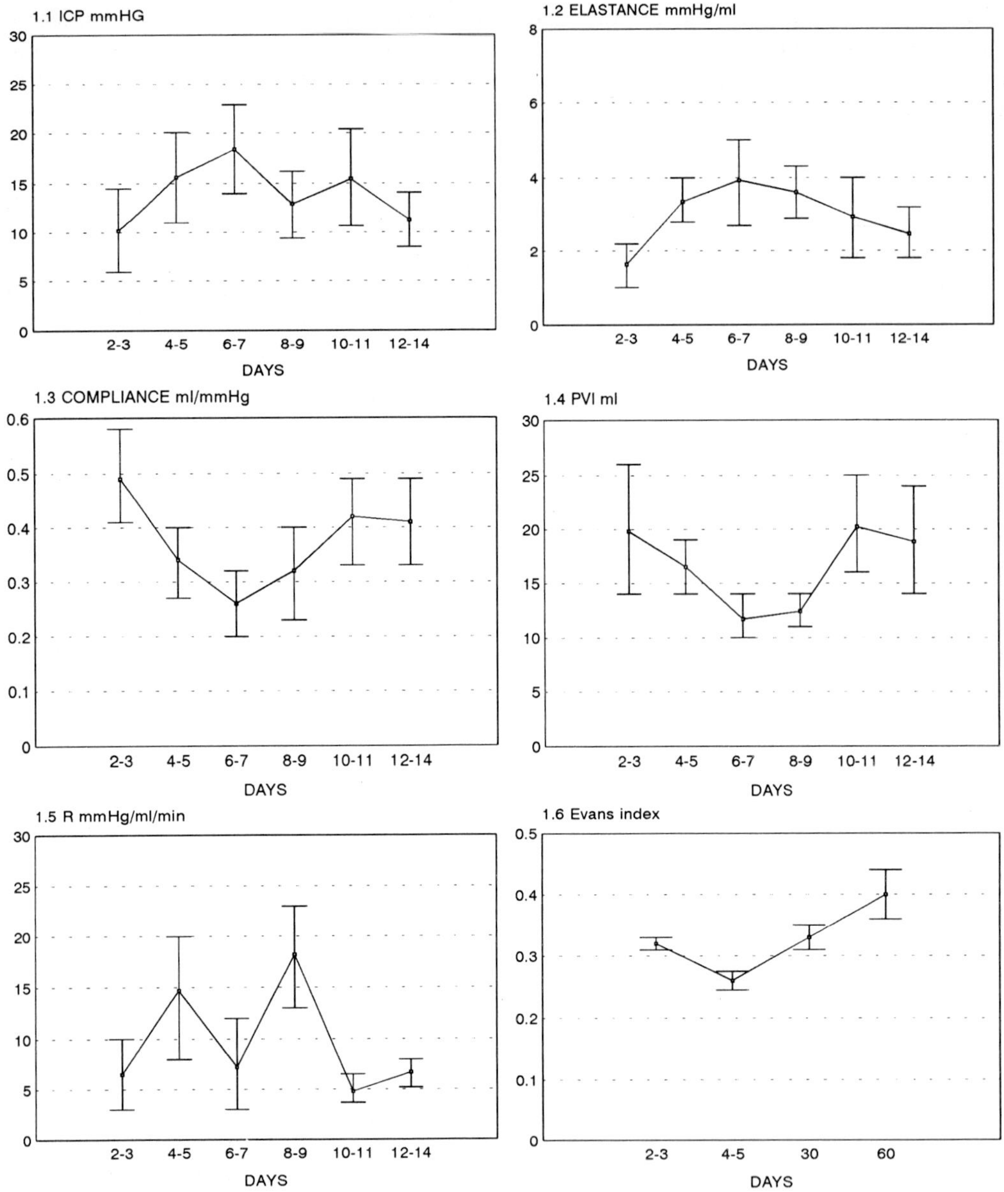

Fig. 1 Time course of ICP, brain elastance, compliance, pressure volume index (PVI), resistance to resorption (R) and Evans index in the patients with spontaneous SAH

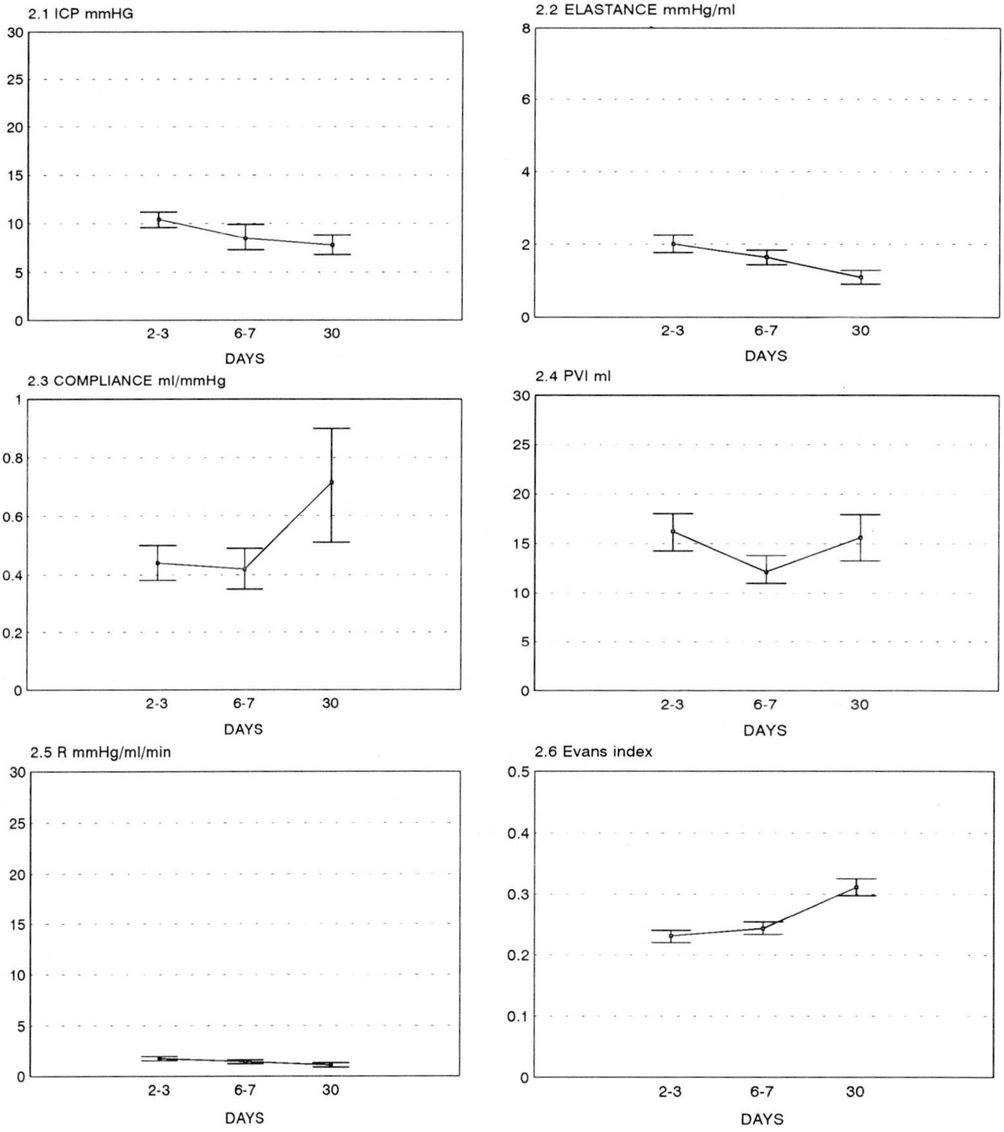

Fig. 2 Time course of ICP, brain elastance, compliance, pressure volume index (PVI), resistance to resorption (R) and Evans index in the patients with severe head injury

resorption after spontaneous SAH and trauma indicates to the brain tissue damage due to primary injury, oedema and ichemia.

References

1. Foltz EL, Ward AA (1956) Communicating hydrocephalus from subarachnoid bleeding. J Neurosurg 13:546-566
2. Ellington E, Margolis G (1969) Block of arachnoid villus by subarachnoid haemorrhage. J Neurosurg 30:651-657
3. Vassillouthis J, Richardson AE (1979) Ventricular dilatation and communicating hydrocephalus following spontaneous subarachnoid haemorrhage. J Neurosurg 51:341-351
4. Granholm L, Svendgard N (1972) Hydrocephalus following traumatic head injuries. Scand J Rehab Med 4:31-34
5. Gudeman S, Kishore P, Becker D, Lipper M, Girevendulis A, Jeffrie B, Butterworth J (1981) Computed tomography in the evaluation of incidence and significance of posttraumatic hydrocephalus. Radiology 141:391-402
6. Eelmäe J, Kuklane M, Tikk A, Asser T (1993) Quantitative Analysis of Different Curves of Lumbar Repetative Bolus Infusion Test in Patients with Ventriculomegaly. In: Avezaat CJJ (ed) Intracranial Pressure VIII. Springer-Verlag. Berlin. pp 824-828
7. Shapiro K, Marmarou A (1982) Clinical applications of the pressure-volume index in treatment of paediatric head injuries. J Neurosurg 56:819-825
8. Marmarou A, Maset A, Ward J, Choi S, Brooks D, Lutz H, Moulton R, Muizelaar P, DeSales A, Young H (1987) Contribution of CSF and vascular factors to elevation of ICP in severely head-injured patients. J Neurosurg 66:883-890
9. Borgesen S, Gjerris F (1987).Relationships between intracranial pressure, ventricular size, and resistance to CSF outflow. J Neurosurg 67:535-539
10. Lobato R, Sarabia R, Rivas J (1986) Normal computerized tomography scans in severe head injury. Prognostic and clinical management implications. J Neurosurg 65:784-789

CSF Dynamics in Spontaneous CSF Rhinorrhea: Clinical Study in 23 Patients

A. Mangiola[1], C. Anile[1], P. Palma[1], A. Vignati[1], and G. Maira[2]

[1] Institute of Neurosurgery, Catholic University, Rome, Italy
[2] University of Perugia, Italy

INTRODUCTION

Ommaya [1] has classified the causes of rhinorrhea by dividing CSF leakage into traumatic and non-traumatic categories. Non-traumatic fistulae are subdivided into high pressure ones, such as caused by tumors or secondary to hydrocephalus, and normal pressure ones. An alternative classification proposed by Spetzler [2] is based on the causes of CSF leakage and the CSF pressure; the juxtaposition of the causes with the evaluation of the CSF dynamics alterations could fournish the bases for an appropriate and rationale treatment in cases of spontaneous CSF rhinorrhea. In this paper we will be presenting the diagnostic protocol and the therapeutic procedures utilized in a group of 23 patients with spontaneous CSF rhinorrhea (Fig. 1).

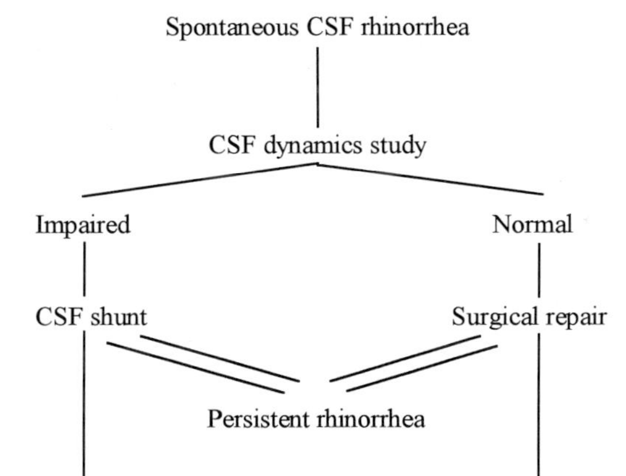

Fig. 1: Diagnostic and therapeutic protocol adopted in spontaneous CSF rhinorrhea.

MATERIALS AND METHODS

Our series consists of 23 patients affected by a spontaneous CSF rhinorrhea with a radiological finding of an intrasellar arachnoidocele (the so-called "empty sella"), that suggested the possibility of a CSF leakage through the sellar floor. In all the cases, a study of CSF dynamics was carried out by means of a 18G needle inserted into the spinal CSF space at the lumbar level. The following parameters were evaluated:

- CSF pressure basal level (normal value $\leq$ 15 mmHg);
- CSF outflow conductance (normal value $\geq$ 0.11 ml/min/mmHg) evaluated by infusing mock CSF at a constant rate into the spinal subarachnoidal space to get a plateau pressure and then calculating the

ratio of the difference between the plateau and resting pressure and the rate of the infusion [3].

RESULTS

An increase in the basal CSF pressure levels and/or an alteration in CSF dynamics were found in 15 cases which were treated by inserting a ventriculo-peritoneal shunt. The operation stopped the fistula in 11 of them and reduced the CSF leakage in the remaining 4; in these latter cases a plasty of the sellar floor definitively stopped the fistula. In the other 8 patients with normal CSF pressure basal levels and dynamics, a surgical repair of the sellar floor was carried out, but only in 2 cases did such a procedure interrupt the CSF leakage . In the other 6 patients the fistula continued and signs and symptoms of increased intracranial pressure appeared in one of them. In all of these last 6 patients an alteration in CSF dynamics became evident after the surgical repair of the sellar floor and the fistula stopped after implanting a CFS shunt (Tab. 1).

Table 1: Treatment for spontaneous rhinorrhea in 23 cases.

Impaired CSF dynamics		15
CSF shunting	11	
CSF shunting + surgical repair	4	
Normal CSF dynamics		8
Surgical repair	2	
Surgical repair + CSF shunting	6*	

* In these patients CSF dynamics disturbances appeared only after sellar repair.

DISCUSSION

Different authors have observed CSF pressure increase in patients with rhinorrhea and empty sella. Woscoboinik [4] suggested the inclusion of such patients in the hypertensive group Ommaya's classification. In our casistic the 91.3% of our patients (21/23) had an alteration of the CSF pressure and/or dynamics, but in 6 cases this was found only after the surgical closure of the fistula. This data suggests that an impairement in CSF dynamics could play an important role in the pathogenesis of the spontaneous CSF rhinorrhea, mainly in patients harbouring a so-called "empty sella". Nevertheless the CSF leakage may act as a safety valve, the closure of which would not be able to stop the leakage or could even worsen the patient's conditions as in one case of our series. The size of the anatomic defect through the sellar floor and the entity of the CSF rhinorrhea could mask the presence of the CSF dynamics disturbance.

REFERENCES

1. Ommaya AK, Di Chiro G, Baldwin M, Pennybacker JB (1968) Non traumatic CSF rhinorrhea. JNNP 31:214-225.
2. Spetzler RF, Wilson CB (1982) Dural fistulae and their repair. In:Youmans JR (ed) Neurological Surgery, WB Saunders Company, Philadelphia, vol. IV pp 2209-2227.
3. Anile C, Maira G, Mangiola A, Rossi GF (1989) Benign intracranial hypertension: CSF dynamics and CSF pulse wave morphology. In: Hoff JT and Betz AL (eds) Intracranial Pressure VII, Springer-Verlag, Berlin Heidelberg, pp 374-378.
4. Woscoboinik D, Remond J, Fisher G, Turjanski L (1988) Les rhinorrhées non traumatiques hypertensives. A propos d'un cas. Neurochirurgie 34:338-341.

The Effect of Subdural Pressure on Traumatic Subdural Hygroma

H.-J. KIM

Department of Neurosurgery, Wonju College of Medicine, Yonsei University, 162 Ilsan-dong, Wonju, Korea

Introduction

The subdural hygroma is still an enigma, especially in older age group and/or diffuse brain injury victims(1-4). Lumbar puncture during isotope cisternography displays various levels of intracranial pressure, from which the author make use of its role as a guideline to anticipate the fate of traumatic subdural hygroma.

Material, Method, and Results

35 operative cases were divided into two groups with 200 mmH_2O as the upper limit of intracranial pressure(ICP). Subdural puncture(Fig. 1) revealed that there was statistical significance between subdural pressure and their space changes in simple - and complex subdural hygroma group, respectively($P < 0.05$)(Table 1).

Table 1 Follow-up CT Scan Findings related to Initial Subdural Pressure

Subdural Pressure (mmH_2O)	Simple			Complex		
	Improved	Plateau	Worsened	Improved	Plateau	Worsened
≦ 50					1	1
51 - 100	1	2	2	1	3	2
101 - 150	1	1			1	1
151 - 200	2	1		1		
201 - 250	1	1		3	1	
251 - 300	4			3		
≧ 301				1		
Total	16(9,	5,	2)	19(9,	6,	4)

★ Improved: decrease of subdural fluid-filled space.
Plateau: no change of subdural fluid-filled space.
Worsensed: increase of subdural fluid-filled space.

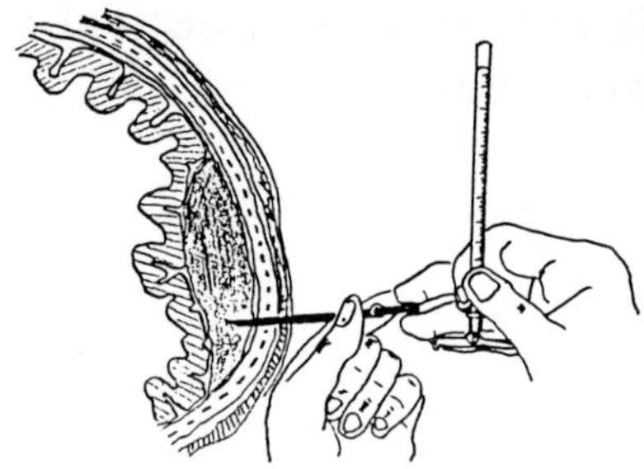

Fig. 1 Illustration of subdural puncture during subdural pressure measurement.

Summary

ICP measurement by lumbar puncture appears to be less accurate than that performed by subdural puncture at operative field. Therefore, it seems more reasonable to use the subdural pressure as a substitute of ICP in order to get a guideline to prevent convertibility of hygroma to hematoma, hydrocephalus and/or reaccumulation. Tentatively, the author proposes a protocol to deal with subdural hygroma(Fig. 2).

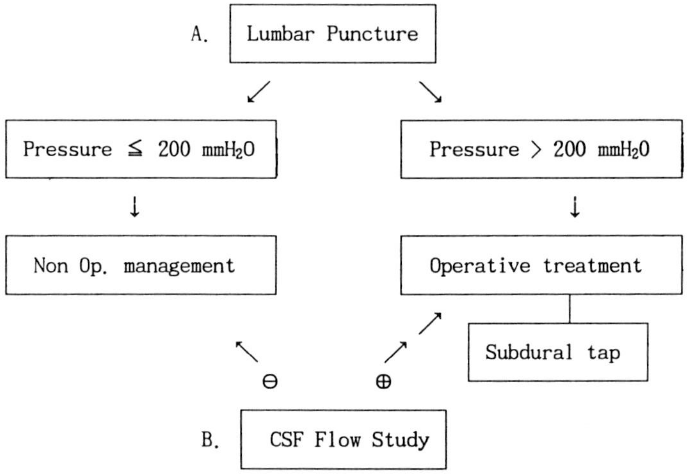

Fig. 2 Protocol to deal with subdural hygroma

REFERENCES

1. Naffziger HE(1924) Subdural fluid accumulations following head injury. JAMA 82:1751-1752
2. Hoff J, Bates E, Barnes B, Glickman M, Margolis T (1973) Traumatic subdural hygroma. J Trauma 13:870-876
3. Stone JL, Lang RGR, Sugar O, Moody RA (1981) Traumatic subdural hygroma. Neurosurgery 8(5):542-550
4. Hasegawa M, Yamashima T, Yamashita J, Suzuki M, Shimada S (1992) Traumatic subdural hygroma : pathology and meningeal enhancement on magnetic resonance imaging. Neurosurgery 31(3):580-585

Intracranial Pressure and Cerebral Blood Flow in Chronic Subdural Hematoma

A. TANAKA, S. KUMATE, Y. NAKAYAMA, M. KIMURA, S. YOSHINAGA, and M. TOMONAGA

Department of Neurosurgery, Fukuoka University, Chikushi Hospital, Chikushino, Fukuoka, 818 Japan

SUMMARY

Chronic subdural hematomas induce neurological dysfunction through a primarily mechanical distortion of deep brain regions such as the thalamus with a secondary influence on remote regions due to transneural depression. The effect of subdural hematomas upon the intracranial pressure (ICP) and /or cerebral blood flow (CBF) are not the major cause of neurological dysfunction in this disorder.

INTRODUCTION

While the cause of neurological dysfunction accompanying chronic subdural hematomas would appear to be due to the rise of ICP and the accompanying lowering of CBF this has not been documented. We have examined the ICP and CBF in 20 patients with chronic subdural hematomas in order to assess the clinical pathophysiology of this disorder.

MATERIALS AND METHODS

All of the patients (male 11, female 9) who ranged in age from 47-88 years with an average of 70 years presented with chronic subdural hematoma defined on CT. All had hemiparesis and/or mental dysfunction like confusion, lethargy or coma. All had a midline shift or a herniation sign on CT. ICP was monitored continuously in all cases with an epidural transducer through a burr-hole 24hours before surgery and then left in place 24 hours following surgery. Xenon/CT CBF studies were obtained prior to surgery, one day following and three to four weeks later. Each baseline CBF study was accompanied by an acetazolamide induced vasodilatory stress test. The type of surgery was one burr-hole and catheter drainage. CBF values in normal controls were obtained from 6 volunteers, aged 50-72 years with an average of 60 years.

RESULTS AND DISCUSSION:

Clinical Changes: Clinical symptoms improved in all cases immediately following drainage of the hematoma.

ICP Changes: Prior to surgery the ICP ranged from 14.6～27.5 with an mean of 20.8$\pm$4.0 mmHg. ICP fell after surgery, but returned to and surpassed preoperative levels in the following day. At 24 hours the ICP measured 13.4～31.7 with a mean of 22.0$\pm$5.6 mmHg.

CBF Changes: The reduction of CBF was most pronouced in the thalamus, while its enhancement by acetazolamide was more pronounced in the hemisphere, cortex and putamen on the side of the hematoma (Table 1). One day after surgery, the CBF stayed at the preoperative level on the side of the hematoma, while the CBF was further reduced on the opposite side. Thus, the CBF reduction became symmetrical on both sides. The CBF enhancement by acetazolamide was homogeneous. Three-four weeks after surgery, the CBF increased up to subnorma levels, ranging from 69.6~81.1% of normal controls. The CBF enhancement by acetazolamide was reduced in each area.

Table 1 Cerebral blood flow (CBF) and its enhancement rate by acetazolamide before and after operation for chronic subdural hematoma[a)]

Regions of interest (CBF in normal controls)	Preope.		Postope. (1 d.)		Postope.(3-4 w.)	
	Baseline CBF	Aceta. en. rate	Baseline CBF	Aceta. en. rate	Baseline CBF	Aceta. en. rate
Hemisphere (45.0 ±2.5)	63.8%[b)] 71.3%	50.8% 38.1%	62.7% 64.2%	54.2% 52.9%	78.4% 81.1%	27.3% 23.7%
Cortex (50.6 ±5.2)	62.8% 67.2%	53.2% 49.8%	63.8% 61.3%	47.4% 56.5%	77.1% 75.5%	17.8% 37.4%
Thalamus (73.4 ±5.3)	55.4% 58.0%	30.1% 36.6%	55.7% 53.4%	43.0% 47.1%	73.7% 75.9%	33.4% 35.9%
Putamen (53.6 ±7.4)	58.6% 66.4%	43.7% 14.5%	58.2% 68.3%	49.4% 49.2%	69.6% 79.1%	18.3% 27.6%

a) CBF, ml/100g/min. b) Upper row of values, reading on the side of the hematoma; Lower row, reading on the opposide side. c) Preope., preoperative; d., day; w., weeks; aceta. en. rate, acetazolamide enhancement rate.

The maximal reduction of CBF within the thalamus in conjunction with reduced cortical flow values but the retension of vasodilatory capacity on the side of the subdural hematoma suggests that the primary injury is to the thalamus. Injury to this region is most likely due to mechanical distortion and to secondary vascular compromise of its blood supply by relatively fixed perforating vessels arising from the posterior cerebral arteries. The reduction of CBF on the side of the hematoma and the opposite side are most likely due to the reduction of metabolic demand secondary to the primary thalamic injury. Consistent clinical improvement despite persistent ICP elevation and CBF reduction provides evidence that they are secondary phenomena. The continued elevation of ICP may be due to an increase of blood volume which follows the improvement of perfusion pressure following hematoma drainage. The delayed return of CBF to more normal levels by weeks 3-4 post surgery also supports the concept of transneurnal dysfunction as a cause of the earlier reduction of CBF.

Theoretical and Physiological Concepts on the Problems Met with Shunted Hydrocephalus

D.A. DE JONG, E.J. DELWEL, and C.J.J. AVEZAAT

Department of Neurosurgery, University Hospital Rotterdam, Dr. Molewaterplein 40, Rotterdam, The Netherlands

SUMMARY

Awareness of the hydrostatic changes due to CSF volume reduction by a shunt is essential to prevent overdrainage. Arguments are presented that overdrainage may occur in the recumbent position and recommendations are given to prevent overdrainage.

INTRODUCTION

Fig. 1 depicts the craniospinal CSF compartment, schematically represented by a rigid cylindrical container closed at both ends by an elastic membrane. The elastic properties mainly depend on the compressibility and distensibility of the surrounding craniospinal veins.

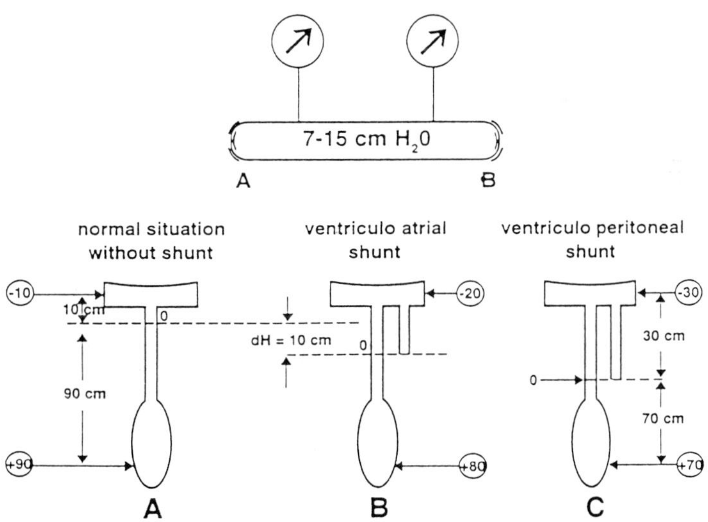

figure 1

In the horizontal (recumbent) position the pressure at A (ventricular pressure) equals the pressure measured at B (lumbar pressure). In the upright position the ventricular pressure will drop to a negative value. Draining CSF by a shunt may lead to an underfilled CSF compartment: on acquiring upright position an exaggerated ventricular pressure drop due to hydrostatic loading by the spinal part of the CSF compartment may lead to complications of overdrainage, expecially subdural effusions. This effect is expected to be worse in peritoneal shunts as compared to atrial shunts because of the lower position of the tip of the catheter.

MATERIAL AND METHODS

In fig. 2 the results of 25 shunted patients with the NPH syndrome are shown. Preoperatively, these patients were randomized for a low or medium-high pressure Codman Hakim valve. From the fact that subdural effusions are strongly correlated with implantation of a low pressure valve ($p = 0.03$) it is concluded that overdrainage in shunted NPH patients takes place in the recumbent position, presumably due to the effect of A- and B-waves. The fact that all patients received a ventriculoperitoneal shunt eliminates the effect of the opening pressure of the valve as the individual differences in negative hydrostatic pressure of the distal catheter will overrule this effect.

figure 2

N = 25	LOW		MEDIUM	
SDE	9	9	2	3
NSDE	4	2	7	9
		IMPROVED		

SDE: Subdural Effusion
NSDE: No Subdural Effusion

DISCUSSION

Overdrainage is not solely confined to the upright position but may as well take place in the recumbent position.

Ventriculo atrial shunts carry less risks of developing overdrainage as compared to ventriculoperitoneal shunts. The Siphon control device (SCD) developed by PS Medical prevents overdrainage in the upright position and benefits restoration of the CSF volume in the upright position by eliminating the negative hydrostatic pressure of the distal catheter in the upright position. Preoperative assessment of the elasticity of the surrounding structures of the CSF compartment, like the Ayala index measured by withdrawal of a fixed amount of CSF, may be helpful in choosing the adequate shunt system. The more profound the CSF pressure drop, the more one has to beware of overdrainage.

Effects of the Hydrocephalic Process on the Cerebral Hemodynamics of Immature Brain with Congenital Hydrocephalus

A. Wakayama[1], K. Morimoto[1], H. Nakamura[1], and T. Hayakawa[2]

[1] Department of Neurosurgery, Osaka Medical Center and Research Institute for Maternal and Child Health, Murodo-cho, Izumi, Osaka, 590-01 Japan
[2] Department of Neurosurgery, Osaka University Medical School, Yamadaoka, Suita, Osaka, 565 Japan

SUMMARY

By color Doppler ultrasonography, blood flow velocity in the anterior cerebral artery and internal cerebral vein was measured serially in neonates with congenital hydrocephalus, who had been delivered in early gestation and treated for hydrocephalus. Cerebral hemodynamic changes after birth in them were reflected in changes in blood flow velocity in basal cerebral vessels as measured by color Doppler sonography, thus indicating the effect of CSF drainage on cerebral circulation. The relationship between blood flow velocity in basal cerebral vessels within a few days after birth and severity of ventricular dilatation suggests impairment of cerebral circulation to be associated with progressive dilatation of ventricle and the entire structure of the brain in fetal hydrocephalus. Immediate surgical treatment may be imperative for progressive fetal hydrocephalus.

INTRODUCTION

Indication of surgical treatment for fetal hydrocephalus has conventionally been based on static data on cranial and ventricular size in neuroimaging study. To determine the most appropriate time for surgical treatment of fetal hydrocephalus, the effects of raised intracranial pressure on cerebral circulation in neonates, delivered intentionally in early gestation, were examined.

CLINICAL MATERIALS AND METHODS

By color Doppler ultrasonography, blood flow velocity in the anterior cerebral artery (ACA) and internal cerebral vein (ICV) was measured serially after birth in neonates, who had been diagnosed as hydrocephalus by maternal transabdominal ultrasonography. Mean gestational age at birth was 36.3 $\pm$ 3.4 weeks gestation. Mean body weight at birth was 2563 $\pm$ 574 g, and mean head circumference 36.0 $\pm$ 3.4 cm. Mean cranial volume was 478 $\pm$ 152 ml, mean CSF space 242 $\pm$ 154 ml, giving a CSF space-to-intracranial space volume ratio of 48 $\pm$ 25 %. Intracranial pressure was measured following the implantation of a miniature Ommaya's reservoir for intermittent CSF drainage. The CSF ventriculocatheter reservoir was implanted in the frontal subcutaneous space with the ventricular catheter placed in the anterior horn of the lateral ventricle at 3.4 $\pm$ 1.5 days. By this reservoir, CSF was drained intermittently until a ventriculo-peritoneal shunt was obtained at 36.8 $\pm$ 15.6 days [1, 2, 3].

RESULTS

1. The results of Doppler studies within 24 hours after birth, at the implantation of miniature CSF reservoir and at the ventriculoperitoneal shunting are given in Table 1. The resistance Index (RI) in ACA within 24 hours after birth was within the normal range for neonates of the same age without hydrocephalus . Reduction in RI in ACA and increase in mean peak flow velocity (MV) in ACA and ICV following establishment of the ventriculo-peritoneal shunt were statistically significant (paired T test, $P < 0.05$).

2. The volume ratio of CSF space to total cranial volume was correlated positively with RI in ACA (r^2=0.42) and negatively with MV in ACA (r^2=0.53) [3].

3. Intracranial pressure (ICP) in the steady state at the time of implanting CSF reservoir was 9.5 ± 3.2 mm Hg. ICP was correlated with total cranial volume [2]. Cerebral perfusion pressure was correlated positively with MV in ACA (r^2=0.66) and negatively with RI in ACA (r^2=0.32).

Table 1 Mean peak flow velocity (cm/sec) and resistant index as determined by color Doppler sonography in neonates with congenital hydrocephalus after birth .*: Reduction in RI and increase of MV following treatment were statistically significant (paired T test, $p < 0.05$)

	day 1	CSF drainage (day 3.5 ±1.5)		V-P shunt (day 36.8 ±15.6)	
		pretreatment	posttreatment	presurgery	postsurgery
ACA					
Mean peak flow velocity	20.4 ± 8.29	19.5 ± 9.47	28.7 ± 17.28*	34.4 ± 10.53	50.0± 10.70*
Resistance Index	0.62 ± 0.07	0.71± 0.19	0.64 ± 0.04	0.79 ± 0.09	0.65 ± 0.07*
ICV					
Mean peak flow velocity	6.1 ± 2.99	6.3 ± 3.30	6.7 ± 2.34	7.7 ± 1.80	9.6 ± 3.97

DISCUSSION

Serial measurements of flow velocity in basal cerebral vessels by color Doppler ultrasonography should provide important data on cerebral circulation in neonate with hydrocephalus after birth. In the present study, cerebral circulation could be understood in greater detail by measurement of flow velocity in ICV. One drawback of Doppler sonography for evaluating cerebral hemodynamics is the lack of accuracy in blood flow volume. Change in cerebral circulation associated with CSF drainage and ventriculoperitoneal shunting was shown by increase in mean peak flow velocity in ACA and ICV and decrease in resistance index in ACA, indicating cerebral circulation in hydrocephalic infants to clearly be hindered by increase in intracranial pressure due to hydrocephalus.

It was not possible by the present Doppler study to demonstrate impaired cerebral circulation within a few days after birth in neonates with congenital hydrocephalus. Cerebral circulation of neonates within a few days after birth may be seriously affected by several factors such as dehydration, which significantly decrease CSF production, and unstable cardiac and respiratory function. The environment in which neonates are placed is different from that in the uterus. This result in the present study may be explained by the unique biomechanical properties of fetal brain and its container, which allows ventricular and cranial enlargement without developing marked elevation of ICP, although the intracranial pressure in congenital hydrocephalus in neonatal period was previously shown to be correlated with the severity of ventricular enlargement [2,3]. However, the relationship between blood flow velocity in basal cerebral vessels and severity of ventricular dilatation and cerebral perfusion pressure in the present study suggests impairment of cerebral circulation to be associated with progressive dilatation of ventricle and the entire structure of the brain in fetal hydrocephalus.

Immediate surgical treatment may be concluded from the present results to be imperative for progressive fetal hydrocephalus, and careful management of hydrocephalus after birth to be required.

REFERENCES

1). Morimoto K, Hayakawa T, Yoshimine T, Wakayama A, Kuroda R (1993) Two-step procedure for early neonatal surgery of fetal hydrocephalus. Neurol Med Chir 33: 158-165
2). Wakayama A, Morimoto K, Nishikuni K, Hayakawa T (1993) Intracranial pressure and CSF dynamic study in neonatal hydrocephalus. Nervous System in Children 18: 213-220.
3). Wakayama A, Morimoto K, Yanagihara A, Hayakawa T (1993) Evaluation of cerebral hemodynamics in neonates with congenital hydrocephalus by color Doppler ultrasonography. Current Tr Hyd 3: 5-10.

A Species Comparing Radiological Study on the Absorption of Cerebrospinal Fluid into the Cervical Lymphatic System

T. BRINKER[1], C. BÖTEL[2], and M. SAMII[1]

[1] Department of Neurosurgery Nordstadt Hospital, [2] Central Laboratory Animal Facility, Hannover Medical School, Germany

INTRODUCTION:

The absorption of cerebrospinal fluid into the cervical lymphatic system was investigated by radiological means. Earlier cisternographic studies have shown that X-ray contrast medium can not leave the cranial subarachnoid space (SAS). On the other hand the opacification of the perineural SAS of cranial nerves (e.g. the optic and the vestibulocochlear nerves) has been shown radiologically after intrathecal injection of contrast medium. The perineural SAS, however, has been recognized as CSF outflow pathways through which CSF and even particles drain into the cervical lymph system [1]. In the present study it is attempted to visualize these pathways by radiological means. Experimental cisternographies were performed in animals but by contrast to earlier studies of others under the condition of an increase in intracranial pressure.

MATERIAL and METHODS:

Following the percutaneous (cats,dogs,monkeys) or the transcranial puncture (rats [2]) of the cisterna magna, the cisternography was performed by a long-term infusion (30 minutes) of X-ray contrast medium (ISOVIST 300, Schering, Berlin). The rate of infusion was adjusted so that the intracranial pressure raised to 40 mmHg in rats (infusion rate 0.02 ml/min), to 50 mmHg in cats and dogs (0.6ml/min), and to 80 mmHg in monkeys (1 ml/min). Serial radiographs (a.p. and lateral view) were taken each 5 minute during the infusion period.

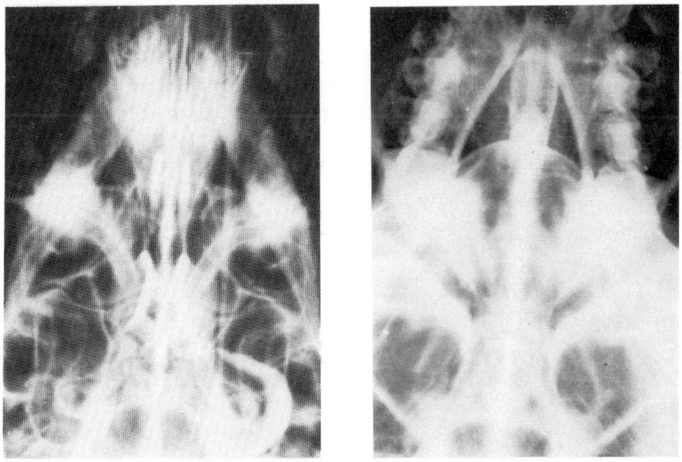

Fig. 1: Leakage of X-ray contrast medium from the optic and olfactory nerve into the orbital and nasal connective tissue of a cat (left) and a monkey (right).

RESULTS AND DISCUSSION:

The SAS of the optic nerve of the animals became opacificated after a 5-10-minute infusion of contrast medium into the cisterna magna. An additional contrast enhancement was found around the olfactory bulb. After 10 - 20 minutes of infusion the contrast material leaked into the orbit as well as into the nasal region (fig.1). Subsequently a diffuse contrast enhancement of skull base structures was observed in rats, cats and dogs. In monkey a deep shadowing of the nasal sinus was seen. In cats and dogs, the deep cervical lymph nodes and some of their afferent and efferent vessels were visualized after a 30-minute infusion (fig.2).

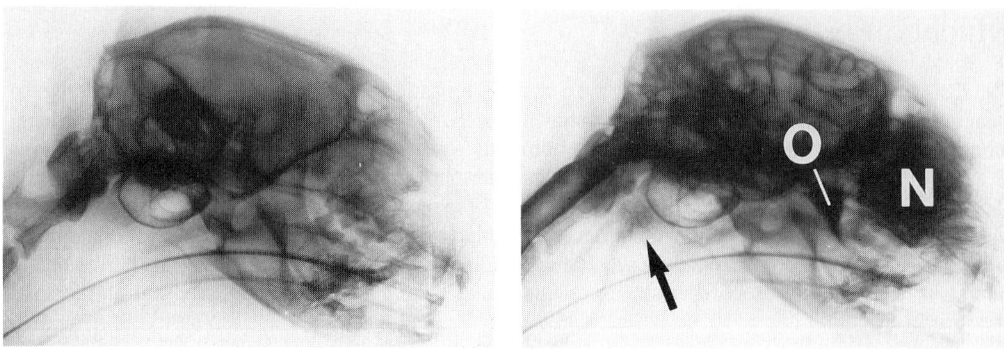

Fig.2: Radiograph (lateral view) of a cat before (left) and after (right) a 30-minute infusion of X-ray contrast medium. The nasal region (N), the orbit (O), and the cervical lymph vessels and lymph nodes (arrow) are visualized.

The study show that CSF drains via the SAS of cranial nerves into the cervical lymphatic system. The lymphatic CSF outflow pathways can be visualized by the means of a long term cisternography which must be performed at an increased ICP. Confirming earlier radiological studies we were not able to visualize these lymphatic CSF outflow pathways under the condition of normal ICP. This finding, however, should not be misinterpreted in a way that those paths are not open under normal ICP as tracer studies have shown the patency also under the condition of normal ICP [1]. According to our results, the absorption of CSF along the SAS of cranial nerves into the cervical lymphatics is not restricted to certain animal species.

LITERATURE:

[1]MC COMB, J. G. (1983). Recent research into the nature of cerebrospinal fluid formation and absorption. *J.Neurosurg.* **59**, 369-383.

[2] BÖTEL, C. & BRINKER, T. (1994). Measurement of the CSF dynamics in the rat. *J Exp Animal Sci* (In Press)

ACKNOWLEDGEMENT:
This study was supported in part by the Deutsche Forschungsghemeinschaft (Grant # Br 1416/1-1)

A Vitalmicroscopic Investigation of Lymphatic Absorption of Cerebrospinal Fluid into the Cervical Lymphatic System

T. BRINKER[1], C. BÖTEL[2], and M. SAMII[1]

[1] Department of Neurosurgery Nordstadt Hospital, [2] Central Laboratory Animal Facility, Hannover Medical School, Germany

INTRODUCTION:

The absorption of cerebrospinal fluid (CSF) is attributed almost completely to the arachnoid villi. However, more recent studies have shown that a considerable amount of CSF drains into the cervical lymphatic system via the perineural subarachnoid space of the cranial nerves. The present study examines the dynamics of the lymphatic pathway for CSF absorption.

MATERIAL AND METHODS:

The study was performed in five anaesthetized rats. A clear nylon catheter (outer diameter 0.9 mm) was placed into the cisterna magna through a drill hole in the interparietal bone (insertion deepness 6 mm). The catheter was fixed waterproofed with tissue acrylate adhesive and connected to a pressure transducer (details of the method see [1]). The cervical lymph vessels and nodes were exposed. After that non toxic filtered india ink was infused into the cisterna magna at a rate of 0.02 ml/min. For the period of ink infusion the cervical lymphatic system was microscopically observed at a 20-fold magnification by video camera. After a 30-minute infusion the animals were killed and the lymph nodes excised for histological examination.

RESULTS AND DISCUSSION:

With the beginning of the infusion the ICP increased within some minutes to a stable pressure plateau at 40-50 mm Hg. During the first 15 minutes of infusion the lymph nodes remained uncolored. After this time, however, a progressive staining was observed and after a 30-minute infusion the nodes were deeply colored.

Video micrographs showed the movement of single particles through the cervical lymph vessels in direction to the lymph nodes (fig.1).
The particles were transported very rapidly and synchronous to the respiratory cycle of the rat: During the inspiratory phase they are moved with a speed of 10-20 mm/sec, during the exspiratory phase the movement ceased (fig.2).
Postmortem the cervical lymph nodes were examined histologically. Transversal cross sections of the lymph nodes showed the sinuses filled with dye particles (fig.3).

The experiments show that the drainage of CSF into the cervical lymphatic system of rats is a fast process. The flow of particles through the cervical lymph system depends on respiratory pressure changes of the thoracic cavity which appears to act as a pump for the lymphatic system. According to the amount of ink, which was retained in the lymph nodes, the lymphatic CSF outflow pathways should contribute in a biological important manner to the clearance of particles from the CSF.

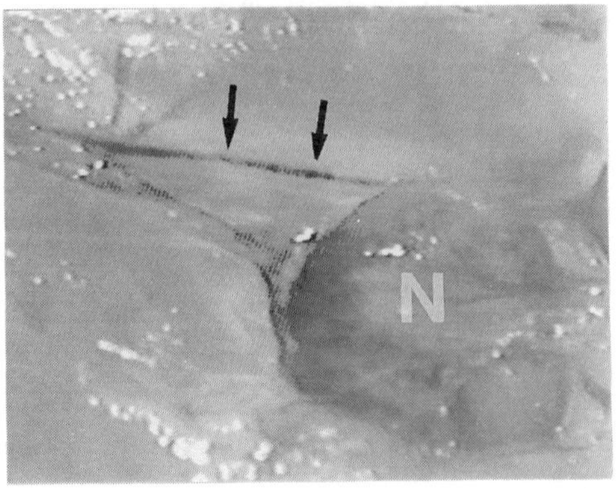

Fig.1: A video micrograph showing the flow of single particles of ink through cervical lymph vessels (arrows) into lymph nodes (N).

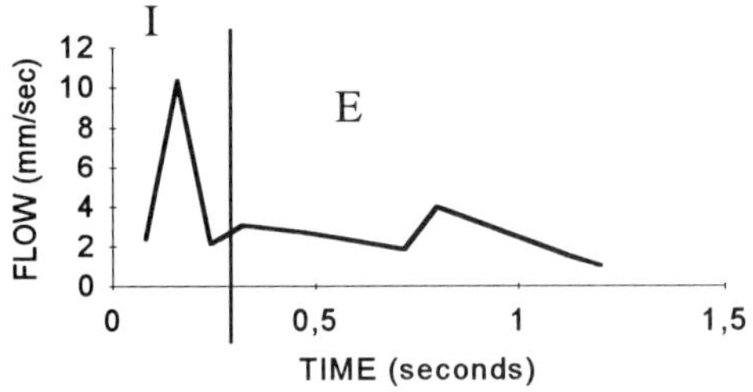

Fig.2: Velocity of the particles versus time. The flow is rhythmic and synchronous to respiratory cycle (I = inspiratory, E = exspiratory phase).

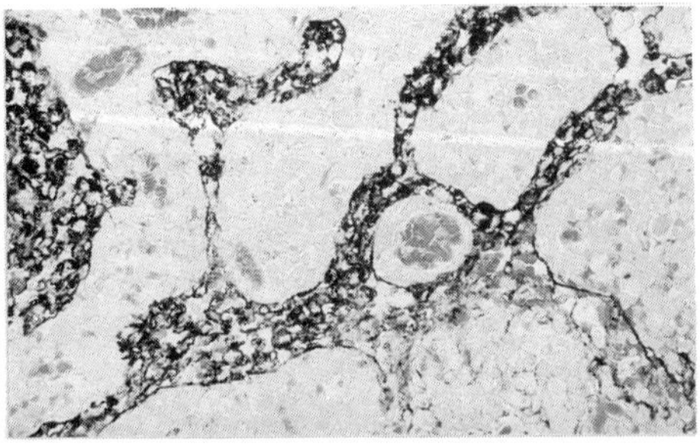

Fig.3: Transversal 5 μm cross section of a cervical lymph node (50-fold magnification, nuclear fast red staining). The sinuses of the node are filled with ink particles.

LITERATURE:

[1] BÖTEL, C. & BRINKER, T. (1994). Measurement of the CSF dynamics in the rat. *J Exp Animal Sci* (In Press)

ACKNOWLEDGEMENTS:
This work is supported in part by the Deutsche Forschungsgemeinschaft (Grant # Br 1416/1-1).

Poster VII: Hydrocephalus and Shunt

Chairman: K. Sato

Experimental Model of Obstructive Hydrocephalus. Part I. Pathogenesis

C. Anile[1], A. Mangiola[1], D. Catapano[1], F.F. Angileri[1], R. Gaspari[2], and G. Maira[3]

Institutes of [1] Neurosurgery and [2] Anesthesiology, Catholic University, Rome, Italy
[3] University of Perugia, Italy

INTRODUCTION

For many years the major part of the authors interested in the intracranial pressure (ICP) field have accepted the idea that the pathogenetic mechanism leading to the ventricular dilation in case of obstructive hydrocephalus was represented by an obstacle to CSF circulation. Few criticisms have opposed this theory; they have mainly pointed out the existence of a ventricular dilation without an obstacle to the CSF circulation (the so-called "communicating hydrocephalus") and the possibility of reproducing experimentally an important hydrocephalus by increasing the intracranial pulsatility (IP) without interfering with CSF circulation [1]. Recently Bulat [2] has published new data that may lead us to reconsider the classical concepts on the CSF circulation and, therefore, the pathogenesis of the obstructive hydrocephalus: if there is no CSF volume circulation within the ventricles, an obstacle to the CSF circulation should not play any role, "de facto", in determining the ventricular dilation. This idea has been recently substantiated by in vivo MRI and radionuclide cisternography studies [3].

MATERIALS AND METHODS

9 pigs were utilized in this study. 3 animals served as control. In 3 animals an intraventricular infusion to raise ICP to about 100 mmHg for a period of 4 to 5 hours was carried out thus producing an overflow through the acqueduct of Silvius in order to simulate a sort of "functional" CSF obstacle (group A). In the remaining 3 animals a balloon was inflated epidurally in the posterior fossa to compress the fourth ventricle for a period of 6 to 7 hours (group B). In groups A and B, arterial blood pressure (ABP), ICP, EKG and EEG were continuously monitored. IP was also evaluated by measuring the ratio between mean and pulse CSF pressure [1]. In the same animals ventriculography was carried out immediately before and after the intraventricular infusion (group A) and the balloon inflation (group B) and thereafter at intervals of 3 hours in order both to confirm the ventricular obstruction and to measure the ventricular dimension before sacrifice. Post mortem ventricular size was analyzed in control and treated animals in formalin fixed slices cut at the same anatomical levels.

RESULTS

In both groups of animals (A and B) no modification in ABP, EEG and EKG basal recordings was observed. In group A, in spite of the conspicuous ICP increase (>100 mmHg), ventricular size always remained as small as those observed in the controls. In this group of animals, the mean IP value at steady state was .117±.0.25. In group B the balloon inflation was followed by an immediate rise of ICP to about 40 mmHg without any further increase (Fig. 1). In these animals serial ventriculographies confirmed ventricular obstruction following the balloon inflation and a progressive increase in ventricular size linearly correlated with the duration of obstruction (Fig. 2). In these animals, the mean IP value after balloon inflation was .132±.021, significantly higher (p<.01) than in group A animals.

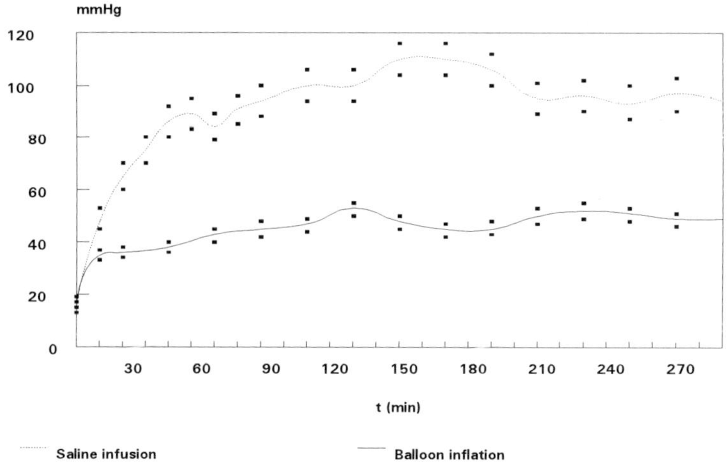

Fig. 1: Mean ICP trends in group A and B animals.

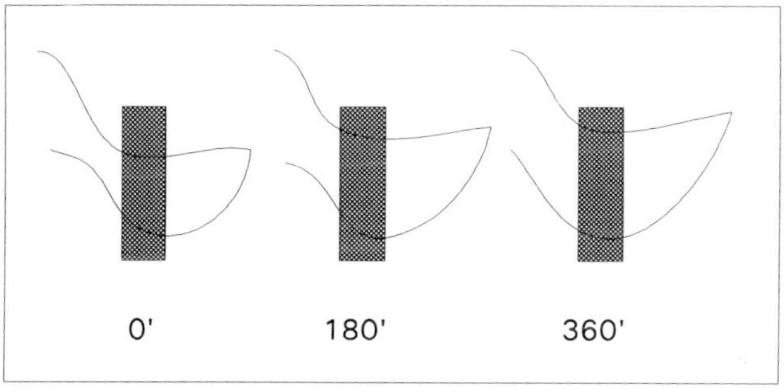

Fig. 2: Example of ventricular dilation in a group B animal. A section of olphactory ventricle is shown.

DISCUSSION

Our findings suggest that the ventricular dilation is not caused by the obstacle to the CSF circulation, occurring in both groups of animals, but, probably, by the increase of the "water hammer" effect [4] determined by the CSF pulse pressure "undamped" within the ventricular space because of the mechanical occlusion in the CSF pathways.

REFERENCES

1. Di Rocco C, Pettorossi VE, Mancinelli R, Caldarelli M, Velardi F (1978) Communicating hydrocephalus induced by mechanically increased amplitude of the intraventricular CSF pressure: experimental studies. Exper Neurol 59:40-52.
2. Bulat M (1993) Dynamics and statics of the cerebrospinal fluid: the classical and a new hypothesis. In: Avezaat CJJ, van Eijndhoven JHM, Maas AIR, Tans JTJ (eds) Intracranial Pressure VIII. Springer-Verlag, Berlin Heidelberg, pp 726-730.
3. Greitz D (1993) Cerebrospinal fluid circulation and associated intracranial dynamics. A radiologic investigation using MR imaging and radionuclide cisternography. Acta Radiol Suppl. 386:1-23.
4. Foltz EL (1984) Hydrocephalus and CSF pulsatility: clinical and laboratory studies. In: Shapiro K, Marmarou A, Portnoy H (eds) Hydrocephalus. Raven Press, New York pp 337-362.

Cerebrospinal Fluid Edema Associated with Shunt Obstruction

H. Sakamoto[1], K. Fujitani[2], S. Kitano[2], K. Murata[3], and A. Hakuba[1]

[1] Department of Neurosurgery, Osaka City University Medical School, Osaka, Japan
[2] Department of Neurosurgery, Children's Medical Center of Osaka, Osaka, Japan
[3] Department of Neurosurgery, Shimada Municipal Hospital, Shizuoka, Japan

INTRODUCTION

Four hydrocephalic children examined by the authors displayed CSF edema along the ventricular catheter in association with shunt obstruction. Three of them had massive CSF edema along the catheter without enlargement of the ventricles in spite of increased ventricular pressure. In this report, the mechanism of development of massive CSF edema at such an atypical site is discussed in relation to ventricular stiffness after shunt installation.

CLINICAL MATERIALS

A clinical summary of the patients is shown in Table 1. CT before the onset of CSF edema showed small or slit-like ventricles in all patients. CT on admission showed that three patients (Cases 1, 2 and 3) had small or slit-like ventricles with a large low density area along the ventricular catheter of the shunt (Fig. 1 left). This low density area was observed predominantly in the white matter from the subependymal site of the lateral ventricle to the subcortical area. The CT findings indicated that the low density area along the ventricular catheter corresponded to CSF edema and that the round lesion with lower density corresponded to a cystic lesion containing CSF. No abnormal enhancement was observed on CT around the CSF edema area after intravenous administration of contrast material. MR image of Case 3 on admission clearly demonstrated a cystic lesion at the center of the massive CSF edema (Fig. 1 right). In Case 4, CT on admission showed a small low density area along the ventricular catheter and enlargement of the ventricles accompanied by periventricular low density. The intraventricular pressure was increased in all patients on admission. CSF analysis of the ventricular fluid revealed no significant increase in cell count or protein content. The obstructed peritoneal catheter was revised with a new one without replacing the patent ventricular catheter previously installed. Symptoms and signs disappeared within one day of shunt revision in all patients.

DISCUSSION

In shunted hydrocephalic patients, ventricular stiffness will exaggerate intraparenchymal CSF migration along the ventricular catheter, inducing massive CSF edema along the catheter. Cases 1, 2 and 3 showed that, in spite of increased intraventricular pressure, the ventricles remained small or slit-like without periventricular CSF edema (Fig. 1). These findings suggest that ventricular stiffness occurred after shunt installation. In Case 4 which displayed ventricular dilatation associated with periventricular CSF edema under increased intraventricular pressure,

CSF edema along the ventricular catheter was much less significant than in the other three patients.

There have been several reports on shunted hydrocephalic children (7 cases) displaying CSF edema along the ventricular catheter.[1,2] Out of these 7 patients presenting with massive CSF edema along the ventricular catheter in association with shunt obstruction, 6 were younger than 17 years old. Pediatric patients develop ventricular stiffness after shunt installation more frequently than adults. This might be one of the reasons why pediatric patients more often show massive CSF edema along the ventricular catheter.

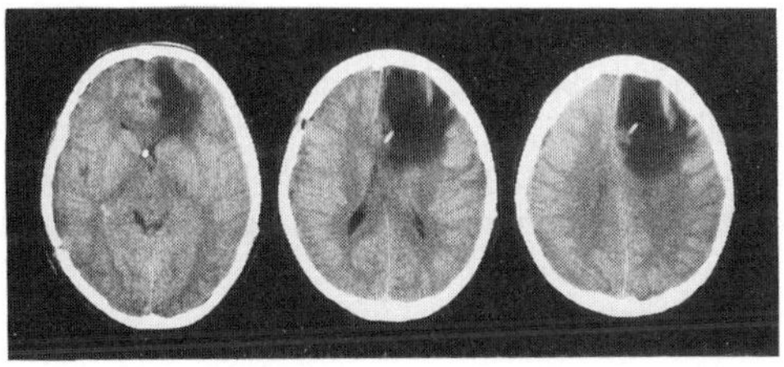

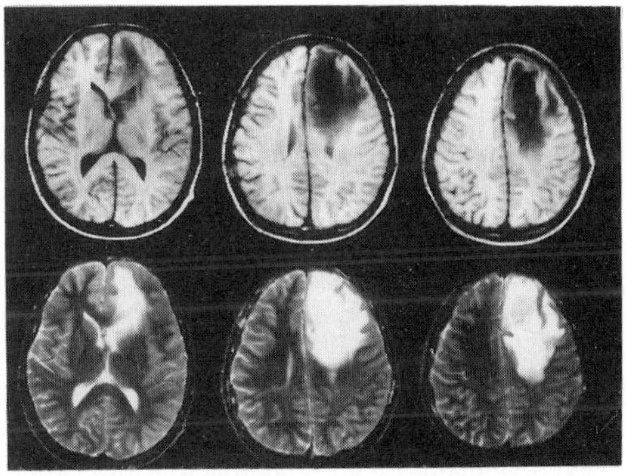

Fig. 1 Neuroimagings of Case 3 on admission Left: CT. Right: T1 (top) and T2-weighted (bottom) MR image.

Table 1 Clinical summary of the patients

Case	1		2		3	4
Present age, sex	7yrs, boy		7yrs, boy		19yrs, boy	6yrs, boy
Associated lesion	myelomeningocele		achondroplasia		NF 1	encephalocele
Age at shunting	10dys	3mos	8mos	17mos	17yrs	2yrs
Shunt system (pressure)	frontal V-P (medium)		frontal V-P (medium)		frontal V-P (medium)	frontal V-P (medium)
Age at onset	3mos (initial)	15mos (second)	15mos (initial)	17mos (second)	17yrs 17mos	3yrs 3yrs
Presentation	S. F. C.	S.F.C.	vomiting S.F.C.	vomiting	headache convulsion	drowsiness vomiting
Shunt patency						
ventricular side	patent	patent	patent	patent	patent	patent
peritoneal side	obstructed	obstructed	obstructed	obstructed	obstructed	obstructed
Ventricular pre.	-	>40cmH2O	>20cmH2O	-	>25cmH2O	>30cmH2O
Ventricular size	small	small	slit-like	slit-like	slit-like	dilated
CSF edema along the catheter	massive	massive	massive	massive	massive	mild

S.F.C.: subcutaneous fluid collection, NF 1: neurofibromatosis type 1

REFERENCES

1) Chiba Y, Takagi H, Nakajima F, Fujii S, Kitahara T, Yagishita S, Itou Y (1982) Cerebrospinal fluid edema: a rare complication of shunt operations for hydrocephalus. Report of three cases. J Neurosurg 57: 697-700

2) Sakamoto H, Fujitani K, Kitano S, Murata K, Hakuba A (1994) Cerebrospinal fluid edema associated with shunt obstruction. J Neurosurg (in press)

Communicating Hydrocephalus Versus Brain Atrophy—Is a Reliable Differentiation Possible?

W. Maksymowicz[1,2], M. Czosnyka[3], W. Zabolotny[4], and W. Koszewski[1]

[1] Department of Neurosurgery, Academy of Medicine, Warsaw, Poland
[2] Department of Neurosurgery, Vojevodship Hospital, Olsztyn, Poland
[3] MRC Cambridge Centre for Brain Repair and Academic Neurosurgical Unit, Cambridge, UK
[4] Department of Electronic, Warsaw University of Technology, Warsaw, Poland

The proper management of patients with enlarged ventricles and signs of dementia, gait disturbance and/or urinary incontinence remains problematic. The main reason being is the difficulty in differentiating between normal pressure hydrocephalus and brain atrophy. However, the clinically relevant aim is to predict which patients may improve after shunting. The authors have analysed data from a group of patients with communicating hydrocephalus to investigate the factors that correlated with outcome after surgery.

MATERIAL

A hundred and two patients with enlarged ventricles (without signs of non-communicating hydrocephalus) were diagnosed in the department of Neurosurgery of Medical Academy in Warsaw in the years 1986-92. The group consisted of 61 males and 41 females aged from 18 to 80 years. The mean age was 45 (range from 10 to 80). Dementia was observed in 92.2 % of the patients. All typical symptoms of the Hakim triad were observed in 50 cases (49%). The aetiology of the syndrome was: SAH 21%, head injury 17%, CNS infection 6%, unknown 56%.

METHODS

All patients were investigated in this prospective study by neurological and psychological examinations, CT scan (Bi-frontal and Bi-caudal indices and the width of the largest cortical sulci and Sylvian sulci were measured), ICP measurements and computerised infusion test [1,2].
Patients with symptoms of communicating hydrocephalus and the resistance to the CSF outflow greater than 9 mmHg/ml/min or ICP higher than 15 mmHg were shunted (N=53). Forty six shunted patients were seen at follow-up more than one year after the surgery. The following "improvement score" was used for the evaluation of the response to shunting:
0- no improvement,
1- slight improvement; behavioural functions not evidently improved,
2- improvement with slight influence on behavioural functions,
3- recovery to state before the disease.

RESULTS AND DISCUSSION

Good outcome after shunting (2 and 3 points in the improvement score) was observed in 60.9% of patients. There was no correlation between improvement and any particular symptom or complete Hakim triad ($p>0.05$). Comparison of the improvement score with the duration of hydrocephalus

showed that the best results were observed when the duration of symptoms was short (not longer than 12 weeks). No patient fully recovered if the history exceeded 24 weeks. The worst outcome after surgery was observed in patients with unknown aetiology. If the CT-scan showed signs of brain atrophy a significantly ($p<0.05$) worse outcome was observed, although in the group of 12 patients with the cortical atrophy, some improvement (but not complete recovery) was observed in 7 cases.
Comparison of ventricular dilatation and the outcome showed that better results were observed in the patients with larger ventricles (however, the difference was not statistically significant $p<0.1$). Better results were observed in the group of patients with visible periventricular lucency in CT scan but the difference was not significant.
Patients with normotensive (ICP<15 mmHg) communicating hydrocephalus had significantly worse outcome after shunting ($p<0.025$) than those with elevated ICP.
The "postshunting degree of the improvement" was higher in the group of patients with the resistance to CSF outflow higher than 12 mmHg/ml/min. This difference had the highest level of the significance ($p<0.0001$). The median improvement score in patients with low resistance was 1 in comparison to 2 in high resistance patients.

CONCLUSIONS

1. CT scan and clinical state are not sufficient for selecting patients with communicating hydrocephalus for shunting.
2. The most important factor in the differential diagnosis of communicating hydrocephalus seems to be an increased value of the resistance to CSF outflow (Rcsf over 12mmHg/ml/min). However some patients do not improve even if Rcsf and ICP are increased.
3. The effective shunting in patients with communicating hydrocephalus was more frequently observed if patients had increased resistance to CSF outflow and increased ICP. Other positive (however not always statistically significant) prognostic factors were: short disease history, known aetiology and signs of periventricular lucency on the CT scan without brain atrophy.

REFERENCES

1. Czosnyka M, Batorski L, Laniewski P, Maksymowicz W, Koszewski W, Zaworski W (1990) A computer system for the identification of cerebrospinal compensatory model. Acta Neurochir (Wien) 105: 112-116
2. Maksymowicz W, Czosnyka M, Koszewski W, Szymanska O, Traczewski W (1989) The role of cerebrospinal compensatory parameters in estimation of functioning of implanted shunt systems in patients with communicating hydrocephalus (preliminary report). Acta Neurochir (Wien) 101: 112-116

ICP Evaluation in Patients Treated by Variable Resistance Valve

G. Salar, R. Mottaran, I. Iob, M. Mattana, G.B. Costella, M. Mazzucco, M. Marcelli, and L. Peserico

Institute of Neurosurgery, University of Padova, Italy

SUMMARY

During the last 3 years, we treated 25 patients with intermittent pressure hydrocephalus by Orbis-Cordis variable resistance devices. The mean pressure values obtained via an implantable telesensor placed in line with the valve showed a reduction of the peaks which are a characteristic of this pathology.

INTRODUCTION

The intermittent pressure hydrocephalus is characterized by cyclic high pressure peaks associated to instable ventricular basal pressure. The latter may depend either on patient's head position or from slow atrophic changes in the cortical structures.

MATERIALS AND METHODS

25 patients (14 males and 11 females, mean age 64) affected with progressive dementia, ataxia and bladder disturbances were examined with CT scan or MRI and prolonged monitoring of the ICP via a lumbar needle.

Each patient was treated by an Orbis-Cordis variable resistance device plus an implantable telesensor. After surgery, every three months the psychic and neurological aspect were examined, while the ventricular size was controlled by repeated CT scan. In addition, ICP monitoring by direct percutaneous registration from telesensor system placed on line with this valve was also examined in all the patients every three months.

In all the patients of this series, the clinical postoperative picture was variable, with evident improvement in 18 cases, while 4 patients were clinically unchanged and 3 showed a progressive worsening of the neurological picture. While the ventricular size resulted unchanged at the CT postoperative examination,all ICP recordings showed the normalization of the mean values and the reduction of the peaks.

CONCLUSION

The postoperative examination of this small series of patients seems to confirm that this variable resistance device is suitable to reduce the characteristic peaks of the so-called normal pressure or intermittent pressure hydrocephalus.

REFERENCES

1. Duplessis E. et al. Traitement de l'hydrocéphalie cronique de l'adulte par dérivation a débit régulé. Neurochirurgie 1991; 37: 40-43.

2. Hakim S. et al. A critical analysis of valve shunts used in the treatment of hydrocephalus. Dev. Med. Child. Neurol.; 15:230-255,1973

3. Cosman E.R. et al. A telemetric pressure sensor for ventricular shunt systems. Surg. Neurol. II;287-294, 1979.

Treatment of Shunt-Resistant Patients with Normal Pressure Hydrocephalus (NPH)

K. TANAKA[1], M. NISHIKAWA[1], H. NARUSE[1], A. NISHIO[1], A. HAKUBA[1], and S. NISHIMURA[2]

[1] Department of Neurosurgery, Osaka City University Medical School, Asahi-machi, Abeno-ku, Osaka, 545 Japan
[2] Osaka City General Hospital, Osaka, 534 Japan

INTRODUCTION

It is known that shunt surgery fails to reverse symptoms in some cases of NPH, even when the patent shunt system has a low pressure differential valve. We have measured various ICP parameters pre- and post-shunt surgery via a ventricular catheter and reported the importance of outflow resistance of the shunt system (*Ro(shunt)*) [1,2]. In this paper, we present the effectiveness not only of a dual shunt (two parallel shunts at a time) but also of a shunt system which has a peritoneal catheter with a larger caliber than usually available in standard commercial catheters.

MATERIALS AND METHODS

Three patients received a dual shunt (group DS), because two patients deteriorated several months after the initial shunt operation and one patient did not improve. In each occasion, patency of the initial shunt system was confirmed radiographically and prior to the installation of a second shunt, ICP parameters were reevaluated by continuous ICP monitoring for 24 hours via a ventricular catheter. ICP parameters included mean ICP for 24h (*mICP24*), peak pressure of B-waves (*BPp*), the percentage of B-waves sampled whose *BPp* exceeded 14.7mmHg (*%B*) and outflow resistance to CSF of the patient (*Ro(h)*) were analyzed as described in the previous papers [1,2]. In this group, Heyer-Schulte's on-off flushing reservoir with anti-siphon device attached to a low pressure Pudenz peritoneal catheter (inner diameter:ID 1.3mm) were used as a shunt system. In five patients with NPH (group PS), considering the importance of *Ro(shunt)* to reduce the post-shunt ICP and to alleviate the magnitude of B-wave activity, a modified Delta valve of low-low pressure with integral siphon control device attached to a peritoneal catheter with a caliber of 1.5mm was used as a shunt system. The *Ro(shunt)* was obtained from the slope of the pressure-flow relationship of the shunt system. The ICP parameters were measured after shunt surgery and compared to their pre-operative values.

RESULTS

The *Ro(shunt)* of the system used in the group DS and in the group PS were 2.02±0.40 (n=5), 1.12±0.16 mmHg/ml/min (n=10) respectively. In the group DS, after dual shunt was installed, a gross *Ro(shunt)* will be established, governed by the following equation:

$$1/Ro(shunt)(gross) = 1/2.02 + 1/2.02 = 1/1.01,$$

where *Ro(shunt)(gross)* is the gross value of *Ro(shunt)* after the dual shunt was installed. The pre-operative values of *mICP24*, *BPp*, *%B* and *Ro(h)* were 10.9±3.1mmHg,

24.0±13.1mmHg, 82.3±16.5%, 4.08±0.59mmHg/ml/min respectively in the group DS, and 10.1±3.0mmHg, 14.7±5.8mmHg, 76.9±34.9%, 7.79±7.00mmHg/ml/min respectively in the group PS. The percent changes due to shunt installations in above four parameters were -53.7, -57.3, -98.8, -77.1% respectively in the group DS, and -53.7, -54.1, -90.6, -82.3% respectively in the group PS (Table 1). The continuous ICP recording

[Table 1] **Pre- & Post-Shunt Changes in ICP Parameters**

		group **DS** (n=3)	group **PS** (n=5)
mICP24	pre-shunt	10.9±3.1	10.1±3.0 mmHg
	post-shunt	5.0±1.2	4.5±2.1
	% change	-53.7±3.1	-53.7±20.9 %
BPp	pre-shunt	24.0±13.1	14.7±5.8 mmHg
	post-shunt	9.2±2.1	6.4±2.5
	%change	-57.3±11.9	-54.1±11.4 %
%B	pre-shunt	82.3±16.5	76.9±34.9 %
	post-shunt	1.2±2.1	9.4±18.8
	%change	-98.8±2.1	-90.6±18.8 %
Ro(h)	pre-shunt	4.08±0.59	7.79±7.00 mmHg/ml/min
	post-shunt	0.89±0.34	0.97±0.40
	%change	-77.06±11.30	-82.26±9.29 %

demonstrated stepwise reduction in ICP when the Heyer-Schulte's on-off flushing reservoirs were opened in group DS although their closing pressures were similar (Fig.1). All patients in the group DS recovered and all patients in the group PS improved.

DISCUSSION

There may be some patients whose *Ro(h)* can not be reduced by a single shunt system. The system used in group PS was as effective as a dual shunt, which could be predicted by calculation using values of *Ro(shunt)*. As an alternative way, the low-low pressure Delta valve in combination with 1.5mm caliber peritoneal catheter appears promising as a treatment of the shunt-resistant NPH patient.

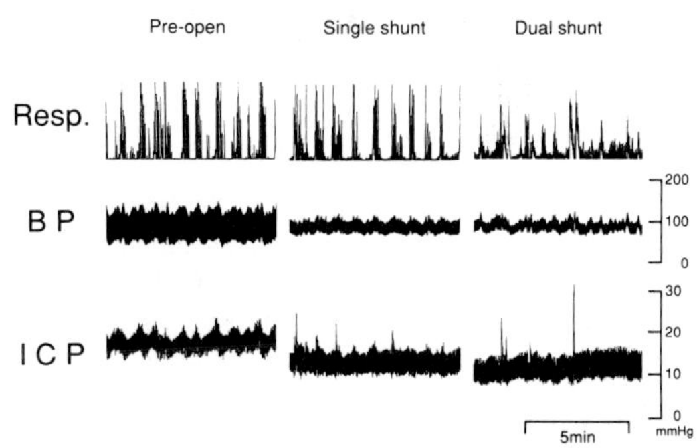

Fig.1 A stepwise reduction in ICP was observed when the on-off reservoirs were opened.

REFERENCES

1. K.Tanaka & S.Nishimura (1989) The importance of outflow resistance of the shunt system for elimination of B-waves. In Hoff JT & Betz AL (eds): Intracranial pressure VII. Springer-Verlag, Berlin Heidelberg New York London, pp 368-373

2. K.Tanaka, H.Naruse, H.Hayashi, Y.Iwai & S.Nishimura (1991) The implications of shunt surgery in the intracranial hydrodynamics of normal pressure hydrocephalus (NPH). In Matsumoto S & Tamaki N (eds): Hydrocephalus-Pathogenesis and Treatment. Springer-Verlag, Tokyo Berlin Heidelberg New York London, pp 611-618

Effect of Cisternal Pumping with a Pulsatile Drainage System in SAH

A. Wachi[1], J. Koike[1], and K. Sato[2]

[1] Neurosurgery, Tamananbu Regional Hospital, 2-1-2 Nakazawa, Tama, Tokyo, Japan
[2] Department of Neurosurgery, Juntendo University, 2-1-1 Hongo, Bunkyo-ku, Tokyo, Japan

INTRODUCTION

The malcirculation of cerebrospinal fluid (CSF) after subarachnoid hemorrhage (SAH) is known to usually result in secondary hydrocephalus, and thus it is important to evaluate the CSF circulation of such patients. Although several methods are available for this purpose, measurement of CSF flow resistance (1, 2) is considered a simple and useful method for partial calculation of how CSF circulates within the subarachnoid space. Congestion of CSF flow within these pathways suggests the patient is suffering from hydrocephalus, and shunt surgery often is necessary.

It is accepted that the shunt procedure basically is a very effective way of reducing CSF outflow resistance by creating bypass-flow and also decreasing abnormally high CSF pressure. Hydrocephalus consequently can be treated by normalizing the abnormally large reservoir. This surgical procedure, however, sometimes associates with such undesirable complications as infection or shunt malfunction. It would then appear best, if possible, not not to use a shunt to avoid these complications. In this regard we developed a theory that a "Cisternal Pumping Method" (3) could to some extent correct CSF malcirculation without resorting to shunt surgery. In this paper, we introduce not only this method, but also a new "Pulsatile Drainage System" which creates artificial intermittent positive pressure in the CSF space, and describe its effects on CSF circulation and intracranial biomechanical environment.

CASES AND METHOD

Seven patients, aged 22 to 57 (mean, 44) with SAH were treated by the cisternal pumping method (CP group). As a control 17 patients, aged 39 to 73 (mean, 57), with SAH were treated by ordinary cisternal drainage method. CSF malcirculation following SAH was suspected in each of these cases. CSF pressure monitoring and the cisternal pumping were conducted through either a lumbar catheter or an intracranial cisternal catheter. Lumbar puncture was accomplished prior to the clipping surgery. Lumbar punctures was achieved prior to clipping surgery. The patient was in a lateral recumbent position during lumbar cannulation, and 18 G (90 mm length) of disposable flexible catheter (Argyle IVH catheter) was inserted into the lumbar subarachnoid space under local anesthesia (0.2% xylocaine). Intracranial cisternal drainage was accomplished with silicone tubes inserted into the basal cistern during aneurysmal clipping. Our Pulsatile Drainage System designed for effective CSF drainage and improvement of CSF malcirculation was connected to either the lumbar catheter or the cisternal tube. This system can raise pressure intermittently within the drainage catheter and subarachnoid space by loading artificial pulse pressure. A pressure transducer (Dynabott Inc.) also was connected to the catheter via T-shape cock, and CSF pressure was recorded on a strip-chart (Nihon Koden Co.). Initial pressure recording and subsequent bolus manipulation test (2) for calculation of PVI and Ro are carried out prior to pumping. The same procedure then is followed after pumping. All these procedures are repeated for 5-7 days.

RESULTS

Values of ICP, PVI, and Ro before and after the cisternal pumping are discribed in Table below. There was no statistical change in ICP before and after pumping (12.1±2.8 mmHg and 13.5±2.1mmHg). However, Ro of 48.4±43.3 mmHg/ml/min finally decreased to 9.1±4.3 mmHg/ml/min ($p<0.01$), and PVI of 15.6±6.1 ml increased to 23.5±5.8 ml ($p<0.05$) after pumping. Sequential changes in CSF absorptive resistance also are demonstrated. Ro gradually decreased by daily pumping. There were significant reduction (effective: Ro < 7 mmHg/ml/min) of Ro in 4 cases, moderate reduction (Ro: 7-15 mmHg/ml/min) in 2 cases, and no significant reduction (Ro >15 mmHg/ml/min) in the remaining one case. VP shunt surgery after SAH was undertaken in 70% of the control cases, but only 28% of the cases in the CP group. Seven-day patency of the drainage tube was achieved in all CP cases, but in only 82% of control cases.

Table Comparison of ICP, PVI, and Ro before and after cisternal pumping

	Pre-pumping	Post-pumping	
ICP	12.1±2.8 mmHg	13.5±2.1mmHg	N.S.
PVI	15.6±6.1 ml	23.5±5.8 ml	($p<0.05$)
Ro	48.4±43.3 mmHg/ml/min	9.1±4.3 mmHg/ml/min	($p<0.01$)

DISCUSSION

Pathophysiologically, it is of significant importance to evaluate CSF absorption capability in hydrocephalus. The choroidal plexus within the ventricular system is considered to daily secrete 400-500 ml of cerebrospinal fluid (4), and this fluid finally is absorbed through the arachnoid villi (5). Since this circulation frequently is disturbed by CSF flow resistance increasing after SAH (6), secondary hydrocephalus often occurs in such patients. Reasonably, they should be treated by reducing CSF flow resistance.

CSF pulsation also is important as an etiological factor which creates ventricular dilatation, and this has been proven by Dirocco (7). He experimentally demonstrated ventricular dilatation by ventricular pulse pressure loading. This observation may indicate that persistent pulse pressure within the CSF space directly forces CSF against such adjacent cerebral structures as ependymal tissue and cerebral mantle, and consequently ventricular dilatation occurs. For this reason, pulse pressure loading in the intracranial cisterns physically functioning to expand CSF space presumably plays an important role in preventing obliteration of CSF pathways after SAH.

Secondary, CSF reportedly is absorbed through several alternative pathways. It is reported that among these pathways, spinal absorption of CSF accounts for about 16% of total CSF absorption (2,8) and also that these pathways may be closed or not fully function in normal persons. However, if there is a possibility that these pathways functionally develop under some hydrocephalic conditions, pulse loading within a lumbar cistern may open and develop such pathways to reduce CSF outflow resistance. From these points of view, there is a possibility that our method, pulse pressure loading through a cisternal tube to the CSF space, can prevent some SAH patients from developing hydrocephalus. Additionally, our Pulsatile Drainage System also was seemed to prevent a tube obstruction with clot or viscous fluid by to-and-fro motion of fluid within a tube, and an effective drainage for SAH is expected.

REFERENCE

1 Bering EA, Sato O: Hydrocephalus: Changes in formation and absorption of cerebrospinal fluid within the central ventricles.
J Neurosurg 20: 1050-1063, 1963

2 Marmarou A, Shapiro K, LaMorgese J: Compartmental analysis of compliance and outflow resistance of the cerebrospinal fluid system.
J Neurosurg 43: 523-534, 1975

3 Effect of Cisternal Pumping on Cerebrospinal Fluid Circulation in Hydrocephalus.
Current tr Hyd(Tokyo) 3:24-26, 1993

4 Welch K: The principles of physiology of the cerebrospinal fluid in relation to hydrocephalus.
In: Friedlander WJ (ed)
Advances in neurology. Raven Press, New York. pp 247-332

5 Davson H: Formation and Drainage of the Cerebrospinal fluid: Hydrocephalus: Shapiro K, Marmarou A, Portnoy H (eds); Raven Press, New York, pp 3-40, 1984

6 Gjerris F, Borgesen SE, Sorensen PS, Boesen F, Schmidt K, Harnsen A, Lester J: Resistance to cerebrospinal fluid outflow and intracranial pressure in patients with hydrocephalus after subarachnoid hemorrhage.
Acta Neurochir (wien) 88: 79-86, 1987

7 Di Rocco C: Hydrocephalus and Cerebrospinal Fluid Pulses
Hydrocephalus: Shapiro K, Marmarou A, Portnoy H (eds); Raven Press, New York, pp 231-249, 1984

8 Welch K, Polly M: The spinal arachnoid villi of the monkeys Cercopithecus aethiops sabaeus and Macaca irus.
Anat Rec 145: 43-46, 1963

Shunt Flow Changes in Postural ICP Alterations: An In Vitro Simulation

SOTARO HIGASHI, MAHMOOD HASSAN, KAZUYA FUTAMI, SHINYA KIDA, KAZUHIKO TOKUDA, and JUNKOH YAMASHITA

Department of Neurosurgery, Kanazawa University School of Medicine, 13-1 Takara-machi, Kanazawa, 920 Japan

INTRODUCTION

Overdrainage problems, in shunted patients with a differential pressure (DP) valve, have stimulated considerable efforts to design new shunt valves and anti-siphon/siphon-control devices (ASD/SCD) to resolve them. Clinical experience has demonstrated a decreased incidence of slit ventricle syndrome, and subdural hematoma.[1] However, an adverse effect has also been reported, that is underdrainage secondary to excessive function of these devices, especially in patients with normal pressure hydrocephalus (NPH).[2] To investigate the mechanism of this underdrainage, we devised a simulation method of shunt flow in which postural ICP alterations are taken into consideration.

MATERIALS AND METHODS

The types of shunt valve examined were as follows: Delta valve (containing a SCD), variable resistance (VR) valve (Orbis-Sigma), and DP valve (PS Medical). Ventricular and peritoneal catheters (PS Medical, Standard, inner diameter = 1.3 mm) were assembled to DP valve or Delta valve. The entire shunt system was placed upon a human dummy. The valves was assembled at the level of vertex, the foramen of Monro, the mastoid process, or the clavicle. Hydrostatic pressure, referred to the level of the foramen of Monro, was used to simulate ICP, and the pressure ranged from 25 cmH_2O to closing pressure of the valves. Flow was measured at the supine, 30 degree lean and upright postures of the dummy in the laboratory.

For the simulation of the driving pressure to the shunt system, ICP was measured in patients with normal and high pressure hydrocephalus (NPH, HPH) at three head positions; supine, 30 degree lean, and erect. Finally shunt flow characteristics of these systems were examined by applying clinical ICP data to the results of flow measurement in the laboratory.

RESULTS

Shunt flow rates of Delta valve correlated with the position in the system: the higher the position of the valve, the lower the flow rate. When positioned on the skull, Delta valve showed underdrainage in NPH. Orbis-Sigma valve showed strictly limited flow irrespective of head positions. DP valves showed overdrainage when the head was elevated above 30 degree (Fig. 1).

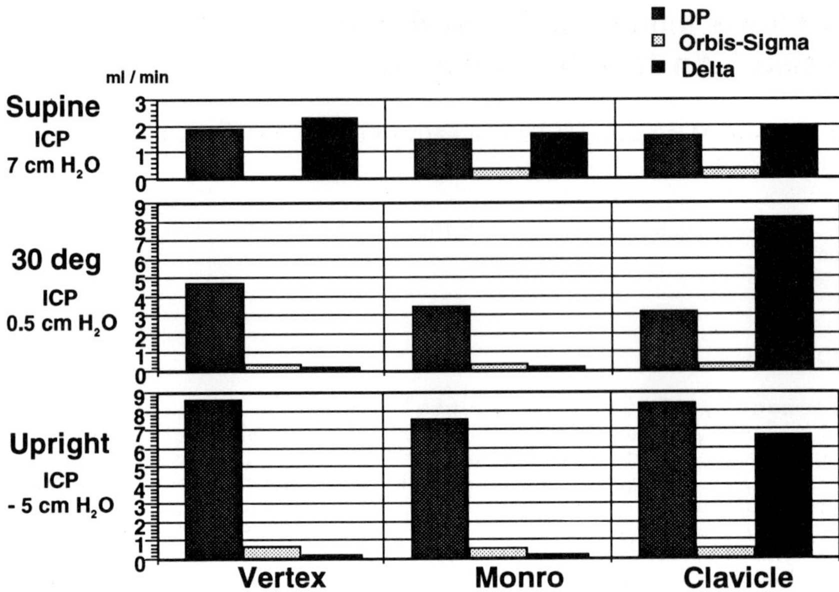

Fig. 1 Shunt flow simulation of three shunt systems in a case of normal pressure hydrocephalus.

DISCUSSION

For the accurate shunt flow simulation, we should remember that VFP is variable according to the patient's posture and to the etiology of hydrocephalus, and that the total shunt resistance is contributed by the resistance of each shunt component. Therefore, to simulate shunt flow in patients as accurately as possible, we took postural ICP alterations into consideration and used an entire shunt system fixed on a dummy.

The present study elucidated the limitation of commercially available shunt systems. Delta valve positioned on the skull may cause underdrainage especially in the case of NPH, because the inlet pressure is too low to overcome the resistance of SCD. Orbis-Sigma valve may also cause underdrainage in bed-laid patients with NPH, because of its high resistance. Shunted patients with DP valve will consistently develop overdrainage with the head elevation.

Our shunt flow simulation seems to be a useful method to predict shunt flow rate in various clinical conditions. It will contribute toward developing new shunt system which can overcome overdrainage or underdrainage in ventricular shunting.

REFERENCES

1. Gruber R, Jenny P, Herzog B (1984) Experiences with the anti-siphon device (ASD) in shunt therapy of pediatric hydrocephalus. J Neurosurg 61:156-162
2. Kremer P, Aschoff A, Kunze S (1991) Therapeutical risks of anti-siphon devices. Eur J Pediatr Surg 1 (Suppl 1):47-48

The Evaluation of Various Flow Control Valves in V-P Shunt System

H. MIYAKE, T. OHTA, Y. KAJIMOTO, and M. MATSUKAWA

Department of Neurosurgery, Osaka Medical College, 2-7 Daigakucho, Takatsuki, Osaka, 569 Japan

INTRODUCTION

Recently, various flow control valves have become available for V-P shunt, which decrease complications due to overdrainage[1-3]. These valves control the shunt flow providing some resistance in V-P shunt system. However, their controllability, especially in the upright position, have not been throughly investigated. In this report, we evaluated their controllability and the differences due to the implantation site.

MATERIALS AND METHODS

The V-P shunt model used was shown in Fig.1. The implantation site of flow control valve was simulated by its setting level in this model. Negative ICP was obtained by turning the cylinder filled with water upside down into the water bath.The differential pressure across the valve(DP) was measured by a differentialpressure meter. The shunt flow(F) was measured by the water volume obtained from the abdominal catheter tip for a minute. Five kinds of valves, the Sophy programmable pressure valve(Sophy valve), the Orbis-Sigma(O-S) valve, the Delta valve, the Medos valve and the MDM valve, were measured their DP and F at three conditions of ICP, -20 cmH2O, 5cmH2O and 20cmH2O.

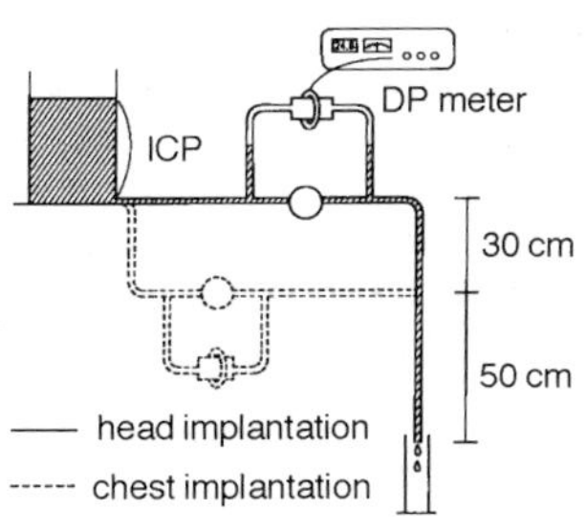

Fig.1 V-P shunt model

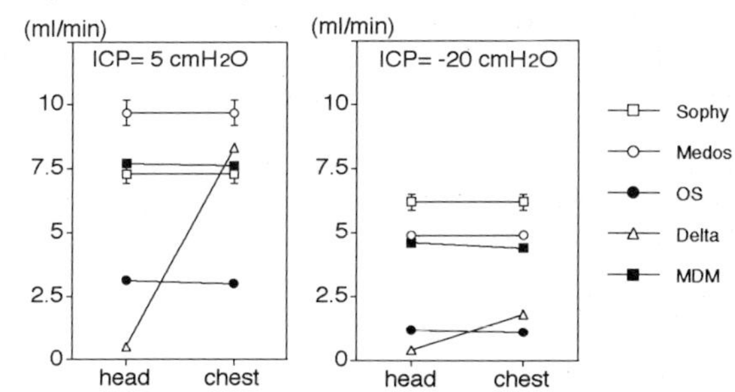

Fig.2 Positional shunt flow change of each valve

RESULTS

1.None of the valves, except the Delta valve, showed any difference in DP or F related to the the implantation site. 2.The resistance value(R) of the Sophy and the Medos valves were less than 50% of total shunt resistance under every ICP condition and also showed a relatively narrow control range.3.The O-S valve demonstrated the lowest flow and more than 70% of the total shunt resistance. 4.The Delta valve showed a marked difference in DP and F due to differences in the implantation site. 5.The MDM valve was situated between the Sophy/Medos valve and the O-S valve.

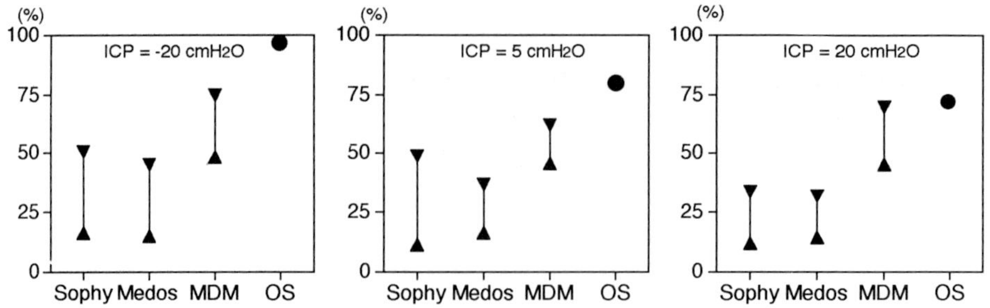

Fig.3 Controllability of each valve(valvar DP/total DP × 100)
▼:high resistance, ▲:low resistance

DISCUSSION

Our investigation revealed that shunt flow and DP were basically the same regardless of the implantation site for all valves except the Delta valve. DP across the valve, which regulates shunt flow, is affected by many factors such as ICP, hydrostatic pressure, siphoning pressure, abdominal pressure and so on. Although hydrostatic pressure and siphoning pressure on the valve are each affected by the implantation site, these are reciprocal factors and the sum of the two should remain constant regardless of the implantation site.Among these four types of valves, the Sophy and the Medos valve, even at the highest pressure settings, demonstrated a non physiologically high shunt flow. Total DP generalized in the standing position is beyond their control and these two valves may be insufficient to prevent the overdrainage. The percentages of valvar DP(Fig.3) was less than 50% of total DP even in the highest setting of the Sophy and the Medos valve in each ICP condition. These values seem to be less than previously thought. Furthermore, the control range of valvar DP in these two valves were relatively narrow. This fact indicates the importance of the tube factor in considering shunt flow. The MDM valve showed the higher DP value but the control range seems to be insufficient too. DP in the O-S valve showed more than 70% of total DP in each ICP condition. This fact indicates the specificity of relatively low shunt flow in the O-S valve[5].Flow controllability of the Delta valve differs with its implantation site, because this has an antisiphon mechanism(delta chamber). In this study, the Delta valve showed the lowest shunt flow with head implantation (Fig.2). This is suitable for preventing overdrainage in the standing position. The disadvantages of this valve are that 1. flow resistance cannot be programmed from outside and 2. the delta chamber can collapse easily by external force.

REFERENCES

1.Miyake H,Ohta T,Nagasawa S,Takatsuka H,Yamashita M,Osaka K(1991) Clinical Experience with a New Ventriculo-Peritoneal Shunt Using a Telemetric Intraventricular Pressure Sensor, an On-Off Flushing Reservoir and a Sophy's Programmable Hydrostatic Pressure Valve. Current Tr Hyd(Tokyo) 1:79-84
2.Nagano Y,Ohta T,Miyake H,Yamashita M,Tanabe H,Tsuzawa S(1990) Chronological Changes in Intraventricular Pressure and CT Findings After Shunt Operation. Progress in Research on ICP:7-13,1990
3.Saint-Rose C,Hooven MD,Hirsch JF(1987):A new approach in the treatment of hydrocephalus. J Neurosurg 66:213-226,

Poster VIII: Head Injury

Chairman: A. Yamaura

Continuous Monitoring of Brain Tissue pO_2 After Severe Head Injury

H. van Santbrink, A.I.R. Maas, and C.J.J. Avezaat

Department of Neurosurgery, Academic Hospital Rotterdam, The Netherlands

Introduction.

Cerebral ischemia is one of the main causes of secondary brain damage after severe head injury. Monitoring cerebral oxygenation is appropriate. We have previously reported on experimental data and preliminary clinical results of continuous monitoring of cerebral tissue pO_2 ($PbrO_2$)[1]. In this report we studied $PbrO_2$ measurements in patients with severe head injury.

Material and methods.

15 patients (11 men and 4 women) with a blunt severe head injury, with a GCS $\leq$ 8 (mean 6.5 $\pm$ 1.0) were investigated. All patients were treated according to a standard protocol, which included artificial ventilation, sedation, ICP monitoring, and treatment of raised ICP according to a staircase model. $PbrO_2$ was measured with a flexible Clark type electrode, connected with a Licox[r] pO_2 device. A special intracranial bolt with three entry points was developed for simultaneously introduction of an ICP sensor and $PbrO_2$ catheter. Measurements started as soon as possible after trauma and continued till day 6. The electrodes were tested for sensitivity and zero drift after the measurement.

Results.

In all 15 patients stable $PbrO_2$ recordings were obtained. No serious complications were encountered during the measurements, especially no microcatheter related infections were seen. $PbrO_2$ measurements started with a mean interval of 7.7 $\pm$ 5.6 hours after trauma (range 3.5 - 23 hours). Initially low $PbrO_2$ values were noted. Within 24 hour after trauma a significant rise till normal or slightly elevated values $PbrO_2$[1] was observed ($p < .003$; Wilcoxon-test) (FIG 1).

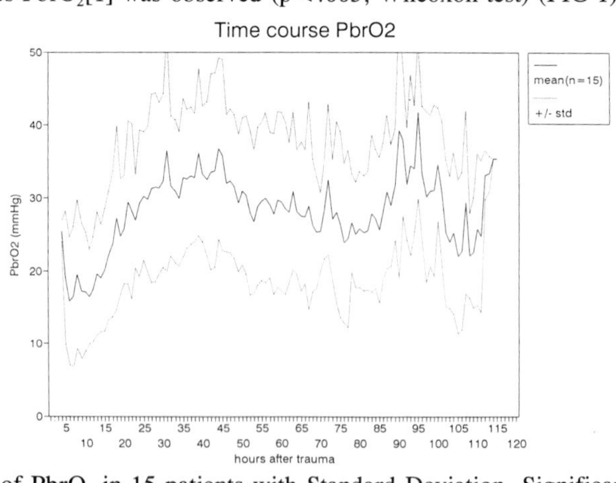

Fig. 1: Time Course of $PbrO_2$ in 15 patients with Standard Deviation. Significant rise during the first 24 hour after trauma ($p < .003$; Wilcoxon test)

In three patients a $PbrO_2$ below 5 mmHg within 24 hour after trauma was observed. Two of these patients died, the third had a GOS of 4 at 6 months after trauma. None of the patients without a $PbrO_2$ below 5 mmHg died or stayed vegetative. The occurrence of $PbrO_2$ values below 5 mmHg within 24 hours after trauma correlated significantly with a GOS of 1 or 2 (equal to dead or vegetative) at 6 months after trauma (Table 1:$p<.03$; Fischer Exact).

$PbrO_2$	GOS 1 or 2	GOS 3,4, or 5	total
< 5 mmHg	2	1	3
> 5 mmHg	-	11	11
total	2	12	14

Table 1: Distribution of patients with and without low $PbrO_2$ (< 5mmHg) values within 24 hour after trauma according GOS at 6 months after trauma (p=.03 Fischer Exact).

The recordings were scrutinized to detect factors which are of influence on $PbrO_2$. The major effect was caused by changes in arterial oxygen pressure (PaO_2). To a much lesser extend influences were detected on changes of CPP and $ETpCO_2$. During ventilatory experiments in which FiO_2 was stepwise increased from 40% till 100% a mean correlation coefficient between $PbrO_2$ and PaO_2 of $.96 \pm .05$ was found, for the total period of observation. O_2 reactivity, defined as:

$$\%PbrO_2 \,/\, PaO_2,$$

differed within a single patient during the period of observation and between patients. Within 24 hours after injury patients with an unfavourable outcome (GOS equal to 1,2 or 3) had an O_2 reactivity of 6.3 ± 3.1 and patients with a favourable outcome (GOS equal to 4 or 5) 1.6 ± 1.0, this was a significant difference (p=.01; Mann-Whitney test)(Table 2).

observation period	O2 reactivity total group mean	std	O2 reactivity if GOS = 1, 2 or 3 mean	std	O2 reactivity if GOS = 4 or 5 mean	std
day 1	3.67	3.20	6.27	3.13	1.59	0.99
day 2	4.54	2.89	5.86	3.29	2.96	1.25
day 3	5.99	2.75	6.34	2.85	5.47	2.92
day 4	4.95	2.13	5.35	2.61	4.28	1.06
day 5	5.09	1.12	4.77	1.34	5.57	0.80

Table 2 shows that mean O2 reactivity is lowest on day 1. On day 1 a significant difference in O2 reactivity was observed between patients with a favourable (GOS equal to 4 or 5) and patients with an unfavourable (GOS equal to 1, 2 or 3) outcome ($p<.01$; Mann Whitney test).

Calibration after finishing the measurement showed a negligible small zero drift (mean 1.1 mmHg) and a mean sensitivity drift of 8.9%.

Discussion and conclusion.

Continuous $PbrO_2$ measurement after severe head injury is a reliable, and easy to measure new parameter. Low $PbrO_2$ values during the first 24 hours after trauma predict a bad outcome, which is probably due to a low Cerebral Blood Flow, this is in good agreement with other investigations[2]. O_2 regulation during the first 24 hours after trauma is disturbed in patients with a bad outcome resulting in a substantial higher O_2 reactivity. Continuous measurement of $PbrO_2$ attributes to a better insight of cerebral oxygenation.

References

1. AIR Maas, W Fleckenstein, DA de Jong, H van Santbrink (1993) Monitoring cerebr Oxygenation: Experimental studies and preliminary clinical results of continuous monitoring cerebrospinal fluid and brain tissue Oxygen tension. Acta Neurochirurgica (suppl) 59:50-57.
2. GJ Bouma, JP Muizelaar, WA Stringer, SC Choi, P Fatouros, HF Young (1992) Ultra-ear evaluation of regional cerebral blood flow in severely head-injured patients using xenon-enhance computerised tomography. J Neurosurg 77:360-368.

Serial Transcranial Doppler Measurements in Patients with Severe Head Injury; The Early Posttraumatic Period

H. VAN SANTBRINK, A.I.R. MAAS, and C.J.J. AVEZAAT

Department of Neurosurgery, Academic Hospital Rotterdam, The Netherlands

Introduction.

Doppler technology for assesing blood flow velocity in intracranial arteries was first used by Aaslid et al[1] in 1982. For clinical practice the Middle Cerebral Artery (MCA) and the Internal Carotid Artery (ICA) and their ratio are used. Several TCD studies[2,3] have shown that mean flow velocity in the MCA increases after trauma and reaches its maximum in about 5 days. In this study we focused attention on the first 24 hours after injury, because ischemia is common in this period, and studied the relation between flow velocity (V) in the Middle Cerebral Artery (MCA) and shift on CT.

Material and methods.

Serial TCD measurements were performed in 40 patients with a severe head injury GCS $\leq$ 8 (mean GCS 6.1 $\pm$ 1.7). All patients were treated according to a standard protocol which included artificial ventilation, sedation, ICP monitoring and treatment of raised ICP according to a staircase model.

The patients were divided into two groups: group I: CT-scan with shift, a Lesion(L)-side and a Non-Lesion(NL)-side could be distinguished (n=26); group II CT-scan without shift (n=14). Ct-scans were also reviewed on the appearance of Subarachnoid Hemorrhage (SAH).

Results.

Mean flow velocity in the Middle Cerebral Artery (mVMCA) within 8 hours after trauma at the L-side in group I (30 $\pm$ 17 cm/s) was significantly lower than mVMCA at the NL-side (46 $\pm$ 19 cm/s) and mVMCA in group II (46 $\pm$ 16 cm/s). mVMCA increased after initial phase after trauma and reached its maximum after 2 till 4 days. However high flow velocities (>100 cm/s) are indicative for vasospasm these values were seldom observed (7/40=18%)(Fig. 1).

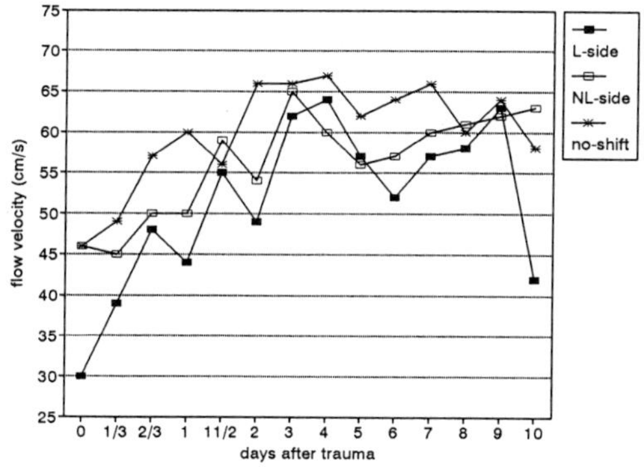

Fig. 1: Mean flow velocity in 40 patients according to CT-scan appearence. Group I: patients with shift, divided into L-side and NL-side and Group II: patients without shift on the CT-scan.

Patients with a VMCA <40 cm/s within 8 h after trauma at the L-side had a significanly lower MCA/Internal Carotid Artery (ICA) ratio than patients with a VMCA >40 cm/s. Pulsatility Index in the MCA (PIMCA) at the L-side was higher in the patients with a VMCA <40 cm/s than patients with a VMCA >40 cm/s. These findings appeared to be characteristic for the early posttraumatic phase and could not be found after 36 hours after trauma. ICP and CPP were not statistical different in these periods for the different "CT"groups, during this time period (Table 1).

		VMCA within 8 hours after trauma							
		< 40 cm/s				> 40 cm/s			
side	PI		MCA/ICA		PI		MCA/ICA		
	mean	std	mean	std	mean	std	mean	std	
Lesion		2.93#	1.74	0.90"	0.57	1.39#	0.35	2.62"	0.37
Non-Lesion	1.76	0.95	1.25	0.57	1.77	0.54	1.81	1.04	

table 1. #p<.03, "p<.002; Mann-Whitney test.

17 out of 40 patients had a flow velocity < 40 cm/s for at least two subsequent measurements in one or both MCA's within 36 hours after trauma(= 'low flow velocity state'). Patients with a 'low flow velocity state' had a significantly lower GCS than patients without a 'low flow velocity state'. 10 patients in the whole group died due to the trauma. 7 out of 10 patients who died had a 'low flow velocity state' (p=.07; Fischer Exact test). No correlation between high flow velocity and SAH on the CT-scan was observed. On the contrary patients with SAH on the CT-scan had a significantly higher frequency (58%) of 'low flow velocity state' than patients without SAH on th CT-scan (14%)(p=.008; Chisq. test).

Conclusions.

TCD measurements in an early phase after trauma at the side of the lesion show a low flow velocity accompanied with a high PIMCA and a low MCA/ICA ratio. This is due to a high peripheral resistance resulting in a low CBF. This is in accordance with reports of CBF after the acute phase of head injury[4,5]. The implication of these results is that patients at risk for ischemia after head injury can be accurately indentified in an non-invasive way with TCD in the very early phase. In this period management should be aimed at increasing cerebral perfusion pressure and cerebral blood flow.

References

1. R Aaslid, ThM Markwalder and H Nornes (1982) Noninvasive transcranial Doppler ultrasound recording of flow velocity in basal cerebral arteries. J Neurosurg 57:769-774.
2. P Grolimund, M Weber, RW Seiler, HJ Reulen (1988) Time course of cerebral vasospasm after severe head injury. The Lancet, may 21:1173.
3. KH Chan, NM Dearden, JD Miller (1992) The significance of posttraumatic increase in cerebral blood flow velocity: A transcranial Doppler ultrasound study. Neurosurg 30(5):697-700.
4. GJ Bouma, JP Muizelaar, SC Choi, PG Newlon, HF Young (1991) Cerebral circulation and metabolism after severe traumatic brain injury: the elusive role of ischemia. J Neurosurg 75:685-693.
5. GJ Bouma, JP Muizelaar, WA Stringer, SC Choi, P Fatouros, HF Young (1992) Ultra-early evaluation of regional cerebral blood flow in severely head-injured patients using xenon-enhanced computerised tomography. J Neurosurg 77:360-368.

Management of Head Injury in Children Showing Diffuse Cerebral Swelling

S. KOBAYASHI[1], H. YOKOTA[2], and S. NAKAZAWA[1]

[1] Department of Neurosurgery, Nippon Medical School, Tokyo, 113 Japan
[2] Department of Critical Care Medicine, Nippon Medical School, Tokyo, 113 Japan

INTRODUCTION

In acute severe head injuries, we reported the existence of special feature called diffuse cerebral swelling which caused comprssion or obliteration of the lateral and third ventrices, as well as of the perimesencphalic cistern despite the absence of focal mass lesions disclosed by bomputerized tomography (CT) within few hours after incurring the trauma [1]. In this study, efficacy of barbiturate overloading therapy (BOT) was evaluated in pediatric patients presenting DCS.

MATERIALS AND METHODS

DCS developes in 16 (24.2%), 11 males and 5 females, of 66 pediatric patients treated recently for acute severe head injury. They renged from 1 to 15 years in ago (mean, 6.9 years). After endotracheal intubation, mild hyperventilation was administered to all patients and, thus, PaCO2 was maintained at 20-25 mmHg. ICP was monitored in 8 of the 16 patients. Intracranial hypertension, if detected, was treated by conventional hypotensive therapy. If this therapy failed to control intracranial hypertension, and the baseline ICP rose to 25 mmHg or higher, barbiturate overloading therapy was begun with a maintenance dose of 3-5 mg/hr of thiamylal of 1-2 mg/kg/hr of pentobarbital.

RESULTS AND DISCUSSION

The ICP upon admission was divided into 3 types as follow; ICP 0-10 mmhg (2 cases), ICP 11-20 mmHg (2 cases) and ICP 21-40 mmHg (3 cases) (Table1).

Table1 Intracraniol pressure (ICP) on admission and outcome.

ICP (mmHg) on Admission	Glasgow Outcome Scale*			Total
	GR/MD	SD/Veg	Dead	
0～10	0	1	1	2
11～20	2	0	1	2
21～40	1	0	2	3
Total	3	1	4	8

*GR=good recovery ; MD=moderate disability
SD=severe disability ; Veg=vegetative

ICP monitoring distinguished 3 groups of DCS (Table2). Namely, ICP remained below 20 mmHg in 1 (Group I). ICP rose to 20 mmHg or higher, but the intracranial hypertension responded to therapy in 4 (Group II) , and rose to 20 mmHg or higher and remained elevated despite the therapy, and, eventually, the cerebral perfusion pressure decreasad to 0 mmHg in 3 (Group III).

Table2 Course of intracranial pressure (ICP) and outcome.

ICP* Group	Glasgow Outcome Scale**			Total
	GR/MD	SD/Veg	Dead	
I	0	1	0	1
II	3	1	0	4
III	0	0	3	3
Total	3	2	3	8

*Group I = ICP remained below 20 mmHg
Group II = ICP rose above 20 mmHg but was controlled by therapy
Group III = ICP rose above 20 mmHg but could not be controlled by therapy
**GR = good recovery ; MD = moderate disability
SD = severe disability ; Veg = vegetative

All patients having Group II and III DCS received the barbiturate therapy. The outcome based on GOS 6 months after injury was as follows : Group I (PVS : 1) Group II (GR : 1, MD : 2, SD : 1), and Group III (dead : 3).

Widespread use of CT in the diagnosis and management of patients with acute severe head injury have ascertained the existence of diffuse cerebral swelling in a very early stage after the trauma. Such evidence has been found commonly in the young patients [2, 3, 4}. Bruce and his colleagues [2] stressed that one of the pathogenic mechanisms producing diffuse cerebral swelling might be vasodilatation and/or cerebral hyperperfusion. Zimmerman and his colleagues [3] measured cerebral blood flow in 4 patients with diffuse cerebral swelling by the technique of Orbist (1975) ultilizing the intravenous injection of ^{131}Xenon. They found that the mean cerebral blood flow was significantly elevated. If these hypothesis would be existed in the pediatric patients showing diffuse cerebral swelling, barbiturato overloading therapy (BOT) may aet on the vesseles of the =brain by means of vasoconstrict effect of barbiturate [5].
In pediatric patients, barbiturate, which produces vasoconstriction, proved efficacious in the treatment of DCS, a condition attributable partly to enlargement of the vascular bed secondary to vasodilation in the brain. Efficacy of early institution of barbiturate overloading therapy for DCS is to be studied.

REFERENCES

1. Kobayashi S, Nakazawa S, Yono M, Yamoto Y, Otsuka T (1983) The value of intracranial pressure (ICP) measurement in acute severe head injury showing diffuse cerebral swelling. In : Ishii S, Nagai H, Brock M (eds) Intracranial Pressure V. Springer-Verlag, Berlin, pp527-531

2. Bruce DA, Alavi A, Bilaniuk L, Dolinskas C, Orbist W, Uzzell B (1981). Diffuse cerebral swelling following head injuries children : the syndrome of "malignant brain edema" J Neurosurg 54 : 170-178

3. Zimmerman RA, Bilaniuk LT, Bruce D, Dolinskas C, Orbist W, Kuhl D (1978) Computed tomography ofpediatric head trauma : scute general cerebral swelling. Radiology 126 : 403-408

4. Aldrich EF, Eisenberg HM, Saydjari C, Luerssen TG,Foulkes MA, Jane JA, Marshall LF, Marmarou A, Young HF (1992) Diffuse brain swelling in severly head-injured children : a report from the NIH traumatic come data bank. J Neurosurg 76 : 450-454

5. Bruce DA, Rephaely RA, Swedlow D (1980) The effectiveness of iatrogenic barbiturate coma in controlling increased ICP in 61 children. In : Shulman K, Marumarou A, Miller JD (eds). Intracranial Pressure JV. Springer-Verlag, Berlin, pp630-632

The Cerebral Thermo-Poolings and Hypothermia Treatment of Critical Head Injury Patients

NARIYUKI HAYASHI, TERUYASU HIRAYAMA, and AKIRA UTAGAWA

Nihon University Critical Care & Shock Trauma Center, Itabashi-ku, Tokyo, 173 Japan

INTRODUCTION

In this paper, we present new secondary injury mechanism after severe head trauma and cerebral hypothermia treatment to these patients based on a new concept of cerebral thermoregulation [4].

MATERIALS AND METHODS

The clinical studies were carried out in 52 critical head injury patients (GCS<8). All of patients were treated with monitoring of intracranial pressure, carotid venous bulb O_2 saturation (SjO_2),SaO_2,SvO_2, cardiac output (CO), brain tissue temperature (BTT), tympanic membrane temperature (TMT). The systemic oxygen metabolisms were evaluated by oxygen extraction ratio (O_2ER). Cerebral oxygen metabolism and circulatory disturbances were estimated by changes of SjO_2, cerebral perfusion pressure (CPP) and cerebral thermal index (CTI=BTT/TMT) which increase inversely correlated to disturbances of cerebral circulation [4].

The effect of mild cerebral hypothermia for the prevention of brain edema and thermal dysregulation was examined in 14 pupils dilated head injury patients (GCS<4). Cerebral hypothermia was produced by whole body cooling throughout a compartment cooling jacket that was developed at our Critical Care Center using a Branketrol and controlled brain tissue temperature to 32-33°C. The optimal brain tissue temperate were estimated with disappearance of cortical loop responses by tibia nerve stimulation.

RESULTS AND DISCUSSION

(l) Cerebral thermo-poolings; The initial pathophysiological changes after head injury included thermo-dysregulation in the brain tissue. The brain tissue temperature elevated to 38-43.8°C until at 17-30 hours after surgery and trauma. Such specific pathophysiological changes, viz, cerebral thermo-poolings, were triggered by insufficient CPP to washout of accumulated brain tissue temperature. The specific thermo-poolings phenomenon could not be controlled successfully by previous ICP management methods. Only elevation of the MABP (> 65 mmHg) could reduce the cerebral thermo-poolings by brain temperature washout with an increased cerebral blood flow. The typical cerebral thermo-poolings phenomenon was observed in patients with post reperfusion stage associated with shock.

(2) Cerebral hypermetabolism in ischemia; Simultaneous monitoring of SjO_2 and CTI indicated that, short period of ischemia and hypoxia followed ischemic hypermetabolism (progressive decrease of SjO_2 and mild reduction of CTI) until at 8-15 hours after surgery. Intracranial hypertension developed with vascular engorgement after these ischemic hypermetabolism. The elevations of ICP with brain edema were started following observation of cerebral thermo-poolings and ischemic hypermetabolism.

(3) Clinical results; In this series of mild cerebral hypothermia treatments of critical acute subdural hematoma who had bilateral dilated pupils, 4 patients died and 10 patients survived. The prognosis was found to be excellent in 9 of the surviving patients. All 9 patients showed a good recovery at 3 months after treatment and the other surviving patient exhibited mild disability after 1 month (Table 1). No speech disturbances were observed with an ordinary life style.

The previous papers revealed high mortality and mobility in this critical head injury patients (GCS<4) [1,2]. Recent studies have demonstrated that glutamate release after cerebral ischemia can be protected against by cerebral hypothermia at 33°C [3]. In our studies, protection against cerebral thermo-poolings, prevention of synaptic excitation, a low metabolic demand, low free radical reactions, stabilization of the vital signs and a low systemic energy transport into the brain were demonstrated as a mechanism of successful treatment by applying mild cerebral hypothermia [4]. The initial pathophysiological change after trauma is progressive increasing of brain tissue temperature. These cerebral thermo-poolings produced elevation of brain tissue temperature at a maximum of 43.8 °C. It could be change or damage of vascular proteins, directly. The changes in brain tissue temperature were influenced basically by four factors; 1) the cerebral metabolism, 2) the systemic excess energy metabolism, 3) the CPP that carries the systemic energy to the brain tissue, and 4) the cerebral blood flow leads to washout of the brain tissue temperature [4,5]. Selective head cooling technique is difficult to control the excess perfusion of systemic energy metabolism into the brain tissue, results in acute elevation of brain tissue temperature vascular engorgement at the rewarming stage. Therefore, systemic whole body cooling technique with stabilization of the brain tissue temperature at exactly 32-33°C and well organized rewarming method by control of systemic O_2ER lower than 30% are more useful than selective cooling of the head. The major issue of this mild cerebral hypothermia treatment is prevention of pulmonary complication and control of acute elevation of intracranial pressure at the rewarming stage. The mild cerebral hypothermia; 32-33°C managed by body compartment cooling technique to the critical conditions of diffuse brain injury patients (GCS <4) produced a good recovery in 9 of 14 patients. The mechanism of this treatment was studied based on the management of cerebral thermo-poolings, synaptic excitation, hypermetabolic demand, and systemic clinical condition of metabolic reserve.

REFERENCES

1. Becker DP, Miller JD, Ward JD, Greenberg RP, Young HF, and Sakalas R (1977) The outcome from severe head injury with early diagnosis and intensive management. J. Neurosurg. 47: 491-502
2. Bricolo A, Turazzi S, and Feriotti G (1980) Prolonged post-traumatic unconsciousness. J Neurosurg. 52: 625-634
3. Busto R, Deitolich WD, Glogus MY-T Deitolich WD, Martinez E, Valdes 1, and Ginsberg MD (1989) Effect of mild hypothermia on ischemia-induced release of neurotransmitters and free fatty acids in rat brain. Stroke 20: 904-910
4. Hayashi N, Hirayama T, Udagawa A,Daimon W and Ohata M (1993) The systemic management of cerebral edema by new concept in severe head injury patients.In: Ito U et al (eds) Acta Neurochirurgica Supplement 60, Springer-Verlag Wien New York. pp 541-543 (The Brain Edema IX)
5. Hayashi N and Hirayama T (1993) Computed cerebral hypothermia management of critical head injury patient in ICU. Medical Postgraduates 31(3): 59-70

Table 1. The prognosis of acute subdural hematoma & diffuse brain injury with a condition of no reactive bilateral dilated pupils

Authors	Year	Cases	GR / MD	SD/VS	D
Becker et al.[1]	1977	23	5 (22%)	3(13%)	15(65%)
Bricolo et al.[2]	1980	59	-	-	45(76%)
Hayashi et al.	1993	14	9/1 (72%)*	0(0%)	4(28%)

GR, Good recovery, D, Mild disability, SD, Severe disability, VS,Vegetable state
D, Death. * No speech disturbances were observed at ordinary life style in 90% of patients

Prospective Validation of Risk Factors for Prediction of Acute Traumatic Intracranial Haematoma After Paediatric Head Injury

K.H. CHAN, S.C.P. NG, Y.W. FAN, and C.F. FUNG

Division of Neurosurgery, Department of Surgery, The University of Hong Kong, Queen Mary Hospital, Hong Kong

INTRODUCTION

Different stages of skull bone development in children has been shown to be related to development of acute intracranial haematoma (ICH) after traumatic brain injury (1). The paediatric patients should therefore be regarded as a heterogenous population instead of a homogeneous group. Children can be subdivided into three groups according to skull bone development; group I: ≤ 2 years, group II: 3-10 years and group III: 11-15 years. The aim of the study is to define the risk factors for development of acute ICH after head injury in children during different stages of skull changes.

MATERIAL & METHOD

Between January 1987 and June 1993, 802 children below the age of 16 years hospitalized for closed head injury were studied. All patients were admitted directly from the Accident & Emergency Department to the neurosurgical ward. Patient's level of consciousness was assessed according to the Glasgow Coma Score (GCS) and all had skull X-ray (anteroposterior, lateral and Towne's views) performed. After admission, all cases were managed according to a standard protocol that included hourly neurological observation and liberal computerized tomography (CT) scanning policy. Indications for CT scanning included GCS < 15 points, presence of skull fracture and whenever clinically indicated. Patients discharged were followed up and deaths had post-mortem examination. The end-point of the study was development of acute ICH within 48 hours of admission, documented by CT, surgery and/or post-mortem.

Patients were subdivided into three groups according to developmental skull changes; group I: ≤ 2 years, group II: 3-10 years and group III: 11-15 years (1). Eleven potential risk factors for predicting of ICH were collected prospectively. Univariate analysis was first used to define significant parameters. Multivariate logistic regression analysis was then used to identify factors of independent significance in the three age groups.

RESULTS

Of the 802 patients, 83 had road traffic accident, 366 fell from height, 206 fell at level ground, 105 were hit by object, 3 had sport-related injury, 24 were assaulted and in 15 cases the mode of injury was unknown.

There were 189, 466 and 147 patients in group I, II and III respectively. Eleven, 23 and 17 patients developed ICH in group I, II and III respectively. In group I, 4 (36%) patients with ICH required operative treatment, the corresponding number of cases in groups II and III were 11 (48%) and 11 (53%) respectively.

Eleven risk factors analyzed included loss of consciousness, vomiting, epilepsy, neurological complaints, blood from nose or ear, cerebrospinal fluid from nose or ear, neurological sign, neck stiffness, admission Glasgow coma score and skull fracture. Univariate analysis identified the following significant factors:

group I : post-traumatic epilepsy ($p=0.0005$)
group II : history of loss of consciousness ($p=0.0005$)
blood discharge from nose ($p=0.02$)
Glasgow coma score on admission ($p<0.0001$)
Skull fracture ($p<0.0001$)
group III: vomiting ($p=0.0008$)
admission Glasgow Coam Score ($p<0.001$)
skull fracture ($p<0.0001$)

Multivariate analysis revealed the following factors of independent significance in the three groups:

Group	risk factors	coefficient	standard error	p value
I	post-traumatic epilepsy	3.6721	1.2715	0.0039
II	GCS < 15	3.5154	0.7784	<0.0005
	skull fracture	3.5837	0.6151	<0.0005
	neurologic signs	3.5067	1.7654	0.047
III	Skull fracture	4.8537	1.2727	0.0001

CONCLUSION

Children should be regarded as a heterogeneous group after head injury. Different age groups have varying risk factors for development of intracranial complications. Guidelines for management of paediatric head-injured patients should be formulated accordingly.

REFERENCE

(1) Mann KS, Chan KH, Yue CP: Skull fractures in children: their assessment in relation to developmental skull changes and acute intracranial haematomas. Child's Nervous System, 2:258-261, 1986.

Assessment of the Autoregulatory Reserve Using Continuous CPP and TCD Blood Flow Velocity Measurement in Head Injury

M. CZOSNYKA, P. KIRKPATRICK, E. GUAZZO, H. WHITEHOUSE, P. SMIELEWSKI, and J.D. PICKARD

MRC Cambridge Centre for Brain Repair and Academic Neurosurgical Unit, Addenbrooke's Hospital, P.O. Box 167, Cambridge CB2 2QQ, UK

Specific changes in the transcranial Doppler (TCD) blood flow velocity waveform in ventilated head injured patients are mainly due to variations in cerebral perfusion pressure (CPP). Our aim was to investigate how convergent TCD waveform indices were in a heterogeneous group of patients and whether they were correlated with the outcome after head injury.

MATERIAL AND METHOD

Forty-two patients suffering severe head injuries with a mean Glasgow Coma Scale of 6 (range from 3 to 13, only three patients had GCS higher than 8 after resuscitation) were assessed. ICP was monitored continuously using a Camino transducer placed intra-dural or by a subdural catheter connected to external pressure transducer. Systemic blood pressure (ABP) was measured using an arterial line. TCD blood flow velocity in the middle cerebral artery was recorded daily for periods from 10 to 120 minutes along with ICP and ABP on a bedside computer and then analysed. A hundred and ninety examinations were recorded and almost four thousand one minute averages of the following parameters were considered:

- systolic, diastolic and mean blood flow velocity (FV_s, FV_d, FV)
- mean ICP, ABP, CPP
- pulsatility indices: Gosling pulsatility index ($PI_g=(FV_s-FV_d)/FV$), spectral pulsatility index ($PI_s=FVa/FV$, where FVa is a fundamental harmonic of the flow velocity pulse waveform) and standardised pulsatility index ($SPI=PI_s/ABPa$, where ABPa is a fundamental harmonic of the ABP pulse waveform)
- gradients of systolic and diastolic FV with CPP varying spontaneously during recording (GFV_s and GFV_d, relatively)

Each patient's outcome was assessed using Glasgow Outcome Scale at 4 to 19 months after injury. Mean values of selected parameters from every examination were analysed in three outcome groups: Group I - GOS 1, 2 (good and moderate outcome; N=20); Group II - GOS 3 (severe disable patients; N=11); Group III - GOS 4, 5 (persistently vegetative or dead; N=11).

RESULTS AND DISCUSSION

Averaged flow velocity systolic and diastolic were plotted with 95% confidence bars against CPP in Fig 1. All pulsatility indices exhibited the same trend but ANOVA revealed the best statistical convergence for SPI, therefore this index has been plotted with CPP along x-axis in Fig 1. The threshold below which the diastolic flow velocity started to decrease significantly with CPP ($p<0.05$) was detected at CPP 55 mmHg. The systolic FV did not exhibit statistically significant threshold. Investigated parameters were compared in three outcome groups (mean values with statistically significance of differences at $p<0.05$ are presented in Table 1).

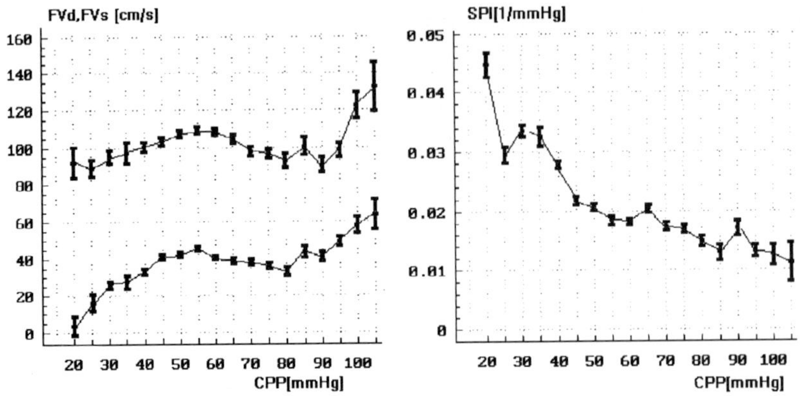

Fig1 Results of ANOVA of selected parameters versus CPP - mean values and 95% confidence limits for means presented as vertical bars. Left- Systolic and diastolic flow velocity. Right- Standardised Pulsatility Index.

Table1. Mean values of calculated parameters in three outcome groups. Significantly different values in rows ($p<0.05$) are denoted by * or **

Parameter	Group 1	Group II	Group III
mean ICP [mmHg]	16*	26	28
mean ABP [mmHg]	81	91*	81
mean CPP [mmHg]	65	65	53*
mean FV [cm/s]	69	66	58*
PI	1.18	1.35	1.78*
PIs	0.51	0.64*	0.93**
SPI [1/mmHg]	0.018	0.02	0.026*
GFV_d [cm/s/mmHg]	0.13	0.25	0.53*
GFV_s [cm/s/mmHg]	-0.10	0.001	0.14*

ICP was increased in Groups II and III. However, because of a higher ABP, CPP in Group II was similar to Group I. The worst outcome can be expected when ICP is elevated and ABP is unable to compensate for it. Patients in Group III were usually not autoregulated, therefore the lowest FV was implicated by the lowest CPP. All pulsatility indices were increasing with worse outcome. However, only the spectral pulsatility index allowed significant differentiation among all three outcome groups. The Gosling and Standardised indices were not so sensitive. The different gradients of systolic and diastolic flow velocities with varying CPP were observed in different outcome groups, justifying our methodology for continuous monitoring of autoregulatory reserve [1]. In well autoregulated patients diastolic FV is not correlated to CPP, systolic FV has a tendency to increase with falling CPP. When mean FV is falling and systolic- diastolic FVs are divergent with decreasing CPP, which causes an increase in FV pulsatility, autoregulatory reserve is weakening . When both systolic and diastolic FVs are decreasing with CPP, autoregulation is severely disturbed.

REFERENCE

1. Czosnyka M, Guazzo E, V.Iyer, Kirkpatrick P, Smielewski P., Whitehouse H , Pickard JD (1994) Testing of Cerebral Autoregulation in Head Injury by Waveform Analysis of Blood Flow Velocity and Cerebral Perfusion Pressure. Acta Neurochirurgica [Suppl 60]: 468-471

Poster IX: Edema and Others

Chairman: M. Brock

Multimodality Monitoring as a Guide of Intracranial Vasospasm After Severe Subarachnoid Haemorrhage

R. Massei[1], F. Lusenti[1], G. Vendrame[1], P. Fumagalli[1], E. Calappi[2], and L. Monolo[3]

[1] Department of Anaesthesia and Intensive Care, Lecco Hospital, Italy
[2] Department of Anaesthesia and Intensive Care, University of Milan, Italy
[3] Department of Neurosurgery, Lecco Hospital, Italy

Summary

We monitored twenty-four patients with SAH (Grades IV-V in the WFNS Scale) to prevent secondary cerebral ischemia. Cerebral extraction of oxygen and arteriojugular lactate difference have been used to evaluate cerebral oxygenation. A total of 483 observations were carried out and a total of 66 episodes of jugular desaturation were documentated. Most of these episodes were determined by a not optimized hyperventilation (33 episodes). Five prolonged episodes of desaturation were correlated with pulmonary disease. Monitoring of jugular venous oxygen saturation is a valuable tool for detecting and treating insufficient cerebral oxygenation in patients with severe brain damage.

Introduction

The rupture of an aneurysm is associated with high morbidity and mortality. Of those patients that survive the initial subarachnoid hemorrhage (SAH), delayed cerebral ischemia from vasospasm remains the major cause of death and disability. Numerous factors have been found to influence the incidence of vasospasm. Among these, an impaired autoregulation and a marked decrease of CBF were seen in patients with worse outcomes. Meyer et al. (1) found that cerebral blood flow (CBF) declined during the first week, reached the maximum during the second week, and began to rise slightly during the third week. Prevention of secondary ischemia is one of the objectives in the management of patients with SAH. Recently monitoring the Cerebral Extraction of Oxygen (CEO2) as the difference between the SaO2 and the SjO2 has been shown to be able to evaluate cerebral oxygenation and to estimate the CBF (2). The aim of the present study was to investigate cerebral oxygenation in comatose patients due to SAH with special emphasis on the influence of hyperventilation in order to avoid episodes of jugular desaturation and production of cerebral lactates.

Materials and Methods

Twenty-four patients with SAH (Grades IV-V in the WFNS Scale) were admitted to the study. The age was between 45 and 69 years. Patients were managed according to a standard protocol that included nasotracheal intubation, artificial ventilation to obtain a PaO2 greater than 100 mmHg and a PaCO2 of 35 mmHg, sedation and, if necessary, muscle paralysis. Surgery was performed as soon as possible and a CT scan was repeated few hours later. Mean arterial pressure, SaO2 and ICP by intraventricular catheter were continuously recorded. SjO2, PaO2, PaCO2, PjO2, arteriojugular lactate difference (AJLD) were monitored every four hours. To measure SjO2 in the jugular bulb, a catheter (G17, L 15 cm) was percutaneously inserted in the right side as described by Cruz (2). Correct placement of the catheter tip in the jugular bulb was confirmed by x-ray. CPP was monitored as the difference between MAP and mean ICP. Global cerebral ischemia was graded according to whether the jugular oxyhemoglobin saturation fell to the ranges of 50% to 54% (Grade 1), 45% to 49% (Grade 2), or lower than 45% (Grade 3) (2). Normal values of AJLD was considered -0,17± 0,2 mmol/L (3).

Results

Four patients had ICP values greater than 30 mmHg , despite moderate hypocapnia. The remaining twenty patients had initial ICP values within the normal range. A total of 483 observations were carried out during a total of 2565 multivariate monitoring hours. Jugular desaturations were documentated in 66 episodes (13,6%). All the patients developed at least one or more episodes of jugular desaturation. All but five were brief, well responding to management. Different types of desaturation were found: neurogenic desaturation due to sudden ICP increases (11 episodes); idiopathic desaturation (5 episodes); desaturation associated with lung disease (17 episodes) and desaturation due to non optimized ventilation (33 episodes). The five, prolonged episodes were associated with arterial hypoxia due to lung pneumonia and the patients suffered neurological deterioration. The jugular oxyhemoglobin saturation was within the Grade 2. All but four AJLD measurements were within normal limits.

Discussion

The monitoring of the jugular venous oxygen saturation as a measure of cerebral oxygenation has been widely studied by several Authors (2) (4). The method could be considered safe and no complications were reported. A. von Helden (5) described 49 desaturation episodes in patients with SAH. Almost 30% of the desaturation episodes were most probabily caused by hyperventilation. This corresponds to our study, where the 50% of desaturation episodes were associated with hypocapnia. Cerebral oxygenation may also be compromised by cerebral vasospasm. Earlier determinations of CBF have shown a general depression of flow in patients with SAH and a correlation between rCBF and neurological status and impairment of consciousness (6). The patients are aggressively treated with hypertensive hypervolemic hemodiluition at the first sign of clinical vasospasm. CEO2 monitoring may avoid iatrogenic damage due to non optimized ventilation and too low values of PaCO2 could be corrected.

In conclusion these findings indicate that hyperventilation should be done cautiously and always during oxymetric monitoring in order to avoid signs of cerebral ischemia.

References

1. Meyer CHA, Lowe D, Meyer M et al (1993) Progressive change in cerebral blood flow during the first three weeks after subarachnoid hemorrhage. Neurosurgery 12:58-76

2. Cruz J, Miner ME, Allen SJ et al (1990) Continuous monitoring of cerebral oxygenation in acute brain injury: injection of mannitol during hyperventilation. J Neurosurgery 73:725-730

3. Gibbs EL, Lennox WG, Nims LF et al (1942) Arterial and cerebral venous blood. Arterial-venous differences in man. J Biol Chem 144:325-332

4. Robertson CS, Narayan RK, Gokaslan ZL et al (1989) Cerebral arteriovenous oxygen difference as an estimate of cerebral blood flow in comatose patients. J Neurosurg 73:725

5. von Helden A, Schneider GH, Unterberg and Lanksch WR (1993) Monitoring of jugular venous oxygen saturation in comatose patients with subarachnoid haemorrhage and intracerebral haematomas. Acta Neurochir (Suppl) 59:102-106

6. Voldby B, Enevoldsen EM and Jensen FT (1985) Regional CBF, intraventricular pressure, and cerebral metabolism in patients with ruptured intracranial aneurysms. J Neurosurg 62:48-58

Cerebral Anaerobic Metabolism After Head Injury

R. Massei[1], F. Lusenti[1], G. Vendrame[1], C. Martini[1], A. Parma[2], and E. Troina[3]

[1] Department of Anaesthesia and Intensive Care, Lecco Hospital, Italy
[2] Department of Anaesthesia and Intensive Care, University of Milan, Italy
[3] Department of Clinical-Chemistry, Lecco Hospital, Italy

Summary

Cerebral extraction of oxygen, ICP, PaCO2, AJDL were monitored in 26 patients with severe brain injury. Jugular desaturation was evaluated and managed. A total of 97 episodes of jugular desaturation were documented. Prolonged episodes occurred 22 times, the remaining 75 episodes promptly responded to treatment. No signs of cerebral ischemia were detected. Desaturation was not associated with neurological deterioration.

Introduction

Ischemic brain damage could contribute to morbidity in patients who suffered severe head injury (1). A great effort has been addressed to monitoring and maintaining an adequate level of arterial oxygen saturation in all the patients admitted to Neurointensive Care. The main purpose of the therapeutic interventions could be to avoid the secundary ischemia due not only to the increased intracranial pressure (ICP) but also to iatrogenic damage. It has been described the risk to induce cerebral ischemia during hyperventilation therapy in order to decrease raised ICP (2). Thus to identify patients at risk from cerebral ischemia could be very important: when CBF is critically reduced in relation to the brain's metabolic need, a wide AVDO2 is obtained (the ratio of CMRO2 to CBF is calculated by the Fick equation as the arterial-jugular oxygen difference: AVDO2 = CMRO2/CBF). Recently it has been reported that, under circumstances of anemia, the AVDO2 is an inaccurate measurement of inadequate cerebral perfusion and oxygenation (3); that is, a more reliable indicator of the ratio of CMRO2/CBF would be the cerebral extraction of oxygen (CEO2) as the difference between SaO2 and SjO2. Moreover global measurements of the arteriojugular lactate difference (AJDL) have been reported as indicators of regional cerebral ischemia (4).

The purpose of the present study was to assess the value of CEO2 in severe head-injured patients in order to avoid cerebral ischemia during therapeutic hyperventilation.

Materials and Methods

Twenty-six patients (median age 40 years) admitted in coma (GCS ≤ 8) due to severe head injury had been studied. Admission computerized tomography scans revealed diffuse brain injury (20 cases) or focal lesions (6 cases). All patients were positioned at an 30° head tilt and underwent continuous monitoring of electrocardiogram, rectal temperature, mean arterial pressure, intracranial pressure (ICP), arterial oxyhemoglobin saturation (SaO2). Right jugular bulb oxyhemoglobin saturation (SjO2), PaCO2, PaO2 and AJDL were obtained every four hours and during spontaneous ICP elevations in the presence of constant MAP, SaO2 and EtCO2. The jugular bulb catheter (G 17, L 15 cm) was inserted percutaneously into the internal jugular vein and positioned so that the tip was in the jugular bulb. The correct position of the catheter was confirmed by x-ray. It was estimated a normal CEO2 range of 31,6± 7,8%. Based on these values, an abnormally increased cerebral extraction of oxygen may allow identification of "oligemic cerebral hypoxia" (CEO2 > 40%) (5).Whole blood lactate concentrations were measured by an enzymatic method (Abbot TDx Analyzer). The normal range of AJDL measurements was considered -0.17± 0.2 mmol/L (6). The ICP was monitored by lateral ventricular catheter in 4 patients and by the subarachnoid catheter in 22 patients. Global cerebral hypoxia was defined according to whether the SjO2 fell lower than 50%. Our treatment protocol for ICP below 20 mmHg included naso-tracheal intubation, mechanical ventilation, sedation, muscle paralysis, hyperventilation avoiding jugular venous desaturation, mannitol intravenous boluses.

Results

Nineteen patients had initial ICP values greater than 30 mmHg (mean 34 mmHg) despite moderate hyperventilation (mean PaCO2 = 33 mmHg). The remaining seven patients had initial ICP values close to 20 mmHg. A total of 507 observations were carried out during the acute phase of injury (1-11 days postinjury). An abnormally increased CEO2 (oligemic cerebral hypoxia) was found in 97 observations (19,13%): 75 episodes of jugular desaturation were brief, rapidly responding to management and 22 were prolonged, not rapidly responding to management. Jugular desaturation was due to: sudden ICP increases (neurogenic desaturation, 35 episodes); desaturation associated with arterial desaturation (18 episodes); idiopathic desaturation (without cause, 7 cases); desaturation due to non optimized hyperventilation (37 episoses).The episodes of desaturation were most common during the first 48 hours after admission (84 episodes), mostly due to non optimized ventilation (48 episodes) and ICP increases (31 episodes). Of the brief jugular desaturation episodes, 69 showed SjO2 between 50% and 40%, 6 were lower than 40%. Of the prolonged episodes, all but one were between 50% and 40%. The hypoxic pattern was not correlated with cerebral ischemia: the cerebral lactate production and all AJDL measurements were well within the normal range. Jugular desaturations were not associated with neurological deterioration: the initial GCS scores prior to desaturation problems were not statistically different from the GCS scores at 2 weeks.

Discussion

The episodes of jugular venous desaturation are common in patients with severe head injury. Two important studies, among the others, by M.Sheinberg (7) and by J.Cruz (8) showed respectevely sixty episodes of jugular venous oxygen desaturation in 45 patients and 121 episodes in 69 patients, during continuous monitoring of the SjO2. We adopted the intermittent monitoring of the SjO2, in order to avoid the incidence of artifactual false jugular desaturation M.Sheinberg et al. (7) reported a very high, clinically unacceptable rate of false desaturation, with a poor correlation between fiberoptic and conventional oximetry. This probably could be minimized by adequate nursing, as indicated by Cruz,1993 (8). It has been shown that jugular desaturation may significantly compromise neurological outcome (7) (8): in our series of patients we were not able to follow up the patients after the dismission from the Intensive Care Unit. However aggressive management of high ICP and arterial desaturation and the best ventilation could have minimized the episodes of desaturation and the subsequent neurological deterioration. Moreover jugular lactate levels showed no evidence of cerebral ischemia.
In conclusion, ideally it would be best to monitor multiple physiological parameters continuously and to understand the cause of desaturation avoiding artifactual readings.

References

1. Gentleman D., Jannett B.(1990) Audit of transfer of unconscious patients to a neurosurgical unit. Lancet 335:330-334
2. Miller JD, Dearden NM, Piper IR, Chan KH.(1992) Control of intracranial pressure in patients with severe head injury. J Neurotrauma 9 (suppl 1): S317-26
3. Cruz J,Gennarelli TA,Alves WM (1992) Continuous monitoring of cerebral hemodynamic reserve in acute brain injury:relationship to changes in brain swelling. J Trauma 32: 629-635
4.Robertson CS, Narayan RK, Gokaslan ZL, et al.(1989) Cerebral arteriovenous oxygen difference as an estimate of cerebral blood flow in comatose patients. J Neurosurg 70:222
5. Cruz J, Miner ME, Allen SJ, et al (1991) Continuous monitoring of cerebral oxygenation in acute brain injury:Assessment of cerebral hemodynamic reserve. Neurosurgery 29:743
6. Gibbs EL, Lennox WG, Nims LF, et al (1942) Arterial and cerebral venous blood:Arterial-venous differences in man. J Biol Chem 144:325
7. Sheinberg M, Kanter MJ, Robertson CS et al (1992) Continuous monitoring of jugular venous oxygen saturation in head-injured patients. J Neurosurg.76: 212-217
8. Cruz J. (1993) On-line monitoring of global cerebral hypoxia in acute brain injury. Relationship to intracranial hypertension. J.Neurosurg. 79: 228-233

Nimodipine in the Treatment of Brain Edema in Neurosurgical Patients

V. Amcheslavskyi[1], E. Sirovskyi[1], M. Demchuk[2], and L. Levchenko[2]

[1] Department of Intensive Care Burdenko Neurosurgical Institute AMS, 125047 Moscow, Fadeev str. 5, Russia
[2] Laboratory of Biochemistry Burdenko Neurosurgical Institute AMS, 125047 Moscow, Fadeev str. 5, Russia

SUMMARY

Influence of Nimodipine (N) on lipid peroxidation in vitro and in vivo examinations was investigated. High antioxidant properties of N were found in experiments on the model system. These properties were also confirmed by clinical investigations in patients with brain edema, where marked decrease of malone dialdehyde (MDA) and increase of antioxidant activity (AOA) in blood serum were determined after the administration of the drug. These firstly discovered antioxidant properties of N allowed us to recommend it in the treatment of brain edema in neurosurgical patients.

INTRODUCTION

Brain edema, belongs to one of the most severe complications of postoperative period in neurosurgery.
It is well known, that activation of lipid peroxidation (LP) plays an important role in the pathogenesis of brain edema[1,2]. That's why antioxidants are traditionally used in brain edema therapy [3].
The aim of our work was to investigate the antioxidant properties of N and the possibility of its usage in the treatment of neurosurgical patients with brain edema.

MATERIALS AND METHODS

62 examinations were made 1–5 days (mean value 2,8 ± 1) after surgery in patients with gliomas of large hemispheres. The clinical condition of patients was evaluated by neurological signs, CT–scan, hemodynamic monitoring. Patients with visceral pathology and postoperative infectious complications were excluded from the examining group.
The indications for N administration were the following: 1)the severe condition of the patient (8–9 GCS); 2) CT– examination, showing a postoperative edema and the absence of haemorrages into the operative wound or subarachnoid space; 3) laboratory investigations revealing activation of LP.
The infusion of the drug was performed as follows: dosage for the first hour at the start of treatment was 50 ml/h (10 mg N per hour), by 50–ml plastic (polypropylene) syringe, through a special fit polyethylene dark tube connected to central venous catheter and with the help of Braun Secura FT syringe pump. In an hour the infusion rate was decreased to 5 ml/h and N injection was continued during 23 hours.
We estimated the level of one of the most stable LP products MDA and total AOA in blood taken from internal jugular bulb, peripherial vein and artery three times: 1)before the N injection; 2) an hour after the start of treatment; 3) 24 hours after the start of treatment.
MDA was determined spectrophotometrically [4]. For determination of AOA of drugs and blood serum we worked out a new modification of the model system where alcohol–water emulsion of linolenic acid was the substrat of oxidation [5].

RESULTS AND DISCUSSION

In the experimental conditions it was found out, that N possessed high AOA (20 mg N revealed 87% AOA). In clinical investigations during the first hour of N injection insignificant changes in haemodynamics were observed. 30% of patients showed transient decrease of arterial blood pressure (on 10–15 mm Hg); 25% of patients showed transient increase of arterial blood pressure, as well as changes of heart rate. But all these alterations were not statistically reliable. Improvement of neurological functions was observed in 90% of patients. The control CT performed 24 hours after beginning of treatment didn't show any changes of brain edema. But biochemical investigations revealed stable decrease in MDA content in dynamics (2,9 ±0, 4 nmol/ml; 1,65 ± 0,33 nmol/ml; 1,5 ± 0,17 nmol/ml);($p<0,01$),r= –0,41, n=62. At the same time the statistically reliable increase of total AOA was observed in a 24 hours ($p<0,01$), r=0,29 in all examined blood samples (72±0,7%; 85±5,9%; 92±6,2%). The results of One–Way Analysis of Variance showed reliable differences between the levels of MDA and AOA in dynamics. Regression analysis showed statistically significant increase of total AOA and decrease of the MDA level.

According to the literature the N –is one of the most powerfull Ca^{2+} antagonists, one of the Bayer's dihydropiridine derivatives, which possesses the principle action on brain vessels [6]. As it is known the effect of N action is connected with its direct influence on the vessel muscular layer (the blocking of Ca^{2+} influx) and also with its action on tromboxane synthesis, cellular energetic potential, ect.. During last years there appeared some new data about more profound N action on metabolic processes [7].

So the main result of our investigations is the discovery of the antioxidant properties of N, previously unknown. The advantage of N, in comparison with other antioxidants is the possibility of its intravenous administration. That's why it can be recommended for the intensive treatment of brain edema in neurosurgical patients.

REFERENCES

1. Demopoulos H.B., Milvy P., Kakari Sophia, and Ransohoff J. (1982) Molecular aspects of membrane structure in cerebral edema. In: Reulen H.J., Schurman K. (ed) Steroids and Brain Edema. Springer–Verlag,. Berlin–Heidelberg–New–York, pp 29–39

2. Ikeda Y., Andersen D.M. (1989) Oxygen free radicals in the genesis of traumatic and peritumoral brain edema. Neurosurgery 24: 679–685

3. Chan P.H.,Longer S., Fishman R.A. (1987) Protective effects of liposome enrapped superoxide dismutase on postraumatic brain edema. Ann Neurol 21: 540–547

4. Gavrilov V.,Gavrilova A., Magul L. (1987)The analysis of lipid peroxidation assays in blood serum based on 2–thiobarbituric tests. Vopr Med Him 33: 118–122

5. Promyslov M.Sh., Demchuk M.L. (1990) Modification of the method of total antioxidant activity determination of blood serum.Vopr Med Him 36: 90–92

6. Auer L.M. (1984) Acute operation and preventive Nimodipine improve outcome in patients with ruptured cerebral aneurysms. J Neurosurg 15: 57–66.

7. Held K., Hohlweck P. (1985) Effects of cerebral–active drugs on the reduced brain functiuons during hypoxic hypoxia. In: E.Betz, K. Deck, F. Hoffmeister. (ed) Nimodipine: pharmacological and clinical properties proceedings of the 1st International Nimotop Symposium. Munich, Stuttgart,New York pp 239–247

Relationships Between Brain Edema, ICP and Motor Performances After Cryogenic Lesion in the Motor Area

G. Gambardella, S. Toscano, G.na Caruso, D. Collufio, D. d'Avella, and F. Tomasello

Neurosurgical Clinic, University of Messina School of Medicine, Messina, Italy

INTRODUCTION

The outcome of neurosurgical lesions located in the critical areas is strongly influenced by the evolution of the secondary damage associated with the surgical approach. In the present experiments the relationships between secondary damage and neurological function were investigated in a rabbit model of cryogenic injury by means of the evaluation of blood-brain barrier (BBB), cerebral edema and brain tissue pressure changes.

MATERIALS AND METHODS

Twenty-eight New-Zealand albino rabbits (1.5 kg b.w.) were used. The cryogenic lesion was created at the level of the right motor area. The experimental procedures adopted are described in details elsewhere [1]. Briefly, under ketamine and xylazine anesthesia, a bone flap was fashioned over the right fronto-parietal cortex. A cold injury was applied placing on the dura a steel rod cooled to - 80 °C over 90 sec. The bone flap was replaced and assured to the skull with sutures and sealed with fibrin glue and hydroxyapatite. The animals were divided into three experimental groups of 8 each, and 4 animals were utilized as controls. The size of the lesions was 3 mm in Group I, 6 mm in Group II and 9 mm in Group III, respectively. Control animals underwent sham operation only. In 4 animals of each group the evolution of the neurological deficits was monitored over four weeks employing an adapted version of the Tarlov scale. The other 4 animals of each experimental group were sacrificed after 24 hours. BBB changes were evaluated by injection of Evans blue, the extent of brain edema was determined by the wet/dry weight ratio method, and the changes in intracranial pressure by a Camino minitransducer fiberoptic device. Brain tissue pressure monitoring was performed in the right frontal area ipsilateral to the lesion in all animals for 24 h after injury and every 48 h over the following four weeks in the animals undergoing chronic observation. In a parallel series of experiments we determined employing MEP's the surface area of the motor cortex, and found it 60 ± 5 mm^2.

RESULTS

Hystologic examination of cold injured brains showed that the lesion area occupied $12 \pm 4\%$ of the motor cortex surface area in Group I rabbits, $24 \pm 3\%$ in Group II rabbits, and $42 \pm 2.5\%$ in Group III, respectively.

BBB dysfunction, as evidenced by Evans blue discoloration of the lesioned area, was identified in the motor area in all experimental animals.

The % water content measured 24 hours following cryogenic injury in the different corticall areas is summarized as follows (Student t test statistics: ipsilateral cortical areas statistically significant ($p < 0.05$) from controls):

Frontal, ipsilateral	78,6 ±1	79,1 ±1,2	79,4 ±1,1	79,8 ±1,4
Motor area, ipsilateral	80,6 ±1,3	81,7 ±1	82,4 ±1,3	83,3 ±1,2
Parieto-occ., ipsilateral	76,8 ±3,7	78.0 ±2,5	79,8 ±1,2	82,8 ±0,9
Frontal, contralateral	78,4 ±0,7	76.0 ±1,3	77,6 ±2,1	79,3 ±1,3
Motor area,contralateral	75,5 ±1,1	72,6 ±1,1	76.0 ±1,7	76,2 ±1,1
Parieto-occ., contralateral	76,3 ±1,2	74,4 ±0,8	78.0 ±0,9	79,3 ±1

Brain tissue pressure recording showed in Group I animals a peak of 12 ± 3 mmHg at 24 h following injury. Pressure returned to baseline values within the first week. In Group II rabbits elevated pressure values were recorded over 2 weeks, with pressure waves alterations indicative of a reduced intracranial compliance. Similar results were obtained in Group III rabbits, and these changes persisted for almost 3 weeks.

The clinical examination of injured rabbits, performed according to an adapted version of the Tarlov's scale (1 = normal motor performance; 2 = active antigravitary movement; 3 active movement with gravity eliminated; 4 = muscle contraction; 5 = total paralysis) recorded over 4 weeks after injury is summarized as follows:

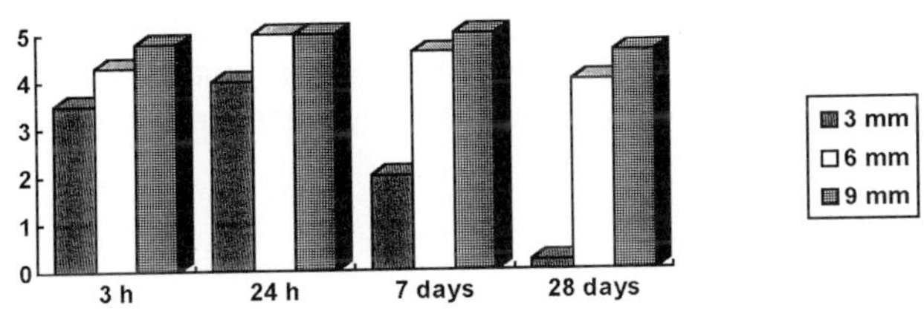

The relationship between neurological deficits and surface area of cold injury is summarized as follows:

Lesion size	Lesion surface in the motor area (mm^2)	Total lesion surface (mm^2)	Perilesional non motor surface (mm^2)	Motor deficit at four weeks (%)
3 mm	7,065	7,065	0	0
6 mm	14	28	14	50
9 mm	24	63	39	~100

DISCUSSION

The data reported here suggest that in this rabbit cold injury model there is a relationship between the extent of motor deficits, BBB changes, brain edema and brain tissue pressure and that the recovery of neurological deficits depends not only on the location of the primary lesion, but also on the extent and severity of perilesional edema and duration of brain tissue pressure changes. These experimental evidences may have clinical implications for neurosurgical approaches to lesions located in critical areas.

REFERENCES

1. Gambardella G, Germanà G, Ciriaco E, Iacopino DG, Muglia U, Tomasello F (1987): Experimental investigations on a model of cryogenic edema. J Neurosurg Sci 31: 133-139

Intracranial Pressure Monitoring in Patients with Spina Bifida and Clinically Arrested Hydrocephalus. Results of a Prospective Study

M.A. Poca[1], J. Sahuquillo[1], A. Cuxart[2], J. Iborra[2], M.D. Calzada[3], and E. Rubio[1]

[1] Neurosurgery Department, [2] Spina Bifida Unit, [3] Neurophysiology Department, Vall d'Hebron University Hospital, Paseo Vall d'Hebron s/n, 08035 Barcelona, Spain

In some patients with spina bifida and with or without non- functioning shunts, moderate or severe stabilized ventriculomegaly is frequently observed in routine control CT scans. These patients can be asymptomatic or have only minor symptoms. The neurosurgeon is then faced with the so-called "Arrested hydrocephalus" (AH). Several authors have warned about the dilemmas that patients with AH can present [1,2]. A wide variety of problems have been described, from slow cognitive deterioration to sudden death attributed to shunt malfunction [3]. AH has not been systematically studied in SB. In this study, we report the results of ICP monitoring in 19 patients with spina bifida and clinically arrested hydrocephalus.

PATIENTS AND METHODS

For admission to this protocol the following criteria were necessary: 1) the patients had no shunt or the shunt was non-functioning at the moment of the study, 2) no evidence of progressive increase in ventricular size and 3) no signs or symptoms of intracranial hypertension. All patients underwent continuous intracranial pressure (ICP) monitoring for at least 72 hours, using a fiberoptic extradural device. According to the ICP recording, all the patients were included in one of the following categories: **Active Hydrocephalus:** Mean ICP $>$ 12 mm Hg, **Compensated hydrocephalus:** Mean ICP $\leq$ 12 mm Hg but with Beta or plateau waves and **Arrested hydrocephalus:** mean ICP $\leq$ 12 mm Hg, without abnormalities in the ICP recording [4].

RESULTS

Twelve females and seven males with a mean age of 18.4 $\pm$ 2.7 years were included in the study. Four patients had a non-shunted hydrocephalus, and 14 had a confirmed or suspected non-functioning shunt. Continuous recording of the ICP demonstrated an Active Hydrocephalus in eleven patients. Six cases were included in the Compensated Hydrocephalus group and in only two patients the diagnosis of Arrested Hydrocephalus was confirmed. Abnormalities in ICP recording were more evident during REM sleep (**Fig.1**).

DISCUSSION

Patients with SB and associated hydrocephalus are difficult to manage. When facing patients with a non-functioning shunt and no neuroradiological evidence of hydrocephalus progression, it is difficult to differentiate between a compensated and an arrested hydrocephalus. On the other hand, the concept of arrested hydrocephalus has always been controversial [1,2]. According to

McLone's recent paper AH "... is defined as adequately shunted hydrocephalus while all other forms of hydrocephalus are at various levels of compensation. Compensation occurs at some cost to the child "[4]. These costs can be subtle (deterioration of school performance, development delay etc.) but excessive if our objective is to obtain an adequate social adaptation and independence of each individual for the daily life activities. In our study, we showed that the majority of patients had an active or compensated hydrocephalus and in only two cases we confirmed the diagnosis of arrested hydrocephalus. We would like to point out that in some of our patients severe intracranial hypertension coexisted with only minor clinical symptoms. In view of our results, we believe that in all cases with a suspected non-functioning shunt or non-shunted ventriculomegaly continuous ICP monitoring is a reasonable method to diagnose arrested hydrocephalus.

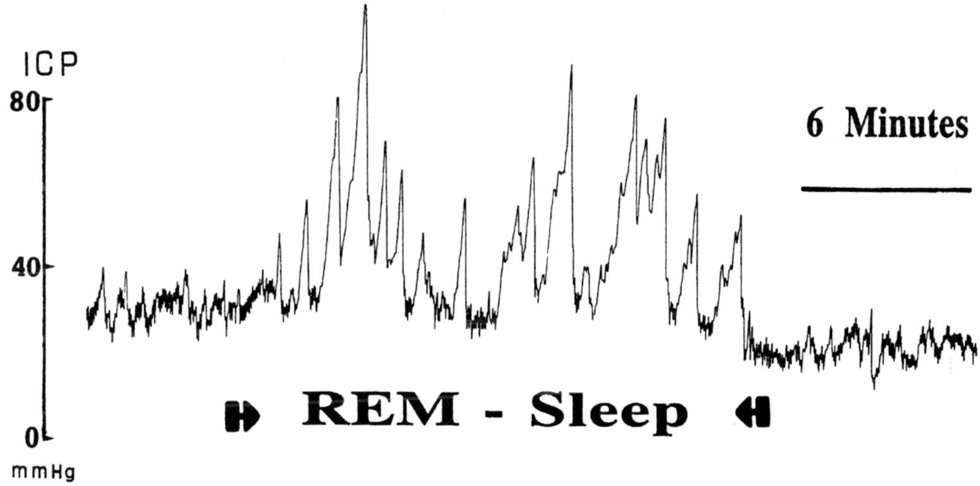

Fig. 1. This 20-year-old girl presented occasional mild headache but with a stable moderate ventriculomegaly. The continuous ICP monitoring showed an active hydrocephalus with B-waves in more than 75 % of the recording time. At night and during REM sleep, B-waves increased in amplitude reaching values of 80 mm Hg.

REFERENCES

1. Schick RW, Matson DD (1961) What is arrested hydrocephalus?. J.Pediatr.58: 791-799.

2. Bird MD, Ratcheson RA, Seigel BA, Fishman MA (1973) The evaluation of arrested communicating hydrocephalus utilizing cerebrospinal fluid dynamics: A preliminary report. Dev. Med. Child Neurol. 15: 474-482.

3. Sahuquillo J, Rubio E, Codina A, Molins A, Guitart JM, Poca MA, Chasampi A (1991) Reappraisal of the intracranial pressure and cerebrospinal fluid dynamics in patients with the so-called "Normal Pressure Hydrocephalus" syndrome. Acta Neurochir. (Wien) 112: 50-61.

4. McLone DG, Aronyk KE (1993) An approach to the management of arrested and compensated hydrocephalus. Pediatr. Neurosurg. 19: 101-103.

Role of Hemicraniectomy in Cold-Induced Brain Edema

K. Kuribayashi, M. Matsuda, and J. Handa

Department of Neurosurgery, Shiga University of Medical Science, Tsukinowa-cho, Otsu, Shiga, 520-21 Japan

INTRODUCTION

The effect of decompressive craniectomy has been controversial [1, 2] . In order to evaluate the effect of the decompressive craniectomy, we measured the water content and tissue pressure, and evaluated neurological function of the brain with cold injury.

MATERIALS AND METHODS

Animals: adult cats, weighing 2.2-4.4kg, divided into two groups, conservative, and decompressive with hemicraniectomy.

Anesthesia: ketamine hydrochloride

Body temperature:37-38°C,

Blood gases: pH 7.33-7.38, pCO_2 33-38 mmHg, pO_2 90-120mmHg

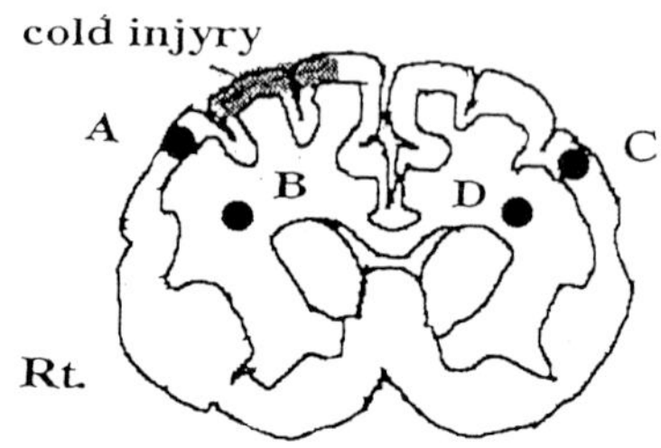

Fig. 1 Coronal view of the brain. The tissue pressure and water content were measured at A, B, C and D .

Cold injury: Gyrus lateralis and Gyrus suprasylvius, application of a metal column cooled with liquid nitrogen for 2 minutes (Fig. 1).

Experimental protocol

Tissue pressure and water content were measured at the sites as shown in Figure 1. One hour after mannitol was administered, tissue pressure was measured again at the same sites. Neurological function was evaluated by the 18-point scale [3] .

RESULTS AND CONCLUSION

Decompressive craniectomy effectively decreased ICP (Fig. 2), and could avoid brain herniation in the acute stage, although brain edema progressed (Fig. 3). There would be no significant difference in neurological state in the chronic stage between the conservative and the decompressive groups (Table 1).

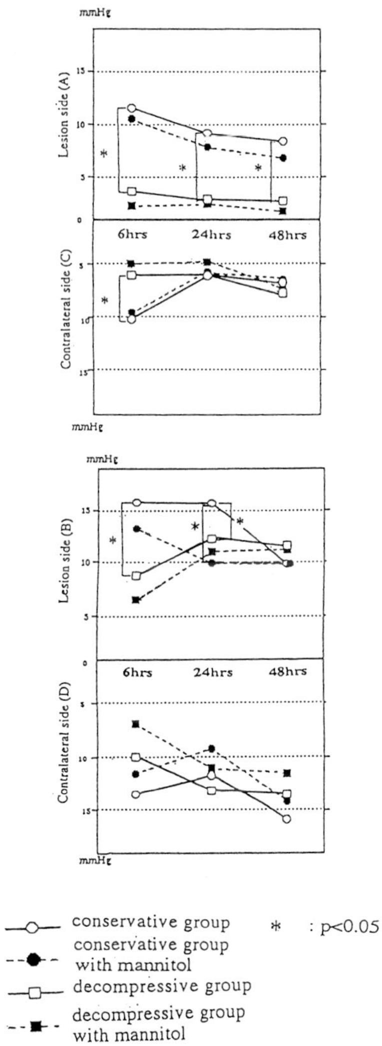

Fig. 2 Tissue pressure. upper: gray matter, lower: white matter

Table 1 Score of Neurological function

group	conservative			decompression		
hours	6	24	48	6	24	48
motor	1	4	5	2	5	6
sensory	2	5	5	3	5	5
consciousness	2	4	5	3	5	5
pupillary	1	2	2	2	2	2
total	6	15	17	10	17	18

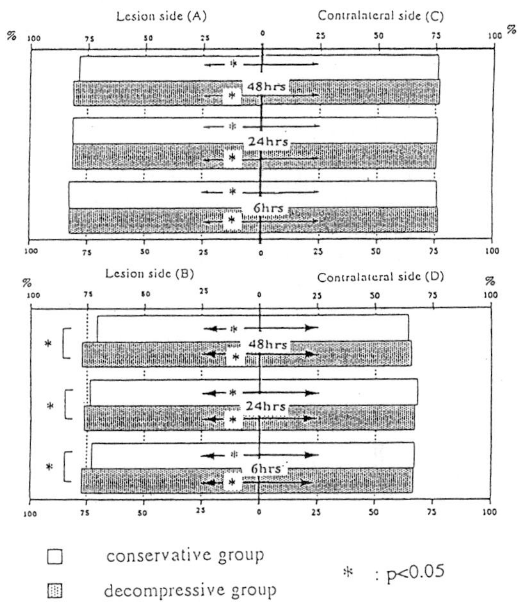

Fig. 3 Water content. upper: gray matter, lower: white matter

REFERENCES

1. Ransohoff J, Benjamin MV, Gage EL, Epstein F (1971) Hemicraniectomy in the management of acute subdural hematoma. J Neurosurg. 34:70-76
2. Cooper PR, Rovit RL, Ransohoff J (1976) Hemicraniectomy in the treatment of acute subdural hematoma : re-appraisal. Surg Neurol 5: 25-28
3. Baskin DS, Hosobuti Y, Loh HH, Lee NM (1984) Dynorphin (1-13) improves survial in cats with focal cerebral ischemia. Nature 312: 551-552

Therapeutical Efficacy of Dietary Vitamin E Supplementation or Depletion in Experimental Vasogenic Brain Edema

M. Stoffel, F. Staub, S. Berger, J. Eriskat, and A. Baethmann

Institute for Surgical Research, Klinikum Großhadern, Ludwig-Maximilians-University, Munich, Germany

SUMMARY

It has become increasingly clear that free oxygen radicals and lipid peroxidation contribute to brain damage after trauma, eventually leading to posttraumatic edema formation. Vitamin E is an important endogenous antioxidant, its administration or depletion was therefore studied in experiments as to its influence on the formation of vasogenic brain edema from a standard insult. Rats were subjected to different vitamin E supplies for 2 weeks, resulting in a decrease of the α-tocopherol level in plasma to 30% of the control value, or increase to 200% of control, respectively ($p<0.01$). For induction of brain edema a cryogenic lesion was made of the left cerebral hemisphere. The animals were sacrificed 24 h later for assessment of hemispheric brain swelling as well as of the tissue water-, Na^+- and K^+-content. Neither depletion nor enhancement of the vitamin E levels were, however, observed to have an effect on swelling of the traumatized hemisphere, or the resulting increase of the cerebral water content 24 h after trauma. Likewise, the increase in Na^+ and decrease in K^+, respectively, of the traumatized brain hemispheres were not affected either. The findings may lead to the conclusion that free radical mechanisms are of limited significance in vasogenic brain edema. It can not ruled out, however, that actual vitamin E levels in the brain, particularly in the traumatized hemisphere, remained unaffected or were only marginally changed by the various regimens.

INTRODUCTION

Free radicals and lipid peroxides may have a mediator function in secondary brain damage following trauma or ischemia [1]. These compounds have a powerful injury potential for structural components of cells and, thus, are likely to be involved in blood-brain-barrier opening, formation of brain edema, and others. Vitamin E is an integral component of cell membranes with antioxidant properties, protecting lipids against free radical induced peroxidation [2]. In the present study the effect of reduced or enhanced α-tocopherol plasma levels was studied on formation of vasogenic brain edema from a cryogenic lesion in rats subjected to dietary vitamin E administration or depletion.

MATERIALS AND METHODS

31 male Sprague-Dawley rats (298±10 g) were fed with different amounts of vitamin E for 2 weeks. 10 animals received a vitamin E-free diet (group I), 11 rats the regular daily need of 5 mg α-tocopherol per 100 g pellet food (group II), whereras another 10 animals 250 mg per 100 g pellet (group III). For the experiments the animals were anesthetized by ether followed by i. p. chloralhydrate. They were spontaneously breathing room air supplied with additional oxygen. Catheters were introduced into the tail artery for determination of blood pressure, blood gases as well as hematocrit and into the right jugular vein for infusion of 0.5 ml saline/h, respectively. Body temperature was maintained at 38.5°C. A circular trephination of the left temporal skull was prepared leaving the dura mater intact. Subsequently, a metal probe (Ø 4.5 mm) cooled to -68°C by a dry ice/acetone mixture was placed onto the exposed brain surface for 15 seconds. 24 h after the trauma the animals were sacrificed by exsanguination. The cerebrum was rapidly removed, separated in the median plane, and the fresh weight was gravimetrically determined. Hemispheric brain swelling was assessed as increase in weight of the traumatized hemisphere over that of the contralateral hemisphere. Water content of the brain specimen

was obtained by the dry/wet weight method (drying at 110°C for 24 h). Na^+- and K^+-contents of dried tissue specimen were measured by flame spectrophotometry.

RESULTS

Dietary vitamin E depletion or supplementation did not affect systemic parameters, such as pO_2, pCO_2 and pH in arterial blood as measured before and after the trauma. Moreover, no differences of the blood pressure, studied from 1 h before up to 1 h after the trauma, were found between the various groups. Vitamin E-free diet (group I) led to a decrease of the α-tocopherol level in plasma to 3.97±2.69 mg/l as compared to 12.32±2.69 mg/l in the controls with normal supply (group II, $p<0.01$). Enhancement of the vitamin E supply (group III) resulted in an increase of the plasma level to 22.89±1.45 mg/l ($p<0.01$). Neither depletion nor enhancement of the plasma level were, however, observed to have an effect on swelling of the traumatized hemisphere, amounting to 7.73±0.6% in group I, 8.41±0.5% in group II and to 8.12±0.5% in group III. Similarly, the resulting increase in cerebral water content by approximately 1% as compared to the contralateral side was neither affected. The cold lesion led also to an increase of the Na^+- and decrease of the K^+-contents of traumatized hemispheres, from uptake of plasma-like edema fluid into the parenchyma. The different vitamin E plasma levels had no effects on either of these parameters.

DISCUSSION

Brain trauma as well as cerebral ischemia are associated with generation of oxygen derived free radicals [1]. Major sources of oxygen radical formation include oxidation of xanthine, hypoxanthine and catecholamines, production by mitochondria and activated neutrophiles as well as degradation of polyunsaturated free fatty acids. Radicals in turn may lead to peroxidation of membrane lipids and accumulation of lipid peroxides by free radical attack and removal of H^+ from unsaturated fatty acids in a radical chain reaction. Free radicals and lipid peroxidation might be responsible for damage of brain parenchyma and capillary endothelium among others, impairing mechanisms that maintain homeostasis of electrolytes and water in the brain. Vitamin E is an important endogenous free radical scavenger, which is integrated into cell membranes. It is a lipid soluble agent and antagonizes lipid peroxyl radicals, thereby breaking the radical chain reaction [2].

The current study was carried out to analyze the effect of a differing vitamin E supply resulting in different plasma levels of α-tocopherol on formation of vasogenic brain edema from a focal lesion. The findings indicate absence of either adverse or protective effects of vitamin E on traumatic brain edema. This may lead to the conclusion that free radical mechanisms and their antagonization by vitamin E, respectively, are of limited significance in vasogenic brain edema. It cannot be ruled out, however, that actual vitamin E levels in the brain, particularly in the traumatized hemisphere, remained unaffected or were only marginally influenced by the various regimens, the lipid solubility of α-tocopherol notwithstanding, allowing penetration of the blood-brain barrier. Since uptake and membrane integration of α-tocopherol in the intact CNS tissue is slow, the two week diet was, although sufficient to raise or decrease plasma levels, probably too short to affect the vitamin E concentration in the brain [3]. Nevertheless, if free radical mechanisms were indeed involved in edema formation, it follows that respective effects were not inhibited by vitamin E at a level as high as 200% of normal, a concentration which had unlimited access to the injured brain through the open blood-brain barrier.

REFERENCES

1. Kontos HA, Povlishock JT (1986) Oxygen radicals in brain injury. Cent Nerv Syst Trauma 3: 257-263
2. Kagan VE, Serbinova EA, Bakalova RA, Stoytchev TS, Erin AN, Prilipko LL, Evstigneeva RP (1990) Mechanisms of stabilization of biomembranes by alpha-tocopherol. The role of the hydrocarbon chain in the inhibition of lipid peroxidation. Biochem Pharmacol 40: 2403-2413
3. Machlin LJ, Gabriel E (1982) Kinetics of tissue alpha-tocopherol uptake and depletion following administration of high levels of vitamin E. Ann NY Acad Sci 393: 48-60

Interstitial Hypertension in Human Brain Tumors: Possible Role in Peritumoral Edema Formation

EHUD ARBIT, JONGBIN LEE, and GENE DIRESTA

Neurosurgical Research Laboratory, Memorial Sloan-Kettering Cancer Center, New York, NY 10021, USA

ABSTRACT

Elevated tumor interstitial fluid pressure (TIFP) is believed to be responsible, at least in part, for the poor penetration and non-uniform distribution of blood-borne therapeutic agents into solid tumors. Measurements of TIFP and peritumoral brain edema were made in 17 patients undergoing craniotomy for tumor resection. Using the Wick-in-Needle (WIN) technique, IFP was measured in human peritumoral cortex and in the tumor's center. Extent of brain edema was estimated from T2 weighted MR images (edema index) and was correlated with TIFP. The mean IFP in cortex was 0.8 ± 0.4 mmHg; central TIFP was 7.2 ± 2.4 mmHg. TIFP was found to highly correlate with the edema index (R^2=0.89, $p < 0.05$).

The results indicate that brain tumors exhibit elevated interstitial fluid pressure and that the extent of peritumoral brain edema correlates with TIFP measured in the tumor center. A casual relationship between TIFP and extent of peritumoral edema is suggested.

INTRODUCTION

The effectiveness of therapies currently in use for solid tumors, including brain tumors, is limited by physiological resistance and by intrinsic or acquired cellular resistance. Physiological resistance implies the impedance to delivery of blood-borne drugs and stems primarily from tumor heterogeneous blood supply, elevated interstitial fluid pressure, and in brain tumors from the existence of the blood brain barrier.

Recently, research interest was focused on understanding the vascular-extravascular molecular exchange in tumors. Elevated TIFP has been observed to be a pathophysiological characteristic of tumors and represents an important barrier for drug exchange at the vascular-tissue level. Transvascular exchange of macromolecular drugs occurs primarily by convection (i.e., solute drag associated with bulk solvent movement), and depends upon a favorable pressure gradient between the intravascular and extravascular spaces. Elevated TIFP reduces the pressure gradient to a less favorable one, resulting in a decrease in drug transport into the tumor parenchyma from the capillaries. (1-4)

Increased IFP is believed to result from tumor growth within a confined space, an increase in tumor vessel permeability, and the absence of a lymphatic drainage system in tumors. A myriad of factors contributing to the extent of peritumoral cerebral edema have been identified, including tumor histology, vascularity, location, dimension, venous compression, and secretory activity of tumors.(5) A relationship between TIFP and edema is logical given that edema is the accumulation of fluid extravasated from leaky tumor capillaries to the surrounding tissue. The degree of edema fluid clearance is related to the hydrostatic gradient between the TIFP and the surrounding interstitium. The higher the TIFP the larger will be the extent of peritumoral edema.

The goals of this study were:

1. Measure IFP "in situ" in brain tumors and peritumoral brain tissue.

2. Establish the relationship between TIFP and extent of peritumoral edema (edema index)

METHODS

WIN IFP measurements were performed in 17 patients undergoing craniotomy for resection of brain tumors in compliance with an IRB approved protocol from our institution. The study included 3 meningomas, 8 metastatic tumors and 6 glioblastomas. Experimental setup is depicted below:

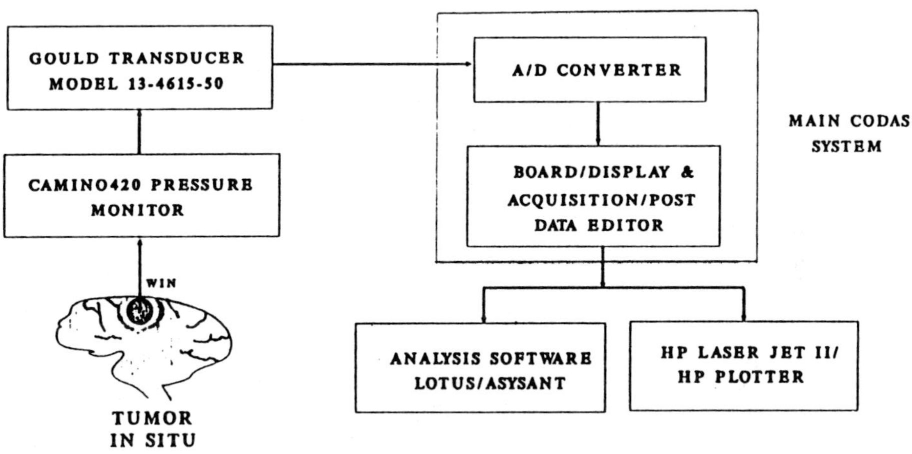

CODAS DATA ACQUISITION SYSTEM

RESULTS

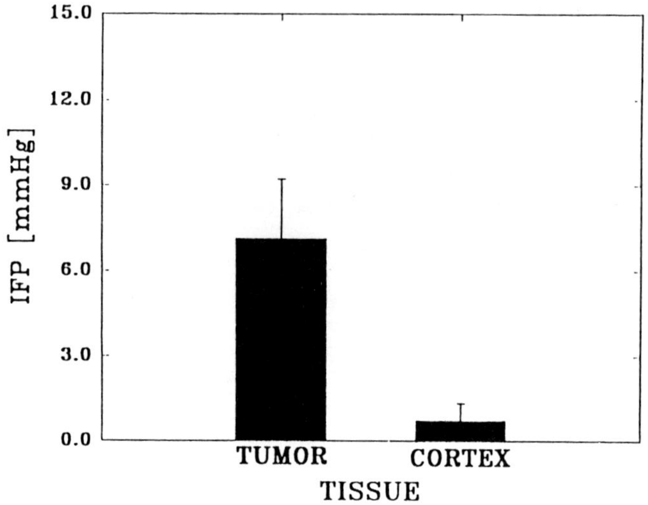

Fig. 1: Interstitial fluid pressure in tumor and cortex expressed as mean and standard deviation.

Tumor IFP: 7.2 ± 2.4 mmHg
Cortical IFP: 0.8 ± 0.4 mmHg

($p < 0.05$)

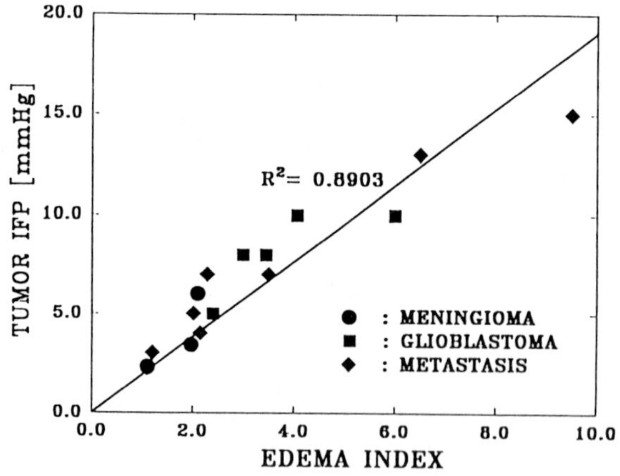

Fig. 2: Correlation between TIFP and extent of peritumoral edema estimated from the edema index ($R2=0.89$, $p<0.05$)

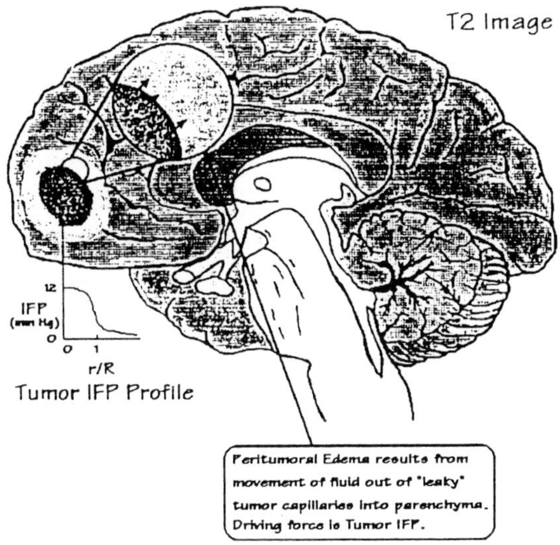

Fig. 3: Pathophysiology of IFP and its proposed role in the formation of peritumoral brain edema:

CLINICAL IMPLICATIONS & CONCLUSIONS

The delivery of blood-borne therapueutic agents to the tumor cell entails the transport of relevant molecules through the tumor microcirculation, across the microvascular wall, and through the interstitial space. Transmural and interstitial transport in tumors are passive processes, occurring predominantly by convection and diffusion. Elevated interstitial fluid pressure, well documented in experimental and several human tumors, would act as a retardant to the convective transport process. Reducing the Starling forces responsible for the extravasation of fluid from a blood vessel, reduces the movement of a solute by convection and leaves the relative slow process of diffusion as the primary transport process.

The present study demonstrates that interstitial fluid pressure in human brain tumors, both primary and metastatic, is significantly higher than that of surrounding brain tissue. Brain TIFP values were widely distributed, however, a wide variation was also observed within tumors of the same histological type. The highest TIFP was recorded in vascular tumors (e.g., metastatic thyroid cancer).

The study also demonstrates a positive correlation between TIFP and extent of peritumoral edema estimated from MR images (edema index). Essentially, fluid extravasated from leaky tumor capillaries is driven by the elevated TIFP outwardly to surrounding brain tissue along pressure gradients. Because the brain lacks a lymphatic drainage system, fluid movement is controlled by the resistance of the interstitial spaces within the parenchyma. Edema results when fluid protection overwhelms the passive drainage capability of the porous network.

The clinical implications of this study includes:

(a) the elevated TIPF observed in brain tumors, acts as a barrier to transport of therapeutic agents, and may be partly responsible for the limited efficacy of chemotherapy

(b) the correlation between TIFP and extent of peritumoral edema is important in that the extent of edema may be an indicator of the magnitude of TIFP and may potentially be useful to predict the response of a specific tumor to antineoplastic agents.

BIBLIOGRAPHY

1. Baxter LT, Jain RK: Transport and macromolecules in tumors: II. Role of heterogenous perfusion and lymphatics. Microvasc Res 40:246-263, 1990

2. Jain RK, Baxter LT: Mechanisms of heterogenous distribution of monoclonal antibodies and other macromolecules in tumors: Significance of elevated interstitial pressure. Cancer Res 48: 7022-7032, 1988

3. Boucher Y, Baxter LT, Jain RK: Interpressure gradients in tissue-isolated and subcutaneous tumors: Implications for therapy. Cancer Res 50:4478-4484, 1990

4. DiResta GR, Lee J, Larson SM, Arbit E: Characterization of neuroblastoma xenograft in flank. I. Growth, interstitial fluid pressure, and interstitial fluid velocity distribution profiles. Macrovasc Res 46:158-177, 1993

5. Inamura T, Nishio S, Takeshita I, Fujiwara S: Peritumoral brain edema in meningiomas - influence of vascular supply on its development. Neurosurgery 31:170-185, 1992

Poster X: Effects of Increased ICP

Chairman: J.T. Hoff

ICP and rCBF After Periacqueduct Gray Matter Stimulation

P.A. Oppido[1], G. Di Giugno[2], G.L. Mattioli[1], E. Sciacca[3], and G. Rosa[2]

[1] Neurosurgery I, Department of Neurological Sciences, [2] Anesthesiology and Intensive Care Institute, [3] General Surgery I Institute, University of Rome "La Sapienza", Rome, Italy

INTRODUCTION

In the last few years some authors [1,2,3,4,5] have been referred that the stimulation of cingulate gyrus,or of the hypothalamus, or of the brain stem make changes in heart rate (HR),blood pressure (BP) and intracranial pressure (ICP) and cerebral blood flow (CBF). These experimental studies have indirectly showed that these hemodynamic changes can be due to a change in cerebral blood volume (CBV) induced by the stimulation [6]. Probably the stimulation of these central areas is involved to mediate the sympathetic activity that modifies the cerebral vessels diameter by A-adrenergic receptors [4]. This neurogenic mechanism works together with the myogenic and metabolic mechanism, better known, to control cerebral hemodynamic [5]. This experimental work was carried out to identify a neurogenic central area in the periacqueduct central gray matter (CGM) [1] that induces changes in ICP,BP,HR and central venous pressure (CVP) rCBF and rCBV in the rabbit.

MATERIALS AND METHODS

Experiments were performed in 25 rabbits,New Zeland,weighing 2.5-3 kg, all anesthetized by ether only for tracheostomy. Once intubated the rabbits were placed on a mechanical ventilator. Intravenous pancuronium bromide (0.1 mg/kg) was used for muscle relaxation and reliable respiratory control. Serial blood samples were obtained for monitoring PaO2, PaCO2, pH and bicarbonate arterial levels,constantly maintained in normal steady state range. Body temperature was maintained at 37 ($\pm$3)°C by a heating pad. Once the rabbit was placed in a stereotactic head holder, a soclet was fixed to the skull,to guide the introduction of electrodes through a cranial window to reach the CGM area according to the coordinates of the atlas of Gangloff and Monnier [7]. Electrical stimulation was applied by giving a train of electrical pulses (duration 1 msec;frequency 100 Hz;intensity 50-200 mA) to a couple of electrodes, spaced themselves 1 mm and insulated except for the tip,that protruded about 1 mm, inserted into the CGM. The electroencephalogram (EEG) was recorded from biparietal electrodes screwed into the skull and referenced to the frontal midline. Electrocardiogram (EKG) was recorded. Intracerebral ICP ,BP from femoral artery, CVP from subclavian vein were continuously recorded by 4F Camino fiber optic transducers. In 5 rabbits rCBF,rCBV and flow velocity (V) per 100 mmc of tissue was monitored by Laser Flou TSI transducer inserted in the right cerebral hemisphere [8].

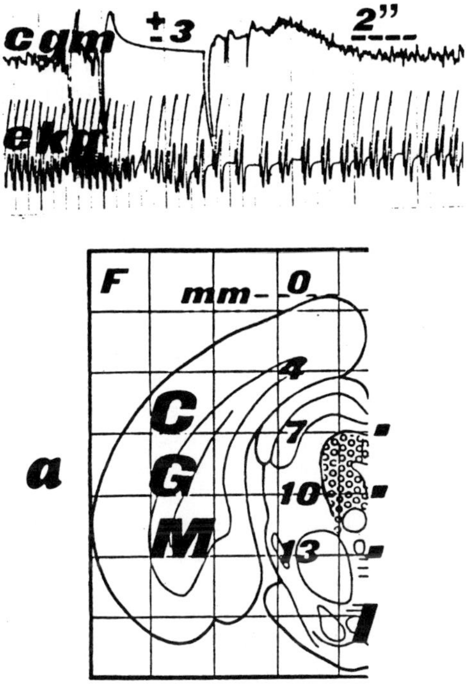

Fig. 1 – After stimulation : CGM electrical activity; EKG decrease in HR.
a : site of stimulation on plane F in atlas of Gangloff and Monnier

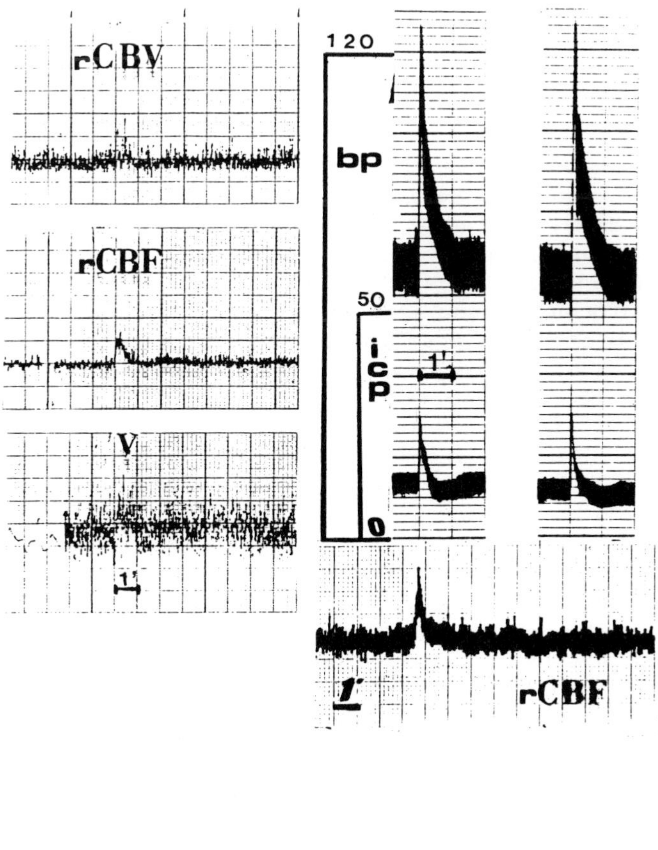

Fig. 2 – After stimulation BP, ICP and rCBF traces are very similar in amplitude and duration.

RESULTS AND DISCUSSION

Electrical stimulation was applied to the CGM,on plane F at a depth of 7-13 mm below the surface of the skull,about 3 mm from the midline [7] (fig. 1a). In each animal stimulation induced a quick rise in BP,CVP,ICP and a fall in HR. The rCBF grew up simultaneously with BP and ICP,too (fig 2). In the same animal BP,ICP and rCBF traces were quite similar in amplitude and their strength was stimulus dependent. These changes followed quickly the CGM stimulation then there was a progressive basal return of rCBF,BP,CVP,ICP and HR. By using the same stimulus the maximum response was obtained applied at depth of 10 mm. Outside this area stimulus was ineffective or required much higher intensity. The rise in rCBV was lower and about 10 sec. later than rCBF and the V did not significantly change (fig.2). Frequency of the EEG and electrical activity in the CGM were altered (fig. 1). Our animals were mechanically ventilated and arterial blood gasses,pH and bicarbonate were maintained within normal range. Thus PaO2,PaCO2 and other metabolic factors did not contribute to modify cerebral hemodynamic during CGM stimulation. Furthermore,CO2 or other vasoactive metabolites require at least 1 sec. to dilate cerebral vessels.Other authors demonstrated [6] that BP is not responsible of changes in ICP and CBF after brain stem stimulation. Thus we interpret the quick rise in ICP and rCBF as evidence of cerebral vasodilatation. Either the stimulation of a cerebral vasodilator area into the CGM could account for the exaggerated rise in rCBF and ICP or a temporary loss of autoregulation could modify ICP and rCBF in response to BP increase. Any way,our data demonstrate a possible role of the CGM in a neurogenic control of cerebral hemodynamic.

REFERENCES

1 - Hanse EL,Pansky B. (1960) Anatomy of brain. In: A functional approach to neuroanatomy,Springer Verlag ,New York,.

2 - Hayashi M,Ishii H,Handa Y,Kobayashi H.(1987) Role of the medulla oblongata in plateau-wave development in dogs. J.Neurosurg 67: 97-101.

3 - Maeda M,Matsuura S,Tanaka K,Nishimura S. (1988) Effects of electrical stimulation on intracranial pressure and systemic arterial blood pressure in cats.Part I: stimulation of brain stem".Neurol Res 10:87-92 .

4- Rosendorf C.,Mitchell G,Scriven DR,Shapiro C. (1976) Evidence for a dual innervation affecting local blood flow in the hypothalamus of the conscious rabbit. Circ. Res. 38 (3):140-145 .

5- Youmans J.R,Chehrazi B.B. (1990) Cerebral blood flow in clinical neurosurgery. In: Neurological Surgery,Youmans,W.B. Saunders ed., Philadelpia, vol. II:697-706,.

6- Maeda M.(1988) Changes in intracranial pressure elicited by electrical stimulation of the brain stem reticular formation in spinal cats with vagotomy. J Auton. Nerv S 25:155-164

7- M. Monnier,H. Gangloff (1961) Atlas for stereotaxic brain research on the conscious rabbit brain research I Elsevier Publ. Company Amsterdam:76

8 - Eyre JA,Essex TJH,Flecknell PA,Sinclair JI. (1988) A comparison of measurement of CBF in the rabbit using laser Doppler spectroscopy and radionuclide labelled microspheres. Clin. Phys. Physiol.Meas. 9: 65-74.

Experimental Papilledema in Cats

KATSUJI SHIMA and HIROO CHIGASAKI

Department of Neurosurgery, National Defense Medical College, Tokorozawa, Saitama, 359 Japan

SUMMARY

A reliable model for producing papilledema in experimental animals is described. Papilledema in increased intracranial pressure (ICP) was produced in cats by kaolin-induced hydrocephalus. Papilledema was found in 76% between the third and sixth days after kaolin injection. The histological changes showed that the axonal swelling and interstitial edema were limited in the prelaminar region. These changes were more marked at the late stage. Abnormal visual evoked potentials were not found even in the chronic stage. Possible mechanisms of papilledema secondary to increased ICP are discused.

INTRODUCTION

Optic dic edema, so-called papilledema, is an important sign of increased intracranial pressure (ICP). Little is known, however, about the mechanism responsible for the development of papilledema following increased ICP. Although many attempts to produce papilledema in animals have been made to clarify the pathogenesis, these studies have been based on the inadequate methods as follows: inflation of subdural balloon [1], block of aqueduct [2], cyclocryotherapy [3] or X-irradiation [4]. Objective of the present study is to find a reliable method of producing papilledema associated with increased ICP in animals.

METHODS

Twenty-one adult cats, weighing 2-4 kg, were anesthetized with ketamine (20 mg/kg). To obtain papilledema in increased ICP, experimental hydrocephalus was induced by injection of a sterile kaolin suspension into the cisterna magna. The neurological status of the animal was evaluated and the optic fundi were photographed with a fundus camera. The ICP from the lateral ventricle was measured before the experiments. The animals were sacrificed at the acute stage between 5 and 8 days or at the chronic stage more than 3 weeks after kaolin injection. The eyes were enucleated and fixed. The tissues were processed for light microscopy (stains of Klüver-Barrera and Bodian) and electron microscopy. Functional changes in the visual system were evaluated by the visual evoked potentials (VEP).

RESULTS

Of the 21 animals, bilateral optic disc developed moderate but definite papilledema in 14% within 3 days after kaolin injection, in 52% within 4 days, and in 76% within 6 days. The mean ICP rose to 15.4 ± 9.3 mmHg (mean ± SD) between the sixth and eighth days after injection. It was 8.2 ± 2.8 mmHg on the 12th day and gradually returned to the normal baseline presure after 3 weeks. On day 6 following the injection, light microscopic studies showed marked elevation of the optic disc and vacuolated axons in the prelaminar region (Fig. 1A). These changes were more prominent in the chronic stage. Electron microscopic studies showed the swollen axons containing scattered large mitochondria, disrupted neurotubules and hydropic degeneration in the anterior part of the prelaminar region (Fig. 1B). The enlarged interstitial space of various sizes were observed between axons in the posterior part of the prelaminar region. Most of the nerve fibers in the retrolaminar region were unremarkable. Changes in the early components of the VEP were not observed even at the chronic stage.

A B

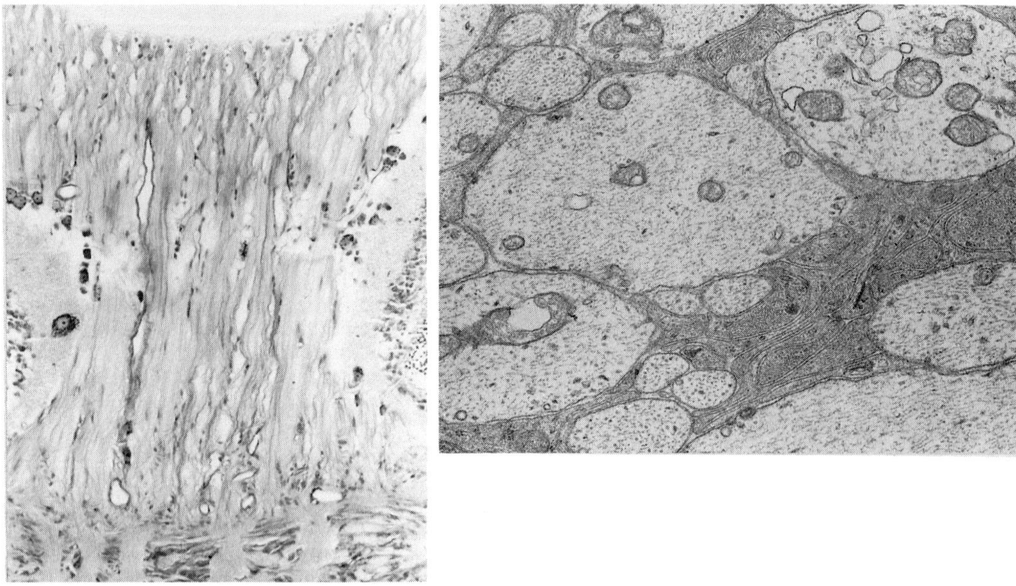

Fig. 1 Papilledema. A Longitudinal section of optic nerve head. × 100 B Electron micrograph showing swollen axons in the prelaminar region. × 20000

DISCUSSION

In the present study, definite papilledema appeared in 76% of eyes when the resting ICP was around 15 mmHg. These findings confirm previous observations that the increased ICP around 15 mmHg was necessary for the development of papilledema [5]. Microscopic findings demonstrated significant axonal swelling and interstitial edema, but no glial swelling. In adition, edematous changes were mostly limited to the prelaminar region. Microscopic tracer studies[1] have shown that the primary cause of axonal swelling is the disturbance of axoplasmic transport in the prelaminar region. Our results support the hypothesis that papilledema in increased ICP is attributed to optic disc swelling [1].

REFERENCES

1. Hayreh SS (1977) Optic disc edema in raised intracranial pressure: V. Pathogenesis. Arch Ophthalmol 95: 1553-1565

2. Kornder LH (1919) Hydrocephalus and choked disc in dogs. Arch Int Med 23: 197-219

3. Minckler DS, Tso MOM (1976) Experimental papilledema produced by cyclotherapy. Am J Ophthalmol 82: 577-589

4. Caveness WF, Tanaka A, Hess KH (1974) Delayed brain swelling and functional derangement after X-irradiation of the right visual cortex in the Macaca mulatta. Radiat Res 57: 104-120

5. Schutta HS, Hedges TR (1971) Fine structure observations on experimental papilledema in the rhesus monkey. J Neurol Sci 12: 1-14

An Experimental Study on Changes in Doppler Flow Pattern and Flow Volume Under Conditions of Intracranial Hypertension

H. NAGAI, K. MORITAKE, M. TAKAYA, and N. MARUYAMA

Department of Neurosurgery, Shimane Medical University, 89-1 Enya-cho, Izumo, 693 Japan

SUMMARY

The effects of increased intracranial pressure on Doppler ultrasonographic findings were studied using an experimental in vitro model. With after-load increases in this model, we obtained four different stages of characteristic flow patterns in the following order : sharp wave, systolic flow, to-and-fro, and spiky flow. This paper describes an in vitro model that approximates cerebral pulsatile flow and illustrates the application of this model to the study of changes that occur in Doppler spectral waveforms in intracranial hypertension.

INTRODUCTION

Transcranial Doppler ultrasonography (TCD) provides useful information on cerebral hemodynamics associated with intracranial hypertension, including brain death [1][2]. However, the interpretation of changes in velocity or waveform is not straightforward, and flow volume cannot be quantitatively measured. Therefore, Doppler ultrasonic recordings were made in an experiment using an in vitro model of intracranial hypertension to investigate the relationship between perfusion pressure, flow volume and TCD pulsatility.

MATERIALS AND METHODS

The in vitro model is illustrated in Fig.1. The tube diameter, flow rate, velocity waveform shape, and Doppler frequency spectrum are nearly identical to those observed in the human middle cerebral artery (MCA). A model of the MCA trunk was constructed from straight silastic tubing (o.d.=4.0 mm, i.d.=2.5 mm, length=120 mm). This MCA trunk was connected to a collapsible tube made from a 0.2 mm latex sheet. Systemic pressure was constituted from gravitational flow (fluid falling from an overhead reservoir into the straight segment) and pulsatile flow, which was generated at a rate of 60 or 40 cycles/min by reciprocal pump. The fluid was made by adding 3 gm of cornstarch to 1 liter of water, as reported by Giller [3]. A 2MHz Doppler probe was mounted at an angle of 45 degrees to the axis of the silastic tube. Several stages of increased intracranial pressure (ICP) were simulated by pressure-loading into a cranium model containing the artificial MCA trunk and a capacitance vessel. In this model, perfusion pressure was calculated by subtracting the pressure in the cranium model (ICP) from extracranial systemic pressure (BP). We investigated the relationship between Doppler wave form and perfusion pressure, after parameters, serial changes in flow velocity(FV), pulsatility index (P.I.), wave form, BP, and ICP, and the influence of the cardiac cycle according to these parameters.

RESULTS

1) Flow patterns: In this model, we observed five different stages of characteristic flow patterns with increases in intracranial pressure (ICP), which appeared in the following order: sharp wave (SW) , systolic flow (SF) , to-and-fro (TOF) , spiky flow (SP) , and no flow (NO).
2) Flow velocity and pulsatility index: Progression of the flow patterns resulted in the reduction of flow velocity. The value of PI increased markedly when TOF was reached.
3) Perfusion pressure: There was a significant correlation between flow patterns and perfusion pressure. At a pulse rate of 60 Hz, the mean perfusion pressure of the TOF pattern was near zero, and at a pulse rate

40 Hz that of the SP pattern was zero.
4) Flow volume: Under normal conditions, flow volume at 60Hz was 222 ml/min and flow volume at 40 Hz was 117 ml/min. Flow volume at 40Hz as well as at 60 Hz was observred to decrease as the flow patterns progressed and was little influenced by pulse rate.

DISCUSSION

We previously reported an intracranial hypertension model [4], but in that model centrifugal zero flow was seen instead of a no-flow pattern. We introduced a collapsible tube in our present model to express the obstruction of distal outflow and obtained a no flow pattern. TCD flow patterns correlate with flow volume. The percent reduction in flow volume was over 90 % for the TOF, SP, and NO patterns. In general, normal cerebral blood flow (CBF) in humans is about 50 ml/100gm of brain/min. The ischemic threshold of CBF in cell membrane failure is approximately 10 ml/100gm of brain/min, corresponding to a reduction of 80 %. Our resultsIt suggest that the stages of TOF, SP, and NO represent ineffective CBF. To analyze the bradycardia observed in brain death, two different pulse rates (40 or 60 Hz) were compared with respect to effects on flow velocity, perfusion pressure, flow patterns, and flow volume. Differences in the correlation between flow velocity and perfusion pressure are minor between these two pulse rates. Irrespective of pulse rate, the TOF stage is associated with a CBF reduction over 90 %. Cardiac cycles may not influence flow volume in TOF, SP, and NO, but may influence mean perfusion pressure (40 Hz is SP, 60Hz is TOF). The results obtained using this simple in vitro model, which consists of only an elastic tube, are not necessarily applicable to clinical situations where more complicated factors must be considered. However, despite these simplifications, the model can improve understanding of the relationship between recorded Doppler signals and intracranial hemodynamic changes. We believed that TCD study can be used to clearly diagnose the absence of cerebral circulation in brain death.

REFERENCES

1. Aaslid R (1986) Estimation of cerebral perfusion pressure from arterial blood pressure and transcranial Doppler recordings. In: Miller JD (eds) Intracranial Pressure VI. pp 226–229
2. Hassler W, Steinmetz H, Pirschel J (1989) Transcranial Doppler study of intracranial circulatory arrest. J Neurosurg 71: 195-201
3. Giller CA, Hodges K, Batjer H (1990) Transcranial Doppler pulsatility in vasodilation and stenosis. J Neurosurg 72: 901-906
4. Takaya M, Moritake K, Fukuma A, Nagai H (1992) An experimental study on the transcranial Doppler ultrasonography in raised intracranial pressure. In: M.Oka (eds) Recent Advances in Neurosonology. Elsevier Science Publishers BV, Hiroshima, Japan, pp 233-237

Fig.1: Illustration of an in vitro model of pulsatile flow in intracranial hypertension.

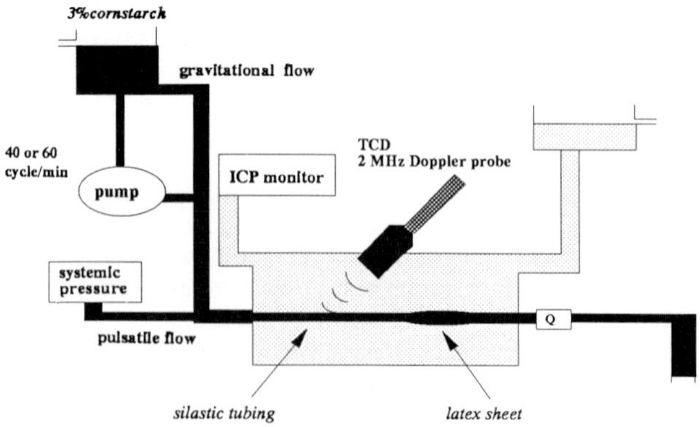

Radionuclide Diagnosis of Cerebrospinal Fluid Abnormalities in Unknown Ethiology Hypertensive Syndrome

E.Ya. Scherbakova, S.S. Gasparyan, V.S. Snigirev, S.V. Kulakova, and E.P. Yurischev

Burdenko Neurosurgical Institute, 5 Fadeeva St., Moscow, 125047, Russia

SUMMARY

Radionuclide cisterno-myelography (RCMG), single photon emission computer tomography (SPECT) and radiometry of tampons (from nose, oral cavity and ears) with 99m-Tc-DTPA were performed in 108 patients with nontumor hypertensive syndrome (benign intracranial hypertension). RCMG and SPECT revealed two variants of radiological picture with "block" of cerebrospinal fluid (CSF) circulation at the level of the cisterna magna, the quadrigeminal plate cistern, or the interpeduncular cistern. In all cases the "block" of the lateral (sylvian) cisterns was found. In our patients disturbed circulation of CSF was always attended by its impaired resorption. Compensatory additional CSF outflow was presented in a form of nasal liquorrhea.

INTRODUCTION

In pathological picture of nontumor genesis hypertensive syndrome the permanent items are cranial and spinal subarachnoid pathways affections. Radionuclide studies (radionuclide cisterno-myelography and single photon emission computer tomography) allows to reveal morphological and liquorodynamic abnormalities. Radiometry of tampons is performed for assessment of degree of basal liquorrhea, which consider as additional compensatory flow of CSF outside the liquor pathways.

MATERIALS AND METHODS

108 patients (90 women and 18 men, age 36-55 years) with benign intracranial hypertension were included in the study. In their life history were notes about brain injury in childhood, sinusitis, about arterial hypertension or renal diseases. Hypertension syndrome in our patients consisted of papilloedema, decpeased visual function, neurological deficits with symptoms of postcranial fossa. The median duration of intracranial hypertension was 3 years (range: 1-5 years). On craniograms were signs of increased intracranial pressure. But cranial computerized tomography and magnetic resonance imaging not revealed a tumorous process.
RCMG followed by the intrathecal injection through a lumbar puncture of 200 MBk of 99m-Tc-DTPA in a volume of 1-2 ml. Multiply views with the planar scintillation camera were obtained at 10 min.-1-3-6 hr. after injection of radiopharmaceutical. To reveal pathology of spinal subarachnoid pathways 3 views were performed and 5 standart views were carry out for study cranial pathways. Tomoscintigrams were performed at 3 hr. using the multidetector SPECT. These studies combined with radiometry of tampons from nose, oral cavity and ears.

RESULTS AND DISCUSSION

Spatial-timely distribution of radiopharmaceutical throughout subarachnoid spaces formed the basis for the formation of radionuclide picture characterizing morphological and liqurodynamic disturbances: presence of lateral and central CSF flow; reabsorption alterations in a form of the accelerated resorption; additional CSF outflow exceeding the bounds of subarachnoid pathways in a form of basal liquorrhea; CSF outflow into the subdural space. RCMG analysis in 108 patients with benign hypertensive syndrome revealed two variants of the radiological picture. The first variant (36 patients) showed the safety of CSF circulation in posterior fossa cisterns, basal cisterns and primary sections of lateral cisterns: besides, the central CSF flow was revealed (from the cisterna magna to the quadrigeminal plate cistern); "obstruction" of subarachnoid space in parasagittal and medial regions was also revealed. There were no abnormalities of spinal CSF pathways but the terminal cistern was enlarged. Circulation disturbances were combined with CSF reabsorption abnormalities - 2/3 of patients showed the accelerated resorption. Together with this presence of compensatory latent nasal liquorrhea was observed. The data obtained showed the parasagittal, convexital and medial CSF pathways lesions the compensatory reactions in a form of central CSF flow, basal liquorrhea in combination with the accelerated resorption were revealed. The second variant of the radiological picture (72 patients) differed from the first one in the following way: radiopharmaceutical was visualized only in the spinal subarachnoid space and in the cisterna pontis. Such CSF circulation alterations only in 1/3 of patients were combined with the accelerated CSF resorption and only in isolated instances the compensatory latent nasal liquorrhea was revealed. This variant of the radiological picture differed from the first one by compensatory reactions decrease in more prominent liquorodynamical disturbances.

REFERENCES

1. Nikolskaya OE, Shcherbakova EYA, Lyass FM (1981) Results of liquoroscintigraphy for the definition of liquorodynamic disturbances. J Med Radiol (in russian) 11:29-37.

2. Shcherbakova EYa, Rakier AYa, Kotelnikova TM, Soboleva OI (1985) Diagnosis of the hypertensive syndrome of unclear genesis. J Vopr Neurosurgery (in russian) 5:25-30.

The Relationship Between the Sagittal Sinus and Intraventricular Pressures of the Dog During Acute Intraventricular Infusion

A.Y. RAZUMOVSKY, G.S.F. LING, M.A. WILLIAMS, M.S. SCHNITZER, and D.F. HANLEY

Department of Neurology, Johns Hopkins Medical Institutions, 600 N. Wolfe Street, Baltimore, MD, USA

The relationship between cerebrospinal fluid (CSF) pressure (P_{csf}) and superior sagittal sinus pressure (SSSP) has been interpreted variously by different authors. Some authors think that P_{csf} variations do not influence SSSP, while others have shown that SSSP was elevated when P_{csf} was increased [1, 2]. Therefore, we investigated the response of SSSP to acute ventricular infusion of artificial CSF.

EXPERIMENTAL MATERIALS AND METHODS

Investigations were performed on 13 beagle dogs weighing from 8-11 kg, anesthetized with pentobarbital (35 mg/kg i.v.), and artificially ventilated. Pressure in the lateral ventricle (IVP) was measured via a silicon polymer catheter and SSSP was measured via a polyethylene catheter connected to strain gauge transducers levelled at the same reference point. Mean arterial blood pressure (MABP), end-tidal CO2, arterial and sagittal sinus blood gases, brain temperature were measured.The animal was placed in the sphinx position with the head in a holder. After surgery, a 45-60 minute period was allowed for the pressures to stabilize before obtaining baseline pressure measurements. IVP was then elevated from resting pressure to 95 mm Hg in 10 mm Hg increments lasting at least 10 minutes by opening a reservoir of artificial CSF into the ventricular system via a 3-way stop-cock. IVP and SSSP were recorded for 10 minutes at each increment. At the conclusion of the experiment the dogs were killed with i.v. injection of saturated KCl solution. Simultaneous datapoints for IVP and SSSP at each IVP level was compared by analysis of variance. The level of significance was set at $p \leq 0.05$.

RESULTS

Baseline IVP ($\pm$SD) and SSSP were equal 15.7 $\pm$ 7.5 mm Hg and 7.7 $\pm$ 4.6 mm Hg, respectively. During step-wise elevations of IVP the response of SSSP was similar in all 13 animals. The value of SSSP was almost the same as that of opening SSSP and there was no change of SSSP associated with an increase of IVP up to 95 mm Hg (Fig 1). The SSSP was stable regardless of initial value and there were no correlations between IVP and MABP, as well as between MABP and SSSP.

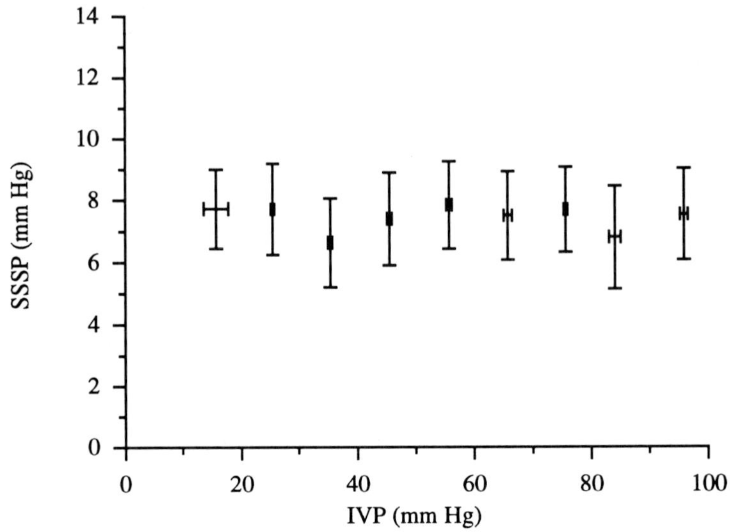

Fig. 1. The SSSP does not change during step-wise IVP increasing.

DISCUSSION

This study demonstrates that the SSS behaves as an isolated vascular compartment within the cranial vault in our model of acute intracranial hypertension. SSSP does not appear to be regulated by the IVP. The SSS is probably not compressed by acute intraventricular hypertension but we did not examine the SSS configuration and it is quite possible that the SSS may change shape under extremely high IVP. Perhaps, the degree and duration of intracranial hypertension determines whether a sinus will collapse. Also, our data suggest that measurement of SSSP as a substitute for ICP in experimental models of brain injury is inappropriate and could seriously overestimate the calculation of CPP.

REFERENCES

1. Martins AN, Kobrine AI, Larsen DF (1974) Pressure in the sagittal sinus during intracranial hypertension in man. J Neurosurg 40: 603-608
2. McCormic JM, Yamada K, Rekate HL, Miyake H. (1992) Time Course of Intraventricular Pressure Change in a canine Model of Hydrocephalus: Its Relationship to Sagittal Sinus Elastance. Pediatr Neurosurg 18:127-133

Supported in part by NS 27795-03 and the Brain Trauma Foundation Fellowship in Neurotrauma and Critical Care.

A Delineator of Neuropsychological Deficits in Following Successfully ICP Managed Severe Closed Head Injuries

C.P. McGraw[1], D. Carden[2], B.M. Baker[2], and A.H. Reese[3]

[1] Department of Neurosurgery, School of Medicine University of Louisville, Louisville Kentucky, USA
[2] Department of Surgery, Division of Speech Pathology, School of Medicine University of Louisville, Louisville Kentucky, USA
[3] Department of Pediatrics, School of Medicine University of Louisville, Louisville Kentucky, USA

INTRODUCTION

The aim of this study was to delineate the long term language and cognitive deficits of severe closed head injured patients one year post incident. The Stroop Color Test is a delineator of a subject's inability to filter two competitive stimuli (words and colors) and to inhibit one, while responding to the other(1). The difficulty of the task involves inhibition of a highly over learned response that would be expected to be produced more quickly and easily.

MATERIALS AND METHODS

These findings were correlated with ICP management during the first 5 days following injury. The methods involved testing 14 patients (mean age 25 years) who had sustained a severe closed head injury. These patients had a Glasgow Coma Score of 8 or below during their initial hospitalization and a mean length of coma of 7 weeks (range 1-32 weeks) and posttraumatic amnesia mean of 11.5 weeks (range 3-32 weeks). The highest ICP's recorded from these subjects averaged 36.3 mmHg (range 19-55 mmHg). These patients had a Glasgow Recovery Score of 4 indicating independence for activities of daily living or 5 indicating resumption of normal life, though with minor neurologic deficits.

Test One Year Post Incident

One year post injury these patients and 9 controls were tested with a modification of the Stroop Color Test (2) which consisted of recording subjects' response times and errors over four consecutive trials. The initial steps required subjects to read the names of colors printed in black ink, recognize colors, and read the names of colors printed in a competing color of ink. The final condition required the subject to ignore the printed word and name the color of ink in which the word was written. This last condition was repeated four times to obtain a total response time and a number of errors for the four trials. These subjects were also evaluated with regard to: audiometrics, language function, learning aptitude, psycho-linguistic ability, aphasia, and the Raven Matrix. An analysis of variance was performed to test the differences between groups.

RESULTS

The Stroop Color Test was the one measure that provided data indicating that a residual cognitive deficit was present one year post incident. The experimental group's performance on the Color Test was different than that of the comparison group in terms of errors made ($p<0.03$), and response time ($p<0.03$). The mean number of total errors for the experimental group was 4.5 (range 0-9) while for the comparison group it was 0.22 (range 0-1). The mean total response time for the experimental group was 100 seconds (range 64-130) while for the normals it was 61 seconds (range 51-72). Mean times did not decrease or increase with repeated trials. A repeated measures analysis of variance indicated a significant difference among the mean error scores across trials for the 14 patients ($p<0.05$). A multiple comparison test found a significant difference between the mean for Trial 1 and Trial 3 & 4, respectively ($p<0.05$).

DISCUSSION

This is a way to measure cognitive deficits one year post incident on subjects who have sustained a severe closed head injury which subsequently requires management based on ICP monitoring. Our experimental patients performed in a manner similar to the controls, without respect to the timed measures, on the other test instruments listed. This may be due to these patients being managed better with respect to treatment based on ICP monitoring(3). This modified version of the Stroop Color Test was the test that elicited the most significant and clinically demonstrable differences between the two groups. While these patients showed skill learning through decreased errors with repetition of trials, the decrease in errors never approached the performance of the control group, nor were these patients able to decrease, in any way, the large difference in time. Thus this test demonstrates the failure of the experimental group to exhibit skill learning with repetition of trials. This test appears to characterize a residual cognizant deficit exhibited by severe closed head injured patients who have been successfully managed with respect to their ICP. They appear to show diminished ability to focus their attention from moment to moment, to inhibit highly automatized response and to respond in a new and flexible manner when presented with competing stimuli. These deficits may surface in complex vocational settings. Therefore, this test may be useful in planning of rehabilitative strategies and determining the timing of interventions.

REFERENCES

1) Stroop JR (1935) Studies of interference in serial verbal reactions. J.Exp.Psy. 18:643-662
2) Reese AH (1990) Reese Adaptation of the Stroop Color Test. Copyright.
3) McGraw CP, Howard G, O'Connor C (1983) Outcome Associated With Management Based on ICP Monitoring. In: Ishii S, Chigasaki H, Handa H, Makino H, Nagai H, Sano K, Yamamoto S, Brock M (eds): Intracranial Pressure V. New York, Springer-Verlag, pp 558-559.

Clinical Features of Benign Intracranial Hypertension

S.S. GASPARIAN, S.V. TANYASHIN, N.A. VLADIMIROVA, and A.A. TUMANOVA

Burdenko Neurosurgical Institute, Moscow, Russia

SUMMARY

95 patients with the syndrome of BIH were examined by standard neurological method with special attention to etiological factors, quantitative papillometric method, carotid or MRI angiography data, CT, lumbar punction for estimation CSF pressure. The analysis of etiological factors, clinical features, CT, CSF pressure was performed as well as correlative analysis between them. As a result of investigation we found more often appearance of the BIH syndrome in patients with hormonal and postinfection disorders. The most significant failure of visual function and severe PO were found after 3 years of papilloedema duration. Patients with disorders of venous outflow circulation had more severe and fast decrease of visual function. We found raised Pcsf in range of 17-49,5 mm Hg, correlations between Pcsf, PO and POD, PO and VF, no correlations with CT data.

INTRODUCTION

The syndrome of BIH or pseudotumor cerebri is very polyetiological state, which leads to important deficits in visual function up to blindness. This syndrome is manifested by papilloedema, raised CSF pressure with normal or low range of protein concentration in CSF without marked neurological deficits and normal ventricular size on CT [1,2].

The aim of current study was to define specific features of evolution of BIH and to analies etiological factors to clear up the possible correlations between etiology, clinical features, level of CSF pressure and CT data.

Abbreviations. BIH-benign intracranial pressure; Pcsf-csf pressure; PO-papilloedema; POD-papilloedema duration; VF-visual function; VI-ventricular bicaudate index; PVO-periventricular oedema.

MATERIAL AND METHODS

The study was carried out in 95 patients with the syndrome of BIH (17 men and 78 women, aged 16-66 years).
All patients were examined by standard neurological method, qantitative papillometric method, CT, carotid or MRI angiography, lumbar punction in order to determine the degree of PO, POD and VF; VI; PVO; Pcsf. Correlation analysis between these characteristics was performed.

RESULTS AND DISCUSSION

The main clinical signs of the syndrome of BIH in our patients were papilloedema , raised CSF pressure low or normal protein concentration in CSF, absence of marked neurological deficits, except paralysis of n.abducens in 38 cases. The etiological factors were different. More frequently BIH manifestated after viral and tuberculosis infection (58%), hormonal endocrinological disorders(29%), head injury (10%) and was rare after chronic intoxications (2%) and neck surgery (1%). Only 4 patients with thrombosis of sagittal sinus and 3 patients with arteriosinus fistula showed more severe and fast decrease of visual function in period of 1-3 weeks up to blindness. Mild decrease of VF was found in 22 cases. The severe PO was determined in 60 patients , moderate PO -32 patients and PO of low degree was in 3 cases. The most significant impairment of VF was found after 3 years of POD (in one case to 13 years). CT was carried out in all patients. Narrow ventricles (bicaudate index 12,2+1,3%) were found in 33% of cases and half of them had severe intracranial hypertension and collapsed basal cysterns. Periventricular oedema manifested in 52% of cases; 77% of patients had normal ventriular size."Empty sella" syndrome was found in 23 women, 17 of them had endocrinological dysfunctions.
P csf was significantly increased in 81 patients: 17-49,5 mm Hg. In 13 patients Pcsf was more than 30 mm Hg. In 75% of cases Pcsf was 18-30 mmHg. We found correlations between Pcsf and PO ($r=0,4$, $p<0,01$); P csf and POD ($r=0,3$, $p<0,02$); VF and PO ($r=0,2$, $p<0,05$); no correlations with CT data.
The obtained results will be useful for future analysis of clinical findings in complex with parameters of CSF dynamics to define compensative capacity of cerebrospinal system, that will allow to improve treatment of patients with the syndrome of BIH.

REFERENCES

1.Jonston I.,Paterson A.,Besser M.(1981) The treatment of benign intracranial hypertension: a review of 134 cases. Surg.Neurol.16, 218-224.
2.Rousseux P.,Vieillart A.,Scherpereel B.,Bernard M.H.,Motte J.,Guyot J.F.(1985) Hypertension intracranienne benigne et thromboses veineuses cerebrales.Neurochirurgie,1985,31,381-389.

Poster XI: Imaging and Others

Chairman: K. Uemura

Computerised Transient Hyperaemic Response Test—A Method for the Assessment of Cerebral Autoregulation and Its Relationship to Outcome

P. Smielewski[1], M. Czosnyka[1], V. Iyer[1], S. Piechnik[2], H. Whitehouse[1], P. Kirkpatrick[1], and J.D. Pickard[1]

[1] MRC Cambridge Centre for Brain Repair and Academic Neurosurgical Unit, Addenbrooke's Hospital, P.O. Box 167, Cambridge CB2 2QQ, UK
[2] Institute of Electronics Fundamentals, Warsaw University of Technology, Poland

INTRODUCTION

Testing of cerebral autoregulation by examining the hyperaemic response following brief carotid compression was first described by Giller [1] and then theoretically analysed by Czosnyka *et al* [2]. Reduction in cerebral perfusion pressure **(CPP)** during carotid artery compression should cause autoregulation-induced vasodilatation of the cerebral resistive vessels. Therefore, after release of the compression the transient increase in cerebral blood flow is seen (fig. 1a). With impaired autoregulation the flow passively comes back to the level recorded before compression without any hyperaemic episodes (fig. 1b). Theoretical analysis has shown that the ratio of mean flow velocity just after release of compression to the pre compression value **(THRR)** is a good indicator of autoregulation [2]. The test is simple and safe but unfortunately cannot be graded mainly because the fall in perfusion pressure in the ipsilateral middle cerebral artery **(MCA)** during carotid compression cannot be measured. The aim of the study was to show that despite this drawback the transient hyperaemic response test **(THRT)** may be considered as a useful non-invasive technique for testing autoregulation.

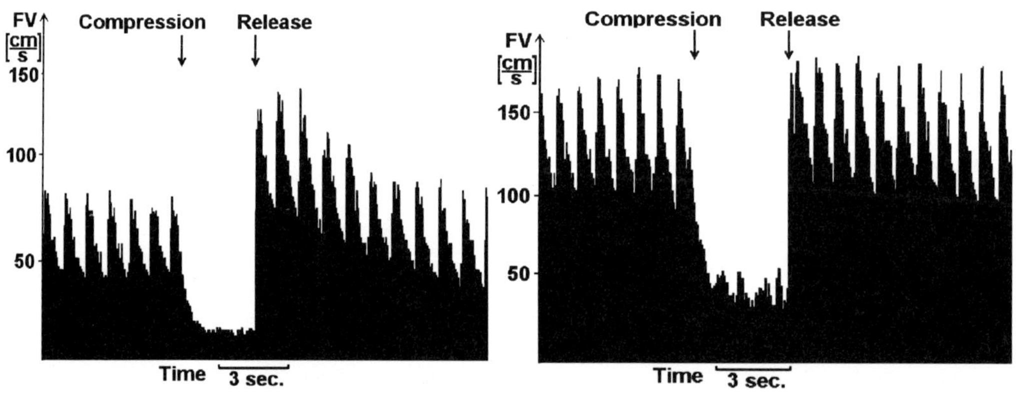

Fig. 1 The typical MCA blood flow velocity response to short compression of common carotid artery in a healthy volunteer (A), and in a patient with impaired autoregulation (B).

MATERIAL AND METHODS

Fifty two patients after subarachnoid haemorrhage **(SAH)** were examined. There were 30 men and 22 women. The age range was 23 to 73 years. Patients were graded using World Federation of Neurological Surgeons **(WFNS)** grade [3] (worse state of the patient is described by higher WFNS grades) , and the numbers of patients per grade were distributed as follows : 3 -grade I, 16 - grade II, 15

- grade IIIa, 5 - grade IIIa, 10 - grade IV, 3 grade V. Outcome was graded according to the Glasgow Outcome Score (1 - good outcome, 5 - dead) and was distributed as follows : 29 - grade 1, 3 - grade 2, 11 - grade 3, 9 - grade 5. A total number of 614 tests were performed on daily basis starting from the day of admission. Flow velocity signal from the middle cerebral artery was measured using transcranial Doppler (PcDop 842, SciMed, Bristol, UK) and recorded digitally on an IBM PC using a program for biological signal recording written by W. Zabolotny (Warsaw University of Technology). Once a good quality flow velocity signal had been obtained a brief carotid compression (4-5 sec.) was performed.

RESULTS

Statistical analysis of the recorded tests showed that correlations of the test results with clinical grades were highly significant when the tests were classified using the ratio of post-compression to pre compression systolic flow velocity. A positive result was assumed when this ratio was higher or equal to 1.09 and negative otherwise. Using this criterion, 247 tests were classified as positive THRT and 367 as negative THRT. WFNS grade was found to be significantly higher ($p < 0.000001$) in a group classified as negative THRT (median 3b) than in group classified as positive THRT (median 2). Also outcome graded using the Glasgow Outcome Score was significantly worse ($p < 0.0003$) in the negative group (median 3) than positive (median 1). Time trend analysis of THRT showed that the frequency of positive results was significantly lower ($p < 0.02$) during the second week after bleeding, the period considered to have the highest risk of vasospasm [4].

DISCUSSION

The test has also been used for testing cerebrovascular reactivity in severely head injured patients. The results of the THRT has been compared in group of 12 patients with another method of assessing the autoregulatory reserve, which is based on the analysis of correlation between spontaneous changes in cerebral perfusion pressure and TCD flow velocity [5]. The study showed a significant correlation ($p<0.01$) between these two methods.

The transient hyperaemic response test is a very simple, non-invasive test of autoregulation, which may easily be performed on a regular daily basis. Despite the fact that the test result may be either positive or negative it correlates strongly with clinical status of the patient. The software developed to support the test performs automatic analysis of the results and make the examination easier. The program automatically recognises carotid compression and release and immediately displays the tests results. Additionally raw TCD flow velocity signal data (sampled with frequency 50 Hz) is recorded digitally on the computer disk and the analysis results together with patients personal data are stored automatically in a data-base for further statistical analysis.

REFERENCES

1. Czosnyka M, Pickard JD, Whitehouse H, Piechnik S: The Hyperaemic Response to a Transient Reduction in Cerebral Perfusion Pressure. Acta Neurochirurgica 115: 90-97, 1992.

2 Giller CA: A bedside test for cerebral autoregulation using Transcranial Doppler Ultrasound. Acta Neurochirurgica 108: 7-14, 1991.

3. Drake CG, Report of World Federation of Neurological Surgeons Committee on universal subarachnoid grading scale J. Neurosurgery 68, 985-986; 1988 (letter to the editor).

4 Kassel NF, Torner JC, Haley EC, Jane JA, Adams HP, Kongable GL et al: The international co-operative study on timing of aneurysm surgery - overall management results. J Neurosurgery 73: 18-36, 1990.

5. Czosnyka M, Guazzo E, Iyer V, Kirkpatrick P, Smielewski P, Whitehouse H, Pickard JD: Testing of cerebral autoregulation in head injury by waveform analysis of blood flow velocity and cerebral perfusion pressure. Acta Neurochirurgica [Suppl] 60: 468-471, 1994.

Intracranial Pressure, Cerebral Circulation and Metabolism in Severe Head Injury

TAKASHI YAMAMOTO, TAISUKE KIKUTI, TAKASHI TOKUTOMI, and MINORU SHIGEMORI

Department of Neurosurgery, Kurume University School of Medicine, 67 Asahi-machi, Kurume, Fukuoka, Japan

INTRODUCTION

It is well known that brain ischemia adversely affect recovery following traumatic brain injuries. But the difference of hemodynamic events between focal and diffuse brain injurie is still unclear. We then studied the intracranial hemodynamic differences between in both groups of patients.

MATERIALS AND METHODS

We studied 20 patients with severe head injury whose Glasgow Coma Scale score of 8 or less on admission. They included 7 of diffuse and 13 of focal brain injuries. Diffuse brain injuried-patients were 5 of type-2 and 2 of type-3 according to Traumatic Coma Data Bank CT classification[2]. Other 13 patients included 10 of subdural hematoma and 3 of epidural hematoma. The age of patients ranged 17 to 88 years with mean age of 35. The intracranial pressures(ICPs) were recorded by subdural transducers on the right frontal region of the patients. The cerebral perfusion pressures(CPPs) were calculated by difference between mean arterial blood pressure and mean ICP. Continous monitoring of jugular bulb venous oxygen saturation(SjO2) was performed by percutaneous retrograde insertion of the fiberoptic catheter via the right internal jugular vein. The position of the tip of the catheter in the jugular bulb was confirmed on X-ray film. Arterial oxygen saturation and the mean flow velocity on the middle cerebral arteries(MCA-FV) were also recorded contineously.

RESULTS

In the time course of CPP and SjO2 in diffuse and focal brain injury of survived patients, the values of CPP and SjO2 were relatively high and stable in both groups compared with dead patients. This tendency was more definite in patients with focal brain injury than those with diffuse brain injury. Fig.1 shows the relationship between CPP and SjO2 in survived cases with diffuse and focal brain injury. In most of these patients, CPP and SjO2 were maintained more than 50mmHg and 50% respectively. In the time course of CPP and SjO2 in diffuse and focal brain injury of dead cases, CPP and SjO2 were low compared with survived cases. Fig.2 shows the relationship of them in dead patients . In the patients with focal injury, we could not find any relationship between CPP and SjO2. On the other hand, both CPP and SjO2 in diffuse brain injuried-patients were maintained at more higher levels. There were no relationship between MCA-FV and SjO2 in both groups of patients.

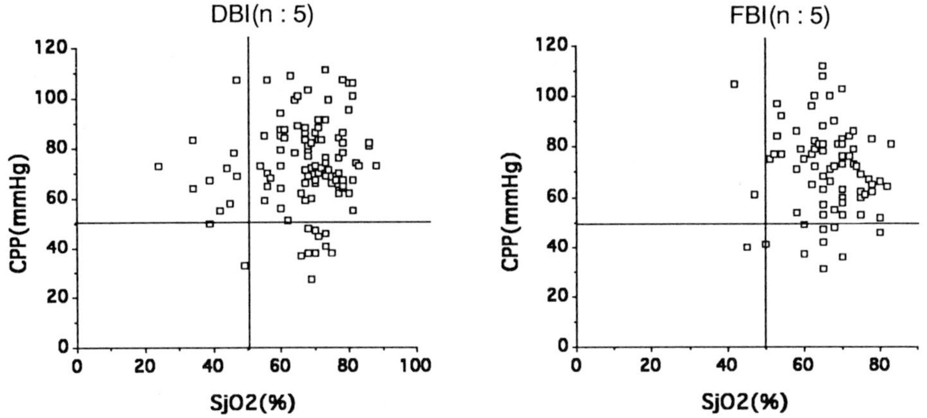

Fig . 1 Relationship between CPP and SjO2 in survived cases

DBI : diffuse brain injury
FBI : focal brain injury

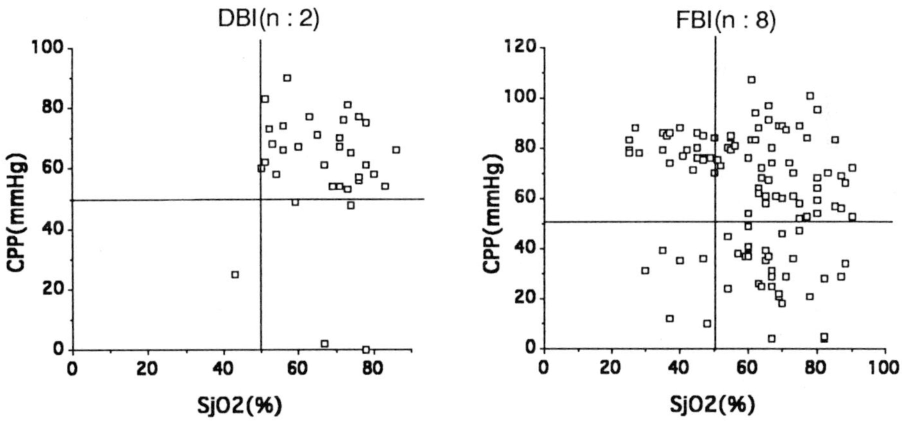

Fig . 2 Relationship between CPP and SjO2 in dead cases

DBI : diffuse brain injury
FBI : focal brain injury

DISCUSSION

In our previous studies, we measured MCA-FV in diffuse and focal brain injury. MCA-FV decreased progressively depending on the elevation of ICP and reduction of CPP. When ICP increased more than 30mmHg and CPP decreased less than 40mmHg, MCA-FV decreased significantly in focal brain injury.However, there was no relationship between ICP level or CPP level and MCA-FV in diffuse brain injury[3)4)]. The decrease of MCA-FV in focal brain injury might be caused by the increase of the peripheral vascular resistances. On the other hand, many complicated factors, such as hyperemia, arterial narrowing, crerbral ischemia, have to be considered in diffuse brain injury[3)4)5)].

Recent studies have demonstrated that TCD can identify state of reduced CPP and decreases in SjO2 with the fall of CPP, these results suggested progressive failure of cerebral blood flow to meet metabolic demands[1)]. But, in our study, the such relationship could not be found.

In focal brain injury, compression ischemia is possibly main factor to induced early mortality after injury. The present study also indicated that brain ischemia is more severe in focal brain injury compared with that in diffuse brain injury in the survivors. In fatal patients, hemodynamic events in diffuse brain injury are not severe than those in focal brain injury and other factor seems to play a important role for their poor outcome.

CONCLUSION

Intracranial hemodynamics changes in focal brain injuried patients are more variable compared with those in diffuse brain injury . In diffuse brain injury, diffuse damage to axons other than hemodynamic events are also considered as an important factor to determine the outcome.

REFERENCES

1) Chan K. , Miller J. D. , et al (1992). The effect of changes in cerebral perfusion pressure upon middle cerebral artery blood flow velocity and jugular blub venous oxygen saturation after severe brain injury.
In: J Neurosurg 77 : 55-61

2) Marshall L. F. , Marshall S. B. , et al(1991). A new classification of head injury based on computerized tomography.
In: Traumatic Coma Data Bank, 1991.

3) Shigemori M. , Moriyama T. , et al(1990). Intracranial hemodynamics in diffuse and focal brain injuries. Evaluation with transcranial Doppler(TCD) ultrasound.
In: Acta Neurochir(Wien) 107 : 5-10

4) Shigemori M. , Kikuchi N. , et al(1992). Monitoring of severe head injured patients with transcranial Doppler(TCD) ultrasound.
In: Neurotraumatology Progressive and Perspective. A. Martins da Silva, A. Tocha Melo, F. Lowe(eds)

5) Shigemori M. , Tokutomi T. , et al(1991). Diffuse axonal injury and early intracranial sequelae in severe head injury.
In: Neuro Med Chir(Tokyo) 31: 390-395

Transcranial Doppler Sonography for Intracranial Hypertension—The Evaluation of the Pulsatility Index in Basilar Artery

Y. Kubota, Y. Nishimura, T. Andoh, N. Sakai, and H. Yamada

Department of Neurosurgery, Gifu University School of Medicine, 40 Tsukasa-machi, Gifu, 500 Japan

INTRODUCTION

Transcranial Doppler Sonography (TCD) has been used for the detection of intracranial blood flow signals[1], and most of its reports have focused on the evaluation of flow signals mainly in middle cerebral artery (MCA). In current study, a major limitation of TCD in the artery is the relatively high frequency of failure to record signals. The clinical utility in basilar artery (BA), however, may be noticed[2], because its signals can be detected irrespective of the presence of bone window. Further, the relationship between BA flow signals and intracranial hypertension is investigated.

MATERIALS AND METHODS

The blood flow of MCA transtemporally and BA through the foramen magnum was sequentially measured by TC2-64 (EME, berlingen, Germany). Subsequently the Gosling's PI[3], [systolic flow velocity - diastolic flow velocity] / mean flow velocity, was analyzed. Sixty volunteers (17 to 71 years of age) were selected for control group, while 55 patients with raised intracranial pressure (ICP) were studied in the early clinical stage; 15 cases with severe head injury (Glasgow Coma Scale < 8 points) and 40 cases with subarachnoid hemorrhage (SAH) or hypertensive intracerebral hemorrhage. Some of those cases were also continuously monitored for ICP by subdural probes (Camino Laboratories, San Diego, USA). Outcome was assessed at discharge and 6 months after admission using the Glasgow Outcome Scale (GOS)[4].

RESULTS

1) The rate of successful recording of MCA flow signals was 69.1%, 38 of 55 cases, while that of BA was 100% of all cases. 2) In control group, PI values of the BA were 0.79±0.11 (mean±SD). When normal range of PI values was defined under 1.01, patients were divided into 4 groups according to sequential changes of PI values: Group I; maintaining within normal range, Group II; higher PI in the early stage returns to normal range sequentially, Group III; PI within normal range in the early stage raises progressively, and Group IV; continually higher PI from the early stage. 3) In general, outcome was favorable in Group I and II, whereas unfavorable in Group III and IV (Table 1). 4) There was a tendency that increment of PI correlatively reflects elevation of ICP. Such a representative case of 45 -year-old male with SAH was shown in Fig. 1, in which MFV and CPP simultaneously were recorded.

DISCUSSION AND CONCLUSION

Suboccipital recordings in BA have been showed to be less valuable because of considerable anatomical variation[5]. However, our study resulted in not only successful TCD recordings in BA than MCA on advantage it can be measured without bone window, but also significant correlations between PI and clinical outcome[6][7]. Moreover, PI in BA was closely correlated with ICP in the early stage. The problem is that evaluation of the flow velocity in BA is less reliable than MCA, but PI may be able to exclude this demerits because of angle-independent parameter[3]. Those results suggested that PI mainly depends on intracranial hypertension.

In conclusion, PI in BA using TCD was considered to be useful parameter for non-invasive monitoring of ICP and prognosis.

Table 1 Relationship between pulsatility index (PI) value and outcome.

A

Group	initial PI	outcome (cases)			
		GR	MD	SD,V	Dead
I	<1.01	1	1	0	0
II	>1.01	4	1	0	2
III	<1.01	0	0	1	0
IV	>1.01	0	0	1	4

B

Group	initial PI	outcome (cases)			
		GR	MD	SD,V	Dead
I	<1.01	9	1	3	2
II	>1.01	4	8	2	0
III	<1.01	0	0	0	2
IV	>1.01	0	2	0	7

A: head injury series, B: SAH, HICH series.
Group I: maintaining within normal range, Group II: higher PI in the early stage returns to sequentially normal range,
Group III: PI within normal range in the early stage raises progressively, Group IV: continually higher from the early stage.
normal range of PI values: < 1.01
GR; good recovery, MD; moderate disability, SD; severe disability, V; vegetative state, SAH; subarachnoid hemorrhage, HICH; hypertensive intracerebral hemorrhage.

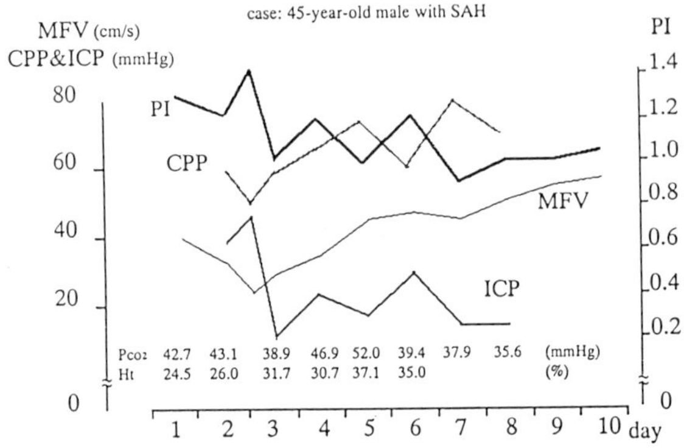

Fig. 1 Sequential changes of PI, ICP, MFV, CPP and laboratory data, in which PI was well-correlated with ICP. MFV; mean flow velocity, PI; pulsatility index, ICP; intracranial pressure, CPP; cerebral perfusion pressure, SAH; subarachnoid hemorrhage.

REFERENCES

1. Aaslid R, Markwalder TM, Nornes H (1982) Noninvasive transcranial Doppler ultrasound recording of flow velocity in basal cerebral arteries. J Neurosurg 57: 769-774
2. Cantu C, Yasaka M, Tsuchiya T, Yamaguchi T (1992) Evaluation of the Basilar Artery Flow Velocity by Transcranial Doppler Ultrasonography. Cerebrovasc Dis 2: 372-377
3. Gosling RG, King DH (1974) Arterial Assessment by Dopple-shift Ultrasound. Proc. roy. Soc. Med. 67: 447-449
4. Jennett B, Bond M (1975) Assessment of outcome after severe brain damage. A practical scale. Lancet 1: 480-484
5. Hassler W, Steinmetz H, Gawlowski J (1988) Transcranial Doppler ultrasonography in raised intracranial pressure and in intracranial circulatory arrest. J Neurosurg 68: 745-751
6. Arita K, Uozumi T, Kuwabara S, Oki S, Nakahara T, Kohno H, Muttaqin Z (1991) Transcranial Doppler Sonography in Intracranial Hypertension and Brain Death. Neurosonology 4: 60-65
7. Cardoso ER, Kupchak JA (1992) Evaluation of Intracranial Pressure Gradients by Means of Transcranial Doppler Sonography. Acta Neurochir 55: 1-5

Cerebral Circulation in Communicating Hydrocephalus Evaluated by TCD and SPECT Studies

A. OKURA, M. SHIGEMORI, and N. KIKUCHI

Department of Neurosurgery, Kurume University School of Medicine, 67 Asahi-machi, Kurume, Fukuoka, 830 Japan

INTRODUCTION

In patients with communicating hydrocephalus after subarachnoid hemorrhage (SAH), various methods have been used preoperatively to predict the result of shunting operation. We studied pre- and postoperative single photon emission CT (SPECT) and transcranial Doppler (TCD) ultra sonographic findings to determine the relationship between the cerebral circulation and effect of shunting operation.

MATERIALS AND METHODS

We operated on 204 patients with ruptured cerebral aneurysms during the last 5 years, and subsequently carried out V-P shunting in 74 patients (36.3 %) of them. All of them presented with all or part of the clinical symptoms of normal pressure hydrocephalus (NPH) such as gait disturbance, mental symptoms, urinary incotinence. They all had progressive dilatation of the ventricular system with 0.4 or more of Evan's index. 16 out of 74 patients without intracerebral hemorrhage, past history of cerebrovascular disease, and vasospasm were selected for this study. Typical NPH signs was found in 9 patients (56.2 %). But mental symptoms including memory disturbance, hypoactivity and decreased intellectual function developed in all 16 patients. SPECT and TCD were done in 13 patients before and after shunting procedures. These findings were evaluated retrospectively with the postoperative outcome. Mean flow velocity of the middle cerebral artery (MFV) and pulsatility index of Gosling and King (PI) were collected from each TCD data.

RESULTS AND DISCUSSION

Of the 16 patients, 5 showed a marked response to shunting operation and had excellent result. But other 6 showed only some response, and had fair or poor results. Preoperative mean PI values in 16 patients were 1.00 and 0.96 on the right and left sides. In patients with excellent result after shunting operation, increase of MFV and decrease of PI values (0.79 and 0.78 on the right and left side respectively) were commonly seen.

Fig.1 showed the relationships between MFV and PI preoperatively in these patients. Fig.2 showed postoperative change of this relationships indicating decreased PI and increased MFV. Preoperative SPECT findings commonly showed focal or lobar decrease of cerebral blood flow (CBF) in the frontal lobes. Postoperative SPECT however showed bilateral increase of CBF in the frontal lobes and basal ganglia in patients with excellent operative result. Improvement of SPECT findings in these patients were well correlated with the clinical symptoms. PI is known to indicate the state of peripheral vascular resistance of the MCA. The decrease of PI value and increase of MFV therefore indicate reduced peripheral vascular resistance and increased CBF by the reduction of CSF pressure following V-P shunt. These results also showed the functional improvement of the patient was caused by the improvement of the cerebral microcirculation after shunting operation.

CONCLUSION

The TCD and SPECT study are thus useful clinical measures in the prediction of shunting operation and its result.

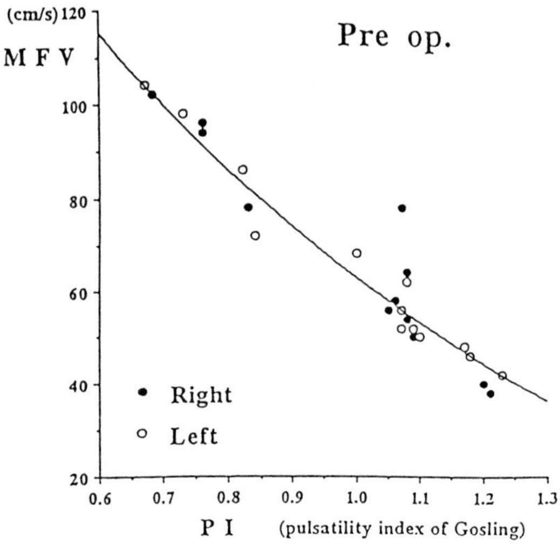

Fig. 1

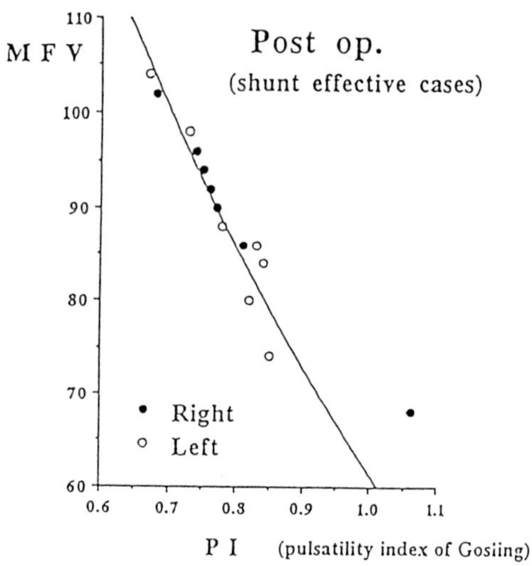

Fig. 2

Key Words ; Communicating hydrocephalus, TCD, SPECT

Anaerobic Change of Glucose Metabolism in Experimental Hydrocephalus Rat

YASUKO HARA, REIZO SHIRANE, SHINYA SATO, and TAKASHI YOSHIMOTO

Department of Neurosurgery, Tohoku University School of Medicine, 1-1 Seiryo-machi, Aoba-ku, Sendai, 980 Japan

INTRODUCTION

We reported characteristic pattern of CBF and rCMRO2 in infantile hydrocephalus. OEF does not increase as CBF decrease on PET scan[1]. However, in experimental hydrocephalus rat, rCMRglc increased independent of decreased CBF in early stage[2]. rCMRglc was measured by DG method, developed by Sokolloff[3]. DG, which is glucose analogue, does not enter the TCA cycle and accumulated in the brain cells. Therefore, DG method indicates the value of glucose-uptake, which is equal to the sum of aerobic and anaerobic metabolism. We speculated that rCMRglc measured by DG method may contain the value of anaerobic metabolism which is involved in the pathophysiology of hydrocephalus[4]. In the present study, we tried to clarify the anaerobic changes of glucose metabolism in experimental hydrocephalus rat by comparison of rCMRglc measured by DG method and 6-labeled glucose method which represents only aerobic metabolism[5].

MATERIALS AND METHODS

We used hydrocephalus rat model made by Kaolin suspension injection. The phase of hydrocephalus was devided into acute phase of 2-weeks after the injection and chronic phase of 6-weeks after the injection. Saline was injected as control.

In each phase, double label semiquantitative autoradiography was made by injection of [3H]DG and [6-14C]glucose intravenously. Each autoradiographic image of DG and glucose was taken from the same brain section using Fujix Bio-Imaging Analizer BAS3000 (Fuji Photo Filum) . In this method, regional difference of uptake of tracers indicate anaerobic glucose metabolism[2]. Difference of uptake ratio of tracers in each brain region was calculated and corrected using the cerebellum as control in order to exclude the effect of difference of rate constants.

RESULTS

In acute phase image, the DG metabolism was higher than that of glucose. It was recognized mainly in the cerebral cortices, thalamus, hypothalamus and corpus callosum. There were significant differences in sensorymotor cortex and thalamus.

However, notable deifference of images was recognized only in sensorymotor cortex in chronic phase model. There was no significant difference in control. (Fig. 1)

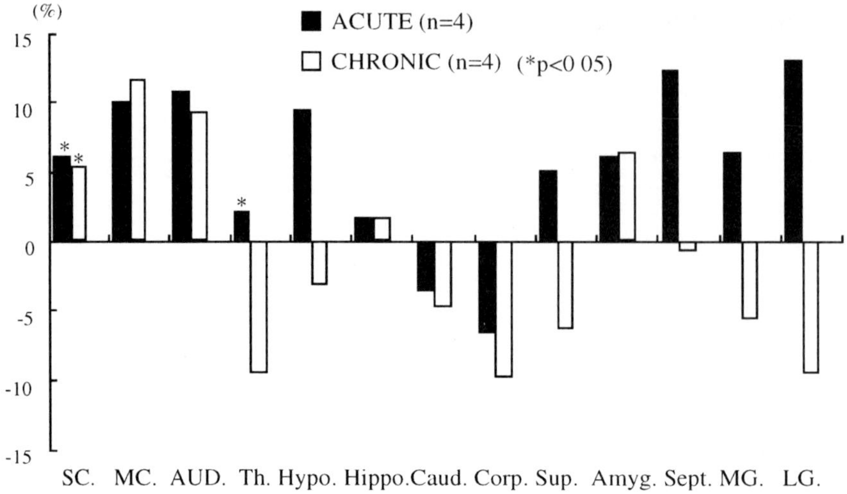

Fig.1. Regional difference of tracer concentration (%) $= \frac{\text{regional [DG]}}{\text{cerebellar [DG]}} - \frac{\text{regional [glc.]}}{\text{cerebellar [glc.]}}$

DISCUSSION

These results suggest that anaerobic change of metabolism exists in the early stage of hydrocephalus. Activation of anaerobic metabolism, dominant in acute phase, may compensate for shortage of the energy. The decrease of anaerobic and aerobic metabolism in chronic phase may suggest the irreversible tissue damage. Therefore the prompt treatment for hydrocephalus is recommended.

REFERENCES

1. Shirane R, Sato S, Sato K (1992) Cerebral blood flow and oxygen metabolism in infants with hydrocephalus. Child's Nerv Syst 8:118-123
2. Satoh S, Shirane R, Yoshimoto T (1992) Regional cerebral blood flow and regional cerebral metabolic rate of glucose in experimental hydrocephalus measured by double tracer method of autoradiography. Current Tr Hyd (Tokyo) 2: 1-4
3. Sokoloff L, Reivich M, Kennedy C (1977) The [14C]deoxyglucose method of local cerebral glucose utilization: Theory, procedure, and normal values in the conscious and anesthetized albino rat. J Neurochem 28: 897-916
4. Ackermann R, Lear J (1989) Simultaneous measurement of cerebral anaerobic and aerobic metabolism. J Cereb Blood Flow Metab. 9, suppl. 1: 238
5. Lear J, Ackermann R (1988) Comparison of cerebral glucose metabolic rates measured with fluorodeoxyglucose labeled in the 1, 2, 3-4, and 6 positions using double label quantitative digital autoradiography. J Cereb Blood Flow Metab 8: 575-585

Transcranial Doppler CO2 Test as an Indicator of Cerebral Vasoreactivity and Prognosis in Patients with Regional CBF Alterations After Head Injury

MYUNGHYUN KIM[1], KYUMAN SHIN[1], and JUNGHWA CHU[2]

[1] Department of Neurosurgery, Ehwa womans University Hospital, Mokdong, Yangcheon-ku, Seoul, 158-056, Korea
[2] Department of Neurosurgery, Korea University Hospital, Ahamdong, Sungbuk-ku, Seoul, Korea

INTRODUCTION

Ischemia is thought to be one of the key secondary detrimental factors after traumatic brain injury, which may be due to intracranial hypertension and the subsequent reduction of the cerebral perfusion pressure or to arterial spasms as a consequence of traumatic subarachnoid hemorrhage.

It is believed that hemodynamically compromised tissue is supplied by maximally, or near maximally, dialted arterioles, which showed reduced or absent regional cerebral blood flow, easily detected by SPECT.

The accessment of the cerebral vasoreactivity measured with TCD provides information regarding to the reserve capacity of the cerebral circulation in patients with acute head injuries, which has important therapeutic consequencies because it allows for the diagnosis of impending ischemia and for the control of the effect of initiated corrective measures. The aim of this study was to correlate the Doppler data with the findings of SPECT, the type of injury and prognosis.

METHODS

Fourteen patients (11 males and 6 females) with cerebral contusion were studied. The initial management of all patients included controlled ventilation and computed tomographic scanning, which was performed in all patients during the first 24 hours after hospital admission and repeated when clinically indicated (table 1).

Case	Sex	age	CT diagnosis	ROI	ROI(locat)	GCS	GOS	CO2	RMIratio	LMIratio
1	F	20	Bifrontal Ct	25	diffuse	8	2	9	1.21	3.08
2	M	20	R Frontal Ct	7	Rt ACA	14	5	14	1.14	1.17
3	M	20	DAI	20	Lt MCA	6	2	12	0.79	0.98
4	M	20	DAI	14	diffuse	7	2	12	0.94	1.03
5	F	23	R Frontal Ct	21	Rt A,MCA	8	4	12	1.61	2.54
6	F	23	DAI	19	diffuse	7	2	9	4.08	1.11
7	M	27	L Frontal Ct	4	Rt ACA	14	5	15	1.09	1
8	M	29	R Frontal Ct	25	Rt>Lt ACA	11	4	14	1.24	1.09
9	M	40	L SDH	20	diffuse	6	2	14	1.02	1.47
10	M	48	R Frontal Ct	53	Rt A,Mca	12	4	16	1.35	1.77
11	M	49	R Frontal Ct	6	Rt ACA	14	5	16	1.4	1.44
12	M	60	R frontal Ct	4	Rt MCA	13	4	13	0.94	1.04
13	M	60	R T ICH, SAH	20	both ACA	13	5	14	1.2	1.35
14	M	68	Bifrontal Ct	5	diffuse	14	4	13	1	1.24

Table 1. Clinical findings of 14 cases with head injury

The control group consisted of 30 healthy age-matched subjects (14 males and 16 females).

In all patients arterial blood pressure was measured with a radial pressure transducer. End-tidal CO2 concentration was monitored in both patient and control group using the mask or trachestomy cannula.

In all patients, SPECT and TCD evaluation was done 5-7 days after trauma.

For the SPECT, patients received 15 to 20 mCi of 99mTc-HMPAO intravenouly. Scannining was performed a half to 1 hour after injection using a single headed movable gamma camera. For analysis, four transverse images (each of 8 mm thickness) were chosen that included a sizable portion of the cerebral cortex and white matter. These were consecutive images beginning just above and excluding the cerebellum posteriorly and the inferior temporal lobe anteriorly. High vertex images were not included. Computer software was used to outline 16 truncated wedges on each transverse image for a region of interest (ROI) analysis . Each wedge in each slice represented one ROI, so that there were a total 32 ROIs from each hemisphere. Asymmetry in isotope uptake was calculated by dividing the counts from a single ROI in the symptomatic hemisphere by counts in the comparable contralateral ROI. A difference of 10% or greater (ratio less than or equal to 0.90) was chosen as a significant asymmetry. Each ROI received a score from 0 to 10, with 0 corresponding to a ratio greater than 0.91 (signifying no abnormality), 1 corresponding to a ratio of 0.81 to 0.90, etc. The scores for all individual ROIs were added for a total score (SPECT graded scale) .

The TCD studies were performed using EME 2MHz pulsed, pseudocontinuous TCD to entire basal cerebral arteries. Time mean velocities were measured from at least 10 cardiac cycles at the sample depth giving the highest values in the supine, resting state with the eye closed. Subjects first breathed room air through the apparatus until a steady expiratory end-tidal CO2 concentration was obtained. Then subjects hyperventilated for 2 minutes, and the MBFV, PI and end-tidal CO2 were recorded with TCD parameters, then breathed room air normally for 4 minutes. The percentage decrease in MBFV of each cerebral artery occuring during hyperventilation was divided by the absolute decrease in end-tidal CO2. These results were statistically analysed with SAS (Statistical Analysis System).

RESULTS

In control group, MBFV, CO2 reactivity and CO2 index were decreased and PI index was increased with increasing ages. There were no significant side-toside differences. The hemispheric indexes were not affected by age or sex. Men showed higher MBFV than men.(P=0.0208)(table 2) (Graph 1)

Age (decade)	side	Mean Blood Flow Velocity				PI index			
		ACA	MCA	PCA	ICA	ACA	MCA	PCA	ICA
3rd	Rt	57.7+4.6	69.3+3.3	64.3+4.7	59.1+3.6	0.73+0.08	0.75+0.06	0.73+0.04	0.72+0.05
	Lt	67.1+9.7	70.1+4.3	47.5+3.4	68.3+7.8	0.72+0.06	0.88+0.08	0.71+0.05	0.63+0.04
5th	Rt	50.1+8.5	67.4+7.9	52.9+5.9	57+7.5	0.86+0.05	0.83+0.06	0.76+0.04	0.98+0.07
	Lt	45.7+5.6	73.9+9.6	50.4+6.4	68.7+7.5	0.85+0.07	0.72+0.04	0.82+0.04	0.85+0.06
7th	Rt	45.9+4.4	53.3+6.7	44.2+5.2	40.2+5.4	0.91+0.05	0.97+0.07	0.93+0.05	0.88+0.07
	Lt	42.5+4.7	48.3+6.6	39.2+5.1	49.9+5.5	0.91+0.05	0.91+0.04	0.96+0.04	0.92+0.06
Age	**side**	**CO2 reactivity**					**M/I ratio**		**CO2 index**
		ACA	**MCA**	**PCA**	**ICA**				
3rd	Rt	4.4+0.3	4.7+0.2	4.0+0.4	4.4+0.3		1.22+0.32		15.9+0.3
	Lt	3.9+0.4	4.0+0.3	4.3+0.3	3.9+0.3		1.08+0.28		
5th	Rt	5+0.4	4.7+0.5	4.5+0.5	3.9+0.6		1.21+0.23		15.1+1.4
	Lt	3.9+0.4	4.5+0.5	4.7+0.4	4.3+0.4		1.15+0.67		
7th	Rt	4.1+0.6	4.3+0.8	3.9+0.4	3.4+0.6		1.37+0.34		13.9+1.5
	Lt	3.9+0.4	3.6+0.4	3.9+0.4	3.3+0.5		0.96+0.22		

Table 2. Mean values of TCD parameters in age-adjusted control group

At 3 months after the injury, 3 patients showed a good recovery(GOS 5), 5 patients were moderately disabled(GOS 4), 5 remained in a vegetative state(GOS 2). Eight patients showed hemorrhagic of non-hemorrhagic contusion mainly in frontal region, 4 patients were diffuse axonal injuries, 1 was traumatic temporal ICH with SAH, 1 was subdural hematoma. Doppler sonographic vasospasm with an average MCA/ICA ratio of more than 3 was identified in 2 patients, and CO2 indices were decresed also. Both remained as vegetative state after 3 months (GOS 2). The patients with head injury showed no significant differences in MBFV, increased PI index, decreased CO2 reactivity especially in ACA territory and CO2 index (P=0.002), compared with age-adjusted controls.

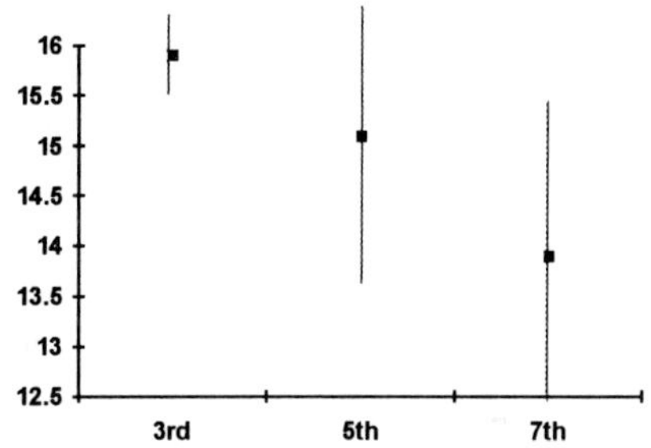

Graph 1. CO2 index in age-adjusted control group

There were close positive correlations between CO2 index and clinical status (r=0.72, P=0.004) or acute prognosis (r=0.71, P=0.004), but ROI has no correlation with both variables (graph 2)(table 3).

The arteries which had abnormal CO2 reactivity showed increased MBFV, decreased PI index. This means the vessels which autoregulation had been paralysed were dilated.

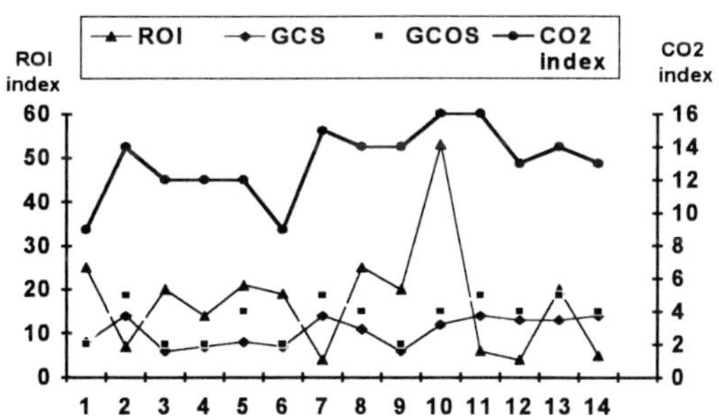

Graph 2. Correlation of various clinical variables in 14 cases of head injury

	CO2	ROI	GCS	GCOS	RMIR	LMIR
CO2	1					
ROI	0.02	1				
GCS	0.72	-0.33	1			
GCOS	0.71	-0.25	0.91	1		
RMIR	-0.5	0.12	-0.25	-0.23	1	
LMIR	-0.12	0.39	-0.24	-0.16	0.01	1

Table 3. Pearson correlation matrix of prognostic factors in head injuries

CONCLUSION

1. In control group, as age increased, MBFVs and CO2 reactivities declined, PI indices increased in all basal cerebral arteries. There was no significant side-to-side difference.
2. The vascular territory with decreased CO2 reactivity showed low perfusion state on SPECT, increased MBFV and decreased PI index on TCD.
3. Doppler vasospasm may correlate with poor prognosis.
4. Doppler CO2 reactivity may well correlate with acute outcome in subacute period after head injury.

REFERENCE

1. Arve Dahl, Karl fredric lindegaard. A comparison of TCD and CBF studies to assess cerebral vasoreactivity. stroke, 23:15-19 1992.
2. Bode H, Wais U. Age dependence of flow velocities in basal cerebral arteries. Arch Dis Child 1988;63:606-611
3. Brouwers P, Vriens EM,Musbach M, Wieneke GH, van Huffelen AC. Transcranial pulsed Doppler measurements of blood flow velocity in the middle cerebral artery : reference values at rest and during hyperventilation in healthy children and adolesecents in relation to age and sex. ultrasound Med Biol 1990;16:1-8
4. Bullock R,Mendelow AD,Bone I,P atterson J, Macleod WN, Allardice G:Cerebral blood flow and CO2 responsiveness as an indicator of collateral reserve capacity in patients with carotid arterial disease. Br J 1985;72:348-351
5. Enevoldsen EM, Jensen FT: Autoregulation and CO2 responses of cerebral blood flow in patients with acute severe head injury. J Neurosurg 1978;48:689-703
6. Hans Tacob Steiger, Rune Aaslid : TCD monitoring in head injury. Neruosurgery, 34:79-81, 1994
7. Targen Klingelhofer, Dirk Sander : Doppler CO2 test as an indicator of cerebral vasoreactivity and prognosis in severe intracranial hemorrhage, Stroke 23:962-966,1992
8. Kirkham FJ, Padayachee TS,Parsons S,Sergeant LS, House FR,Gosling RG. Transcranial measurement of blood velocities in the basal cerebral arteries using pulsed Doppler ultrasound : velocity as an index of flow. Ultrasound Med Biol 1986;12:15-21:62-71
9. Muizelaar JP, Lutz HA, Becker DP: Effect of mannitol on ICP and CBF and correlation with pressure autoregulation in severely head-injured patients. J Neursurg 1984;61:700-706 10.SK Hfansm,TC GroHa Value of SPECT in acute stroke therapeutic trials. Stroke 24:1305-1309,1993.

Outcome Prediction in Severe Closed Head Injury: Magnetic Resonance Versus Evoked Potentials

M. Cenzato[1], A. Ducati[1], N. Anzalone[2], L. Beretta[3], A. Dell'Acqua[3], G. Citerio[3], L. Sacchi[3], and S. Acerno[1]

[1] Department of Neurosurgery, [2] Department of Neuroradiology, [3] Chair of Anesthesiology, University of Milano, H. San Raffaele, Milano, Italy

INTRODUCTION

A correct prediction of survival expectancy, in the acute phase, does change the clinical management of severely head injury patients as demonstrated by Murray, Jennet and Teasdale in a recent paper[1] Concentrating the therapeutical resources ameliorates the prognosis of patients with a possibility to return to social life, while it does not worsen the prognosis of the other patients.
The predictive value of Glasgow Coma Score, of CT scans and of Multimodality Evoked Potentials as well as ICP collected in the acute phase is already part of the cultural background of everybody dealing with severe head injury patients.
Narayan[2] in 1981 emphasize the value of Multimodality Evoked Potentials in predicting the prognosis, underlining the absence of false pessimistic prediction, which means no risk of underestimation of the patient's possibility of survival.
The predictive value of Evoked Potentials is based, as far as survival is concerned[3], on the possibility to reveal a brainstem lesion and to quantify its severity with the recording of Brainstem Acoustic Evoked Potentials (BAEPs) and of Short Latency Somatosensory E.P. (s.l.SEPs). At the opposite, brainstem lesions are not always recognizable on CT scan.
MRI evaluation of head injured patients may demonstrate brainstem lesion even when CT evaluation is negative. MRI may therefore give a new informations to predict outcome.
The unquestionable higher sensitivity and accuracy of MRI as compared to CT scan suggested that the former will assume a primary role in the management of patients with closed head injury[4].
It is not clear, however, whether the signal changes shown by MRI in the acute phase of head injured patients correspond to an anatomical lesion or may at least justify a functional impairment of the involved structure. Which value, in terms of prognosis, do we have to attribute to a signal seen acutely on MRI and in particular to brainstem lesions? We approach this problem comparing MRI and BAEPs data in patients with brainstem lesions in closed head injury.

MATERIALS AND METHODS

We studied 14 (12 males, 2 females) patients with severe closed head injury with an admission Glasgow Coma Score less or equal to 8 (mean 5.33), for at least 8 hours, and no evidence of surgical lesions (Diffuse Injury type 1 and type 2)[5] on admission CT scan. Mean age was 22.8 (range from 5 to 44 years). All these patients were admitted to our Neurosurgical Intensive Care Unit.
In these patients we carried out a Magnetic Resonance (Siemens Magnetom, 1.5 Tesla) within 72 hours from trauma. Multimodality Evoked Potentials (MEPs) were carried out on day one, day three and day seven post-trauma. ICP was measured for a mean monitoring time of 4±2 days with intraparenchymal (Camino fiber optic transducers)(4 patients), intraventricular (fluid filled catheter)(4 patients) and subdural catheter (1 patient).

RESULTS AND DISCUSSION

In all these patients ICP never exceeded 20 mm Hg longer than 15 min.
All these patients had at least one supratentorial lesion, on MRI evaluation within 72 hours, and 65% of them, i.e., 9 patients (7 males, 2 females), had brainstem lesions as well.
Brainstem lesions seen on MRI ranged from 2 mm to 3 cm in diameter and were mostly distributed, as expected in DAI [6], in the dorsolateral part of the upper brainstem.

In three cases the extent of the lesion shown on MRI occupies more than one third of the sagittal section of the brainstem (see pictures). It is remarkable that all these lesions were not evident or not correctly evaluable on CT scans. All these 9 patients showed various degrees of brainstem involvement as judged on clinical ground, varying from an altered oculocephalic response to a bilateral fixed pupil. The association of MRI brainstem lesion and of clinical signs of brainstem involvement would therefore suggest a negative prognosis. On the other hand, EP recordings in day one in these 9 patients showed a complete although somewhat delayed and reduced, BAEPS responses in 8 case, an incomplete (lacking wave 5) response in one case. Moreover, 4 out of 9 patients had normal s.l.SEPs responses, while in the other 5 patients s.l.SEPs were abnormal presenting a prolonged latency of the cortical N20 response, that however was present at least on one side in all patients. The probability of survival, based on EP evaluation, was therefore higher, ranging from 88% to 100%, despite the lesions of the brainstem seen on MRI, which in some cases appeared to be impressive.
All the described patients survived: 3 had good outcome, 5 had moderate disability and 1 patient remained with a severe disability. Follow up for these patients is greater than 6 months.
We therefore conclude that evaluation of prognosis of the traumatic patient using MRI might be excessively pessimistic. MRI might infact overestimate the severity of the lesions.
In evaluating traumatic patient, along with the great anatomical detail that MRI gives, functional testing as Evoked Potentials are still an essential prognostic index for what concerns survival, at least until a better understanding of the prognostic value of the lesions seen on MRI is achieved.

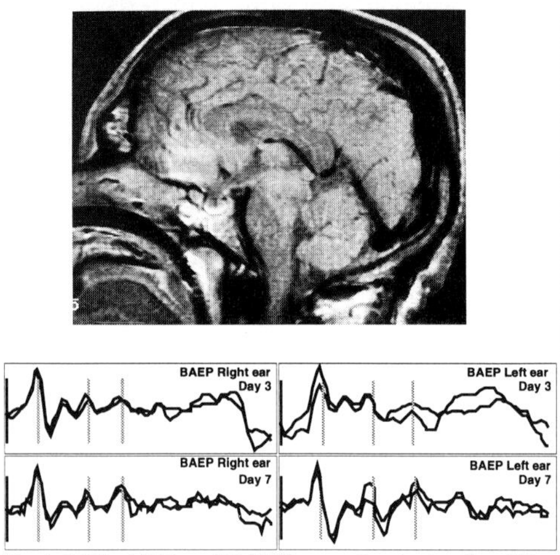

Fig. 1: MRI at 24 h and BAEPs recording in day 3 and 7 of patient with extensive lesion of the upper brainstem. BAEPS recordings show a complete response in the upper traces that becomes almost normal in day 7

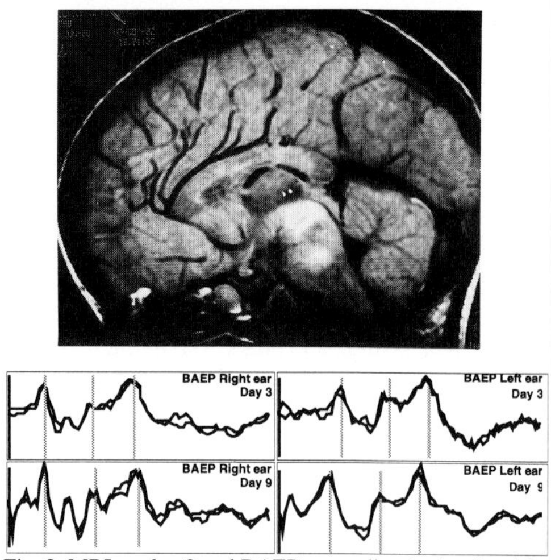

Fig. 2: MRI on day 3 and BAEPs recording in day 3 and 9 of patient with extensive lesion of the upper brainstem In the upper traces BAEPs recording within normal limit which persisted within normal limits on day 9

REFERENCES

1 Murray L.S., Teasdale G.M.,Murray G.D., Jennet B. et al. (1993) Does prediction of outcome alter patient management? Lancet 341: 1487-1491.

2 Narayan R.K., Greenberg R.P., Miller J.D. et al. (1981) Improved confidence of outcome prediction in severe head injury. A comparative analysis of the clinical examination, multimodality evoked potentials, CT scanning and intracranial pressure - J.Neurosurgery 54:751-762

3 M. Cenzato, A. Ducati, M. Fava, A. Landi, E. Sganzerla and G. Signoroni (1988), Evaluation of traumatic coma by means of multimodality evoked potentials - In: B. Grundy, R. Villani eds: "Evoked potentials: intraoperative and ICU monitoring" Springer Verlag, Vienna, 169-176

4 Salcman M., Pevsner P (1992). The value of MRI in head injury. Comparison with CT. Neurochirurgie,38,329-332

5 Marshall L.F., Marshal S.B., Klauber M.R., Clark M.V.B., Einsenberd H.M., Jane J.A., Luerssen T.G., Marmarou A., Foulkes M.A. (1991) A new classification of head injury based on computerized tomography. - J. Neurosurgry, 75, S14-S20.

6 Adams J.H., Graham D.I., Murray L.S., Scott G. (1982) Diffuse axonal injury due to non missile head injury in humans: ana analysis of 45 case - Ann. Neurol. 12:557-563

Experimental Analysis of Brain Surface Elastance and Its Clinical Application

T. Fukuhara[1], S. Nishio[1], M. Kawauchi[1], S. Asari[1], T. Ohmoto[1], and T. Akioka[2]

[1] Department of Neurological Surgery, Okayama University Medical School, 2-5-1 Shikata-cho, Okayama, 700 Japan
[2] Mizushima Central Hospital, Mizushima, Kurashiki, Okayama, 712 Japan

SUMMARY

To examine the relationship between brain stiffness and expansion, we measured brain surface elastance in cats and subsequently in patients with chronic subdural hematoma. In the cats, a stiff brain expanded poorly. In the clinical study, patients with high brain surface elastance tended to have an enlarged subdural space 1 month after surgery. Measuring brain elastance may help predict the degree of brain expansion in patients after the removal of a chronic subdural hematoma.

INTRODUCTION

As a mechanical property related to brain stiffness, the pressure needed to compress the brain surface [1], *brain surface elastance*, was investigated experimentally and clinically. The ophthalmodynamometer was adapted to compress the brain surface.

MATERIALS AND METHODS

In the experimental study, brain surface elastance was measured in 6 cats using three burr holes on each side. Measurements were taken before an intracranial mass was inserted, 10 and 70 minutes after removal of the intracranial mass (which was placed in each burr hole on the right side for 3 hours) and 60 minutes after cardiac arrest. After the mass was removed, the depression of the cortex was observed and the degree of depression was categorized into two groups: more than 1 mm (poorly expanded group) or 0-1 mm (well expanded group). The mean values of the elastance were compared. In clinical study, the brain elastance of 14 patients with chronic subdural hematoma was measured and analyzed in relation to the patient's age, symptoms on admission, hematoma density and volume, and brain expansion 1 month after surgery.

RESULTS AND DISCUSSION

In the experimental study, brain surface elastance did not change between sides, but could change among regions, the parietal region having the highest elastance ($p<0.05$)(Fig. 1). Furthermore, elastance increased after compression ($p<0.05$) but not after cardiac arrest (Fig. 1). Finally, the poorly expanded region had higher elastance than the well expanded region ($p<0.05$). The results of the clinical study appear in Table 1. The patient's age and symptoms and the hematoma's density and volume had no significant effect on elastance. The elastance of patients having an enlarged subdural space 1 month after surgery was significantly higher than those without an enlarged space ($p<0.05$). These results indicate that a stiff brain tends to result in an enlarged subdural space, which sometimes causes symptoms [2] or reaccumulation of the hematoma [3]. Measuring the brain surface elastance during surgery may make it possible to predict the persistence of an enlarged subdural space.

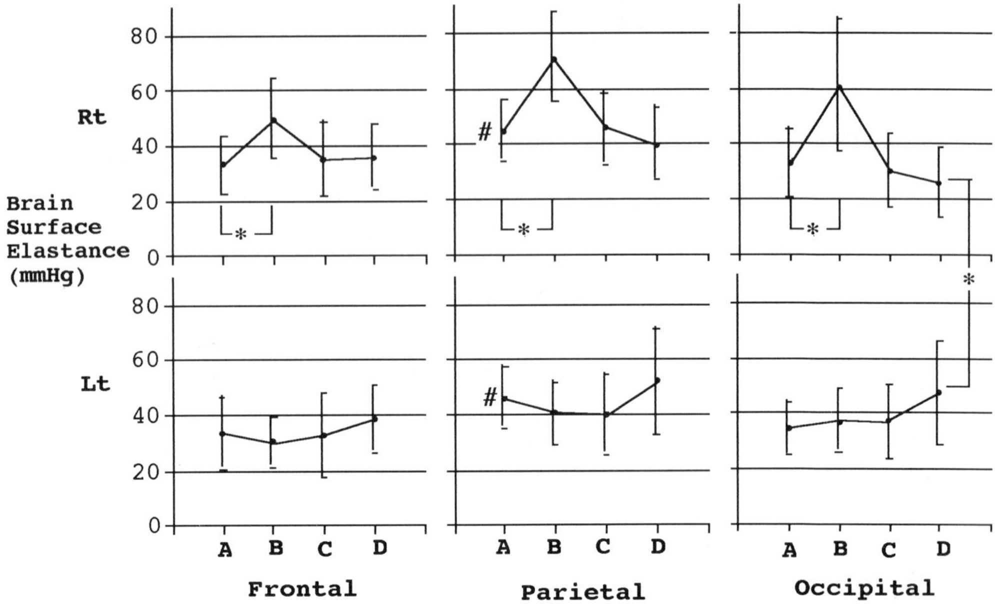

Fig. 1. Changes of brain surface elastance in each region. A; before the intracranial mass was inserted, B; 10 minutes after the intracranial mass was removed, C; 70 minutes after the intracranial mass was removed, D; 60 minutes after cardiac arrest, *; p<0.01, #; elastance in the parietal portion was significantly higher than that in the frontal and occipital portions on both sides.

Table 1. Brain surface elastance

Age		Symptoms on Admission		CT Findings of Hematoma		Hematoma Volume		Subdural Space 1 Month After	
<70	≥70	Minor	Major	Low	High	<100	≥100	(-)	(+)
19.8 ±9.7	26.3 ±6.9	20.2 ±8.4	24.9 ±9.5	20.1 ±9.0	25.8 ±8.6	22.6 ±6.8	22.6 ±10.4	18.6 ±7.7	27.9* ±8.1

*p<0.05

REFERENCES

1. Walsh EK, Schettini A (1990) Brain tissue elasticity and CSF elastance. Neurol Res 12: 123-127
2. Tanaka Y, Mizuno M, Kobayashi S, Sugita K (1987) Subdural fluid collection following craniotomy. Surg Neurol 27: 353-356
3. Robinson RG (1984) Chronic subdural hematoma: Surgical management in 133 patients. J Neurosurg 61: 263-268

Theoretical Model and Computer Simulation of ICP and Its Related Problems Based on Continuum Mechanics and Thermodynamics

TATSUYA NAGASHIMA[1], NORIHIKO TAMAKI[1], SEIJI HAMANO[1], and YUKIO TADA[2]

[1] Department of Neurosurgery, School of Medicine, [2] Department of Computer and Systems Engineering, Faculty of Engineering, Kobe University, 7-5-1 Kusunoki-cho, Chuo-ku, Kobe, 650 Japan

Since 1985, continuum mechanical and thermodynamical understanding of intracranial pressure has been developed. The purpose of the present study is to establish a theoretical framework to describe the interrelationship among many parameters that are related to intracranial pressure.

THEORETICAL FRAMEWORK

The intracranial phenomenons are described by "continuum mechanics" and "non equilibrium thermodynamics". "Continuum mechanics" describes mechanical behavior of continuum such as brain, cerebrospinal fluid, blood, interstitial fluid, dura, and bone. Intracranial pressure, energy, temperature and trans-membrane movement of substances are described by "non equilibrium thermodynamics".

(1) Field equations: Mass and energy conservation and mechanical equilibrium are described by three field equations; equation of continuity which describe mass conservation law(Eq. 1); equation of mechanical equilibrium(Eq. 2), and equation of energy conservation which describes the first law of thermodynamics(Eq. 3).

(2) Constitutive equations: Constitutive equations describe the specific mechanical properties of the brain tissue. Elastic(or viscoelastic) theory describe stress-strain relationship of the brain tissue(Eq. 4). Darcy's law describes the movement of interstitial fluid depending on tissue hydrostatic pressure gradient(Eq.5). The relationship between interstitial fluid pressure and intracerebral stress is described by Terzaghi'sprinciple(Eq.6); that is a difinition of tissue pressure.

$$\frac{D\rho}{Dt} + \dot{q} = 0 \quad (1)$$

$$\frac{\partial \sigma_{ij}}{\partial x_j} + X_i = 0 \quad (2)$$

$$dE = dQ - P\,dV + \psi\,d\varepsilon + \Sigma \mu_i\,dn_i \quad (3)$$

$$\sigma_{ij} = C_{ijkl}\,e_{kl} \quad (4)$$

$$q_{,i} = \left(\frac{k_{ij}}{\mu}\right) \phi_{,\iota} \quad (5)$$

$$\sigma_{ij} = <\sigma_{ij}> + \phi\,\delta_{ij} \quad (6)$$

Where, ρ is mass of the brain, q dot is mass flux into and from the brain, σij is internal force(stress in the brain), Xi is external force to the brain, E is internal energy, V is volume of the brain, Q is heat, ψ is electrical potential, ε is electric charge, μi is chemical potential, ni is molar, Cijkl is elastic modulus, ekl is strain tensor, ϕ,i is interstitial pressrue gradient, m is viscosity of the interstitial fluid, kij is parenchymal fluid conductivity, δij is Kronecker delata, q,i is flow vector through the brain parenchyma. Comma denotes partial deferentiation. P is intracranial hydrostatic pressure itself.

(3) Kedem-Katchalsky(K-K) equations: The nonequilibrium thermodynamical description of the coupled movement of fluid, non-electrolytes and, electrolytes through capillaries and other cell membranes are described by K-K equation. The description of electrolyte movement by K-K equation links the theoretical description of energy metabolism to change of the brain volume and intracranial pressure.

COMPUTER SIMULATION

Computer simulation of several pathological conditions(brain edema, hydrocephalus, hematoma) was conducted by finite element method. Several finite element models were constructed from horizontal and coronal slices of the brain. The results of the computer simulation indicated that the theoretical model based on continuum mechanics represented the intracerebral stress, the movement of interstitial fluid, the deformation of the brain. The result of the simulation were evaluated bu comparing them with clinical cases with subdural hematoma, hydrocephalus, or brain edema.

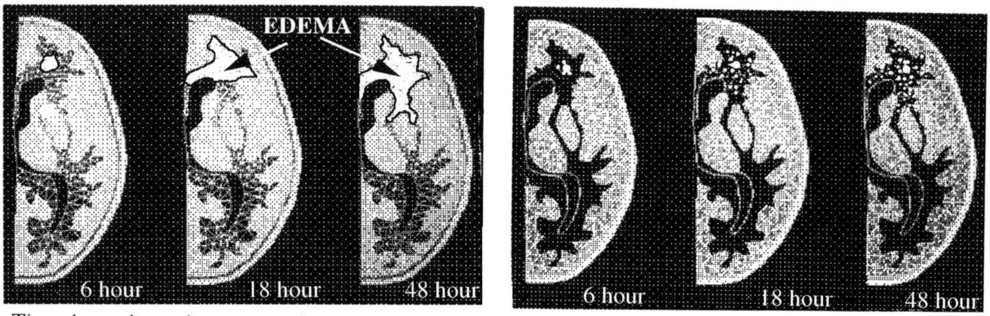

Time dependent edema extension   Interstitial pressure change

Fig.1 Computer simulation of the extention of vasogenic brain edema. Edema fluid extends throught the white matter depending on the tissure pressure gradient. The simulation coincides with the the distribution of the edema observed by MRI. Left: edema extension is expressed by white area. Right: interstitial pessure is presented by the size of circles.

CONCLUSIONS

A theoretical model is recognized valid(or useful) when it describes rationally the known phenomenon or it predicts unknown phenomenon. The result of computer simulation indicated that the theoretical model could describe intracranial phenomenon which was observed by MRI and CT scans. At present, the model is the most comprehensive one which bases on continuum mechanics and thermodynamics. The further theoretical study should be focused on the complete unification of thermodynamical description to the continuum mechanical description. It is necessary to develop a new experimental model to test the nonequilibrium-thermodynamical part of the model.

REFERENCES

(1) Kedem O, Katchalsky A,. Biochim Biophys Acta 27;229-238, 1958
(2) Nagashima T, Shirakuni T, Rapoport SI. A two dimensional finite element analysis of vasogenic brain edema. Neurogia medico-chirugica 30;1-9, 1990

A Non-Invasive Inshunt ICP Sensor

C. KADOWAKI[1], M. HARA[2], K. TAKEUCHI[2], and I. SAITO[2]

[1] Division of Neurosurgery, Kugayama Hospital, Kita-Karasuyama, Setagaya, Tokyo, 157 Japan
[2] Department of Neurosurgery, Kyorin University School of Medicine, Shinkawa, Mitaka, Tokyo, 181 Japan

SUMMARY

To clarify the changes in ICP after CSF shunting in hydrocephalus, we have applied a non-invasive ICP measurement with fully implantable pressure measuring device in a ventriculo-peritoneal shunt. It can measure ICP non-invasively and repeatedly, and evaluate the changes in ICP affected by CSF shunting in hydrocephalus.

INTRODUCTION

Cerebrospinal fluid [CSF] shunt has been widely adopted in the treatment of hydrocephalus. It is very important for neurosurgeons to evaluate the changes in intracranial pressure [ICP] to prevent complications in CSF shunting such as over-drainage or other malfunctions. In order to clarify the physiological changes in the intracranial space after CSF shunting, we applied a non-invasive simple technique for postoperative measurement of ICP with a fully implantable inshunt pressure measuring device in a ventriculo-peritoneal shunt.

PRESSURE SENSOR AND PRESSURE MEASUREMENT

The fully implantable pressure measuring system consists of a thin silicon dome reservoir [MDM ICP reservoir, MPS-301, originally designed to be placed on the chest wall] implanted under the skin, a pressure detector placed over the skin and a display system with a micro-computor developed by Japan MDM, Ltd [Tokyo, Japan]. The principle of this system is based on a collapsing technique [1].

METHODS

Basic studies:

To clarify the accuracy of the estimated pressure values obtained with this system, we compared the estimated pressure with the actual hydrostatic pressure affected to the pressure measuring device within the model of CSF shunt. We measured these pressures at every 5 cmH_2O of hydrostatic pressure ranging from 0 to 40 cmH_2O, while either the CSF shunt is patent or occluded.

Clinical trials:

Four hydrocephalic patients, 3 normal pressure hydrocephalus following subarachnoid hemorrhage and 1 aqueductal stenosis, were examined; their ages ranged from 8 to 63 years. The pressure measuring device was arranged in an in-line series connection between a ventricular catheter and a CSF flow control valve, and placed under the scalp at the level of the foramen of Monro [Fig. 1].

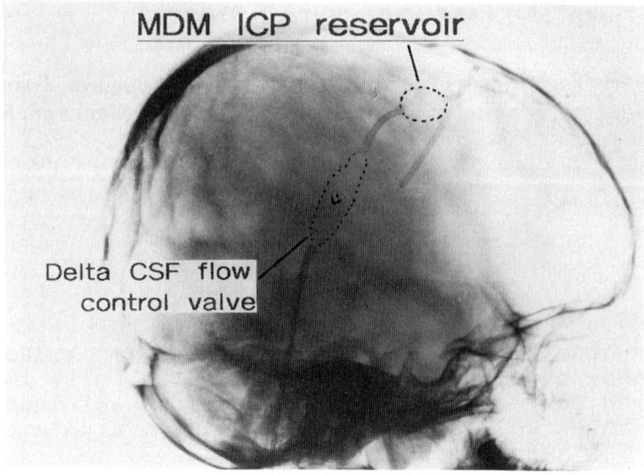

Fig. 1. X-ray of the pressure measuring device [MDM ICP reservoir] in an in-line series connection between a ventricular catheter and a CSF flow control valve.

We measured ICP by the pressure measuring system after CSF shunting, and evaluate the changes in the ICP corresponding to the postural changes while CSF shunt is either patent or obstructed by pressing a shunt occluder. The time on investigation elapsed from the CSF shunting was between 8 days and 6 months.

RESULTS

Basic studies:

Between 5 and 35 cmH_2O, the estimated values obtained had a good correlation with the actual values of hydrostatic pressure when the CSF shunt was either occluded or patent as shown in Fig. 2. However, the pressure values could not be estimated, because the silicon dome was not inflated enough resulting from inadequate pressure below 5 cmH_2O, and was too inflated to be collapsed over 35 cmH_2O.

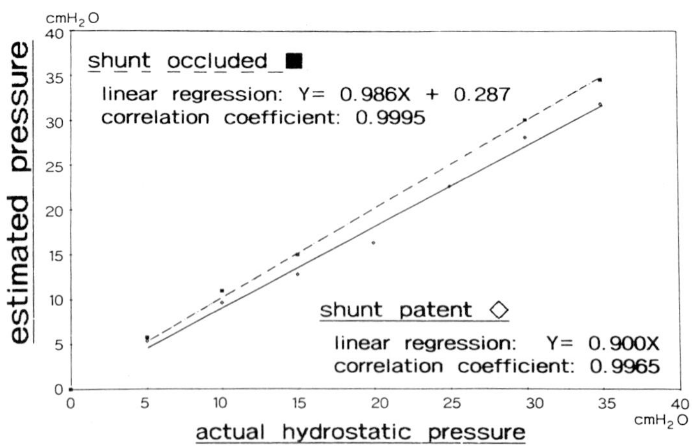

Fig. 2. Comparison of the estimated pressure and the actual hydrostatic pressure, while either the CSF shunt is patent (■) or occluded (◇).

Clinical trials:

While the CSF shunt was patent, the estimated ICP values in supine position were related to the opening pressure of the CSF flow control valve in each case. When the CSF shunt was occluded in supine, the estimated ICP values increased slightly to almost the individual ICP values measured prior to CSF shunting. Head elevation immediately led to decrease the estimated ICP values in each case, occasionally to negative as shown in Fig. 3.

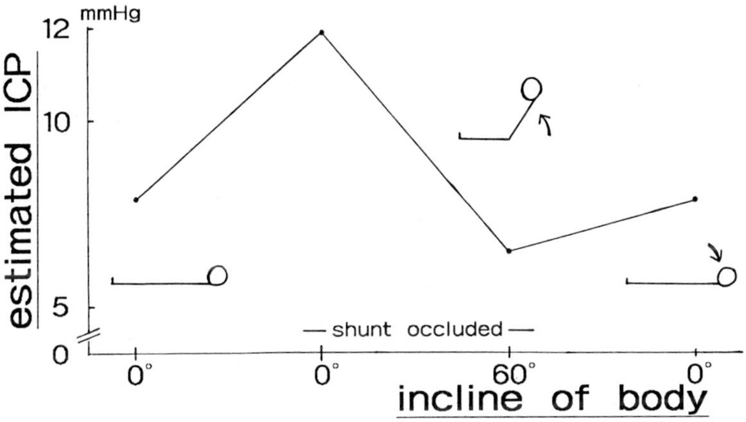

Fig. 3. Changes in ICP with head elevation.

DISCUSSION

There is no neurosurgeon who has never had unexpected complications such as malfunctions of the CSF shunt, over-drainage, low pressure syndrome and slit ventricle syndrome after the CSF shunting [2, 3]. In spite of the great deal of researchs to evaluate the unsolved problems regarding the CSF shunt impanted in hydrocephalus such as the changes on ICP [4, 5, 6, 7, 8, 9], CSF shunt physics and it's effects on intracranial physiology including ICP have yet to be clarified well, and should further investigated to prevent unfortunate accidents.
We have tried to clarify the intracranial physiology after the CSF shunting including the CSF shunt physics [10, 11]. We have applied a simple technique to measure the ICP with a fully implantable ICP measuring system after the CSF shunting. The results in vitro showed that the estimated values obtained with this system had a good correlation with the actual values.
In clinical trials, furthermore, the results obtained with this non-invasive measuring system after CSF shunting provided important informations about the intracranial physiology after CSF shunting as well as the CSF shunt function.

CONCLUSION

This inshunt ICP monitoring system, a simple technique for estimating ICP after CSF shunting, can measure ICP non-invasively and repeatedly. The changes in ICP obtained by this monitoring system indicate not only the shunt patency but also the effects of CSF shunt on ICP and intracranial physiology.

REFERENCES

1. Hashimoto T, Nakamura N, Shimazu H, Gondoh M, Tamai T (1993) Non-invasive measurement of ICP in shunt system by collapse technique. In: Avezaat CJJ, van Eijndhoven JHM, Maas AIR, Tans JTI (eds) Intracranial pressure Ⅷ. Springer-Verlag, Berlin-Heidelberg, pp 916-920.
2. Fried AH, Epstein MH (1994) Childhood hydrocephalus: Clinical features, treatment, and the slit-ventricle syndrome. Neurosurg Quarterly 4: 51-66.
3. Di Rocco C (1987) The treatment of infantile hydrocephalus, Vol.2. CRC Press, Florida, pp 79-154.
4. Fox JL, McCullough DC, Green RC (1973) Effect of cerebrospinal fluid shunts on intracranial pressure and on cerebrospinal fluid dynamics. J Neurol Neurosurg Psychiat 36: 302-312.
5. Cosman ER, Zervas NT, Chapman PH, Cosman BJ, Arnold MA (1979) A telemetric pressure sensor for ventricular shunt system. Surg Neurol 11: 287-294.
6. Haraoka J, Nakajima S, Takeda Y, Miki T, Miwa T (1993) Changes of ICP after shunt surgery for hydrocephalus-long time evaluation by telemetric sensors. In: Avezaat CJJ, van Eijndhoven JHM, Maas AIR, Tans JTI (eds) Intracranial pressure Ⅷ. Springer-Verlag, Berlin-Heidelberg, pp 896-900.
7. Ohta T, Miyake H, Nagasawa S, Nagano Y, Tanabe H (1993) Cholonological changes in intraventricular pressure and ventricular size after ventriculo-peritoneal shunt - Telemetric measurement using Osaka telesensar (NS-20). In: Avezaat CJJ, van Eijndhoven JHM, Maas AIR, Tans JTI (eds) Intracranial pressure Ⅷ. Springer- Verlag, Berlin- Heidelberg, pp 889-895.
8. Reilly PL, Savage JP, Doecke L (1989) Isotope transport studies and shunt pressure measurements as aguide to shunt function. Br J Neurosurg 3: 681-690.
9. Aschoff A, Benesch C, Kremer P, von Haken MS, Klank A, Osterloh M, Fruh K (1993) The solved and unsolved problems of hydrocephalus valves: A critical comment. In: Lorenz R, Klinger M, Brock M (eds) Advances in Neurosurgery Vol.21. Springer-Verlag, Berlin-Heidelberg, pp 103-114.
10. Kadowaki C, Hara M, Numoto M, Takeuchi K (1987) Factors affecting cerebrospinal fluid flow in a shunt. Br J Neurosurg 1:467-475.
11. Kadowaki C, Hara M, Numoto M, Takeuchi K, Saito I (1994) Inshunt physics: factors affecting cerebrospinal fluid flow in a shunt. Child's Nerv Syst (in press).

Poster XII: Drugs and Others

Chairman: K.M. Shin

Treatment of Elevated Intracranial Pressure in an Experimental Awake Model of Focal Cerebral Injury: Comparison Between Mannitol and Hypertonic Saline

D. DENCHEV[1], M. SCHNITZER[2], M. MIRSKI[2], and D. HANLEY[2]

[1] Department of Neurology and Neurosurgery, Medical University, Pleven, Bulgaria
[2] Departments of Neurosurgery, Neurology and Anesthesiology/Critical Care Medicine, The Johns Hopkins Hospital, Baltimore, MD, USA

INTRODUCTION

Current pharmacological approach toward treatment of acute elevations of intra-cranial pressure (ICP) following head injury is the employment of osmotically active agents, most commonly mannitol. Experimental data, however, suggests that the use of mannitol has several disadvantages, including a short duration of action, rebound ICP elevation, and disturbances in intravascular volume. The present study was conducted to compare the effectiveness of equiosmolar doses of hypertonic saline (HTS) and mannitol to reduce elevated ICP in an awake model of focal cerebral injury.

MATERIALS AND METHODS

Two hundred male Sprague-Dawley rats were divided into six groups: 1) unlesioned, untreated; 2) unlesioned, treated with HTS; 3) unlesioned, treated with mannitol; 4) lesioned, untreated; 5) lesioned, treated with HTS; and 6) lesioned, treated with mannitol. The animals in groups 2-6 were briefly anesthetized with 2% halothane/oxygen for placement of catheters monitoring ICP, central venous pressure (CVP), and mean arterial pressure (MAP), and (where indicated) for production of unilateral cerebral lesions induced by application of liquid nitrogen to the parietal skull for 90 sec.[1,2,3]. Thereafter, the animals were maintained under minimal sedation (0.25-0.5 % halothane in oxygen via face mask) to retard gross movements. Sixty min. after injury, equiosmolar doses of mannitol (25%) or HTS (NaCl 23.4%) were infused over 10 min. Changes in ICP and other physiological parameters were recorded and compared between lesioned and unlesioned groups, each having either no treatment or treatment with HTS or mannitol (2.2-27.5 mOsm/kg). Following the experiment, animals were sacrificed and brain water content and lesion size were determined.

RESULTS

In unlesioned animals, decreases in ICP were observed in both mannitol and HTS-treated groups at doses of 5.5 mosm/kg (equil. to 1 gm/kg mannitol). Maximal decreases in ICP occurred following 11.0 mosm. Following acute injury, maximal ICP elevation occurred by 1 hr to a mean of 28.4-30.6 mm Hg between the three groups. Mannitol ($n=28$) caused a maximal decrease in ICP of $31.5\% \pm 2.9\%$ 10-20 min after injection. The duration of effect before ICP returned to pretreatment levels was 97.5 ± 6.7 min. In the HTS group ($n=28$), ICP decreased by $45.6\% \pm 2.7\%$ ($p<0.01$ compared to mannitol) and the effect lasted 280. ± 52.8 min before returning to pretreatment levels ($p<0.01$). Cortical brain water content, although higher in the lesioned hemisphere, did not change significantly following treatment with either mannitol or saline. Neither mannitol nor HTS significantly changed the CVP although the hematocrit was significantly decreased in both. Serum sodium was significantly decreased in the mannitol treated group and significantly increased in the HTS treated groups but both resulted in an increase in serum osmolarity. MAP and arterial blood gas measurements did not vary between groups and remained well within the physiologic range.

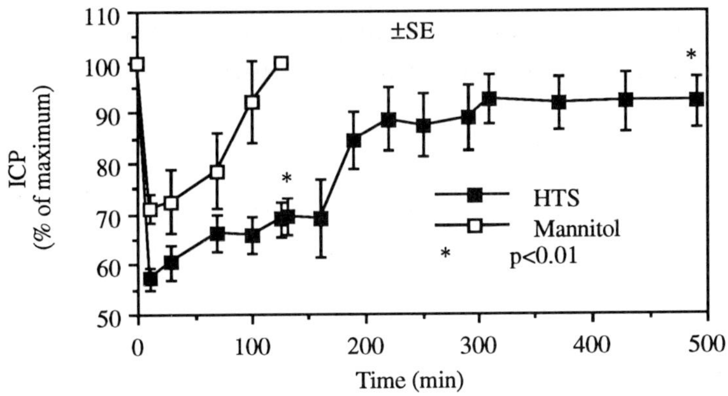

Fig. 1. ICP After Treatment

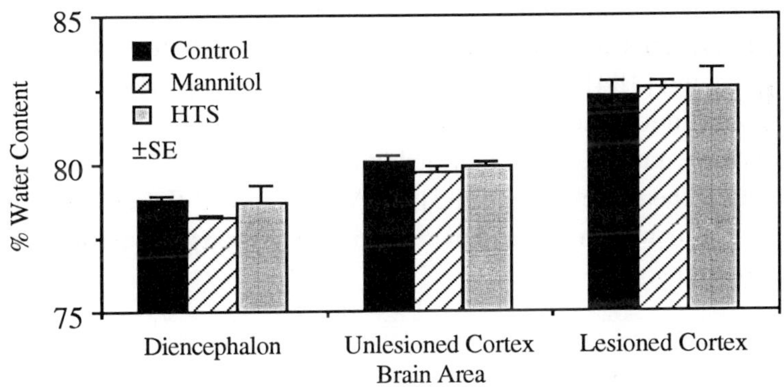

Fig. 2. Percent Water Content by Brain Region

DISCUSSION

In clinically relevant doses, HTS is more effective than mannitol for decreasing elevated ICP in both the magnitude of reduction as well as duration of action. In addition, the reduction of elevated ICP following acute head injury does not correlate with changes in water content. These data support the rationale for the use of hypertonic saline over mannitol for treatment of traumatically-induced elevations in ICP. The mechanism of its effect is not simply via dehydration of brain but is more complex and requires further investigation.

REFERENCES

1. Scheller MS, Zornow MH, Oh YS (1991) A comparison of the cerebral and hemodynamic effects of mannitol and hypertonic saline in a rabbit model of acute cryogenic brain injury. J Neurosurgical Anesthesia 3: 291-296
2. Zornow MH, Scheller MS, Shackford SR (1989) Effect of a hypertonic lactated Ringer's solution on ICP and cerebral water content in a model of traumatic brain injury. J Trauma Vol 29: 484-488
3. Zornow MH, Scheller MS, Todd MM, Moore SS (1988) Acute cerebral effects of isovolemic crystalloid and colloid solutions following cryogenic brain injury in the rat. Anesthesiology 69: 180-184

Prevention of ICP Elevation During Endotracheal Suctioning: Effect of Intravenous Lidocaine

A. YOSHIDA[1], T. SHIMA[2], Y. OKADA[2], and K. YAMANE[2]

Departments of [1] Critical Care Medicine and [2] Neurosurgery, Chugoku Rosai Hospital, 1-5-1 Hiro-Tagaya, Kure, 737-01 Japan

INTRODUCTION

Endotracheal suctioning frequently evokes a prominent cough reflex and resultant intracranial hypertension in patients with reduced intracranial compliance [1][2]. Although muscle relaxants and narcotics successfully prevent the ICP elevation during endotracheal suctioning [3][4], these drugs can not be used if patients had been weaned from controlled ventilation and were spontaneously breathing.

Intravenous lidocaine, known as an anti-arrhythmic agent, potently suppresses cough reflex during endotracheal suctioning [3][5][6]. We examined the effect of intravenous lidocaine on ICP during endotracheal suctioning in sixteen patients who were spontaneously breathing.

MATERIALS AND METHODS

Clinical materials were sixteen patients with intracranial hypertension (nine closed head injuries, four subarachnoid hemorrhages and three intracerebral hemorrhages). The mean age was 49 years and the GCS scores ranged from 3 to 7. All patients were intubated and spontaneously breathing after weaning from controlled ventilation. A frontal epidural transducer was used for monitoring ICP. An indwelling radial artery catheter was placed for measurement of blood pressure and analysis of blood gasses.

We examined the changes in epidural pressure (EDP) during the two successive endotracheal suctionings: one after saline i.v. and the other after lidocaine i.v. First, we suctioned trachea one minute after 5 ml saline i.v. and recorded EDP changes as a control. After the recovery of EDP to its baseline value, we subsequently suctioned trachea one minute after 1.5 mg/kg lidocaine i.v. in the same patient. The two successive suctionings were performed by the same nurse, and trachea was aspirated for 15 seconds following adequate oxygenation. We compared ΔEDP, defined as the peak minus baseline EDP, between the two suctionings.

RESULTS

There was no significant difference between the baseline values of EDP before saline i.v. (31.8 ± 9.3 mmHg) and lidocaine i.v. (31.9 ± 9.5 mmHg) [mean ± SD].
EDP exhibited no significant change following saline i.v., while EDP decreased from 31.9 ± 9.5 mmHg to 25.9 ± 9.1 mmHg one minute after lidocaine i.v. ($p<0.01$).
A prominent cough reflex and EDP elevation was evoked (ΔEDP= 43.9 ± 20.0 mmHg) when trachea was suctioned after saline i.v., whereas cough reflex was markedly suppressed and ΔEDP was reduced to 22.0±12.4 mmHg when endotracheal suctioning was performed after lidocaine i.v. ($p<0.01$).
No statistical difference was observed between the baseline value of $PaCO_2$ (35.0 ± 4.4 mmHg) and the value of $PaCO_2$ one minute after lidocaine i.v. (35.5 ± 5.3 mmHg). The mean arterial pressure decreased from 97.8 ± 12.6 mmHg to 91.6 ± 21.6 mmHg one minute after lidocaine i.v., however there was no statistical difference between the two values. No nuerological deterioration was observed following lidocaine i.v.

DISCUSSION

Our results suggested that intravenous lidocaine could prevent the hazardous ICP elevation during endotracheal suctioning by the two mechanisms: the suppression of cough reflex and the direct reduction in ICP. It was considered that intravenous lidocaine (1.5 mg/kg) was especially useful for patients who are spontaneouly breathing, because lidocaine did not suppress respiratory, circulatory or neurological function.

REFERENCES

1. Fisher DM, Frewen T, Swedlow DB (1982) Increase in intracranial pressure during suctioning-stimulation vs. rise in PaCO2. *Anesthesiology* 57: 416-417
2. Rudy EB, Baun M, Stone K, Turner B (1986) The relationship between endotracheal suctioning and changes in intracranial pressure: A review of the literature. *Heart & Lung*15: 488-494
3. Donegan MF, Bedford RF (1980) Intravenously administered lidocaine prevents intracranial hypertension during endotracheal suctioning. *Anesthesiology*52: 516-518
4. Yano M, Nishiyama H, Yokota H, Kato K, Yamamoto Y, Otsuka T (1986) Effect of lidocaine on ICP response to endotracheal suctioning. *Anesthesiology* 64: 651-653
5. Poulton TJ, James FM (1979) Cough suppression by lidocaine. *Anesthesiology* 50: 470-472
6. Steinhaus JE, Gaskin L (1963) A study of lidocaine as a suppressant of cough reflex. *Anesthesiology* 24: 285

The Effect of Atrial Natriuretic Peptides on Crude and Cultured Endothelial Cells of Cerebral Microvessels

H. NAKAMURA, T. NAGASHIMA, WU S., H. KURATA, H. TOMITA, K. FUJITA, and N. TAMAKI

Department of Neurosurgery, Kobe University School of Medicine, Chuo-ku, Kobe, Hyogo, 650 Japan

SUMMARY

The effect of atrial natriuretic peptide(ANP) on cultured brain capillary endothelial cells was studied by the cyclic guanosine monophosphate(c-GMP) production method. In the cultured endothelial cells, ANP stimulated c-GMP production with concentration dependent manners. In this study, it was recognized that there are ANP receptors on the cultured brain capillary endothelial cells. Cultured brain capillary endothelial cells will provide an excellent model for the investigation of the physiological role of ANP involvement in the volume regulation of the brain.

INTRODUCTION

Atrial natriuretic peptides(ANPs) are a family of peptides which cause natriuresis, diuresis, and vascular smooth-muscle relaxation[1]. ANPs regulate water and electrolyte homeostasis by a series of complex actions. The strong action of ANP on blood vessels and choroid plexus suggests that these peptides play an important role in the volume regulation of the brain. Binding sites of ANP on endothelial cells are identified[3], but it is controversial whether there are ANP receptors on cultured endothelial cells. One of the earliest events following binding of ANP to receptors on target cells is an increase in cyclic guanosine monophosphate(c-GMP) concentration, indicating that this nucleotide is a second messenger of the physiological effects of the hormone[4]. In this study, we established a invitro experimental model to study the effect of ANP on cultured brain capillary endothelial cells.

MATERIALS AND METHODS

(1) The brain capillary endothelial cells were isolated from Sprague-Dawley rats' brain cotices by the method of two step enzymatic treatment and cultured in the collagen-coated dishes.
(2) The cultured brain capillary endothelial cells were identified by positive immunoperoxidase stain of factor VIII and PGI_2 production.
(3) The intracellular c-GMP was measured by enzyme immunoassay after endothelial cells were exposed to various concentrations of rat ANP(8-33).

RESULTS AND DISCUSSION

(1) ANP stimulated c-GMP production in the cultured brain capillary endothelial cells with concentration dependent manners. (Fig. 1)

(2) ANP induced time-dependent increases in c-GMP levels in the cultured brain capillary endothelial cells until 5 minutes and there was no change in c-GMP levels after that. (Fig. 2)

(3) C-type natriuretic peptide(CNP) didn't effect the c-GMP production.

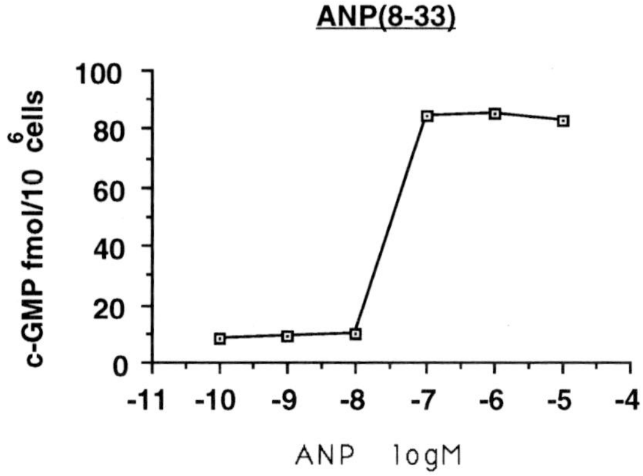

Fig. 1 Relationship between the ANP concentration and the c-GMP level.

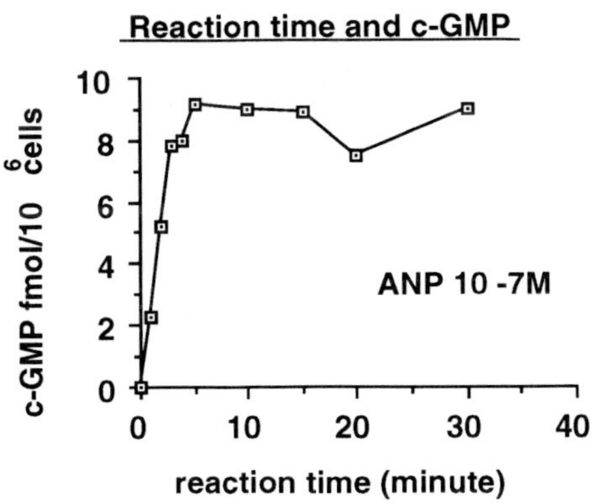

Fig. 2 Relationship between the reaction time and the c-GMP level.

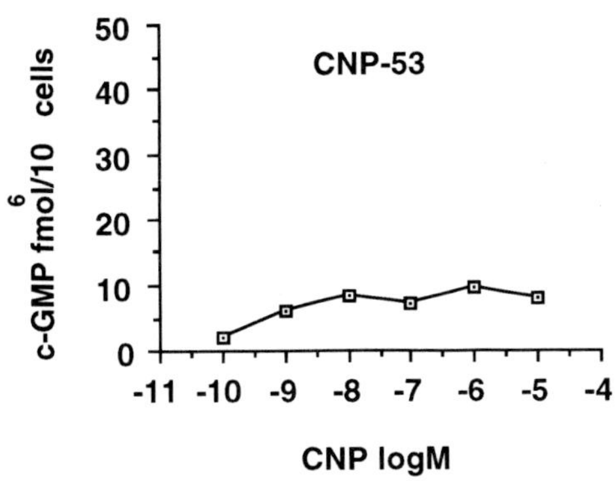

Fig. 3 Relationship between the CNP concentration and the c-GMP level.

Several investigators reported that ANP reduced cold inury or hemorrhagic brain edema[5]. However, the mechanism of brain volume regulation by ANP is still controversial. ANP stimulates the production of the intracellular c-GMP in the cultured brain capillary endothelial cells and choroid plexus, suggesting that these cels must have effects on the volume regulation of the brain. In the cultured endothelial cells, c-GMP production stimulated by ANP suggests the presenc of the ANP receptors. In this study, it was recognized that there are ANP receptors on the cultured brain capillary endothelial cells. Cultured brain capillary endothelial cells well provide an excellent model for the investigation of the physilogical role of ANP involvement in the volume regulation of the brain. Five thousands greater surface area of the brain capillary as compared to regions not protected by the blood-brain-barrier(i.e. choroid plexus) indicated an important role of endothelial cells in the volume regulation of the brain by the central neuro-endocrine system.

REFERENCES

1. Genest J (1986) The atrial natriuretic factor. Br Heart J 56: 302-316
2. Inagami T (1989) Atrial natriuretic factor. J Biol Chem 264: 3043-3046
3. Quirion R (1989) Receptor sites for atrial natriuretic factors in brain and associated structures: an overview. Cell Mol Neurobiol 9: 45-55
4. Beaumont K,Tan PK (1990) Effects of atrial and brain natriuretic peptides upon cyclic GMP levels, potassium transport and receptor binding in rat astrocytes. J Neurosci Res 25: 256-262
5. Nakao N, Itakura T, Yokote H, Nakai K, Komai N (1990) Effect of atrial natriuretic peptide on ischemic brain edema: changes in brain water and electrolytes. Neurosurgery27: 39-44

Cerebral Hemodynamic Effects of Flumazenil

Gabriel P. Lu, Clifford Gevirtz, John A. Gibson Jr., and Carmelo Monell

Department of Anesthesiology, Albert Einstein College of Medicine/Montefiore Medical Center, 1300 Morris Park Avenue, Bronx, NY 10461, USA

INTRODUCTION

Flumazenil (F), a benzodiazepine antagonist, has been reported to reverse the effect of Midazolam.[1] In human volunteers, F (R015-1788) study demonstrates the absence of effect on cerebral blood flow (CBF) with or without Midazolam.[2] Other study in dogs showed F given in the presence of Midazolam may increase cerebrospinal fluid (CSF) pressure and impairing contraction of CSF volume, but the effect is not clinically important.[3] However, there is little information concerning its effect on intracranial hemodynamics. This study is designed to evaluate the effect of F by monitoring changes in internal diameter (ID) of single pial microvessels, intracranial pressure (ICP) mean arterial pressure (MAP), cerebral perfusion pressure (CPP) and regional CBF.

MATERIAL AND METHODS

Fifty female Wistar rats (230-270 gm) were anesthetized with intraperitoneal pentobarbital (25 mg/kg). The femoral arterial pressure was recorded and blood gases and pH maintained within normal limits by controlled ventilation via a tracheostomy. A left parietal craniotomy with an encapsulated cranial window was prepared for biomicroscopy.[4] Changes in arteriolar ID were measured by image shearing. ICP was measured through an outlet port of the cranial window. Percent change of CPP was calculated based on the differences between MAP and ICP. Each rat received intravenous bolus injection of F (0.1, 0.2, 0.3, 0.4, 0.5, 0.6 mg/kg) via cannulated femoral vein with dosing interval of 60 minutes. CBF was measured by a laser Doppler Flowmetry.[5]

RESULTS

Flumazenil at all 6 test doses resulted in transient decreases in MAP (27%, 34%, 39%, 41%, 45%, 46%, $P<0.01$) and CPP (29%, 37%, 42%, 43%, 47%, 48%, $P<0.01$) up to 40 seconds. At 0.1 mg/kg of F, there are no changes in ICP and ID. At doses of 0.2 and 0.3 mg/kg, F significantly increased in ICP (11%, 12%, $P<0.05$) and ID (6%, 8%, $P<0.05$). At higher doses (0.4, 0.5 and 0.6 mg/kg), F also significantly increased in ICP (9.5%, $P<0.05$, 12.3%, 16.9%, $P<0.01$) and ID (10.5%, 13.0%, 13.4%, $P<0.01$). CBF also increased significantly in all doses tested (4.8%, 7.5%, 9.2% $P<0.05$; 11%, 16%, 20% $P<0.01$) (Fig. 1).

DISCUSSION

Our results indicated that under normocapnic conditions, F transiently causes dose related hypotension and decreases in CPP. Also intracranial hypertension and arteriolar dilation as well as increase in CBF are noted at higher doses which is in contrast to Midazolam findings.[6] If the above results can be extrapolated to humans, appropriate hemodynamic support must be given clinically to patients with critical blood brain perfusion.

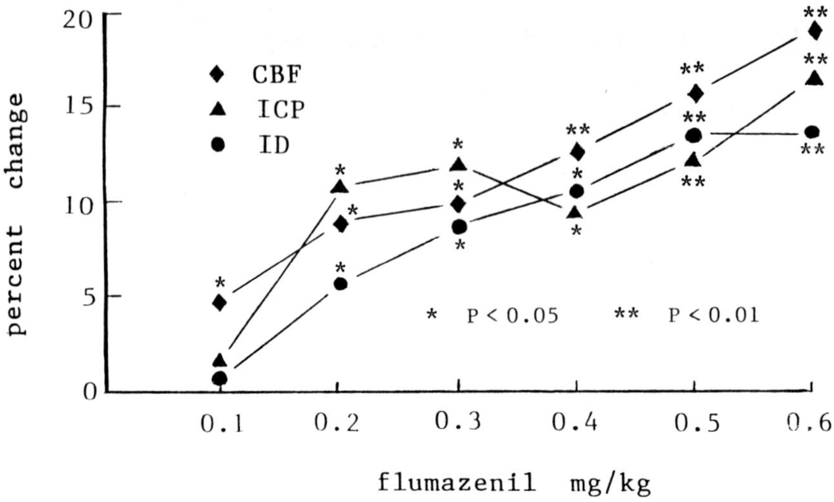

Fig. 1 Represents the changes in arteriolar diameter (ID), intracranial pressure (ICP) and regional cerebral blood flow (CBF) with different doses of Flumazenil.

REFERENCES

1. Sage DJ, Close Ak, Boas RA. (1987) Reversal of midazolam sedation with Anexate. Br J Anaesth 59:459-464
2. Forster A, Juge O, Louis M, Nahory A. (1987) Effects of a specific benzodiazepine antagonist (RO 15-1788) on cerebral blood flow. Intl Anes Res Soc 66:309-13
3. Artru, A. (1990) The rate of CSF formation, resistance to reabsorption of CSF, and aperiodic analysis of the EEG following administration of flumazenil to dogs. Anesthesiology 72:111-117
4. Lu GP, Kaul DK, Feldman SM, Orkin LR, Baez S. (1990) Sodium nitroprusside (SNP) hypotension: intracranial pressure (ICP) and hemodynamics in pial arteriole in the rat. Microcirc Endoth Lymphatics 6:315-341
5. Dirnagl U, Kaplan B, Jacewicz M, Pulsinelli W. (1989) Continuous measurement of cerebral cortical blood flow by laser-Doppler flowmetry in a rat stroke model. J Cerebr Bl Flow and Metabol 9:589-596
6. El-Sheikh AM, Lu GP, Frost EAM, Gibson J, Shamloula MF. (1992) Cerebral microcirculatory effects of midazolam in rat model of intracranial hypertension. Anesthesiology 77:3A, A746

Contribution of Probenecid-Sensitive Anion Transport Processes at the Brain Capillary Endothelium and Choroid Plexus to the Efficient Efflux of Valproic Acid from the Central Nervous System

K.D.K. ADKISON[1], A.A. ARTRU[2], K.M. POWERS[2], and D.D. SHEN[1]

[1] Department of Pharmaceutics, BG-20, School of Pharmacy, [2] Department of Anesthesiology, RN-10, School of Medicine, University of Washington, Seattle, WA, USA

INTRODUCTION

This study examined the relative contribution of the probenecid (PBD)-sensitive transport systems located at the choroid plexus and at the brain capillaries to the overall efflux of valproic acid (VPA) from the CNS of rabbits. The present method involves simultaneous iv infusion of VPA and ventriculocisternal (VC) perfusion with artificial CSF containing the radiotracer ^{3}H-VPA. The kinetic data on VPA concentration in plasma, VC perfusate outflow, and brain tissue were subjected to compartmental modeling to yield estimates of the blood-brain-CSF distribution parameters. Parallel experiments were conducted during co-treatment with PBD to assess the quantitative role of organic anion transporter(s) in the translocation of VPA across the blood-CNS barriers.

METHODS

Sixteen rabbits were anesthetized and surgically prepared for VC perfusion. At the start, rabbits in the control group (n=6) received a priming dose of VPA (7.5 mg/kg) followed by a constant rate iv infusion (125 μg/kg/min) to quickly achieve and maintain a steady-state plasma VPA concentration of approximately 65 μg/ml. Blank VC perfusion was continued for 120 min, at which point it was switched to a mock CSF containing ^{3}H-VPA at a concentration of 0.3 μCi/ml or 6 nM. VC perfusion with ^{3}H-VPA and iv infusion of unlabeled VPA were continued for another 105 min. Serial perfusate samples were collected from the cisternal outflow catheter at 5 min intervals for the first 30 min of each study phase. Thereafter, perfusate outflow was sampled at 15 min intervals. The outflow rate was determined by gravimetric analysis of the perfusate samples. Blood samples were obtained at the midpoint of each perfusate collection interval during the first phase and at the midpoint during the last three perfusate collection intervals of the second phase. Arterial blood samples were centrifuged immediately, and a portion of the plasma was quickly frozen in acetone/dry ice for subsequent VPA protein binding determination. Animals in two PBD-treated groups received identical dual input of VPA via iv infusion and ^{3}H-VPA via VC perfusion. In addition, the animals in the PBD-VCP group (n=4) received PBD in the VC perfusate (200 μl/ml) for the duration of the experiment. Animals in the PBD-IVI group (n=6) received a priming dose of PBD (30 mg/kg) at time zero followed by a continuous iv infusion of PBD (0.5 mg/kg/min) for the duration of the experiment. At the end of each experiment (225 min), the rabbit was euthanized and the brain was immediately removed from the cranium, dissected into halves, rinsed with saline to remove residual perfusate, and frozen in a dry ice/acetone mixture.

RESULTS

In the control group, 59±7% of ^{3}H-VPA in the inflow perfusate was removed during its passage through the ventricles. PBD treatment either by iv infusion or by direct addition to the VC perfusate did not significantly alter the VC extraction of ^{3}H-VPA (56±9, 53±10%, respectively). The mean concentration of ^{3}H-VPA in the ten brain tissue regions was no more than 4% of the estimated average ventricular concentration in all three groups. The steady-state plasma concentrations of VPA did not differ among the three groups. Intravenous infusion of PBD increased the concentration of VPA in all areas of the brain, some by as much as 2-fold (e.g., frontal cortex). In contrast, no significant difference in the mean brain concentrations was observed between the PBD-VCP group and the control group. The steady-state brain-to-plasma concentration ratios were very low, ranging from 0.056 to 0.089 in the control group. The increase in brain-to-total plasma concentration ratio in the PBD-IVI group was statistically significant. A slight, but not statistically significant, increase in the brain-to-total plasma concentration ratio of VPA was observed in the PBD-VCP group. Iv infusion of PBD significantly reduced the rate constant from brain-to-plasma efflux (K_{bo}) by 60% compared with control animals. Iv PBD tended to decrease the rate constants for brain-to-ventricle (K_{bv}) flux and ventricle-to-brain (K_{vb}) flux by 55% (NS) and 32% (NS), respectively. The rate constant for plasma-to-brain flux (K_{pb}) and the ventriculocisternal transit rate constant (K_{out}) remained unchanged by the various treatments. No statistically significant differences were observed between the PBD-VCP group and either of the other two groups. However, the estimates of K_{bo}, K_{bv}, and K_{vb} lay between the estimates for the control and PBD-IVI group, *i.e.*, addition of PBD to VC perfusate did lead to small changes in distribution parameters along the same direction as was observed in the PBD-IVI group.

DISCUSSION

The first major observation of this study was the remarkably high steady-state VC extraction of ^{3}H-labeled VPA (57%) compared to the reported VC extraction of several prototype organic anions, such as para-aminohippurate (17%), thiocyanate (37%), penicillin (40%), and PBD (26%) (present study). Neither iv infusion of PBD nor the addition of PBD to the VC perfusate had a significant effect on the mean VC extraction of ^{3}H-VPA. Another major finding of this study was the significant increase in the brain concentration of unlabeled VPA administered iv when PBD was co-infused. In view of our earlier conclusion that the choroid plexus is not a major site for the efflux of VPA, the elevation in brain tissue concentration of VPA following PBD treatment is best explained by a preferential inhibition of VPA transport from brain into blood. The results of our compartmental modeling are consistent with the preceding proposal of a PBD-sensitive transport of VPA at the capillary endothelium and neural cell membrane. In the PBD-IVI group, the rate constant for brain-to-blood efflux, K_{bo}, decreased by 60% when compared with controls, which strongly supports the idea of inhibition of an efflux pump for VPA at the vascular endothelium. In addition, the rate constants for the exchange of VPA between the brain tissue and the ventricular compartment, K_{bv} and K_{vb}, showed a decrease in the PBD-IVI group, although this change did not reach statistical significance. The translocation of VPA from the tissue sites into the perfusate is a multi-step process involving efflux of VPA from the intracellular sites, diffusion or convective transport through the extracellular space, and, finally, passage across the ependyma.

The Effects of Alfentanil Anaesthesia on Local Cerebral Blood Flow and Intracranial Pressure in the Rat

I.R. Piper, M.J. Souter, P.A.T. Kelly, I.M. Ritchie, D. Weir, P. Andrews, and J.D. Miller

Department of Clinical Neurosciences, Edinburgh, Scotland, UK

Alfentanil is a synthetic opioid analgesic with a shorter half-life and more rapid emergence than its parent compound Fentanyl. These properties are valuable for anaesthesia and sedation. Alfentanil has, however, been reported to cause raised intracranial pressure (ICP) in head injured patients [1]. The mechanism underlying this apparent action is unclear. Reports in the literature on the cerebrovascular effects of Alfentanil conflict. Further study is warranted in view of the current use of Alfentanil within neuro-intensive care for sedation of patients at risk of raised ICP. This paper reports on the effects of Alfentanil anaesthesia on cerebral blood flow (CBF) and ICP in an experimental study in rats.

METHODS

Sprague-Dawley rats (n = 32) were allocated to 2 groups:

Group A contained 3 equal sized (n = 5) subgroups receiving: i) Alfentanil anaesthesia (500 mcg/kg/hr IV), ii) Fentanyl anaesthesia (100 mcg/kg/hr IV) or iii) Chloralose/Urethane anaesthesia (80 mg + 800 mg/kg IP). The Alfentanil and Fentanyl groups included anaesthetic maintenance with intravenous Midazolam (3 mg/kg/hr). Continuous IV anaesthesia was maintained for 50 minutes before measurement of focal CBF using [^{14}C]iodoantipyrine quantitative autoradiography.

Group B received either a sham(n=5) or severe head injury(n=6) using Marmarou's Impact acceleration model of global closed head injury [3]. Animals in this group received Chloralose/Urethane anaesthesia and were instrumented for intraventricular ICP measurement and regional CBF using the hydrogen clearance technique. ICP was then measured before, during and after rapid infusions of 250, 500 and 750 mcg/kg of Alfentanil. CBF was measured before the rapid infusions and then at 30 minute intervals after the start of a subsequent slow intravenous infusion of 500 mcg/kg/hr of Alfentanil. A further group(n = 6) received a severe head injury with no Alfentanil. Mean arterial pressure (MAP) was measured continuously and blood gas samples taken at intervals through a femoral cannula. All animals were paralysed with Pancuronium (2mg/kg), ventilated under positive pressure ($PaCO_2$ 40 - 45 mmHg) and maintained physiologically stable.

RESULTS

Group A: Focal CBF was measured in 11 brain regions. In all brain regions, except brain-stem and sub-cortical white matter, CBF was significantly lower in the Chloralose/Urethane anaesthesia group compared to either the Alfentanil or Fentanyl groups **(TABLE 1)**. There was no significant difference between the Fentanyl and Alfentanil groups CBF in any brain region. When compared with CBF data obtained from similar brain regions in conscious but lightly restrained animals, the focal CBF values during Alfentanil and Fentanyl anaesthesia were not elevated in any brain region compared with the conscious animal.

Group B: Bolus doses of Alfentanil produced rises in ICP and drops in MAP in both sham and injury groups.**(FIGURE 1)** ICP rises were clinically unimportant and were only statistically significant in the sham group. MAP drops in response to rapid i.v. infusion were highly significant throughout. There was no correlation with the dose of Alfentanil. There were no significant differences between the sham and injury groups. Cerebral blood flows were similar for both groups, with no significant differences before and after slow infusion, nor between groups. Further comparison with an injured group receiving no Alfentanil, showed no significant differences in CBF.

DISCUSSION & CONCLUSIONS

The evidence for a direct effect of Alfentanil upon the cerebral vasculature is poor. There have been no direct assessments of CBF. This study has shown that both rapid and slow i.v. infusions of Alfentanil have no significant effect on either global or regional cerebral blood flow. ICP is increased, but not beyond treatment levels. Of more significance is the effect of rapid i.v. infusions of Alfentanil on MAP. This has a greater contribution to decreases in CPP than ICP changes. This is not seen in slow i.v. infusion. We suggest that haemodynamic factors are the important determinant in CPP changes due to Alfentanil, and would not use rapid i.v. infusions in patients with neurotrauma. However slow infusions, as practised for sedation in ITU, appear entirely safe.

REFERENCES

1. Hanowell LH, Thurston JD, Behrman KH, Disbrow E (1993) Alfentanil administered prior to endotracheal suctioning reduces cerebral perfusion pressure. J. Neurosurg. Anaesth. 5:31-35.
2. Marmarou A, Foda M, Van den Brink W, Campbell J, Kita H, Demetradou K (1994) J Neurosurg. 80: 291-300.

Table 1 **Focal CBF vs Anaesthesia Type**

	Anaesthesia Type				
Brain Region Focal CBF (ml/100g/min)	Chloralose	Alfentanil	Fentanyl	Conscious	p
Cerebellum	94±19^{c}	130±21	150±34^{d}	110±26	0.0189
Nucleus Ambiguans	94±18	127±37	145±40	126±19	0.1014
Occipital Cortex	70±15^{c,d}	122±36^{d}	141±42	184±57	0.0041
Temporal Cortex	71±15^{b,c,d}	139±37	127±27	252±47^{b,c}	0.0001
CA2 Hippocampus	62±15^{b,c,d}	96±22	92±23	100±17	0.0309
Dentate Hippocampus	55±15^{b,c,d}	88±16	84±23	96±23	0.0356
CA1 Hippocampus	56±14^{b,c,d}	98±20	92±23	93±19	0.0132
Sensori-Motor Cortex	83±20^{b,c,d}	157±38	160±38	202±67	0.0052
Lateral Striatum	101±20$^{b,c.}$	188±57	177±46	136±18	0.0118
Medial Striatum	64±26	99±9	116±39^{a}	90±12	0.0323
Corpus Callosum	28±9	39±20	46±11	42±8	0.2069

Anova: Duncans: The effect of anaesthetic type on CBF

Note: Multiple range tests:
a=sign. diff. from chloralose; b=sign. diff from alfentanil; c=sign. diff. from fentanyl; d=sign. diff. from concsious

Figure 1 **Alfentanil ± Head Injury: Effect upon ICP and MAP**

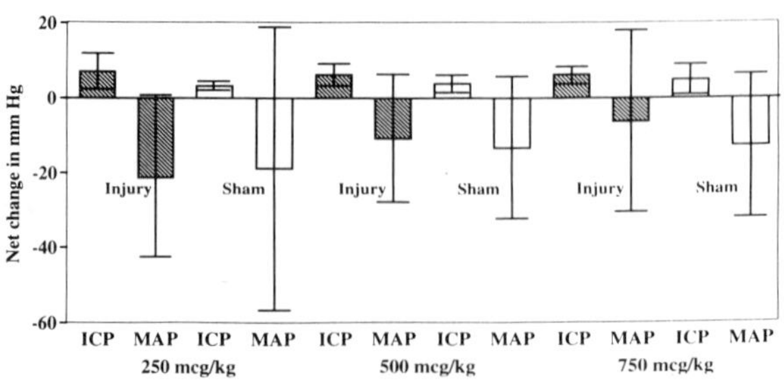

Delayed Impairment of Cerebral Perfusion Pressure After Head Injury: Role of Infection and Sepsis

ALBERTO BIESTRO[1], MARIO CANCELA[1], RICARDO ALBERTI[2], HORACIO PANZARDO[1], and BERNARDO BOROVICH[2]

[1] Intensive Care Unit, [2] Department of Neurosurgery, Hospital de Clínicas, Montevideo, Uruguay

INTRODUCTION.

In clinical field, intracranial pressure (ICP) monitoring with subdural methods (screw or catheter) have shown to be reliable and safe with very low risk of infection [1]. Consequently, we and other investigators have extended the duration of ICP for longer than five days. Under these circumtances, it has been possible to study different patterns of the temporal course of ICP after head injury [2]. Severe infection or sepsis are not infrequent delayed complications of head injury. They might influence long term ICP course. The purpose of this clinical study was to determine the effects of infection, other than cranial, and sepsis on ICP and cerebral perfusion pressure (CPP) after head injury.

Material and Methods

Between June 1989 and December 1993, 80 severely closed head injuries (Glasgow Coma Scale score <8) were admitted to our unit. Of this group, 8 patients were identified that developed severe respiratory infection during ICP monitoring. Their ages ranged from 15 to 69, with a mean of 35. Cranial computed tomogrphy (CT) were performed in all cases at admission and posteriorly according to clinical and ICP evolution. Mean arterial pressure (MAP), was measured by intraarterial cannula. Mean ICP was monitorized by subdural methods. The mean duration of ICP monitoring was 7.6 days with a range of 6 to 10 days, beginning between the first and fifth day postrauma with a mean of 2.2 days. MAP and Mean ICP recordings were taken from hourly measurement on the bedside monitor by a nurse according to Coma Data Bank methodology [3]. CPP was calculated from the above parameters. Daily highest rectal ttemperature (RT) were recorded. A modified therapeutic intensity level (TIL) [4], was used. Indomethacin was scored 2, like hiperventilation < 30 mm Hg. A vasopressor index (VI) was created to assess the need of vasocontrictor (Table 1).

Table 1. VASOPRESSOR INDEX.

DRUG	DOSE	SCORE
Dopamina	< 36 mg/h	1
	36-72 mg/h	2
	>72 mg/h	3
Nora or adrenalina	< 1 mg/h	2
	1-2 mg/h	3
	> 2 mg/h	4

Infection was demonstrated in all cases by bacteriologic studies. In four of these patients a Swan-Ganz catheter was inserted. All showed a septic pattern: high cardiac output, low arterial resistance and low oxygen consumption. ICP, CPP, TIL, VI, and RT were studied the day before and the day after that infection was suspected. This time was named zero time in the evolution of each patient. Daily mean value of each variable was taken. Comparison between both group of values before and after zero time ware tested by t test. P values less than 0.05 were considered statistically significant.

Results.

Respiratory infection was initially suspected between 72 and 168 hours, with a mean of 93 hours postrauma in these patients. Figure 1 shows our findings.

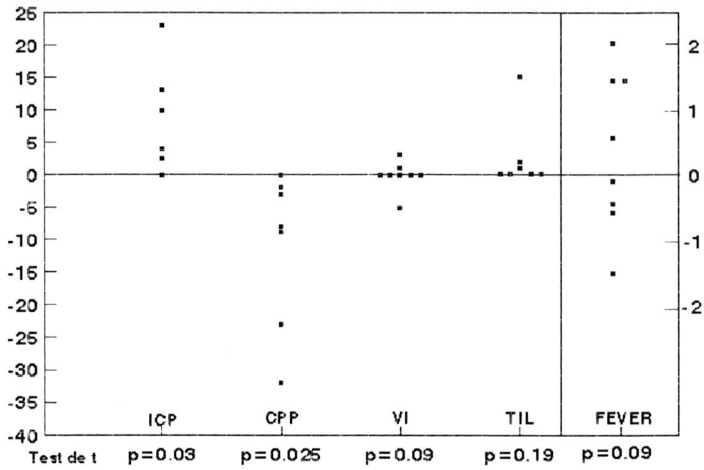

Figure 1. Illustration showing the change of each variable analysed at zero time. The values are: mm Hg for ICP and CPP, absolute values for TIL and VI and °C for RT.

In all cases a mass lesion was discarded by CT. No one case had hypoxemia < 60 mm Hg or hyponatremia. Four patients died from sepsis with uncontrollable ICP. Four patients survived and improved with control of infection.

Discussion.

No other fector but infection could be recognized as a cause of delayed changes in intracranial dynamics of our patients. These findings are different from Unterberg`s [2] who could not demonstrate infection in his patients with secondary rise of ICP and hyperleukocytosis. Although fever has been identified as a factor increasing ICP [5], the temperature changes were very variable and not significative to be the explanation. As well as Maset [4], developed TIL to assess ICP course, and Tsutsumi [6] , showed that different MAP with identical ICP do not represent similar conditions of ICP, we consider necessary to create the VI to compare CPP better. As a group, our patients showed, around the fourth day, a secondary rise of ICP with important deterioration of CPP. The absence of a significant change in TIL and VI may be due to low resolution of these variables and because some patients showed persistent ICP increase from the start. The important changes in vascular reactivity induced by sepsis could be the most prtobable explanation to our findings [7]. However the response of intracranial dynamics can not follow the same pattern, depending upon early or late stage of the sepsis. We conclude that infection or sepsis after head injury should be considered as a cause of persistent ICP increase or secondary rise of ICP around the fourth day, above all when there are in addition deterioration of CPP and a mass lesion is discarded by CT. These findings preceded the confirmation of infection.

References.

1 Aucoin PJ, Kitilainen HR, Gantz NM et al, (1986) Intracranial Pressure Monitors. Epidemiologic study of Risk Factors and Infections. Am J Med 80: 369-376.

2 Unterberg A, Kiening K, Schmiedek P, et al, (1993) Long Term Observations of Intracranial Pressure after Head Injury. The Phenomenon of Secondary Rise of Intracranial Pressure. Neurosurgy 32: 17-24.

3 Marmarou A, Anderson RL, Ward JD, et al; (1991) NINDS traumatic Coma Data Bank: Intracranial Pressure Monitoring Methodology. J Neurosurgery 75 (Suppl): S21-S27.

4 Maset AL, Marmarou A, Ward JD, et al, (1987) Pressure-Volume Index in Head Injury. J Neurosurgery 67: 832-840.

5 Malkinson TJ, Veale WL, Cooper KE (1993) Intracranial Pressures and Fever in the Rat, Rabbit and Cat. In: CJJ Avezaat (Ed) Intracranial Pressure VIII Springer, BErlin, pp 198-202.

6 Tsutsumi H, Ide K, Mizutani T, et al (1986) The Relationship betwwen Intracranial Pressure, Cerebral Perfusion Pressure and Outcome in Head-Injured Pateints: The Critical Level of Cerebral perfusion. Pressure In: Miller JD, Teasdale GM, Rowan JO, et al, (Eds) Intracranial Pressure VI, Springer- Verlag pp 661-666.

7 Sibbald WJ, Fox G, Martin C (1991) Abnormalities of Vascular Reactivityin the Sepsis Syndrome. Chest 100 (Suppl) 3, 155S-159S.

Changes of ICP, CBF-Velocities and Systemic Hemodynamics After Raising of the Upper Trunk in Neurointensive Care Patients

G. CUNITZ and W. SCHREGEL

Department of Anesthesia and Intensive Care, Knappschaftskrankenhaus Ruhr-University, D-44892 Bochum, Germany

Introduction

Treatment of neuro-intensive care patients with increased intracranial pressure (ICP) requires some elevation of the upper trunk. Postural changes of that kind reach a limit when no further ICP reductions can be achieved and cerebral perfusion pressure (CPP) may be reduced to a critical level. By using a transcranial doppler device it is possible to investigate the cerebral circulation in that situation.

Clinical Material and Methods

After approval of the Ethic Commitee of the university in 10 sedated patients of our ICU, suffering from various cerebral diseases (GCS <7 points), in 9 cases mechanically ventilated, changes of ICP (Gaeltec ICTB), BP (blood pressure), CPP, HF (heart frequency) and mean maximum blood flow velocity v (EME TC 2/64) in the middle cerebri artery (MCA) were studied after raising the upper trunk to 30° and 60° from horizontal. Also the pulsatility index (PI) was calculated. 8 healthy volunteers served as controls for v, PI and BP and HF. A paired t-test (Wilcoxon) was used for statistics.

Results

An elevation of the patients (s.fig.) from 0 to 30° produced an effective ICP drop from 25.6 +/- 5.7 to 18.5 +/- 6.1 mmHg (x +/- SEM, P <0.01) and to 15.6 +/- 5.7 when going on to 60°. Mean BP, calibrated to the level of acoustic meatus, changed from 95 +/- 5 to 89 +/- 5 (P <0.05) and finally to 83 +/- 5, whereas CPP remained nearly constant (>65 mmHg) HF did not change. v in MCA fell significantly from 49.6 +/- 4.8 cm/sec (horizontal) to 44.3 +/- 4.5 (30°) P <0.05 and finally to 42 +/- 4.4. PI ranged from 3.4 to 3.7 and to 3.8. In the controls v showed some tendency to drop, from 41.4 (0°) to 36 maximum after 60°.The differences, however, could not be verified. PI did not change (2.4.-2.3-2.4) BP clearly fell if an ear was chosen as zero point, HF did not show significant increases.

Discussion

Providing that the diameters of the basal cerebral arteries remain nearly constant, and there is a lot of evidence that they do under various conditions, changes in blood flow velocities to a certain degree reflect concomitant blood flow alterations. Based on these results it can be assumed that, when raising a patient with cerebral disorders, cerebral blood flow (CBF) may be depressed to some degree. Our supposition is that in our controls some quick way of compensation occured, because autoregulation was intact.Feldman and coworkers (1), however, were unable to demonstrate alterations in real CBF (Kety-Schmidt N2O technique) when elevating head injured patients to 30°. Improved venous outflow from the brain and a redistribution of cerebrospinal fluid are the main reasons why postural changes have an ICP lowering effect.Our results also showed that a position of 30° resulted in an effective ICP drop and that continuing to 60° had only a slightly greater effect.Rosner and Coley (2), however, do not recommend head elevation, because a CPP reductuion may stimulate pressure waves.Yoshida et al (3) stressed that changes of CPP may be different in each patient. In conclusion: When raising a neurointensive care patient`s upper trunk, especially when going on to more than 30°, it seems useful to monitor brain blood supply. This can easily be done by a transcranial doppler.

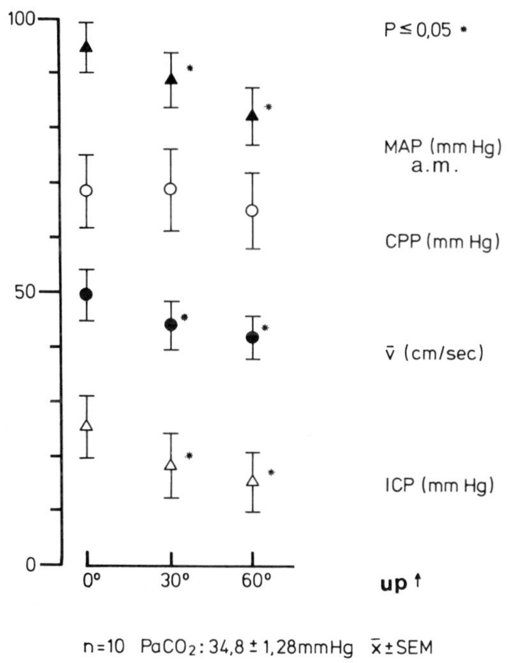

Fig.
Raising of the upper trunk of ICU patients from horizontal to 60° produced a drop in mean blood pressure(MAP, zeropoint acoustic meatus), mean maximum blood flow velocity in MCA (v) and intracranial pressure (ICP). Cerebral perfusion pressure (CPP) did not change significantly.

References

1. Feldmann Z, Kanter MJ, Robertson CS, Contant CF, Hayes C, Steinberg MA, Villareal CA, Narayan RK, Grossman RG (1992) Effect of head elevation on intracranial pressure, cerebral perfusion pressure, and cerebral blood flow in head-injured patients.J Neurosurg 76:207-211.
2. Rosner MJ, Coley IB (1986) Cerebral perfusion pressure, intracranial pressure, and head elevation. J Neurosurg 65:636-641.
3.Yoshida A, Shima T,Okada Y, Yamada T, Kurino H (1993)Effects of postural changes on epidural pressure and cerebral perfusion pressure in patients with serious intracranial lesions. In:Avezaat CJJ, van Eijndhoven JHM, Maas AIR, Tans JTHJ (eds) Intracranial Pressure VIII. Springer.Berlin Heidelberg. pp433-436.

Experimental Study on Motor Evoked Potential with Increased Intracranial Pressure

M. KUSUNOSE, M. NISHIJIMA, M. NISHIKATA, N. HAYASHI, and A. TAKAKU

Department of Neurosurgery, Toyama Medical and Pharmaceutical University, Sugitani, Toyama, Japan

SUMMARY

Motor evoked potential (MEP) and pathological change were investigated during acute progressive elevation of intracranial pressure (ICP) in 20 anesthetized dogs. Various degree of ICP was observed by extradural balloon inflation for a certain period of time. ICP and MEP were monitored while the balloon was inflated or deflated.

The short latency response (D-response) and the following two responses (I-responses) were observed in MEP. When ICP increased, the latency of I-responses was delayed more significantly than that of D-response, and they did not recovered rapidly. If ICP is between 40-60 mmHg, D-response disappeared when balloon was inflated but reappeared after balloon was deflated. Various degree of morphological damage was correlated with the recovery of D-response.

I. Introduction

Motor evoked potential (MEP) monitoring is a relatively new technique to assess motor function. The purpose of this experimental study was to assess MEP changes related to various degrees of intracranial hypertension. Furthermore, correlations between electrophysiological changes and morphological change were evaluated after return to the baseline pressure level.

II Material and method

A)***Anesthesia*** thiopental sodium under artificial respiration with pancronium

B)***Condition of stimulation & recording of MEP***

stimulation area	motor cortex		recording electrode	C3
	intensity	7mA	reference electrole	paravertebral muscle
	duration	0,2msec	bandpass	10-3000Hz
	frequency	5Hz		
	repetition	200		

C)***The method to increased ICP*** A latex balloon was inserted into the left temporal extradural region, and ICP was monitored at the contralateral side(FIG.1.). Various degree of ICP was produced with gradual balloon inflation for less than three minutes, and it was kept for various period of time. Then the balloon was deflated quickly.

D) ***Materials*** Mild compression group (<40mmHg)--- 6 dogs
Moderate compression group(40-60mmHg)---9 dogs
Severe compression group(>60mmHg)---5 dogs

FIG.1. Schematic drawing of experiment

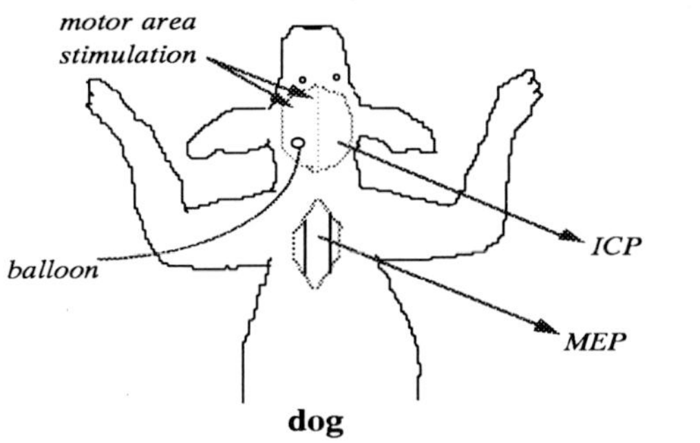

FIG.2. Alteration in MEP

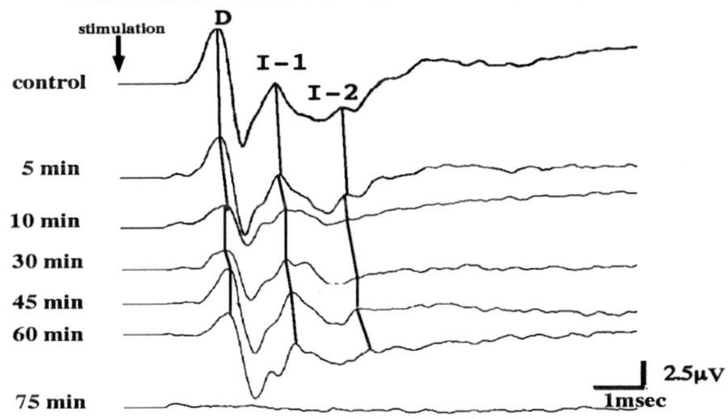

Ⅲ Result

A) ***Typical MEP wave form*** (FIG. 2.)

MEP recorded from the epidural space of the spinal cord. D-response (D) and two I-responses (I-1,I-2) were observed. Peak latency, from stimulus onset to peaks, was measured. Mean latency of D, I-1 or I-2 before inflation was 2.11, 3.44 or 4.80msec, respectively .

In this case, D and I-response were suppressed during compression, subsequently disappeared 75 minutes after the initiation of compression.

B) ***Sequential change of MEP amplitude***(FIG.3.)

mild compression

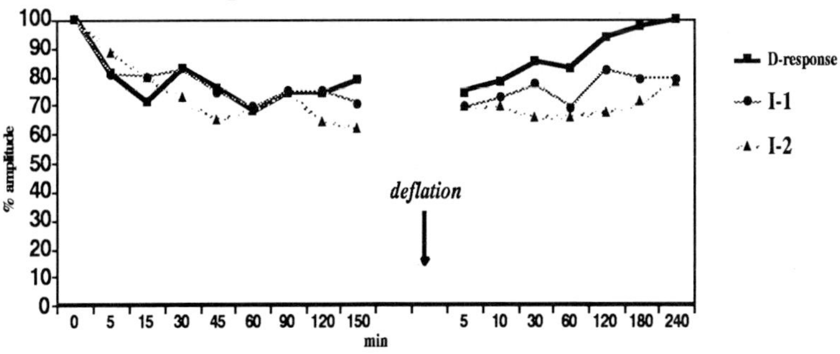

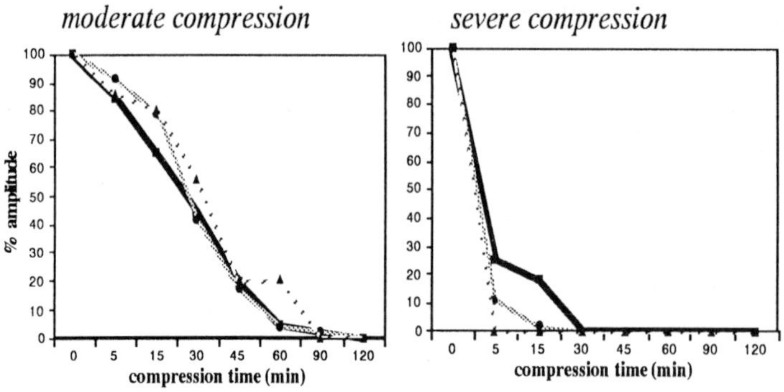

During mild compression, D, I-1 and I-2 wave were only suppressed but not disappeared. During moderate and severe compression, each wave was disappeared.

They recovered after the decompression in order of the mild, moderate and severe compression. The recovery of D-response was more rapid than those of I-responses.

C)*Sequential change of MEP latency* (FIG. 4.)

FIG.4 Sequential changes of MEP latency in *mild* compression group

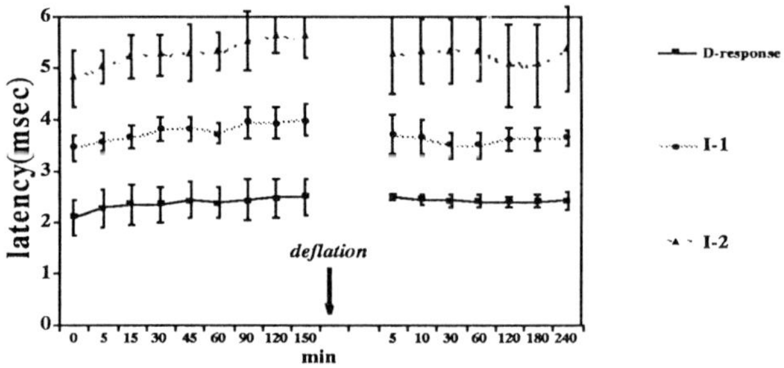

During mild compression, the latency of I-responses was more significantly delayed than that of D-response. After decompression, they did not recovered rapidly. During moderate and severe compression, the latency of each wave was significantly delayed, and all waves disappeared.

D)*Correlation between absent time of D-response and recovery ratio* (FIG. 5.)

Fig. 5. Correlation between absent time of D-response and recovery ratio

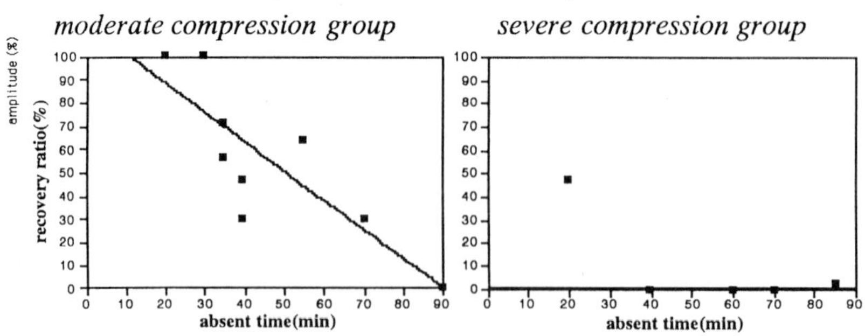

The absent time means the period from disappearance of the wave to balloon deflation. Recovery ratio means percent change of amplitude four hours after deflation.

In mild compression group, D-response was suppressed, but never disappeared and recovered completely.

In moderate compression group, if absent time was short, the amplitude of D-response sufficiently recovered. In severe compression group, it did not sufficiently recovered.

E)*Morphological change*

A: Mild compression group. No marked change.

B: Moderate compression group, in which D-response sufficiently recovered after deflation. Various degree of subcortical petechial hemorrhages were observed on the side of compression.

C: Moderate and severe compression group, in which D-response did not sufficiently recovered after deflation. Severe intracerebral hematomas were observed.

Ⅳ Conclusion

Our data suggest that observation of the MEP wave form is a useful method to anticipate the following brain dysfunction after the insult by intracranial hypertension.

V References

1) Amassian VE, Stewart M, Quirk GJ, Rosenthal JL: Physiological bases of motor effects of a transient stimulus to cerebral cortex. Neurosurg 20: 74-93, 1987

2) Hoerlein BF: Canine Neurology. Chapter2 Anatomy and physiology. W.B.Saunders company: 7-52, 1978

3) Nagao S, Roccaforte P, Moody RA: Acute intracranial hypertention and auditory brain stem responses. Part 1: Change in the auditory brain stem and somatosensory evoked responses in intracranial hypertention in cats. J. Neurosurg 51: 669-676, 1979

4) Patton HD, Amassian VE: Single multiple unit analisis of cortical stage of pyramidal tract activation. J. Neurophysiol 17: 345-357,1954

5) Shimoji K, Higashi H, Kano T: Epidural recording of spinal electogram in man. Electroenceph. Clin. Neurophysiol. 30:236-239, 1971

6) Stone JL, Ghaly RF, Subramanian KS, Roccaforte P, Kane J: Transtentorial brain herniation in the monkey : Analysis of brain stem auditory and somatosensory evoked potentials. Neurosurgery 26: 26-31, 1990

7) Tsubokawa T, Katayama Y: Cortical direct (D) response in humans. Rinsho Noha 29:510-516, 1987

Cerebral Hemodynamic Reserve During Nursing Procedures

N. Stocchetti[1], M. Barbagallo[1], C. Mattioli[1], A. Paparella[1], and P. Mainini[2]

[1] First Department of Anesthesia and Intensive Care, Hospital of Parma, Italy
[2] Division of Neurosurgery, Hospital of Parma, Italy

Introduction

One of the main goals of intensive care for head injured patients is the preservation of an adequate cerebral perfusion. Perfusion is a function of cerebral perfusion pressure (CPP) but recently it has been suggested that a normal or even high CPP does not imply adequate coupling of flow to the cerebral metabolic rate of oxygen consumption [2]. During routine nursing procedures such as suctioning, some reduction of CPP is often unavoidable. This may lead to a situation of impending ischemia which may be detected by measuring the Cerebral Hemodynamic Reserve (CHR)[1]. We have investigated CHR during routine nursing in order to 1) detect and minimise potentially dangerous situations of cerebral ischemia 2) identify the relationships between CHR and other clinical parameters such as ICP, CPP and Cerebral Extraction of Oxygen (CEO_2).

Methods

20 head injured patients, 3 female, with a mean age of 40.6 years (14-64), were included in the study. Mean admission motor Glasgow Coma Score was 3.15 (sd 1.56). CT scan showed 4 cases of epidural hematoma, 8 subdural hematomas, and 8 contusions. All patients were artificially ventilated. ICP was recorded through a ventricular catheter in 11 cases, and through a subdural catheter in the remaining patients. In cases monitored through ventricular catheters Pressure Volume Index (PVI) was determined twice a day using the bolus technique [4].
CEO_2 was measured as the difference between arterial (SaO_2) and jugular oxyhemoglobin saturation (SjO_2) sampling blood from the radial artery and from the jugular bulb of the right internal jugular vein (the position of the catheter was confirmed by radiological examination). Arterial and venous hemoglobin saturations were measured using a Co-Oxymeter (Instrumentation Laboratory 482 Co-Oximeter). In sixteen patients artero-jugular difference of lactate (AJDL) was measured using a discrete clinical analyzer (ACA IV Dupont Medical Products).
Twice a day, during scheduled suctioning and cleaning of patients, CHR was tested in case of reduction of CPP caused by ICP rise [3]. CHR was determined according to the following equation:

$$CHR=[(CEO_2 \text{ after nursing} - CEO_2 \text{ baseline})/CEO_2 \text{ baseline}]/[(CPP \text{ after nursing} - CPP \text{ baseline})/CPP \text{ baseline}]$$

By definition, a preserved reserve is indicated by a positive number, while an exhausted reserve is detected where negative values occur. After baseline sampling, the second couple of blood samples was obtained at least five minutes later, allowing time for changes in CBF to be reflected in IJ saturation measurements [3]. CEO_2 after nursing was corrected according to the CO_2 measured at the baseline by assuming a 3% change in CEO_2 per mmHg change in arterial CO_2 tension. Mean comparisons were calculated using the Student t-test and a one-way ANOVA when necessary. Correlation was assessed calculating the Pearson Product-Moment value.

Results

Mean ICP was 24 mmHg (sd 9.7) while mean CPP was 73 mmHg (sd 13). Mean CEO_2 was 30 Vol % (sd 11).
CHR was tested 92 times, the average value was -0.91 (sd 6.65). Only two patients demonstrated a

preserved CHR during all measurements and seven had a mean value of CHR greater than zero. The time course of CHR showed the worst values during the fourth and fifth day after trauma, while ICP and CPP were more severely disturbed during the third day.
There was no correlation between CHR and GCS, ICP or CPP.
Six patients with a PVI lower than 15 ml had a mean CHR of -0.75 (sd 1.88), while the others had a mean value of -0.09 (sd 5.8) (not significant).
We hypothesized that in cases of reduced CBF, as suggested by a wide CEO_2, CHR would be less effective than in cases with normal CBF. In the former situation, in fact, maximal vasodilation of the cerebral vessels may occur and, therefore, a reduced capability of further increasing the vascular diameter is suspected. The scatterplot shows mean data of CHR against CEO_2. By subdividing patients according to outcome, a good correlation between the two variables is found for patients with good recovery (GR) or moderate disability (MD) (Correlation coefficent of 0.95) while no correlation is detected for patients with poor outcome. The chart suggests that in patients with GR or MD a reduction of CHR is associated with an increase of CEO_2.

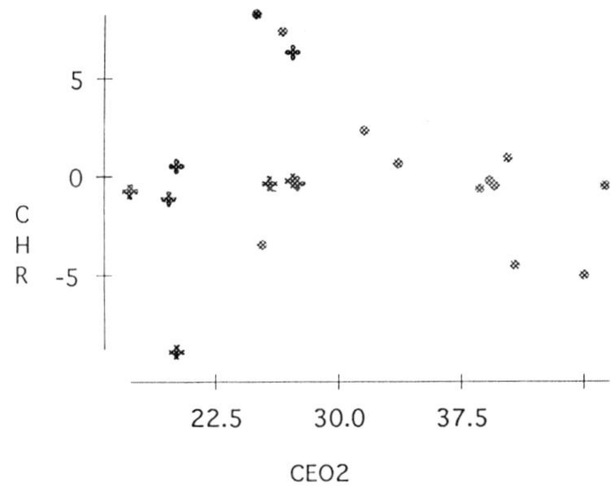

Fig. 1: Mean values of corrected Cerebral Hemodynamic.Reserve.(CHR) against mean values of Cerebral Extraction of Oxygen (CEO_2) are plotted. Patients with good outcome are showed as filled circles while patients with poor outcome are indicated by crosses.

The mean AJDL measured during reduced or abolished hemodynamic reserve was -0.13 (sd 0.1), while in cases of preserved CHR, mean AJDL was 0.06 (sd 0.1)($p<0.01$)
Six months after trauma, twelve patients showed a favourable outcome (good recovery or moderate disability), five were still severely disabled and three died. Mean CHR in patients with good outcome was 0.37 (sd 3.9), while in patients with poor outcome it was 1.20 (sd 2.9); patients who died showed a mean CHR of -3.36 (sd 4.7). These differences were not significant.

Discussion

During routine nursing procedures reductions of CPP are common and probably dangerous. In cases of adequate autoregulation patients may accomodate for reduction of CPP as showed by a stable level of CEO_2. Patients with impaired autoregulation, instead, may present episodes of cerebral ischemia. Since one of the main goals of intensive treatment is the avoidance of such a situation, detection of patients at risk of suffering from nursing-induced cerebral ischemia is of paramount importance. That may be achieved measuring CHR.
The occurrence of reduced CHR is quite high, since only two patients in 20 showed a normal CHR in each study. Patients with reduced intracranial compliance, as indicated by a PVI < 15 ml, had a CHR lower than patients with greater PVI. The time course of CPP and ICP was not correlated with the values of CHR, which, therefore, may not be estimated by looking at these two parameters.
CHR is inversely proportional to CEO_2 in patients with good recovery and moderate disability. When it is measured in patients with poor outcome there is no correlation with pressure autoregulation, probably because low CEO_2 values in these cases are more related to a reduced $CMRO_2$ than to a true increase of

CBF. During episodes of inadequate CHR, cerebral production of lactate was detected, suggesting anaerobic cerebral metabolism.

In conclusion, CHR can be easily measured at the patient's bedside and is an inexpensive way of assessing autoregulation. When CHR is abnormal a nursing technique capable of preserving CPP is mandatory.

References

1. Cruz J, Miner ME, Allen SJ, Alves WM, Gennarelli TA (1991) Continuous monitoring of cerebral oxygenation in acute brain injury: assessment of cerebral hemodynamic reserve. Neurosurgery 29:743-749.

2. Cruz J, Raps E,Hoffstad O, Jaggi JL, Gennarelli TA (1993) Cerebral Oxygenation monitoring. Crit Care Med 21:1242-1246

3. Fortune JB, Feustel JP, Weigle CGM, Popp, AJ (1994) Continuous measurement of jugular venous oxygen saturation in response to transient elevation of blood pressure in head-injured patients. J Neurosurg 80:461-468

4. Maset AL, Marmarou A, Ward JD, Choi S, Luts HA, Brooks D, Moulton RJ, Desalles A, Muizelaar JP, Turner H, Young HF (1987) Pressure-volume index in head injury. J Neurosurg 67:832-840

CO_2-Reactivity, Autoregulation and Hemodynamic Reserve in the First 24 Hours After Severe Head Injury: Bedside Assessment by Relative Changes in $AVDO_2$

J. SAHUQUILLO[1], M.A. POCA[1], A. GARNACHO[2], A. ROBLES[2], A. CHASAMPI[2], E. CANDELA[3], and E. RUBIO[1]

[1] Department of Neurosurgery, [2] Neurotraumatology Intensive Care Unit and [3] Anesthesiology, Vall d'Hebron University Hospital, Barcelona, Spain

When cerebral metabolic rate of oxygen ($CMRO_2$) is constant, changes in arterio-jugular differences of oxygen ($AVDO_2$) reflect changes in CBF. Our aims in this paper are to use relative changes in $AVDO_2$ after manipulations of mean arterial blood pressure and arterial pCO_2 to assess CO_2-reactivity and autoregulation in severe head injury patients.

PATIENTS AND METHODS

In 48 consecutive severe head injury patients (post-resuscitation prehospital or admission GCS ≤ 8) with a mean age of 30 $\pm$ 18.4 years and a diffuse brain injury, cerebrovascular response to changes in pCO_2 was tested within the first 24 hours after injury. In 28 of the above mentioned cases autoregulation was also assessed. After admission, a catheter was inserted in the internal jugular bulb and $AVDO_2$ calculated by the following equation: $AVDO_2 = 1.34 \times Hb\,[SaO_2 - SjO_2]$. To test CO_2-reactivity arterial and jugular blood samples were extracted to establish baseline values for pCO_2 and $AVDO_2$. Manipulations in the ventilator settings were made to change the basal arterial pCO_2. After 15 minutes of the ventilator manipulations, $AVDO_2$ were recalculated. Two different indexes were used: 1) Absolute CO_2-reactivity (**CO_2R_{ABS}**) and 2) Percentage reactivity (**CO_2R %**). **CO_2R %** is the percentage increase or decrease of estimated CBF per mm Hg change in pCO_2. Pressure reactivity coefficient to changes in arterial pCO_2 (PRC_{CO2}) was also calculated as the change in steady state ICP per torr change in arterial pCO_2 [1]. Patients with $CO_2R_{\%}$ above 1 % were considered to be in the intact CO_2-reactivity group and patients in whom $CO_2R_{\%}$ was below or equal to 1 % were included in the impaired/abolished CO_2-reactivity group. To test autoregulation phenylephrine was used to increase MABP by about 25 %. Arterial and jugular blood samples were obtained before and after increase of MABP. All $AVDO_2$ values were corrected for changes in pCO_2. The percent change of $1/AVDO_2$ relative to the resting value was evaluated. In those patients in whom rising MABP provoked an increase of ICP, cerebral hemodynamic reserve (**CHR**) was calculated by a modification of Cruz's method and according to the following equation : $(AVDO_2H - AVDO_2B)/AVDO_2B$ [2]. According to Enevoldsen's criteria [3], those patients with changes in $1/AVDO_2$ less than or equal to 20 % were included in the intact autoregulation group. Patients with CBF changes above 20 % were classified in the impaired autoregulation group.

---

[1] **Supported by Grants 93/1257 and 94/0688 from the Fondo de Investigaciones Sanitarias de la Seguridad Social (FISS).**

RESULTS

The mean age of our series was 28 ± 16.7 years. The mean absolute induced change in arterial pCO_2 was 4.6 ± 2.4 mm Hg. The results of CO2R% are plotted in **Fig.1.** According to the above mentioned criteria, only 5 cases (12.8 %) presented an impaired/abolished CO_2 reactivity. The mean change in MABP in the patients in whom autoregulation was tested, was 26 ± 9.5 mm Hg. In 12 patients (43 %) changes in estimated CBF were below the 20 % margin defined to consider autoregulation as intact. In the remaining 16 patients (57 %) autoregulation was impaired. In 15 of the 28 cases ICP increased when increasing BP. Nevertheless, in all but 2 cases the net result was an increase of the CPP. Only one patient had a compromised CHR. Of the 28 cases, CO_2-reactivity was impaired in 5 and all patients with an impaired CO_2-reactivity also had an impaired autoregulation.

DISCUSSION

The approach of using $AVDO_2$ as an estimate of CBF changes, has been widely used by different authors and recently put forward as an accepted and reliable method to study the effects of drugs on autoregulation [4]. According to our criteria, only 12.8 % of the studied patients presented an impaired CO_2-reactivity in the first 24 hours after injury. Following the above-mentioned criteria, 57 % of our series had an impaired/abolished autoregulation. Our data are in agreement with other studies in that autoregulation is a very vulnerable mechanism and that impaired autoregulation is highly prevalent in head injury. Monitoring relative changes in $AVDO_2$ permits the reliable study of CO_2-reactivity and autoregulation at the bedside. This can increase our knowledge of these parameters and their dynamic changes in the evolution of the head injury patient. Introducing these variables on a day-to-day management basis should be considered in the treatment protocols. A consensus of the range of normality for CO_2-reactivity and autoregulation would be desirable in order to standardize methods and to compare patients from different series.

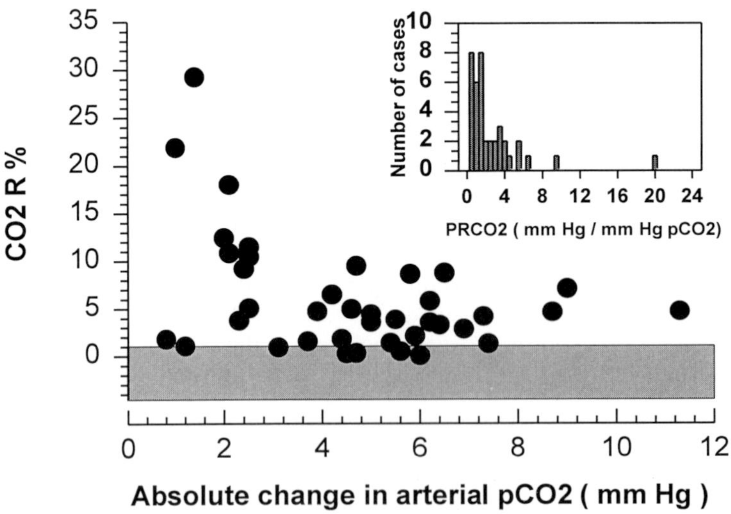

Fig.1: Absolute change in arterial pCO_2 plotted against CO_2R %. The grey box defines the zone of impaired/abolished CO_2-reactivity. Inset: Histogram showing the distribution of $PRCO_2$.

REFERENCES

1. Marmarou, A., Wachi, A. (1989): Blood volume responsivity to ICP change in head injured patients. In: *Intracranial Pressure VII*, edited by J.T. Hoff, et al, pp. 688-690. Springer-Verlag, Berlin.Heidelberg.

2. Cruz, J., Miner, M.E., Allen, S.J., Alves, W.M., Gennarelli, T.A. (1991): Continuous monitoring of cerebral oxygenation in acute brain injury: Assessment of cerebral hemodynamic reserve. Neurosurgery 29:743-749.

3. Enevoldsen, E.M., Jensen, F.T. (1978): Autoregulation and CO2 responses of cerebral blood flow in patients with acute severe head injury. J.Neurosurg. 689:698-703.

4. Olsen, K.S., Videbaek, C., Agerlin, N., Kroll, M., Bogerasmussen, T., Paulson, O.B., Gjerris, F. (1993): The effect of tirilazad mesylate (U74006F) on cerebral oxygen consumption, and reactivity of cerebral blood flow to carbon dioxide in healthy volunteers. Anesthesiology 79:666-671.